1.20

Medical Problems in Dentistry

Medical Problems in Dentistry

Fourth Edition

Crispian Scully
MD PhD MDS FDSRCPS FFDRCSI FDSRCS FRCPath

Dean, Director of Studies and Research;
Professor of Special Needs Dentistry,
Eastman Dental Institute for Oral Health Care Sciences,
University of London

Roderick A. Cawson
MD BDS FDSRCS FDSRCPS

Emeritus Professor of Oral Medicine and Pathology,
Eastman Dental Institute for Oral Health Care Sciences,
and United Medical and Dental Schools of Guy's and
St Thomas's Hospitals (UMDS), University of London

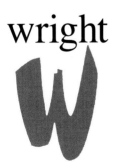

wright

Wright
An imprint of Butterworth-Heinemann
Linacre House, Jordan Hill, Oxford OX2 8DP
225 Wildwood Avenue, Woburn, MA 01801-2041
A division of Reed Educational and Professional Publishing Ltd

A member of the Reed Elsevier plc group

OXFORD AUCKLAND BOSTON
JOHANNESBURG MELBOURNE NEW DELHI

First published 1982
Second edition 1987
Third edition 1993
Reprinted 1993, 1994 (twice), 1995
Fourth edition 1998
Reprinted 1999, 2000, 2001, 2002

British Library Cataloguing in Publication Data
Scully, C.M. (Crispian Michael)
    Medical problems in dentistry. – 4th ed.
    1 Oral manifestations of general diseases
    I Title   II Cawson, Roderick A.
    616'.0024'6176

ISBN 0 7236 1056 8

Library of Congress Cataloguing in Publication Data
Scully, Crispian
    Medical problems in dentistry/Crispian Scully, Roderick A.
    Cawson. – 4th ed.
        p.   cm.
    Includes bibliographical references and index.
    ISBN 0 7236 1056 8
    1 Sick – Dental care.   2 Oral manifestations of general diseases.
    I Cawson, R.A.   II Title.
    [DNLM: 1 Medicine.   2 Dental Care.   WB 100 S437m 1998]
    RK55.S53S38   97–51176
    617.6–DC21   CIP

For more information on all Butterworth-Heinemann
publications please visit our website at www.bh.com

Composition by Scribe Design, Gillingham, Kent
Printed and bound in Great Britain by The Bath Press, Bath

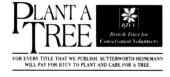

Contents

Drug doses must always be checked in a formulary before administration. Doses must be reduced for children. Doses may need to be reduced in the elderly or in some medical conditions. Contraindications must always be checked and the patient warned of any possible adverse effects.

The author and publishers cannot be responsible for any errors herein.

Preface to the fourth edition

This text covers the general medical and surgical conditions relevant to the oral health care sciences. In providing a basis for the understanding of how these disorders influence oral health and oral health care, it appears to have become widely recognized as a useful source of information for all dental staff who are aware of the possibility that they may have to contend with a variety of medical problems. They should also be aware that they face a growing risk of litigation if they do not keep themselves familiar with current knowledge, in line with the increasing acceptance of the need for continuing professional education. This new edition has therefore been very extensively revised, and is as up-to-date as the rapid advances in knowledge allow.

When *Medical Problems in Dentistry* was first published, approximately 15 years ago, we appeared to be among the few aware both of the importance of oral health to those with medical problems and also of the hazards in operative intervention in some. We therefore tried to focus the attention of the dental profession towards these areas of difficulty. We have subsequently done our best to develop this area of expertise, established units to provide oral health care for problem patients, appointed specialists to undertake and direct such care, and initiated Masters courses in the specialty of Special Needs Dentistry. We are gratified to see the area becoming rightfully recognized as a specialty bridging both hospital and community practice.

The extent of the sales of the previous editions of this book has encouraged our interest and efforts to stay abreast of the understanding of diseases, and developments in medical and surgical care relevant to the oral health care sciences. The fact that this text had become a best-seller and provided probably the most comprehensive coverage available has, in the face of the changing world, stimulated us into renewed efforts. The extensive revision of this fourth edition incorporates much new relevant material, a feat that has been considerably helped by the fact that we now work in the same department in a postgraduate institute with excellent facilities. We have strengthened further those areas of particular, almost day-to-day, concern to *all* dental staff, particularly the problems associated with a bleeding tendency, cardiac disease, diabetes, drug use and abuse, fits, general anaesthesia and sedation, hepatitis and other transmissible diseases including HIV, immunosuppressive treatment, and malignant diseases and their management.

Meanwhile, the world has changed dramatically. In the developed world, the population is ageing. Political changes have resulted in changes in lifestyles of many people and many have acquired a new degree of mobility. New diseases have been emerging and are being recognized. HIV has spread relentlessly throughout the world. Infections, particularly tuberculosis, have re-emerged, and there has been a resurgence of diphtheria in Eastern Europe as a consequence of neglect of immunization. Vast numbers of people now travel between continents daily, so that diseases are being imported into areas where they were previously unknown. On the other hand, new technologies and drugs have been developed, many of which have resulted in complications to oral health care. An increased range of medical problems has thus become relevant to dentistry.

Thus this edition now includes much more detail on a number of diseases that have come into the limelight. A further fifteen years' experience has also enabled us to incorporate additional practical advice and to update information and references. Also added have been the management of some problems such as odontogenic infections previously omitted, and drugs that have been recently introduced.

A new chapter has been added to cover socioeconomic, ethnic and geographical aspects of oral health care. This chapter therefore includes many otherwise exotic diseases which may be imported from across the world, as well as coverage of a number of new problems that have become evident and drugs that have been introduced since the last edition.

Thus this edition now includes for the first time socioeconomic, ethnic and geographical issues, occupational hazards, nutrition, latex allergy, hormone replacement therapy, anabolic steroids, necrotizing fasciitis, hypercoagulability states, short bowel syndrome, liver transplants, Burkitt's lymphoma, idiopathic CD4 lymphopenia, lipoid proteinosis, antiphospholipid syndrome, Castleman's disease, angiolymphoid hyperplasia with eosinophilia, chronic paroxysmal hemicrania, pica, glycogen storage diseases, familial dysautonomia, psoriasis, Kimura's disease, Kikuchi–Fujimoto disease, a number of disorders relevant because of HIV disease (such as the deep mycoses, cytomegalovirus, papillomaviruses, non-tuberculous mycobacteria, cat scratch disease, epithelioid angiomatosis, and toxoplasmosis) and several syndromes (Sweet's, Carney's, William's, Romberg's, hypereosinophilic syndrome, syndrome X, and oral allergy syndrome).

New illustrations have also been added, some in colour, and the text has been restructured, to appear in a more digestible and accessible form, with key points highlighted. To incorporate the new material, the number of chapters has risen from 19 to 27, and we have endeavoured to make the guidance applicable in all parts of the world.

This book has never purported to be a comprehensive textbook of *oral* medicine, though a considerable amount of material relevant to that subject is discussed herein. Further detail on oral medicine can be found in recent texts, such as:

Color Atlas of Oral Disease (Cawson R.A., Binnie W., Eveson J.W., 1995, Mosby)
Colour Guide to Oral Medicine (Scully C., Cawson R.A., 1998, Livingstone)
Oral Diseases in Children and Adolescents (Scully C., Welbury R., 1994, Wolfe)
Surgical Pathology of the Mouth and Jaws (Cawson R.A., Langdon J.D., Eveson J.W., 1995, Butterworth-Heinemann)
Oral Pathology (Eveson J.W., Scully C., 1995, Mosby-Wolfe)
Oral Diseases (Scully C., Flint S.F., Porter S.R., 1996, Dunitz)

We are grateful to Dr Roger Davies and Mr St John Crean (Eastman) for helpful comments on parts of this edition and to Professors Stephen Porter and Joel Epstein for some illustrations. Any comments or criticisms from readers will be gratefully received, though we hope that the improvements in this edition, together with the dearth of criticism of previous editions, means that we have fulfilled our aims as best we can.

C.S.
R.A.C.
The Eastman
London

Preface to the third edition

When this text was first written, HIV infection had not been recognized. Within a mere decade the epidemic of AIDS has spread worldwide with explosive rapidity. As a consequence, of this infection particularly, dental clinicians have been forced to review their practices. Another consequence has been that the public has become increasingly concerned about medical problems in dentistry, especially after media publicity given to the transmission of AIDS in an American dental practice.

This third edition cannot therefore avoid considerable emphasis on HIV infection as well as the risks from the different types of viral hepatitis and other infections such as endocarditis. All of these problems create health hazards for patients or dental workers but increasingly are having medico-legal implications. With such considerations in mind, the whole of this text has been updated and we hope that any errors or ambiguities in the previous editions have been eliminated. We welcome any comments but hope that the very few thus far received – less than a handful in ten years – truly reflect the accuracy of the contents.

C. S.
R. A. C.

Preface to the second edition

In the relatively short time since the first edition of this book there has been a substantial increase in the awareness among dental surgeons of the importance of medical problems in dentistry. A second edition is therefore long overdue, especially now that the Acquired Immune Deficiency Syndrome (AIDS) has appeared since the preparation of the previous edition.

Although reviews of the first edition were very generous and we have received virtually no suggestions for improvements we have not only included new systemic diseases, particularly AIDS, recent diseases of increasing importance such as delta agent infection, new oral complications of disease and therapy such as cyclosporin-induced gingival hyperplasia, and relevant newly recognized diseases such as the MAGIC syndrome, Legionnaire's disease and Lyme disease, but also some aspects omitted from the first edition, such as some causes of bleeding tendency, myelodysplastic syndromes, antral and nasopharyngeal carcinoma, premature infants, and points relevant to anaesthesia.

We have tried to avoid too great an increase in size by eliminating much excess verbiage, especially in the chapters on Cardiovascular disease and on Neurological disease, and by eliminating the lists of drug names. We have updated the whole text, added new figures and tables and, hopefully, corrected the few printing errors.

This text is not designed to cover all aspects of *oral disease* but rather to highlight systemic diseases that influence dental care or treatment. Standard oral medicine texts should be consulted for fuller details of oral diseases.

In relation to this edition we are grateful to Mrs M. Seward, Editor of the *British Dental Journal*, for permission to include material from the *Hospital Dental Surgeon's Guide* (Scully C., *Br. Dent. J.*, 1985) and from papers we have published in the Journal. We are also most grateful to Stephen Porter, Karen Porter and Stephen Flint for stimulating discussions and for their help in reading the proofs.

C. S.
R. A. C.

Preface to the first edition

Unless he is quite unusually oblivious to potential consequences, the dentist who discovers that a patient has a disease of any of the major organ systems is likely to be made anxious by the possibility that complications might result from dental treatment. It is often worse when the patient has some uncommon syndrome with a bizarre name. Such anxiety may well be justified, and may be increased by doubt as to which aspects of dental treatment may be hazardous for such a patient.

There are three basic problems regarding the dental treatment of patients with significant systemic disease. The first is to detect such patients. This is a difficult task but an attempt at medical assessment of the patient must always be made, especially when a general anaesthetic has to be given – even if that anaesthetic is euphemistically termed sedation with methohexitone. Very often, however, there are severe limitations on what can be discovered about a patient who may have no significant symptoms or, if under medical treatment, may have only the haziest of ideas of what it is all about. The problem is even greater with patients who speak poor or little English and with those of low intelligence or who are unable to give a clear history for any other reason.

It has to be accepted that, largely as a result of current drug treatment, the days are past when it was reasonable to assume that a patient walking in from the street was as fit as he appeared. There is no doubt therefore that it is the dentist's responsibility at least to attempt to make a medical assessment of his patients. Apart from the fate of the patient, neglect of the medical history can result in unpleasant medico-legal complications.

Secondly, if a patient is found to have a systemic disease, it then becomes necessary to determine what implications the disease or its treatment have for dental management.

Finally, once this has been decided, it then remains necessary to discover how best to deal with the problem.

It is easy to exaggerate the frequency with which systemic disease can seriously complicate dental treatment. The very rarity of such an emergency as cardiac arrest makes it likely that at some time it may catch the dentist by surprise and sometimes, as a consequence, powerless to do anything to help the patient significantly. Nevertheless, the fact is that cardiovascular disease, the most frequent underlying cause of cardiac arrest and other emergencies, is very common.

These considerations aside, hospital dental staff can find themselves in the difficult position of having to manage the total initial care of patients with maxillofacial injuries who may also be comatose for one or more of a variety of reasons.

Unfortunately it is difficult to discover, from any one of the standard texts, the great variety of dental implications of systemic diseases and how any such problems should be managed. The aim of this book was therefore to try to ease this task for the dentist, but the writing of this text made it only too apparent how wildly ambitious we had been in setting our sights on such a target.

Some areas of medicine are particularly difficult. Many dentists have a mental block about the subject of immunology. We thought it worth while therefore to review briefly the working of the immune system before considering how disorders of this system are related to disease. In practice, however, few immunologically mediated diseases, apart from Sjögren's syndrome, are of major relevance for dentistry. By contrast, treatment of many such diseases with immunosuppressive drugs, particularly corticosteroids, is relatively common and can cause serious complications in dental practice.

Another traditionally difficult area of medicine is neurology, and unfortunately the neurology of the head and neck region is by no means the easiest part of this subject. Some trouble has therefore been taken to delineate the disorders affecting the cranial nerves and the clinical features that help to differentiate them. This aspect is particularly important in the case of maxillofacial injuries where cranial nerve lesions can be extracranial or the result of brain damage.

Perhaps most difficult of all is the subject of psychiatric disease. Nevertheless, dentists are perhaps insufficiently aware of how frequently psychiatric disease can cause difficulties with their patients. In addition, oral symptoms probably have a psychiatric basis more frequently than is generally realized.

Overall, therefore, this book is intended for hospital dental staff, for those studying for the Fellowship and for interested general practitioners.

The structure of this book is as follows. First, we have tried to provide sufficient background information about systemic diseases and their management to make their effects understandable. Secondly, we have outlined the relevance of these diseases and their treatment for dentistry. Thirdly, we have tried to suggest, wherever possible, how these problems should be dealt with. In some cases, as indicated in the text, the only satisfactory solution is to refer the patient for specialist care.

Our original intention was to be very brief, but there are few conditions that do not have *some* dental implications, however slight. Moreover, though rare diseases are unlikely to be encountered in routine dental practice, it is typically these, or unusual aspects of common diseases, which can cause most difficulties. Moreover, the rarity of a disease in statistical terms does not mean that it cannot be a source of trouble. It is of no comfort to tell someone who has been struck by lightning that it shouldn't have happened! Therefore, to avoid overloading the main body of the text even further, many of these rare syndromes have been summarized in tabular form as appendices. Tropical diseases are not included, neither is detailed coverage of oral diseases.

We have unavoidably had to be dogmatic about many things. However, it is impossible to cater exactly for all the variables in dental practice, such as the facilities provided and the calibre or availability of medical advice and assistance, let alone the different types of patient encountered at different clinics. Inevitably also, there is no general agreement as to how best to manage some problems.

All we can hope therefore – whether too much or too little information has been provided – is that this book will help to answer some of the many questions that have been put to us over the years.

C. S.
R. A. C.

1

Medical history and assessment

Key points

- A medical history is essential in order to:
  assess the fitness of the patient for the procedure;
  decide on the type of pain control required;
  decide how treatment may need to be modified;
  warn of any possible emergencies that could arise and determine any effect on oral health;
  warn of any possible risk to staff.
- The most relevant conditions are allergies, bleeding tendencies, cardiac disease, immune defects, or where the patient is on drugs acting on the endocrine or central nervous system (CNS).
- Relevant systemic disease is more common in the elderly, those with disability and inpatients.
- The medical history should elicit any systemic disease relevant to dentistry, in particular:
  Anaemia
  Bleeding disorders
  Cardiorespiratory disorders
  Drug treatment and allergies
  Endocrine disease
  Fits and faints
  Gastrointestinal disorders
  Hospital admissions and attendances
  Infections
  Jaundice or liver disease
  Kidney disease
  Likelihood of pregnancy, or pregnancy itself.
- The history must be reviewed before any surgical procedure or general anaesthetic, and at each new course of dental treatment.
- Examination of the patient's appearance, behaviour and speech, and inspection of the face, neck and hands can reveal many significant conditions.
- Investigations may be helpful but must always be interpreted in the light of the history and clinical findings.
- Confidentiality must be respected with regard to the history, investigational and examination findings (Chapter 2).

Provided that the patient is fit, local anaesthesia is used, and the procedure is not dramatically invasive, dentistry is a safe procedure. Risks arise when these conditions do not apply and dental staff attempt anything overambitious in terms of their skill or knowledge.

It was said many years ago that 'Dentists are now concerned not with the treatment of teeth in patients but the treatment of patients who have teeth' (Morris, 1967); we hope very much that this is true. While local analgesia (anaesthesia) is a remarkably safe procedure in most situations, the same is not true of general anaesthesia, and at one time any patient who could climb a flight of stairs without distress was judged fit for dental general anaesthesia. Today, many patients with life-threatening diseases survive as a result of advances in surgical and medical care. One result of this is that an apparently fit patient, coming for dental treatment, can have a serious systemic disease and be under drug treatment. Either or both can significantly affect the dental management or even the fate of the patient. The risk is greatest when general anaesthesia or sedation is going to be given. These problems may be compounded by the fact that patients are seen briefly and medical support is lacking in the dental surgery.

MEDICAL HISTORY

It is therefore essential to try to obtain as much relevant information as possible about the dental patient, especially when invasive procedures or the use of potent drugs such as general anaesthetic agents, are being considered. The objective of the medical history and patient assessment is, first, to determine whether the patient is fit to undergo the particular treatment in question; second whether any drugs or general anaesthesia are contraindicated, and third, to exclude oral disease. No patient should suffer any deterioration of health as a result of treatment.

The medical history should thus be directed towards eliciting anything that might:

1. result in an emergency – examples include epilepsy, diabetes, allergies;

2. need medical care *before* dental treatment – examples include bleeding tendencies or a susceptibility to endocarditis;
3. require modification of dental care – examples include allergies, sickle cell disease, corticosteroid treatment or recent myocardial infarction;
4. pose risks to other patients or staff – examples include the violent or intoxicated patient, or those with an infectious disease;
5. assist the diagnosis of oral and peri-oral disease.

Unfortunately, both patients and dentists often fail fully to appreciate the relevance of the medical history. Some patients may even resent being questioned; this is particularly so in the *more* educated, and in the case of transmissible disease or drug abuse. In one study, 10 per cent of patients believed dental staff did not need to know about a patient's medical status (McDaniel et al., 1995). Some patients, especially those with learning disability or from overseas, may have particular language, cultural or communication difficulties in giving their medical history (Chapter 26). Thus it is best always to check the history with a patient-completed questionnaire and, where possible, with the patient's usual medical adviser and/or relatives. However, communication between doctors and dentists is sometimes also poor, despite studies showing that dental treatment plans are altered in nearly one-third of cases where there has been medical consultation (Jainkittivong et al., 1995).

The prevalence of medical disorders that might affect dental treatment can be relatively high. Surveys from different dental settings have shown medical problems in up to 75 per cent, though typically in general practice most are ambulant, relatively fit individuals. Cardiovascular disease and allergies are by far the most common relevant medical histories seen in most studies. The prevalence of medical problems appears to be rising (Rhodus et al., 1989) and several relevant conditions can be latent. For example, blood and urine glucose levels may be abnormal in 5 per cent or more of dental patients (Falace, 1978) and screening may detect unsuspected diabetes mellitus. Nevertheless, it is important not to undertake testing that may cause unnecessary trauma, delay, worry or expense; many studies have shown the disadvantages of 'routine' and 'screening' tests carried out with little focus. Too often, trivial or inexplicable findings are revealed and most evidence shows that the history and physical examination usually provide all the clinically useful data.

The prevalence of many of the more relevant systemic diseases is much higher in certain groups, particularly the elderly, those with disability and inpatients. However, there are other medical problems, particularly blood-borne viral infections, that are more prevalent in younger and otherwise apparently healthy individuals attending for dental care. Infections with the human immunodeficiency virus (HIV) and with the various hepatitis viruses are seen mainly in younger adults, particularly those from metropolitan areas, and are transmitted primarily sexually or by intravenous drug abuse. They pose a risk to other patients and staff unless all body fluids are regarded as infective, and adequate infection control procedures are invariably followed.

The magnitude of the problem of drug use or drug interactions in dental practice is unknown but, in view of the relatively limited prescribing habits of dentists, it must fall well below that experienced in medical practice. Dental patients with pain often self-medicate with paracetamol, or aspirin. The latter can induce a bleeding tendency. Oksas (1978) reported that 30 per cent of a group of 2418 dental hospital patients had a history of chronic systemic disorders that could contraindicate some drugs used in dentistry. Of these patients, 23 per cent also admitted to having drug-related reactions, many of which involved drugs commonly used in dentistry. In the hospital under study, adverse drug reactions were theoretically possible in about one in every 24 prescriptions given.

It is therefore essential to establish as clearly as possible, within the practical limitations of dental practice, the presence and significance of medical problems likely to affect dental management, and especially whether general anaesthesia or sedation may be particularly hazardous. Good preoperative assessment endeavours to anticipate and prevent trouble. Morbidity and mortality following dental operations is even less excusable than when it follows more serious

surgery. Morbidity or mortality are significantly less when local anaesthesia is used than in any other technique.

By contrast, with intravenous or inhalational general anaesthesia, control of vital functions is impaired or lost to the anaesthetist. The evidence suggests that there will remain a need for dental treatment under general anaesthesia in a minority.

The first principle must be to 'do no harm'.

PRACTICAL ASPECTS OF ASSESSMENT

Adequate assessment is essential if the patient is to have general anaesthesia or even sedation. The criteria of 'fitness' are not absolute but depend on the health of the patient, the degree of urgency of the procedure and the skill and experience of the anaesthetist and operator. Overall, sedation is considerably safer than general anaesthesia, but even so, must be carried out by adequately trained personnel and with due consideration of the possible risks, as indicated by the General Dental Council (*see* Chapter 2, Appendix 1). Further details of perioperative care have been provided by Carter (1988).

Since medical examination of the routine dental outpatient is neither always feasible nor appropriate, the most useful aspect of assessment is the medical history. This must be accurate but also concise and systematically applied to ensure that the maximum information is obtained. Many systems are available, but each should have a preamble to explain why the questions are being asked and, in particular, to make it clear that the purpose of the questions is to ensure the patient's safety. In one such system the history is reduced to 12 routine questions (**A** to **L**) as follows:

Anaemia
Bleeding disorders
Cardiorespiratory disorders
Drug treatment and allergies
Endocrine disease
Fits and faints
Gastrointestinal disorders
Hospital admissions and attendances
Infections
Jaundice or liver disease
Kidney disease
Likelihood of pregnancy, or pregnancy itself.

Further enquiry should be made about any positive answers. Each answer should be recorded as Yes or No to ensure accuracy. Some centres use a questionnaire that the patient answers in the waiting room. This saves time, reminds the patient about their history, and allows the patient to write about things they might not wish to speak openly about. It also provides documentary evidence that proper enquiries have been made, if any complications lead to medicolegal claims. Answers from such a questionnaire should always be confirmed by the dental surgeon, as quite serious disease is sometimes neglected by both the patient and the dentist (Scully and Boyle, 1983; Dunne and Clark, 1985). Indeed, only 68 per cent of patients provided valid data in one study (Brady and Martinoff, 1980); by contrast, some overestimate their problems (Mohammad and Ruprecht, 1983).

One limitation of such questionnaires is the delicate matter of sexually transmitted diseases and, in particular, that of HIV infection. There is no easy answer. If direct questions are asked, the patient is likely to be offended; there also is no guarantee that answers are honest or even that the patient is aware of having been infected. However, it is worthwhile to have a final section headed 'Please add anything else about your health or medication which may be relevant'. In the writers' experience, a very 'conventional-looking' young businessman admitted, in this last section, that he had or had had an impressive list of sexually transmitted diseases and was infected with HIV.

A few patients bring a list of their medical complaints and histories with them. Whilst these may sometimes be accurate and helpful, they are occasionally a sign of neuroticism (Chapter 18).

CLINICAL ASSESSMENT – THE FACE AND GENERAL APPEARANCE IN DIAGNOSIS

Although it has been stressed above that even very ill patients can look remarkably well, much can sometimes be learned simply by listening to, looking at and examining the patient. Conditions which may suggest an immediate diagnosis include the following.

Pallor (anaemia or an imminent faint), cyanosis (cardiac or respiratory disease), jaundice (liver disease), prominent cervical lymph nodes (HIV and other infections particularly), hyper- or hypothyroidism, prognathism and thickened facies (acromegaly), Cushing's disease or cushingoid facies due to corticosteroid treatment, emaciation (possibly due to anorexia, malignant disease or HIV), Parkinson's disease, myotonia, tardive dyskinesia, myasthenia gravis, pupil abnormalities, facial and other cranial nerve palsies, Down's or Turner's syndromes, congenital syphilis, hereditary haemorrhagic telangiectasia, pigmentation (Addison's disease and other causes), systemic sclerosis, lupus erythematosus, dermatomyositis, hypertrichosis, bullous erythema multiforme, salivary gland swellings and other swollen faces, eye disorders (such as uveitis or Sjögren's syndrome), osteogenesis imperfecta, dyspnoea, herpes labialis or zoster, candidosis (angular stomatitis in HIV and other diseases), pregnancy, finger clubbing (cardiorespiratory disease) and neurotic or psychotic behaviour. Oral manifestations of systemic disease such as thrush secondary to HIV infection should also be looked for.

Speech may be defective as a result of drug intoxication, severe xerostomia, neurological or muscle diseases such as Parkinson's disease, motor neurone disease or myasthenia gravis.

INVESTIGATIONS: THE VALUE AND LIMITATIONS OF INTERPRETATION

Investigations are useful only when the appropriate tests are requested, and interpreted in the light of the history, clinical findings, knowledge and experience. It is useless to ask for investigations, the results of which will have no influence on the diagnosis or management. The interpretation of biochemical results is shown in Appendix 1 to this chapter, and that of haematological results is summarized in the Appendix to Chapter 5.

RELEVANCE OF THE MEDICAL HISTORY AND ASSESSMENT

Anaemia

Anaemia is often a contraindication to general anaesthesia, particularly if the haemoglobin is less than 10 g/dl. Lassitude, weakness, pallor, breathlessness or swelling of the ankles are signs of severe anaemia but may be seen in other conditions. Racial origins may be important, especially in the case of sickle cell disease or thalassaemia (Chapters 5 and 26).

Bleeding disorders

Though the history is of paramount importance in assessing bleeding disorders, enquiries about abnormal bleeding produce more vague answers than do most other questions. Specific questions should therefore be asked, as suggested in Chapter 4. Bleeding disorders are a significant hazard and any such possibility must always be taken seriously. A history of involvement of other members of the family or of admission to hospital for control of bleeding is particularly important.

Cardiorespiratory disorders

Cardiac disease is often a contraindication to general anaesthesia or it may necessitate antibiotic cover as prophylaxis against infective endocarditis, or both. Inquiry must be made about a history of rheumatic or congenital heart disease, ischaemic heart disease, cardiac operations and previous attacks of infective endocarditis.

Respiratory disorders also significantly influence the choice of anaesthesia. Asthma, bronchitis and emphysema are the most common problems (Chapter 8) but even the common cold can be a contraindication to general anaesthesia.

Chest pain, dyspnoea, swelling of the ankles, palpitations and hypertension are all significant features suggesting cardiovascular disease. Wheezing, cough or dyspnoea are common symptoms of respiratory disease.

Drug treatment and allergies

Drugs may not only influence dental disease or treatment but their nature may be the only indication of serious underlying disease. Corticosteroids, antihypertensives, anticonvulsants, anticoagulants, antibiotics and antidiabetics are all important drugs in this respect.

In order to get useful answers about drug treatment it is often necessary to phrase the question 'Do you ever take any injections, drugs, pills, tablets or medicines of *any* kind?' Many patients neglect to mention such drugs as analgesics, hypnotics or contraceptives (*Plate 1*). Smoking and drinking habits must also be asked about and, in some cases, the possibility of drug abuse must be considered. Drug or other allergies or atopic disease should be carefully noted. All drugs taken by the patient should be checked. The type of drug, potential side-effects and possible interactions should then be established (*see* Appendix to Chapter 25). If, as is often the case, the patient does not know or cannot recall the name of medicines, treatment should be deferred until the drug is identified by checking the drug itself, by consulting the patient's doctor or, in hospital, the Drugs Information Unit or Pharmacy.

The most serious drug interactions in dentistry are with general anaesthetic agents (intravenous or inhalational), monoamine oxidase inhibitors and antihypertensive agents. There are many other contraindications for drugs. For example, aspirin may be a hazard in anticoagulated, diabetic or pregnant patients, or those with peptic ulcer (*see* Appendix to Chapter 25).

Allergies can be important; the most relevant are those to **a**naesthetics, **a**nalgesics, **a**ntibiotics or **a**ntiseptics. Common allergies are to aspirin, codeine, penicillin, iodine, latex and sticking plasters (Band aids) (Chapter 25).

Endocrine disorders

Diabetes mellitus and thyroid disease are common. Hypoadrenocorticism is rare but also important (Chapter 14).

Fits or faints

Epilepsy and other causes of loss of consciousness can disrupt dental treatment and may result in injury to the patient. The type and severity of epilepsy should be noted; treatment is best carried out during a stable phase (Chapter 17).

Gastrointestinal disorders

Some gastrointestinal disorders, such as Crohn's disease or coeliac disease, may lead to oral complications, and gastric disorders

DETAILS OF RELEVANT MEDICAL HISTORY (Please date and sign each entry)

Date		Date	
17·9·8	– 1984 HEPATITIS ; probably HBV. –1985 HEPATITIS; ? type – 1986 March ; known HIV positive – Previous STD ; NSU : several episodes Gonorrhoea · 1980 Syphilis : 1981		

Fig. 1.1 Medical history from a male promiscuous homosexual

may increase the risk of vomiting during general anaesthesia. Questioning should be directed towards the presence of abdominal pain, frequency and type of stool, bleeding and weight loss (Chapter 9).

Hospital admissions and attendances

Operations are good indicators of the possible reactions to general anaesthesia and surgery. A patient who has had a tonsillectomy, for example, without complications is most unlikely to have a congenital bleeding disorder. Hospital admissions may also indicate underlying disease, and past operations may suggest the possibility of future complications that can influence dental treatment.

Infections

The possibility of transmissible infections and their sequelae must be considered, particularly in at-risk groups. Infection with HIV, for example, is a growing problem throughout the world in those who are sexually active or exposed to infected blood or blood products. Promiscuous male homosexuals and abusers of intravenous drugs, and patients who have attended sexually transmitted disease clinics, are more likely to have a history of infection with HIV, hepatitis viruses, herpes simplex, syphilis, gonorrhoea and many other infections (*Fig 1.1* and Chapters 10, 11 and 20). Patients who are carriers of *Staphylococcus aureus*, which is then often present in the anterior nares, may be a hazard to others,

as may be those who carry *Neisseria meningitidis* in their pharynx. Methicillin-resistant *S. aureus* (MRSA) is the cause of severe infections in some hospitals. Thus patients may need to be screened for these organisms when there are concerns about, or outbreaks of, infection.

Jaundice and liver disorders

A history of jaundice may imply carriage of hepatitis viruses, although jaundice is by no means always infective. A prolonged bleeding state and impaired drug metabolism can result from liver disease (Chapter 10). Jaundice after an operation may have resulted from halothane hepatitis, and if this is suspected, a different anaesthetic – such as isoflurane, desflurane or sevoflurane – should be given.

Kidney disorders

Renal disorders can affect dental management, mainly because excretion of some drugs is impaired. Nocturia and hypertension are early manifestations of renal failure, while polyuria, anorexia, vomiting, lassitude and weight loss are late features. Rarely, renal failure or complications of renal transplantation can give rise to oral signs or affect dental management (Chapter 13).

Pregnancy

It is important to know whether a woman is pregnant, since any dental procedure involving drugs, radiography or general anaesthe-

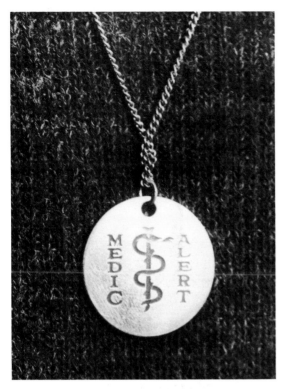

Fig. 1.2 Medic-Alert warning emblem: the patient's main diagnosis or drug treatment is engraved on the reverse, together with the telephone number of the company, which holds details of the medical history

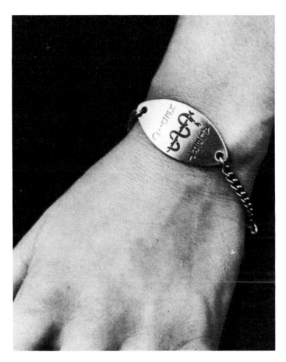

Fig. 1.3 Medic-Alert bracelet

sia is best left until the middle trimester (Chapter 14). Though there is no known risk of teratogenic effects from most drugs used in dentistry, drug administration should be kept to an absolute minimum.

LIMITATIONS OF THE MEDICAL HISTORY

These questions cover most of the important conditions that may influence or be influenced by dental treatment. *However, it is essential that the history be updated before each course of treatment, every sedation session and especially before surgery or a general anaesthetic, as it may radically change.* Ellinger *et al.* (1973) followed a small group of middle-aged and elderly dental patients and reported that nearly 20 per cent developed significant medical disorders (mostly cardiovascular) over a period of 5 years.

Patients should be asked if they carry a medical warning card and careful note should be taken of it, particularly in respect of corticosteroid use, a bleeding disorder or diabetes. Similar attention should be given to any medical warning medallion, such as Medic-Alert (*Figs 1.2, 1.3*).

It is important to emphasize again that the history is of prime importance in outpatient dentistry where physical examination is usually inappropriate. However, as mentioned earlier, it is important to look at the patient for such readily visible signs as pallor, cyanosis or jaundice and dyspnoea or wheezing, and not merely examine the mouth. Inpatients must always have a full physical examination before operation.

Although every care should be taken to identify the unfit patient, it must be appreciated that the means to do so in conventional dental settings are limited and by no means always successful. *It is impossible to legislate for all possibilities and there have been many cases where apparently fit people have dropped dead within a short time of having passed a medical examination.*

BIBLIOGRAPHY

Bedi R. and Crawford A.N. (1982) Assessment of the medical status of Asian immigrant children undergoing dental care. *J. Dent.* **10**, 144–8.

Brady W.F. and Martinoff I.T. (1980) Validity of health history data collected from dental patients and patient perception of health status. *J. Am. Dent. Assoc.* **101**, 642–5.

Carter D.C. (ed) (1988) Perioperative care. *Br. Med. Bull.* **617**, 235–514.

Chambers I. and Scully C. (1987) Medical information from referral letters. *Oral Surg. Oral Med. Oral Pathol.* **64**, 674–6.

Cottone J.A. and Kafrawy A.H. (1979) Medications and health histories: a survey of 4365 dental patients. *J. Am. Dent. Assoc.* **98**, 713–18.

De Jong K.J.M., Abraham-Inpijn L., Oomen H.A.P.C. *et al.* (1991) Clinical relevance of a medical history in dental practice; comparison between a questionnaire and a dialogue. *Commun. Dent. Oral Epidemiol.* **19**, 310–11.

Dunne S.M. and Clark C.G. (1985) The identification of the medically compromised patient in dental practice. *J. Dent.* **13**, 45–51.

Ellinger C.W., Kanner I., Wesley R. *et al.* (1973) Are your patients as healthy as you think they are, doctor? *J. Am. Soc. Prev. Dent.* **3**, 36–8.

Evans B.E. (1978) Dental care for patients with systemic health problems. *NY J. Dent.* **48**, 313–19.

Falace D.A. (1978) An evaluation of the clinical laboratory as an adjunct to dental practice. *J. Am. Dent. Assoc.* **96**, 261–5.

Fast T.B., Martin M.D. and Ellis T.M. (1986) Emergency preparedness, a survey of dental practitioners. *J. Am. Dent. Assoc.* **112**, 499–501.

Halpern I.L. (1975) Patient's medical status – a factor in dental treatment. *Oral Surg. Oral Med. Oral Pathol.* **39**, 216–26.

Hampton J.R., Harrison M.J.G., Mitchell J.R.A. *et al.* (1975) Relative contributions of history-taking, physical examination and laboratory investigation to diagnosis and management of medical outpatients. *Br. Med. J.* **2**, 486–9.

Jainkittivong A., Yeh C-K., Guest G.F. *et al.* (1995). Evaluation of medical consultations in a predoctoral dental clinic. *Oral Surg. Oral Med. Oral Pathol.* **80**, 409–13.

Kaplan E.B., Sheiner L.B., Boeckman A.J. *et al.* (1985) The usefulness of preoperative laboratory screening. *J. Am. Med. Assoc.* **253**, 3576–81.

Luker J., Matthews R. and Scully C. (1993) Radionuclide imaging in dentistry. *Postgrad. Dentistry* **3**, 204–8.

Matthews R.W, Peak J.D and Scully C. (1994) The efficacy of management of acute dental pain. *Br. Dent. J.* **176**, 413–16.

McDaniel T.F., Miller D., Jones R. *et al.* (1995) Assessing patient willingness to reveal health history information. *J. Am. Dent. Assoc.* **126**, 375–9.

McLundie A.C.,Watson W.C. and Kennedy G.D.C. (1969) Medical status of patients undergoing dental care. *Br. Dent. J.* **127**, 265–71.

Miller C.S., Kaplan A.L., Guest G.F. *et al.* (1992) Documenting medication use in adult dental patients: 1987–1991. *J. Am. Dent. Assoc.* **123**, 41–8.

Mohammad A.R. and Ruprecht A. (1983) Assessment of dental patients' comprehension of health questionnaire. *J. Oral Med.* **38**, 74–5.

Morris A.L. (1967) The medical history in dental practice. *J. Am. Dent. Assoc.* **74**, 129–37.

Nery E.B., Meister F., Ellinger R.F. *et al.* (1987) Prevalence of medical problems in periodontal patients obtained from three different populations. *J. Periodontol.* **58**, 564–8.

Oksas R.M. (1978) Epidemiologic study of potential adverse drug reactions in dentistry. *Oral Surg. Oral Med. Oral Pathol.* **45**, 707–13.

Osman F., Scully C., Dowell T.B. *et al.* (1986) The reasons for taking radiographs in general dental practice. *Commun. Dent. Oral Epidemiol.* **14**, 146–7.

Osman F., Scully C. Dowell T.B. *et al.* (1986) Use of panoramic radiographs in general dental practice in England. *Commun. Dent. Oral Epidemiol.* **14**, 8–9.

Peacock M.E. and Carson R.E. (1995) Frequency of self-reported medical conditions in periodontal patients. *J. Periodontol.* **66**, 1004–7.

Porter S.R. and Scully C. (1996) *Innovations and Developments in Non-invasive Oral Health Care.* Northwood, Science Reviews.

Porter S.R., Scully C., Welsby, P. and Gleeson, M. (1992) *Colour Guide to Medicine and Surgery for Dentistry.* Edinburgh, Churchill–Livingstone.

Rhodus N.L., Bakdash M.M., Little J.W. *et al.* (1989) Implications of the changing medical profile of a dental school patient population. *J. Am. Dent. Assoc.* **119**, 414–6.

Rose L.F., Steinberg B.J. and Atlas S.L. (1995) Periodontal management of the medically compromised patient. *Periodontology 2000* **9**, 165–75.

Scully C. (1979) Orofacial manifestations of disease. 1: Normal appearances. *Hosp. Update* **5**, 817 (*Dent. Update* **6**, 443).

Scully C. (1980) Examination of the head and neck – Part I. *Student Update* **2**, 159.

Scully C. (1980) Examination of the head and neck – Part II. *Student Update* **2**, 197.

Scully C. (1980) Examination of the head and neck – Part III. *Student Update* **2**, 228.

Scully C. (1988) *The Dental Patient.* Oxford, Heinemann.

Scully C. (1989) *The Mouth and Perioral Tissues.* Oxford, Heinemann.

Scully C. (1989) *Patient Care: a Dental Surgeon's Guide.* London, British Dental Association.

Scully C. (1993) Diagnosis and diagnostic procedures: general and soft tissue diagnosis. In: *Pathways in Practice*, London, Faculty of General Dental Practice, Royal College of Surgeons of England, pp. 25–33.

Scully C. (1993) The new professional role of the dentist:

internal medicine. In: *Interprofessional Cooperation in Dental Care*, Koln, Institute der Deutschen Zahnarzte, pp. 167–206.

Scully C. (1993) The new professional role of the dentist under aspects of internal medicine. *Int. Dent. J.* **43**, 323–34.

Scully C. and Boyle P. (1983) Reliability of a self-administered questionnaire for screening medical problems in dentistry. *Commun. Dent. Oral Epidemiol.* **11**, 105.

Scully C. and Prime S. (1980) Acute dental problems in medical practice. *Dent. Update* **21**, 1239.

Scully C. and Prime S. (1980) Acute dental problems in medical practice. *Dent. Update* **21**, 1511.

Scully C., Cawson R.A. and Griffiths M.J. (1990) *Occupational Hazards to Dental Staff.* London, British Dental Journal.

Sigvard P. (1991) Self-assessment of dental conditions: validity of a questionnaire. *Commun. Dent Oral Epidemiol.* **19**, 249–51.

Sonis S.T., Fazio R., Setkowicz A. *et al.* (1983) Comparison of the nature and frequency of medical problems among patients in general speciality and hospital dental practices. *J. Oral Med.* **38**, 58–61.

Suomi J.D., Horowitz H.S. and Barbano J.P. (1975) Self-reported systemic conditions in an adult study population. *J. Dent. Res.* **54**, 1092.

Wagner J.D. and Moore D.L. (1991) Preoperative laboratory testing for the oral and maxillofacial surgery patient. *J. Oral Maxillofac. Surg.* **49**, 177–82.

Wessberg G. (1978) Role in screening for hypertension in patient management. *J. Am. Dent. Assoc.* **96**, 1040–4.

APPENDIX 1 TO CHAPTER 1: INVESTIGATIONS

PROCEDURES FOR SUBMITTING SPECIMENS FOR LABORATORY INVESTIGATIONS

1. Haematology Specimens

Blood for film and red cell indices must be collected into a tube containing potassium EDTA (4 ml into an EDTA or sequestrene tube). The blood must be gently mixed to ensure that the anticoagulant is well distributed; clotted samples are useless. Blood for assay of corrected whole blood folate levels is also collected in an EDTA tube. Most other necessary investigations are performed on serum.

Blood film Red cell indices White cell count and differential Platelet count 6 Corrected whole blood or red cell folate Serum vitamin B_{12}	EDTA tube
Serum iron Total iron binding capacity Serum ferritin 6 Paul–Bunnell test	Plain tube
Erythrocyte sedimentation rate (ESR)	Citrated tube (*contact haematologist*)
Clotting studies Prothrombin time	Citrated tube
Blood grouping	Plain tube
Cross-matching	Plain tube + EDTA tube (as red blood cells are also required for testing)

2. Biochemistry Specimens

There is currently some variation as to whether serum or plasma are needed for certain biochemical tests depending on the laboratory involved. Special containers may be required for automated multichannel analysers which give a full biochemical profile on a single blood specimen. However, most biochemical estimations can be carried out on serum (collect blood in a plain container), although plasma (collect in a lithium heparin tube) may be needed for estimation of electrolytes, cortisol and proteins. Blood glucose assays are carried out on a sample in a fluoride bottle.

3. Immunology Specimens

Most tests of humoral immunity and complement components are carried out on serum (plain tube). Autoantibodies are determined on serum. In order to prevent the rapid decay of complement compo-

continued

nents the serum should be separated as soon as possible and frozen at least at –20 °C and prefer-ably at –70 °C. Serum for immune complexes and cryoglobulins may need special handling, details of which can be obtained from the relevant laboratory.

Tests of cell-mediated immunity are expensive and can often only be carried out once special preparations have been made (consult the laboratory).

See below for direct immunofluorescence specimens.

4. Histopathology Specimens

A biopsy of adequate size and representative of the lesion should be taken, placed in a fixative such as formol saline, and sent to the pathology laboratory carefully labelled and with the appropriate form of request for histopathological examination.

1. Specimens for routine histological examination: these should be fixed in a 10 per cent formol saline; at least 10 times the volume of the biopsy is needed for adequate fixation.
2. Specimens for immunofluorescent investigations: these are not usually carried out on formol saline fixed tissue but should be sent for immediate freezing at –70 °C and direct immunofluo-rescence. Serum should also be sent for indirect immunofluorescence.

If tuberculosis or a deep mycosis is suspected a tissue specimen should be sent for culture.

5. Microbiology Specimens

Specimens should be collected before antimicrobials are started. If pus is present a sample should be sent in a sterile container, in preference to a swab. Requests for culture and antibiotic sensitivity should indicate possible aetiology, present antimicrobial therapy and any drug allergies. If tubercu-losis is suspected this must be clearly indicated on the request form.

If the microbiological specimen cannot be dealt with within 2 hours, the swab should be placed in transport medium and kept in the refrigerator at 4 °C (not a freezer) until dealt with by the micro-biology department.

Actinomycosis: Preferably send pus for culture but in the absence of adequate pus send a dressing that has been in contact with the wound for several hours.

Candidosis: Swabs from the lesions and from the fitting surface of the denture should be sent for Gram stain or culture.

Viral hepatitis or HIV infection: Many centres have defined protocols for the collection of specimens from patients with suspected hepatitis or HIV infection. Particular care must be taken to avoid needlestick injuries and contaminating the outside of the containers and to indicate the hazard of the infection. Special coloured plastic bags (usually red) to indicate this hazard should be used for transporting the specimen.

Other viral infections: Swabs must be sent in viral transport medium: dry swabs are no use. Acute and convalescent serum samples (10 ml blood in plain container) should be taken. The convalescent serum is collected 2–3 weeks after the acute illness.

Syphilis: Oral lesions should be cleaned with saline to remove oral treponemes before a smear is made for dark ground examination: 10 ml of serum should be sent for VDRL testing (Chapter 11) .

URINALYSIS

Urinalysis: interpretation of results[a]

	Colour	Protein	Glucose[b]	Ketones	Bilirubin[c]	Urobilinogen[c]	Blood[d]
Health	Yellow	Usually no protein, but a trace can be normal in young people	Usually no glucose, but a trace can be normal in 'renal glycosuria' and pregnancy	Usually no ketones, but keto-nuria may occur in vomiting, fasting or starved patients	Usually no bilirubin	Usually present in normal healthy patients, particularly in concen-trated urine	Usually no blood

continued

	Colour	Protein	Glucose[b]	Ketones	Bilirubin[c]	Urobilinogen[c]	Blood[d]
False positives	Red: beet	Alkaline urine. Container contaminated with disinfectant, e.g. chlorhexidine. Blood or pus in urine. Polyvinyl pyrrolidone infusions	Cephamandole. Container contaminated with hypochlorite	Patients on L-dopa or any phthalein compound	Chlorpromazine and other phenothiazines	Infected urine. Patients taking ascorbic acid, sulphonamides or paraminosalicylate	Menstruation. Container contaminated with some detergents
Disease	Brown: homogentisic acid, bilirubin, urobilin Red: Hb	Renal diseases. Also cardiac failure, diabetes, endocarditis, myeloma, amyloid, some drugs, some chemicals	Diabetes mellitus. Also in pancreatitis, hyperthyroidism, Fanconi syndrome, sometimes after a head injury, other endocrinopathies	Diabetes mellitus. Also in febrile or traumatized patients on low carbohydrate diets	Jaundice, hepatocellular and obstructive	Jaundice, haemolytic, hepatocellular and obstructive. Prolonged antibiotic therapy	Genitourinary diseases. Also in bleeding tendency, some drugs, endocarditis

[a]Using test strips, e.g. Ames Reagent Strips, BM-Test-5L, Diastix or Diabur strips. Normal or non-fresh urine may be alkaline; normal urine may be acid.
[b]Dopa, ascorbate or salicylates may give false-negatives.
[c]May be false-negative if urine not fresh.
[d]Ascorbic acid may give false-negative.

BLOOD TESTS: INTERPRETATION OF HAEMATOLOGICAL RESULTS

Blood	Normal range[a]	Level ↑	Level ↓
Haemoglobin	Male 13.0–18.0 g/dl Female 11.5–16.5 g/dl	Polycythaemia (vera or physiological), myeloproliferative disease	Anaemia
Haematocrit (packed cell volume or PCV)	Male 40–54%; Female 37–47%	Polycythaemia; dehydration	Anaemia
Mean cell volume (MCV) $MCV = \dfrac{PCV}{RBC}$	78–99 fl	Macrocytosis in vitamin B_{12} or folate deficiency; liver disease; alcoholism; hypothyroidism; myelodysplasia; myeloproliferative disorders; aplastic anaemia; cytotoxic agents	Microcytosis in iron deficiency; thalassaemia; chronic disease

continued

Blood	Normal range[a]	Level ↑	Level ↓
Mean cell haemoglobin (MCH) $$MCH = \frac{Hb}{RBC}$$	27–31 pg	Pernicious anaemia	Iron deficiency; thalassaemia; sideroblastic anaemia
Mean cell haemoglobin concentration (MCHC) $$MCHC = \frac{Hb}{PCV}$$	32–36 g/dl		Iron deficiency; thalassaemia; sidero-blastic anaemia; anaemia in chronic disease
Red cell count (RBC)	Male $4.2–6.1 \times 10^{12}/l$; Female $4.2–5.4 \times 10^{12}/l$	Polycythaemia	Anaemia; fluid overload
White cell count (total)	$4–10 \times 10^9/l$	Pregnancy; exercise; infection; trauma; leukaemia	Early leukaemia; some infections; bone marrow disease; drugs; idiopathic
Neutrophils	average $3 \times 10^9/l$	Pregnancy; exercise; infection; bleeding; trauma; malignancy; leukaemia	Some infections; drugs; endocrinopathies; bone marrow disease; idiopathic
Lymphocytes	average $2.5 \times 10^9/l$	Physiological; some infections; leukaemia; bowel disease	Some infections; some immune defects (e.g. HIV, AIDS)
Eosinophils	average $0.15 \times 10^9/l$	Allergic disease; parasitic infestations; skin disease; lymphoma	Some immune defects
Platelets	$150–400 \times 10^9/l$	Thrombocytosis in bleeding; myelo-proliferative disease; chronic inflammatory states	Thrombocytopenia related to leukaemia; drugs; HIV; other infections; idiopathic; autoimmune
Reticulocytes	0.5–1.5% of RBC	Haemolytic states; during treatment of anaemia	
Erythrocyte sedimentation rate (ESR)	0–15 mm/hour	Pregnancy; infections; anaemia; inflammation; connective tissue disease; temporal arteritis; trauma; infarction; tumours	
Plasma viscosity	1.4–1.8 cp	As ESR	

[a]Adults unless otherwise stated. Check values with your laboratory.
MCH: mean corpuscular haemoglobin; MCHC: mean corpuscular haemoglobin concentration.

INTERPRETATION OF BIOCHEMICAL RESULTS

Biochemistry[a]	Normal range[b]	Level ↑	Level ↓
Acid phosphatase	0–13 IU/l	Prostatic malignancy; renal disease; acute myeloid leukaemia	
Alanine transaminase (ALT)[c]	3–60 IU/l	Liver disease; infectious mono-nucleosis	

continued

Biochemistry[a]	Normal range[b]	Level ↑	Level ↓
Alkaline phosphatase	30–110 IU/l (3-13 KA units)	Puberty; pregnancy; Paget's disease; osteomalacia; fibrous dysplasia; malignancy in bone, liver disease; hyperparathyroidism (some); hyperphosphatasia	Hypothyroidism; hypophosphatasia; malnutrition
Alpha$_1$-antitrypsin	200–400 mg%	Cirrhosis	Congenital emphysema
Alphafetoprotein	<12 µg/l	Pregnancy; gonadal tumour; liver disease	Drop in pregnancy indicates fetal distress
Amylase	70–300 IU/l	Pancreatic disease; mumps; some other salivary diseases	
Antistreptolysin O titre (ASOT)	0–300 Todd units/ml	Streptococcal infections; rheumatic fever; drugs[e]	
Aspartate transaminase (AST)[d]	3–40 IU/l	Liver disease; biliary disease; myocardial infarct; trauma; drugs[e]	
Bilirubin (total)	1–17 µmol/l	Liver or biliary disease; haemolysis	
Caeruloplasmin	1.3–3.0 µmol/l	Pregnancy; cirrhosis; hyperthyroidism; leukaemia	Wilson's disease
Calcium	2.3–2.6 mmol/l (*Total* calcium)	Hyperparathyroidism (some); malignancy in bone; renal tubular acidosis; sarcoidosis; thiazides	Hypoparathyroidism; renal failure; rickets; nephrotic syndrome
Cholesterol	3.9–7.8 mmol/l	Hypercholesterolaemia; pregnancy; hypothyroidism; diabetes; nephrotic syndrome; liver or biliary disease	Malnutrition; hyperthyroidism
Complement (C3)	0.79–1.60 g/l	Trauma; surgery; infection	Liver disease; immune complex diseases: e.g. lupus erythematosus
(C4)	0.2–0.4 g/l		Liver disease; immune complex diseases; HANE
Cortisol (*see* steroids)			
Creatine phosphokinase (CPK)	50–100 IU/l (< 130)	Myocardial infarct; trauma; muscle disease	
Creatinine	0.06–0.11 mmol/l	Renal failure; urinary obstruction	Pregnancy
C-reactive protein (CRP)	< 10 µg/ml	Inflammation; trauma; myocardial infarct; malignant disease	
C1 esterase inhibitor	0.1–0.3 g/l		Hereditary angioedema
Ferritin	Adult male 25–190 ng/ml Adult female 15–99 ng/ml Child mean 21 ng/ml	Liver disease; haemochromatosis; leukaemia; lymphoma; other malignancies; thalassaemia	Iron deficiency

continued

Biochemistry[a]	Normal range[b]	Level ↑	Level ↓
Fibrinogen	200–400 mg%	Pregnancy; pulmonary embolism; nephrotic syndrome; lymphoma	Disseminated intravascular coagulopathy (DIC)
Folic acid	3–20 μg/l (red cell folate 120–650 μg/l)	Folic acid therapy	Alcoholism; dietary deficiency; haemolytic anaemias; malabsorption; myelodysplasia; phenytoin; methotrexate; trimethoprim; pyrimethamine; sulphasalazine; cycloserine; oral contraceptives
Free thyroxine index (FTI) (serum T4 × T3 uptake)	1.3–5.1 U	Hyperthyroidism	Hypothyroidism
Gammaglutamyl transpeptidase (GGT)	(5–42 IU/l)	Liver disease; myocardial infarct; pancreatitis, diabetes; renal diseases; tricyclics	
Globulins (total) (see also under protein)	22–36 g/l	Liver disease; myelomatosis; autoimmune disease; chronic infections	Chronic lymphatic leukaemia; malnutrition; protein-losing states
Glucose	2.8–5.0 mmol/l	Diabetes mellitus; pancreatitis; hyperthyroidism; hyperpituitarism; Cushing's disease; liver disease; after head injury	Hypoglycaemic drugs; Addison's disease; hypopituitarism; hyperinsulinism; severe liver disease
Hydroxybutyrate dehydrogenase (HBD)	100–250 IU/l	Myocardial infarct	
Immunoglobulins			
Total	7–22	Liver disease; infection; sarcoidosis; connective tissue disease	Immunodeficiency; nephrotic syndrome; enteropathy
IgG	5–6 g/l	Myelomatosis; connective tissue diseases	Immunodeficiency; nephrotic syndrome
IgA	1.25–4.25 g/l	Alcoholic cirrhosis; Buerger's disease	Immunodeficiency
IgM	0.5–1.75 g/l	Primary biliary cirrhosis; nephrotic syndrome; parasites; infections	Immunodeficiency
IgE	< 0.007 mg%	Allergies; parasites	
Lactic dehydrogenase (LDH)	90–300 IU/l	Myocardial infarct; trauma; liver disease; haemolytic anaemias; lymphoproliferative diseases	Radiotherapy
Lipase	0.2–1.5 IU/l	Pancreatic disease	
Lipids (triglycerides)	50–150 mg%	Hyperlipidaemia; diabetes mellitus; hypothyroidism	
Magnesium	0.7–0.9 mmol/l	Renal failure	Cirrhosis; malabsorption; diuretics; Conn's syndrome; renal tubular defects

continued

Biochemistry[a]	Normal range[b]	Level ↑	Level ↓
Nucleotidase	1–15 IU/l	Liver disease	
Phosphate	0.8–1.5 mmol/l	Renal failure; bone disease; hypopara-thyroidism; hyper-vitaminosis D	Hyperparathyroidism; rickets; malabsorption syndrome; insulin
Potassium	3.5–5.0 mmol/l	Renal failure; Addison's disease	Vomiting; diabetes; diarrhoea; Conn's syndrome; diuretics; Cushing's disease; malabsorption
Protein (total)	62–80 g/l	Liver disease; myelo-matosis; sarcoid; connective tissue diseases	Pregnancy; nephrotic syndrome; malnutrition; enteropathy; renal failure; lymphomas
Albumin	35–55 g/l	Dehydration	Liver disease; malabsorption; nephrotic syndrome; myelomatosis; connective tissue disorders
Alpha$_1$-globulin	2–4 g/l	Oestrogens	Nephrotic syndrome
Alpha$_2$-globulin	4–8 g/l	Infections; trauma	Nephrotic syndrome
Beta-globulin	6–10 g/l	Hypercholesterolaemia; liver disease; pregnancy	Chronic disease
Gamma-globulin	6–15 g/l	(see Immunoglobulins)	Nephrotic syndrome; immunodeficiency
SGGT (see GGT) SGOT (see AST) SGPT (see ALT)			
Sodium	130–145 nmol/l	Dehydration; Cushing's disease	Oedema; renal failure; Addison's disease
Steroids (corticosteroids)	110–525 mmol/l (14 ± 6 μg%)	Cushing's disease; some tumours	Addison's disease; hypopituitarism
Thyroxine (T4)	50–138 nmol/l	Hyperthyroidism; pregnancy; oral contraceptive	Hypothyroidism; nephrotic syndrome; phenytoin
Urea	3.3–6.7 mmol/l	Renal failure; dehydration	Liver disease; nephrotic syndrome; pregnancy
Uric acid	0.15–0.48 mmol/l	Gout; leukaemia; renal failure; myelomatosis	Liver disease; probenecid; allopurinol; salicylates; other drugs
Vitamin B$_{12}$	150–800 ng/l	Liver disease; leukaemia	Pernicious anaemia; gastrectomy; Crohn's disease; ileal resection; vegans; metformin

Note: Values may differ from laboratory to laboratory. For further information, consult R. D. Eastham, *Biochemical Values in Clinical Medicine*, Bristol: Wright, 1975. There are many more causes of abnormal results than are outlined here.
[a]Serum or plasma.
[b]Adult levels; always consult your own laboratory.
[c]ALT = SGPT (serum glutamate-pyruvate transaminase).
[d]AST = SGOT (serum glutamate-oxaloacetic transaminase).
[e]Ampicillin, cephalothin, cloxacillin, erythromycin, indomethacin, methotrexate, opioids.
SI values: 10^{-1} = deci (d); 10^{-2} = centi (c); 10^{-3} = milli (m); 10^{-6} = micro (μ); 10^{-9} = nano (n); 10^{-12} = pico (p); 10^{-15} = femto (f).

continued

SIGNIFICANCE OF THE MORE COMMON ANTINUCLEAR ANTIBODIES

Antinuclear antibodies	Associated with antibodies to	Significance
Diffuse (homogeneous)	Deoxyribonucleoprotein	High titres: SLE Low titres: other connective tissue diseases
Rim (peripheral)	Double-stranded DNA (ds-DNA)	Antibody with the highest specificity for SLE and found in most patients
Speckled	Extractable nuclear antigens (ENA)	
	to Smith (Sm) antigen:	very specific for SLE but only seen in minority of cases
	to ribonuclear protein (nRNP or UIRNP) antigen:	mixed connective tissue disorder, scleroderma, SLE
	to Robair (Ro) A antigen (SS-A):	SLE skin disease; some Sjögren's syndrome
	to: Lattimer (La) B antigen (SS-B):	SLE and primary and secondary Sjögren's syndrome JO-1: polydermatomyositis PM-SC1[a] polydermatomyositis, and scleroderma
	to Centromere:	CREST syndrome
Nucleolar	nucleolus-specific RNA	Scleroderma or Raynaud's
DNA antibodies	ds-DNA (*Crithidia luciliae*)	High titres: SLE
	ss-DNA	Rheumatic diseases and chronic inflammatory disorders (not specific but sensitive)

ss-DNA = single-stranded DNA; ds-DNA = double-stranded DNA; SLE = systemic lupus erythematosus; CREST = calcinosis, Raynaud's, oesophageal, sclerodactyly and telangiectasia.
[a]SC1-70 = anti-topoisomerase 1.

OTHER AUTOANTIBODIES THAT MAY BE USEFUL IN DIAGNOSIS IN DENTISTRY*

Autoantibody	Significance		Positive in
Rheumatoid factor[a]	Latex test SCAT DAT	> 1 in 20 > 1 in 32 > 1 in 16	Rheumatoid arthritis (sometimes systemic lupus erythematosus)
Salivary duct antibody			Sjögren's syndrome, particularly in sicca syndrome
Parietal cell antibody; intrinsic factor antibodies			Pernicious anaemia
Epithelial intercellular cement			Pemphigus
Epithelial basement membrane zone			Some pemphigoid

*The presence of autoantibodies does not always indicate disease.
[a]Agglutination tests. SCAT = sheep cell agglutination test; DAT = direct agglutination test.

continued

RADIOGRAPHY

Radiographs recommended for demonstrating lesions at various sites

Radiography requests: To enable the radiographic staff to give you the best or most appropriate radiographs for the region under investigation:
1. Fill in the request form as fully as possible with full, relevant clinical findings.
2. Request the region required rather than specific views, except for panoral tomography, when OPT or OPG will suffice.

Region required	Standard views	Additional views
Skull[a]	PA 20 Lateral Townes (1/2 axial view)	SMV Tangential
Facial bones	OM OM 30 Lateral	Zygoma Reduced exposure SMV
Paranasal sinuses	OM for maxillary antra	Upper occlusal or lateral SMV OPT, tomography
Orthodontics	OPT/OPG Cephalometric lateral skull	
Pre- and post-osteotomy	OPT/OPG Cephalometric lateral skull Cephalometric PA skull	
Nasal bones	OM 30 Lateral Soft tissue lateral	
Mandible	OPT/OPG	Lateral obliques PA mandible Mandibular occlusal
Temporomandibular joints	Transcranial lateral obliques *or* OPT/OPG (mouth open and closed)	Transpharyngeal Arthrography Reverse Townes Reverse OPT Consider CAT scan/MRI

[a]CAT scanning is valuable in craniofacial injuries. PA = postero anterior; OM = occipito mental; SMV = submento vertex

VENEPUNCTURE

Complications of venepuncture

Complication	Remarks
Failure in a young normal adult	Relax. Check that the syringe and needle *will* aspirate Try the other arm; use a sphygmomanometer cuff at just below diastolic pressure; make sure you can palpate the vein before trying again
Difficult patients Fat arm: veins difficult to locate	Remember that the veins *are* there. Palpate the antecubital fossa over the usual vein site (see text) If unsuccessful, try the veins on the radial side of the wrist or on the back of the hand (painful)

continued

Complication	Remarks
Thin arm: veins move away from needle	Most annoying! Insert the needle deliberately alongside the vein, preferably at a Y-junction and immobilize the vein with your other hand before penetrating vein from the side
Haematoma formation	Most annoying to the patient! May cause venous thrombosis. Try not to penetrate through the other side of the vein. Keep gentle pressure with swab on vein after venepuncture until haemostasis secured In the elderly, maintain this pressure for several minutes

APPENDIX 2 TO CHAPTER 1: SUMMARY OF ANTIBACTERIAL, ANTIFUNGAL AND ANTIVIRAL AGENTS USED IN DENTISTRY

ANTIBACTERIALS*

Beta-lactam	Penicillin
	Cephalosporins
	Carbapenems (Imipenem–cilastin)
	Monobactams (Aztreonam)
Rifampicin	
Metronidazole	
Glycopeptides	Vancomycin
	Teicoplanin
Sulphamides and trimethoprim	
Macrolides	Erythromycin
	Clarithromycin
	Azithromycin
Lincosamides	Clindamycin
Aminoglycosides	Gentamicin
	Tobramycin
	Amikacin
	Streptomycin
Fluoroquinolones	Ciprofloxacin
(4-quinolones)	Ofloxacin
	Norfloxacin
Tetracyclines	Tetracycline
	Doxycycline
	Minocycline

Erythromycin
Similar antibacterial spectrum to penicillin. Often used for penicillin-allergic patients. Avoid erythromycin estolate which may cause liver disturbance.

Erythromycin stearate	Given by mouth, but absorption erratic and unpredictable
	Useful in those hypersensitive to penicillin
	Effective against some staphylococci and most streptococci
	May cause nausea or hearing loss in large doses
	Rapid development of resistance
	Reduced dose indicated in liver disease
	With astemizole, terfenadine and cisaprid may cause dysrhythmias

continued

Cephalosporins, cephamycins and other beta-lactams
These agents are rarely needed in dentistry, they are expensive, and many may cross-react with penicillins, causing hypersensitivity reactions in those allergic to penicillins. They include:

> cephalosporins (cefotaxime, ceftazidime, cefuroxime, cephalexin and cephradine), cephamycins (cefoxitin), monobactams (aztreonam), carbapenems (imipenem and meropenem).

Clindamycin	Mainly reserved, *as a single dose*, for prophylaxis of infective endocarditis in patients allergic to penicillin Given by mouth, very reliably absorbed Mild diarrhoea common Repeated doses may cause pseudomembranous colitis, especially in the elderly and in combination with other drugs
Gentamicin	Reserved for serious infections and prophylaxis of endocarditis Can cause vestibular and renal damage Contraindicated in pregnancy and myasthenia gravis
Metronidazole	Given by mouth Effective only against anaerobes Use only for 7 days (or peripheral neuropathy may develop, particularly in patients with liver disease) Avoid alcohol (disulfiram-type reaction) May increase warfarin effect Available as i.v. preparation but expensive Avoid in pregnancy

Penicillins
This section covers penicillins used in dentistry. Carboxypenicillins (carbenicillin and ticarcillin), and ureidopenicillins (azlocillin and piperacillin) are active against Gram-negative organisms and therefore rarely used in dentistry except amoxycillin.

Amoxycillin	Given by mouth (absorption better than ampicillin) Broad spectrum (effective against many Gram-negative bacilli) *Staphylococcus aureus* often resistant Not resistant to penicillinase Contraindicated in penicillin allergy Rashes, particularly in infectious mononucleosis, lymphoid leukaemia, or during allopurinol treatment May cause diarrhoea
Ampicillin	Less well absorbed than amoxycillin otherwise similar. (Many analogues, such as bacampicillin and pivampicillin – but few advantages) Available with cloxacillin (Ampiclox) or flucloxacillin (Co-fluampicil) Contraindicated in penicillin allergy
Benzylpenicillin	Given i.m. or i.v. Most effective penicillin when organism-sensitive. Not resistant to penicillinase. Contraindicated in penicillin allergy. Large doses may cause K^+ to fall, Na^+ to rise
Co-amoxiclav	Mixture of amoxycillin and potassium clavulanate: inhibits some penicillinases and therefore active against most *S. aureus*; also active against some Gram-negative bacilli Contraindicated in penicillin allergy
Flucloxacillin	Given by mouth Effective against most penicillin-resistant staphylococci Contraindicated in penicillin allergy

continued

Phenoxymethyl penicillin (penicillin V)	Given by mouth Not resistant to penicillinase Contraindicated in penicillin allergy
Procaine penicillin	Depot penicillin Not resistant to penicillinase Contraindicated in penicillin allergy Rarely, psychotic reaction due to procaine
Temocillin	Given by intramuscular or intravenous injection Active against penicillinase-producing Gram-negative bacteria Contraindicated in penicillin allergy
Triplopen	Depot penicillin (benzyl penicillin 300 mg, procaine penicillin 250 mg, and benethamine penicillin (475 mg) Not resistant to penicillinase Contraindicated in pencillin allergy

Rifampicin	Reserved mainly for treatment of tuberculosis May be used in prophylaxis of meningitis after head injury since *N. meningitidis* and *S. aureus* frequently resistant to sulphonamides Safe and effective but resistance rapidly develops. Body secretions turn red May interfere with oral contraception Occasional rashes, jaundice or blood dyscrasias

Sulphonamides	Main indication is for prophylaxis of post-traumatic meningitis but meningococci increasingly resistant Contraindicated in pregnancy and in renal disease Adequate hydration essential to prevent (rare) crystalluria Other adverse reactions include rashes, erythema multiforme and blood dyscrasias
Co-trimoxazole (trimethoprim with sulphamethoxazole)	Given by mouth Broad spectrum Occasional rashes or blood dyscrasias Contraindicated in pregnancy or liver disease May increase effect of protein-bound drugs Use should now be confined to infections in HIV-infected persons

Teicoplanin	Reserved mainly for endocarditis prophylaxis Occasional rashes, nausea, fever, anaphylaxis May cause hearing loss or tinnitus Reduce dose in renal failure and elderly

Tetracyclines

Very broad antibacterial spectrum. Little to choose between the many preparations, but doxycycline and minocycline (*see below*) are safer for patients with renal failure. In children, tetracyclines cause dental discoloration. Absorption impaired by iron, antacids, milk, etc. Use of tetracyclines may predispose to candidosis

Tetracycline	Given by mouth Many bacteria now resistant Contraindicated in pregnancy and children up to at least 7 years (tooth discoloration) Reduce dose in renal failure, liver disease and elderly Frequent mild gastrointestinal upsets
Doxycycline	Given by mouth in a single daily dose Contraindicated in pregnancy and children up to at least 7 years (tooth discoloration) Safer than other tetracyclines in renal failure Reduce dose in liver disease and elderly Mild gastrointestinal effects

continued

Minocycline	Given by mouth	
	Active against some meningococci	
	Safer than tetracycline in renal disease	
	May cause dizziness and vertigo	
	Absorption not reduced by milk	
	Contraindicated in pregnancy and children up to at least 7 years (tooth discoloration). May also cause mucosal pigmentation	
Vancomycin	Reserved for serious infections or prophylaxis of endocarditis, given by slow (100 minutes) i.v. infusion.	
	Extravenous extravasation causes necrosis and phlebitis	
	Effective by mouth for pseudomembranous colitis	
	May cause nausea, rashes, 'red man syndrome', tinnitus, deafness when given i.v.	
	Contraindicated in renal disease or deafness	

*Warn patients on the oral contraceptive to use additional precautions if on antimicrobials for more than a single dose.

ANTIFUNGALS

	Comments	Oral dose
Amphotericin*	Active topically. Negligible absorption from gastrointestinal tract. Given IV for deep mycoses	10–100 mg, 6-hourly
Nystatin*	Active topically. Negligible absorption from gastrointestinal tract. Pastilles taste better than lozenge.	500 000 unit lozenge, 100 000 unit pastille or 100 000 unit per ml of suspension 6-hourly
Miconazole*	Active topically. Also has antibacterial activity. Absorption from gastrointestinal tract. Theoretically the best antifungal to treat angular cheilitis. Interacts with anticoagulants, terfenadine, cisapride and astemizole. Avoid in pregnancy, porphyria	250 mg tablet 6-hourly or 25 mg/ml gel used as 5 ml 6-hourly, for 14 days
Ketoconazole	Absorbed from gastrointestinal tract. Useful in intractable candidosis. Contraindicated in pregnancy and liver disease. May cause nausea, rashes, pruritus and liver damage. Interacts with anticoagulants, terfenadine, cisapride, and astemizole	200–400 mg once daily with meal, for 14 days
Fluconazole	Absorbed from gastrointestinal tract. Useful in intractable candidosis. Contraindicated in pregnancy, liver and renal disease. Interacts with anticoagulants, terfenadine, cisapride and Astemizole	50–100 mg daily for 14 days
Itraconazole	May cause nausea, diarrhoea, rash. Absorbed from gastrointestinal tract. Useful in intractable candidosis. Contraindicated in pregnancy, liver disease. Interacts with terfenadine, cisapride and astemizole. May cause nausea, neuropathy, rash	100 mg daily for 14 days

*Dissolve in mouth slowly.

continued

ANTIVIRALS

At present there are few antiviral agents of proven efficacy. Management of viral infections is therefore predominantly supportive. Most antivirals will achieve maximum benefit if given early in the disease. Immunocompromised patients with viral infections may well benefit from active antiviral therapy, since these infections may spread locally and systemically. Antiretroviral drugs are discussed in Chapter 20.

Antiviral therapy of oral viral infections

Virus	Disease	Otherwise healthy patient	Immunocompromised patient
Herpes simplex	Primary herpetic gingivostomatitis Recurrent herpetic ulcers	Consider oral aciclovir[a] 100–200 mg, five times daily as suspension (200 mg/5 ml) or tablets. 5% aciclovir cream or penciclovir 1% cream every 2 hours	Aciclovir 250 mg/m i.v. every 8 hours. Consider aciclovir as above.
Herpes varicella	Chickenpox		Aciclovir 500 mg/m^2 (5 mg/kg) i.v. every 8 hours
	Zoster (shingles)	3% aciclovir ophthalmic ointment for shingles of ophthalmic division of trigeminal	As above. Or famciclovir 250 mg three times daily, or 750 mg daily

[a]In neonate, treat as if immunocompromised.
Aciclovir: systemic preparations, caution in renal disease and pregnancy, occasional increase in liver enzymes and urea, rashes, CNS effects.
Famciclovir: caution in renal disease and pregnancy. Occasional nausea and headache.

2

Perioperative care

Key points

- The aim of immediate preoperative assessment is to ensure that the:
  correct patient is operated on;
  correct site is operated on;
  outcome of operation is optimal.
- Valid informed consent from the patient is required before any procedure.
- Tens of thousands of dental local anaesthetics (LA) are given daily with no untoward effects. LA is remarkably safe if given in safe doses with an aspirating syringe.
- Allergy to local anaesthetic agents is exceedingly rare, but sulphites or other preservatives may be sensitizing.
- Drug interactions with local anaesthetics are rare.
- Most morbidity and deaths in dentistry have been related to general anaesthesia.
- Before general anaesthesia (GA), the patient must take no food for 6 hours, but clear fluids can be taken up to 3 hours (adult) or 2 hours (child) before operation.
- Premedication should be agreed with the anaesthetist.
- There is no place for the operator–anaesthetist, and neither conscious sedation nor GA should be carried out without well-trained staff and suitable equipment for life support.
- All patients must be monitored perioperatively, clinically and with a pulse oximeter and blood pressure monitor.
- The immediate postoperative period is the most dangerous. Great care of the airway must be ensured.
- A responsible adult must accompany the recovered patient home.
- The patient must not drive or ride any vehicle, operate unguarded machinery, or make important decisions until 24 hours after the operation under GA.
- Gaseous anaesthetics must be minimized in the operatory air by scavenging and good ventilation.

Assessment of the patient is discussed in Chapter 1. The main aims are to ensure that procedures are carried out:

- on the correct patient;
- on the correct site;
- with the best possible outcome.

Although operations are nowadays associated with less morbidity and mortality than previously, there is still considerable room for improvement. The UK National Confidential Enquiry into Perioperative Deaths pointed out in 1996 that consultation between surgeons and other specialists, including anaesthetists, needs to be more frequent in order to promote a team approach, and that surgical operations should not be started in hospitals without critical care services.

CONSENT

Valid consent must be obtained from every patient for all procedures. Patients who undergo procedures performed without their valid consent may be entitled to damages resulting from the charge of assault and battery against the person who provided the treatment. This whole area is fraught with problems, as discussed elsewhere (Applebaum and Grisso, 1988).

Patients *must* be informed appropriately about treatment decisions and they have the right to accept or refuse recommended treatment. Parental or guardian's consent is needed for those under 16 years of age. For those with learning disability it is important to get consent from the carer or, in their absence, from two professionals who should sign in the best interests of the patient.

A signed document, however, is not itself the consent to treatment, but merely indicates that the patient and health care worker have discussed the procedure, and the patient has signed. There are two main forms of consent:

- *Expressed*: where the patient verbally or in writing gives consent in a direct statement.
- *Implied*: where consent appears to be given by inference from the patient's conduct.

Clearly, expressed consent is preferred (Appendix).

CONFIDENTIALITY

Medical records and their information are confidential, and can only be released with the express consent of a competent patient or their legal representative, to a person authorized to receive the information.

ANAESTHESIA AND SEDATION

The choice of the appropriate method of anaesthesia for any particular patient for a specific procedure depends on a number of factors (*Table 2.1*), including:

1. The physical and mental fitness of the patient (*see* Appendix 3).
2. The type of operation or procedure indicated.
3. Social circumstances; for example, is the patient able to be accompanied, and cared for at home.
4. Lack of cooperation, such as at a very young age, or for other reasons.
5. Other factors, such as the urgency and the facilities available at the time.

Attempts have been made to grade patients as to physical fitness for operation (*see* Appendix 3 to this chapter), and these may help the decision-making. However, the fact that serious disease can fail to reveal itself during medical examination should act as a deterrent to the use of general anaesthesia or so-called sedation with intravenous barbiturates, which are a significant cause of morbidity or even mortality. **Local anaesthesia should therefore be used wherever possible for outpatient dentistry** (*Table 2.1*), with conscious sedation if necessary.

LOCAL ANAESTHESIA

In most countries, only the amide local anaesthetics are now used. Those mainly used are lignocaine (lidocaine) and prilocaine, but mepivacaine, bupivacaine, articaine and etidocaine are also sometimes used (*Table 2.2*). Bupivacaine and etidocaine have a prolonged action. Vasoconstrictors such as adrenaline are often used in order to maintain duration of anaesthesia; these solutions may contain bisulphites as preservative. Local anaesthetic injections should be given with an aspirating syringe, to avoid intravascular injection.

Local anaesthetic creams (EMLA; lignocaine plus prilocaine) effectively reduce the pain of needle pricks and are thus useful for children.

Lignocaine

Lignocaine is the most widely used local anaesthetic. It is an amide-type with a rapid

Table 2.1   Relative indications and contraindications of anaesthesia and sedation

Indications	*Contraindications*
General anaesthesia	
Major surgery	Severe cardiac or respiratory disease
Multiple extractions	Severe hepatic or renal disease
Acute local infections (but not Ludwig's angina)	Severe anaemia (especially sickle cell anaemia)
Allergy to LA	Severe infections in floor of mouth
Learning disability or anxious	Unescorted patient
	Pregnancy
Local anaesthesia	
Minor surgery or procedure	Sepsis in field
Poor-risk patient for GA	Uncooperative patient
No GA available	Major surgery
Inadequate facilities for GA	Bleeding tendency
Recent meal	Haemangioma in field
	Allergy
	Pseudocholinesterase deficiency
Sedation	
Patient too anxious to accept treatment under local anaesthesia.	Chronic obstructive pulmonary disease (intravenous benzodiazepines especially)
Many prolonged operations such as removal of third molars or preparation for multiple implants for which GA would otherwise be needed	Airways obstruction or respiratory infections
	Disabling severe heart disease
	Psychotic personalities

Note: For epileptics or those with asthma, myasthenia gravis, or some drug-users, relative analgesia is preferable to intravenous sedation because it provides better control of the patient.

Table 2.2   Local anaesthetic agents[a]

Agents	*Comments*	*Maximum safe dose LA agent for fit adults*
Lignocaine 2% plain	Poor and brief analgesia	200 mg (5×2 ml cartridges)
Lignocaine 2% plus adrenaline 1 in 80 000[b]	Effective analgesia for >90 min	500 mg (12×2 ml cartridges)
Prilocaine 4% plain	Poor and brief analgesia Methaemoglobinaemia	400 mg (6×2 ml cartridges)
Prilocaine 3% plus felypressin 0.03 IU/ml	Usually effective analgesia for 90 min[c] Methaemoglobinaemia	600 mg (10×2 ml cartridges)
Bupivacaine 0.25% plain	Used only for prolonged nerve block (up to 8 h)	

[a]Allergy to amide local anaesthetic agents, if it exists, is *very* rare (supposed 'allergies' are common however).
[b]The total dose of adrenaline must never exceed 500 µg, i.e. not more than 40 ml of LA containing adrenaline in a 1 in 80 000 solution.
[c]No evidence that it is safer than lignocaine with adrenaline for patients on monoamine oxidase inhibitors or tricyclic antidepressants.

onset of action producing anaesthesia of intermediate duration.

• **Metabolism of lignocaine**

Lignocaine rapidly distributes to highly perfused tissues and then to adipose tissue and muscle. In plasma, up to 80 per cent binds to an alpha-1-acid glycoprotein (AAG). Lignocaine has an elimination half-life of 1–2 hours, rapidly undergoing first-pass metabolism in the liver, being dealkylated by mixed-function oxidases to monoethylglycinexylidide and glycinexylidide, which may be further metabolized to monoethylglycine and xylidide. Both monoethylglycinexylidide and glycinexylidide can contribute to the effects of lignocaine as they have half-lives longer than that of lignocaine. Monoethylglycine and xylidide also have local anaesthetic activity.

About 75 per cent of xylidide is excreted in urine as a metabolite 4-hydroxy 2,6-dimethyl-aniline. Less than 10 per cent of lignocaine is excreted in urine unchanged. Lignocaine can cross the placenta, and may enter breast milk.

Alterations in concentrations of AAG may influence plasma levels of free lignocaine. AAG is an acute phase protein which rises after trauma, burns and in chronic inflammatory disorders such as Crohn's disease, and malignancy, whereas in disorders such as nephrotic syndrome there will be a fall in AAG levels. Levels of AAG may also be reduced by oestrogens. Phenytoin may increase production of AAG.

Factors that affect hepatic blood supply and/or enzyme function can significantly influence lignocaine metabolism. Reduced metabolism may be seen in severe cardiac failure and liver disease. Beta-blockers may reduce hepatic blood flow and inhibit hepatic microsomal enzymes. Cimetidine may reduce hepatic blood flow. By contrast, phenytoin, benzodiazepines and barbiturates may induce hepatic enzymes, reducing levels of free lignocaine.

- ### Adverse effects of lignocaine

Systemic signs of lignocaine toxicity are likely when blood levels rise above 5 µg/ml. There may not, however, be a linear relationship between the dose of lignocaine injected and the resultant blood level.

In general, toxicity is more likely in children, the elderly and some acutely ill patients. Early features of toxicity include tinnitus, circumoral paraesthesia, metallic taste, light-headedness, nausea and vomiting, and double vision. At higher levels, nystagmus, slurred speech, auditory and visual hallucinations, localized muscle twitching and tremors of the hands and feet may occur. CNS manifestations include convulsions followed by loss of conciousness, respiratory arrest and eventual cardiovascular collapse. Lignocaine may cause some degree of depression of atrial and atrioventricular nodal activity, intraventricular conductivity and ventricular contraction.

Local adverse effects are more common and include blanching of the facial skin, transient facial palsy (LA misplaced and entering the parotid where it affects the facial nerve), visual disturbance (misplaced LA), persistent anaesthesia or trismus (damage to nerve supply or medial pterygoid muscle), or lip trauma (due to the patient biting an anaesthetized lip).

Prilocaine

Prilocaine is an amide-type local anaesthetic agent of fast onset and intermediate duration of action. Like lignocaine, it binds to AAG. It is rapidly metabolized by the liver and excreted in the urine as o-toluidine, a metabolite that may give rise to methaemoglobinaemia. Prilocaine can cross the placenta.

- ### Adverse effects of prilocaine

The local and systemic side-effects of prilocaine are similar to those of lignocaine, but prilocaine is less toxic. Methaemoglobinaemia may arise if o-toluidine accumulates. O-toluidine oxidizes ferrous iron in haemoglobin to ferric methaemoglobin, resulting in impaired oxygen-carrying capacity. Methaemoglobinaemia manifests as cyanosis, when levels of methaemoglobin exceed 1.5 g/dl, and symptoms of methaemoglobinaemia (e.g. dyspnoea) occur when levels exceed 5 g/dl. Methaemoglobinaemia appears within 1 hour and usually resolves within 2–3 hours. It appears more likely to occur when a vasoconstrictor is not given, when there is anaemia, in newborns and in infants, in patients on sulphonamides or antimalarials, in glucose-6-phosphate dehydrogenase deficiency or the autosomal recessive NADH-dependent methaemoglobin reductase deficiency.

The CNS and cardiac toxic effects of prilocaine are similar to those seen with lignocaine.

Mepivacaine

Mepivacaine is an amide-type local anaesthetic with a more rapid onset and more prolonged duration of action than lignocaine. Mepivacaine binds to plasma proteins, has a plasma half-life of 2–3 hours and is rapidly metabolized in the liver. About 50 per cent of the metabolites of mepivacaine are excreted in bile; less than 10 per cent of the unchanged drug is excreted in urine. Mepivacaine can cross the placenta.

Bupivacaine

Bupivacaine is an amide-type local anaesthetic with a slow onset but long duration of action. Most bupivacaine binds to plasma protein. It has a plasma half-life of 1.5–5.5 hours, and is largely metabolized in the liver.

• Adverse effects of bupivacaine

Bupivacaine is the most cardiotoxic of the local anaesthetics. Bupivacaine inhibits cardiac conductivity and contractility and may induce ventricular fibrillation. The cardiotoxic effects are enhanced by hypoxia, hypercapnoea, acidosis and hyperkalaemia. Bupivacaine should not be used for patients with cardiac disease.

Adrenaline

The inclusion of adrenaline to a local anaesthetic increases haemostasis and anaesthesia: 1 in 100 000 adrenaline enhances pulpal anaesthesia nine-fold, and soft tissue anaesthesia four-fold.

Adrenaline is a potent sympathomimetic having significant beta-adrenergic activity and some alpha-activity. The beta-1 action increases cardiac rate and contraction force while beta-2 activity causes bronchodilatation. Adrenaline is rapidly inactivated by hepatic metabolism via both catechol-O-methyl transferases (COMT) and monoamine oxidases (MAO). Adrenaline is first methylated to metanephrine by COMT then deaminated by MAO to 4-hydroxy-3-methoxymandelic acid (vanillylmandelic acid: VMA), or to 3,4-dihydroxymandelic acid which is then methylated by COMT to 4-hydroxy-3-methoxymandelic acid. The metabolites are excreted in urine, mainly as glucuronides or ethereal sulphate conjugates.

The cardiac effects of adrenaline-containing local anaesthetic solutions are of significant clinical interest. By virtue of its alpha-adrenergic activity adrenaline causes vasoconstriction of vessels of the skin and mucosae, its beta-adrenergic action increases the rate and force of cardiac contraction, hence cardiac output, and together with the raised peripheral resistance there can be an increase in blood pressure.

There is considerable debate as to the possible systemic consequences of the addition of adrenaline. By virtue of the enhanced anaesthesia, adrenaline may reduce the release of endogenous catecholamines, but recent data using tritiated adrenaline suggest that the rise in peripheral blood catecholamine levels associated with intra-oral injection of adrenaline-containing local anaesthetic is mainly due to exogenous adrenaline. Despite the use of aspirating techniques, up to 20 per cent of all local anaesthetic injections made into the highly vascular head and neck region may result in a significant, rapid, albeit transient rise of peripheral blood levels of adrenaline following injection of adrenaline-containing local anaesthetics. In addition there is a slow rise in peripheral blood levels of adrenaline as a consequence of the gradual release of local anaesthetic solution from the site of injection into local blood vessels.

The levels of adrenaline in local anaesthetics are sufficient to increase cardiac output in healthy persons and in those with cardiovascular disease. This is not seen when adrenaline is not used. There is a very small rise in systolic blood pressure (up to 8 mmHg), and a slight fall in diastolic pressure when lignocaine with 1:100 000 adrenaline is used, and up to 14 mmHg with 1:25 000 adrenaline. Patients with hypertension have more marked increases in systolic pressures after the administration of local anaesthetics, but patients with ischaemic heart disease or prosthetic cardiac valves have changes similar to those of healthy persons.

However, patients can have changes in systolic and diastolic pressures and cardiac rate *even before attending for dental treatment* – indeed the mere sight of a clinician can cause a slight rise in blood pressure. Immediately before the injection of local anaesthetic there can be significant rises in cardiac rate, systolic pressure and, to a lesser extent, diastolic pressure. Interestingly, cardiac rate may fall but systolic pressure rises during the administration of the local anaesthetic. Similar cardiovascular changes may be seen when saline is injected or even if a syringe is placed in the mouth but the needle does not touch the mucosa. Anxiety must underlie these changes.

It has recently been shown that adrenaline-containing local anaesthetics may cause a significant, but transient, fall in plasma potassium, an effect particularly notable in patients on non-potassium-sparing diuretics. This hypokalaemic action appears due to a beta-2 adrenergic action on membrane-bound ATPase. The clinical significance *if any*, remains unclear.

Adrenaline-containing local anaesthetics may also cause a transient rise in plasma glucose levels, due to alpha-2 adrenergic inhibition of insulin release. This appears *not* to be of any clinical significance.

Adrenaline-containing local anaesthetics may also *slightly* delay wound healing following dental surgery and may increase the frequency of post-extraction alveolar osteitis.

Felypressin

Felypressin is a synthetic analogue of vasopressin with little of the antidiuretic or oxytocin-like actions. Even if given intravenously in amounts far in excess of those used for local anaesthesia, felypressin has little toxicity. The administration of large amounts of felypressin to patients receiving general anaesthesia with halothane *may* result in cyanosis and a slight rise in blood pressure, but these changes are not serious.

Adverse reactions to local anaesthetic injections

Serious reactions to local anaesthetics are rare and most adverse responses are caused by reactions unrelated to the drug itself (such as fainting), or due to inadvertent entry of the drug into the circulation. Such reactions include:

1. Reactions unrelated to the local anaesthetic agent
   psychomotor responses
   sympathetic stimulation
2. Dose-related toxic responses in normal individuals
   cardiovascular
   CNS
3. Idiosyncratic and allergic responses.

Maximum doses of local anaesthetics

An aspirating technique should always be employed and the local anaesthetic slowly injected. Excessive doses of lignocaine have been followed by death. As discussed above,

lignocaine should be used with caution in cardiac, hepatic or renal disease.

Lignocaine should not be given in a dose exceeding 4.4 mg/kg body weight. *The maximum dose of lignocaine* for the average adult therefore is 200 mg, or 500 mg if given with adrenaline as the vasoconstrictor. A dental local anaesthetic cartridge of 2.2 ml containing lignocaine 2 per cent contains 44 mg of the drug, and thus the maximum safe number of cartridges for a normal adult if the solution contained adrenaline would be four, and certainly no more than seven cartridges. Children, elderly patients and some medically compromised persons (especially patients with liver disease, or after cardiac surgery) should be given less.

The maximum adult dose of prilocaine is 400 mg if used alone, or 600 mg if used with felypressin. Excessive doses can cause methaemoglobinaemia. Thus prilocaine is contraindicated in methaemoglobinaemia, and some advise against the use of prilocaine in children.

Local anaesthetic allergy

It is estimated that at least 50 000 000 cartridges of lignocaine (lidocaine) are used each year in Great Britain. Convincing reports of *authenticated* allergic reactions, or confirmation that lignocaine was the component responsible, cannot be found. The risk of hypersensitivity to other amide local anaesthetics such as prilocaine or mepivicaine is equally low. Mechanisms involved in such allergies, if they exist, may be IgE-mediated immediate-type, immune complex or delayed-type hypersensitivity reactions.

The most sensitizing component of local anaesthetic solutions has been the methyl parabens preservative. As a consequence, this has been replaced in some anaesthetic solutions. Sulphite preservatives may also be sensitizing. Amide local anaesthetics such as lignocaine also far more rarely cause contact dermatitis than the ester-type agents and fewer than 20 cases have been reported worldwide. Esters such as amethocaine, sometimes used in surface anaesthetic preparations, can be potent sensitizers.

Attempts to confirm putative allergy to local anaesthetics by skin testing (prick tests or intracutaneous tests) are time-consuming, usually uninformative, in the rare instances of true allergy can provoke anaphylaxis, and are therefore rarely justified. Specific IgE responses are also rarely demonstrable by radioallergosorbent tests. Challenge tests with the implicated agents are also typically negative and, in those who respond, the mechanism appears to be direct release of histamine rather than an allergy. *In vitro* tests depending on histamine release from sensitized basophils may be more informative but are not readily available.

If a patient claims to be allergic to a local anaesthetic then either a non-cross-reacting agent should be used or an alternative management (such as general anaesthesia), or it may be feasible to skin test with a non-cross-reacting agent first, on the basis that lack of skin reaction probably means the agent will be safe to use. In cases where there are multiple supposed allergies, it may be best to first administer sterile saline subcutaneously as a test to reveal a non-allergic cause, then decreasing dilutions of the local anaesthetic, given at 30 minute intervals. Resuscitation facilities must be at hand.

Drug interactions with local anaesthetic solutions (*see* Chapter 25)

Adrenaline in theory may be potentiated in patients taking tricyclic antidepressants, and in patients on beta-blockers or adrenergic-blocking agents. Other interactions are exceedingly rare.

Deaths associated with local anaesthesia

Local anaesthetics are remarkably safe if given in low doses. Over a 10-year period there were only three deaths in persons receiving dental care under LA in Britain (1980–89). All were related to the use of prilocaine, a fact that does not suggest that prilocaine is dangerous but serves to emphasize that it is not necessarily safer than lignocaine. Overdosage of LA has, however, caused deaths; one recent case was an elderly patient with angina who died after being given 16 cartridges of LA. There should rarely be a need to give more than two cartridges; if more is deemed necessary, cardiac monitoring is indicated.

PRECAUTIONS BEFORE SEDATION OR GENERAL ANAESTHESIA

(*See also* Appendices to this chapter)

Patients quickly forget or fail to take in what they are told. As mentioned earlier therefore, it is important not merely to give instructions verbally as suggested below, but also to give these same instructions in written form when it has been decided that either general anaesthesia or sedation is necessary.

Identification of the patient and operation site

The patient's name and the reason for having general anaesthesia must be confirmed. This apparently obvious precaution avoids embarrassing confusion between patients coming from a crowded waiting room. The operation site should be marked in ink, by the operator, while the patient is conscious, and checked with the patient.

Informed consent

Written consent to general anaesthesia must be obtained before each operation.

Suitable consent forms are supplied by the medical defence societies. It is also helpful, and there is increasing pressure, to provide patients with written information relevant to their treatment.

No food or drink

Adults should not consume food nor take oral medication for 6 hours preoperatively. Food or materials present in the stomach may be vomited and inhaled during anaesthesia with disastrous consequences. Clear instructions must be given that adults should take no food or drink (including tea or alcohol) for 6 hours preoperatively, though clear fluids may be taken up to 3 hours preoperatively (*see* Appendix 4 to this chapter). Clear fluids include still water or fruit squash, *not* tea, coffee, milk, fizzy drinks or alcohol. Vomiting is more likely in a patient who is pregnant or has gastric disease or a head injury, or has taken alcohol or a drug such as erythromycin which may precipitate vomiting.

In the case of children, however, it is important to avoid dehydration, and thus clear fluids *can* be taken up to 2 hours before the anaesthetic. Food, however, should not be taken for 6 hours preoperatively.

Dentures, bladder, bowels and other factors

Dentures should be removed preoperatively. The anaesthetist must be warned of the presence of crowned, fragile or loose teeth, or bridges which could be damaged during intubation, of contact lenses, hearing aids, or a colostomy bag.

The bladder should be emptied preoperatively and it is sometimes necessary to catheterize inpatients. A nasogastric tube should be inserted if required. It may be necessary to shave a skin operation site. Never shave eyebrows.

Psychological preparation and premedication

Most people are apprehensive of general anaesthesia; some are terrified. Dental treatment in general, and oral surgery in particular, is stressful for many patients, and can induce a rise in blood pressure and pulse rate, and ECG changes. Apart from poor cooperation as a result of anxiety, autonomic overactivity can precipitate cardiac dysrhythmias, swings in blood pressure and vomiting.

One of the most effective methods of reducing anxiety is by sympathetic reassurance and brief discussion of a patient's particular anxieties. If this fails, however, premedication with a benzodiazepine may be necessary, though this is not usually feasible in general dental practice as it delays recovery. Benzodiazepines may also be ineffective in children, and persons on long-term medication with psychoactive drugs.

Anaesthetists vary widely in their requirements for premedication which must be discussed with the anaesthetist. The main purpose of premedication is to lessen anxiety, and it is typically given 30–35 minutes preoperatively. For inpatients, benzodiazepines, or opioids (pethidine, morphine or omnopon), are traditional premedicants because of their sedative action. However, opioids increase nausea, vomiting and respiratory depression.

Table 2.3 Preoperative modification of regularly used medications

Medication	Modification before operation under general anaesthesia or sedation
Corticosteroids	*See* Chapter 14. **Increase** dose
Digoxin	Give up to op.
Beta-blockers	Give up to op.
Anticonvulsants	Give until 1 hour before op.
Monoamine oxidase inhibitors or lithium	Stop 3 weeks before op.
Oral contraceptives	Stop and use alternative contraception if long operation
Anticoagulants	*See* Chapter 4; consult haematologist
Insulin or antidiabetics	*See* Chapter 14

Promethazine or trimeprazine may be used for their sedative and anti-emetic effect, for premedication of children, but they have a prolonged action and are often ineffective. They also raise blood sugar levels – a consideration when treating diabetics. Children may be given oral trimeprazine or triclofos, or rectal barbiturates such as thiopentone.

Benzodiazepines are useful because of their anxiolytic and amnesic actions. Their relative freedom from side-effects and wide safety margin have caused diazepam, lorazepam or temazepam to be increasingly widely used. Beta-blockers may also be used and may help to prevent dysrhythmias induced by surgery.

Atropinics such as atropine, glycopyrronium or hyoscine, are anti-emetics and may also reduce the parasympathomimetic effects and dysrhythmias sometimes associated with suxamethonium but are unlikely to be needed for outpatients. However, the effectiveness of atropinics in preventing dysrhythmias other than vagal overactivity is controversial. Glaucoma is a specific contraindication to the use of atropinics and diazepam. Since the maximal effect of atropine is apparent 30–60 minutes after injection, some anaesthetists give the drug during induction of anaesthesia, thus achieving the desired parasympatholytic effect during the operation while sparing the patient the unpleasant dry mouth and thirst during the preoperative period. Hyoscine is best avoided in the elderly, in whom it may cause confusion. Atropinics should not be given to febrile patients.

Table 2.4   Agents for general anaesthesia and sedation

Drug	Proprietary names	Adult dose	Comments
Drugs for intravenous anaesthesia			
Etomidate	Hypnomidate	0.2 mg/kg	Good for outpatient anaesthesia. Pain on injection: use large vein and give fentanyl 200 µg first. After operation give naloxone 0.1–0.2 mg and oxygen. Little cardiovascular effect. Often involuntary movements, cough and hiccup. Hepatic metabolism. Avoid in repeated doses on traumatized patient – may suppress adrenal steroid production
Ketamine	Ketalar	0.5–2 mg/kg	Rise in BP, cardiac rate, intraocular pressure. Little respiratory depression. Often hallucinations. Contraindicated in hypertension, psychiatric, cerebrovascular or ocular disorders. Rarely used in dentistry
Methohexitone	Brietal	1.5 mg/kg 1% solution (10 mg/ml)	Ultra short-acting barbiturate. The most commonly used i.v. anaesthetic in dentistry. No analgesia. Mild hyperventilation or apnoea if given rapidly. Dose-dependent cardiovascular depression. Relatively non-irritant to tissues. Hepatic metabolism. Contraindicated in epilepsy, cardiorespiratory disease, porphyria, barbiturate sensitivity. Rarely: acute allergy, cough, hiccups, sneezing
Propofol	Diprivan	2 mg/kg	May cause pain on injection. Occasional fits or anaphylaxis. Contraindicated in children
Thiopentone	Intraval	2.5 mg/kg (2.5% solution)	Ultra short-acting barbiturate. No analgesia. Danger of laryngospasm. Rapid injection may cause apnoea. Irritant if injected into artery or extravascularly. Contraindications as for methohexitone
Drugs for intravenous sedation[a]			
Diazepam	Valium	Up to 20 mg	Benzodiazepine: gives sedation with amnesia but no analgesia. Give slowly i.v. in 2.5 mg increments until ptosis begins, i.e. eyelids begin to droop (Verril's sign) (rapid injection may cause respiratory depression). Then give local analgesia Disadvantages: 1. May cause pain or thrombophlebitis 2. Drowsiness returns transiently 4–6 h postoperatively due to metabolism to oxazepam and desmethyldiazepam and enterohepatic recirculation 3. May produce mild hypotension and respiratory depression
	Diazemuls	Up to 20 mg	Preferred to Valium since, although it has most of the actions above, it causes less thrombophlebitis and therefore can be given into veins on dorsum of hand. Expensive. Do not give intramuscularly
Midazolam	Hypnovel	0.07 mg/kg (up to 7.5 mg total dose)	Benzodiazepine. Compared to diazepam: 1. Onset of action is quicker (30 s) 2. Amnesia is more profound, starting 2–5 min after administration and lasting up to 40 min (with no retrograde amnesia) 3. Recovery is more rapid. Midazolam is virtually completely eliminated within 5 h, without the recurrence of drowsiness that may follow the use of diazepam 4. Incidence of venous thrombosis is less than with Valium 5. At least twice as potent. Signs of sedation less predictable – very slow injection required. Occasional deaths in elderly.

continued

Table 2.4 *Continued*

Drug	Proprietary names	Adult dose	Comments
Inhalational agents[b]			
Nitrous oxide	—		Analgesic, but weak anaesthetic. Non-explosive. No cardiorespiratory effects. Mainly used as a vehicle for other anaesthetic agents, or for sedation.
Halothane[c]	Fluothane		The most widely used anaesthetic agent. Non-explosive. Anaesthetic but weak analgesic. Causes fall in BP, cardiac dysrhythmias and bradycardia. Hepatotoxic on repeated administration. Post-anaesthetic shivering is common, vomiting rare
Enflurane	Ethrane Alyrane		Less potent anaesthetic than halothane. Non-explosive. Less likely to produce dysrhythmias or affect liver than halothane. Powerful cardiorespiratory depressant
Isoflurane	Forane Aerrane		Isomer of enflurane, which causes less cardiac but more respiratory depression than halothane. Induction and recovery are slower than with halothane
Desflurane	Suprane		Less potent than isoflurane. May cause apnoea or coughing and is contraindicated for children
Sevoflurane	Sevoflurane		Rapid action and recovery. May cause agitation in children
Trichloroethylene	Trilene		Analgesic and anaesthetic. Non-explosive. Bradycardia and dysrhythmias are common as are tachypnoea, nausea and vomiting

[a]Particular caution in pregnancy, the elderly, children and those with liver or respiratory disease. Do *not* give pentazocine with a benzodiazepine. Midazolam is the preferred preparation.
[b]Gas scavenging should be used.
[c]Do not give halothane if patient has had halothane within the previous 6 weeks or has previously had an adverse reaction to halothane.

Cardiac dysrhythmias are common during oral surgical procedures, presumably because afferent impulses via the trigeminal nerve stimulate sympathetic nerve centres; regional anaesthesia (such as with bupivacaine) reduces such dysrhythmias, and also postoperative pain.

Other medication

Patients on regular medication may need to be maintained on this, for example those on digoxin, or it may need to be stopped, for example, monoamine oxidase inhibitors, or increased, for example corticosteroids (*Table 2.3*).

CONSCIOUS SEDATION

Nitrous oxide and oxygen is overall the safest combination for conscious sedation because of its lack of respiratory or cardiodepressant effects, and rapid reversibility. Other agents are available, but the administrator's experience and facilities, and the relative safety of the different agents, must be taken into consideration (*Table 2.4*).

The benzodiazepines are mild respiratory depressants with minimal risk to healthy persons but they are potentially dangerous to those with cardiorespiratory disease and particularly chronic obstructive pulmonary disease. The depth of sedation necessary is established by the patient showing Eve's sign, the inability to touch accurately the end of the nose.

Midazolam is considerably (2 or 3 times) more potent than diazepam and the onset of signs of sedation is less reliable. The maximal effect of midazolam on the brain appears to be about 10–15 minutes after intravenous administration (Greenblatt *et al.*, 1989). As a consequence, there have been a few deaths after administration of midazolam alone in elderly patients. Flumazenil may be used to reverse the effect of midazolam. Cases have been reported of potentiation of midazolam by erythromycin. More dangerous still is the combination of a benzodiazepine with an opioid such as pentazocine. These are both respiratory depressants and deaths have resulted from their combined use.

Propofol appears to have the advantages of a rapid sedative response, with a quicker recovery and better effects on mood compared with midazolam (Stephens *et al.*, 1993).

In conducting sedation in the UK, the requirements of the Code of Practice issued by the General Dental Council must be fulfilled (*see* Appendix 1 to this chapter).

Fantasies of sexual assault during benzodiazepine sedation

It is essential that a dental surgeon does not administer sedation in the absence of a second trained person. The latter is required not merely to assist and help deal with any mishaps but also to act as a chaperone. If the patient makes unjustified allegations that sexual improprieties were committed as a result of fantasies induced by the sedating agent, these can usually be effectively dispelled by the assistant.

OUTPATIENT GENERAL ANAESTHESIA

General anaesthetic agents

It is beyond the remit of this book to discuss anaesthetic agents or intraoperative care in detail, but the main features of anaesthetic agents are summarized in *Table 2.4*. Many of the available general anaesthetic agents are less than ideal for outpatients. Enflurane, isoflurane, desflurane and sevoflurane are useful alternatives for patients at risk from halothane hepatitis (Chapter 10) and cardiac rhythm is more stable, but they are expensive. They cause, however, greater respiratory depression than halothane and induction is less pleasant. Enflurane causes cardiorespiratory depression and can be epileptogenic. Immediate recovery is slower after isoflurane than halothane and there may be some coughing. Recovery after sevoflurane is rapid but it

may agitate children. Desflurane may cause apnoea or breathholding, and increased secretions, and is not indicated for use in children.

Propofol is often used as an intravenous anaesthetic for day cases, and when:

- The anticipated duration of anaesthesia is under 1 hour.
- The use of a laryngeal mask is planned.
- Total intravenous anaesthesia is indicated.

However, several instances of systemic infection arising from bacterially contaminated vials of propofol have now been reported.

Particular hazards of outpatient general anaesthesia

Five aspects of general anaesthesia for ambulant dental patients deserve special consideration.

1. The patient is ambulant, is in the premises for a short period and is observed only briefly postoperatively.
2. The operation site is close to the airway – any inflammatory oedema, haemorrhage or foreign bodies can endanger respiration.
3. Equipment, facilities and technical assistance are rarely of the standard found in a modern operating theatre.
4. Fewer than one in four general anaesthetics in dental practice are given by anaesthetists who have had postgraduate training in dental anaesthesia.
5. Patients may have pre-existing medical disorders.

It has been reported that, after outpatient general anaesthesia, despite instructions to the contrary (Ogg, 1980):

- Thirty-one per cent of patients returned home unaccompanied by a responsible person.
- Thirty per cent of car owners drove within 12 hours of general anaesthesia and 9 per cent even drove themselves home from the surgery.

Patients should therefore be asked to agree:

1. To bring an accompanying responsible adult who will supervise them after discharge from the surgery.

Mark each item with a tick or N/A for *every* sedation given

Patient label

STAFF CHECK   DATE:

Experienced qualified DSA present?					
Another dentist/doctor/nurse/DSA is within easy call?					
Operator and assistants know emergency procedures?					

EQUIPMENT CHECK

Site of emergency equipment known?					

Have the following been checked by the operator?

Oxygen					
Suction – dental unit					
Suction – mobile/back-up					
Positive pressure ventilating bag					
Sphygmomanometer					
Pulse oximeter					
Other automatic monitor (BP/ECG)					
Emergency drugs (Flumazenil)					
Sedation equipment					

Have the following been checked?

Dental equipment					
Dental unit					

PATIENT CHECK

Patient, parent or guardian know what is planned?					
Written consent has been obtained?					
Written pre + postoperative instruction issued?					
Medical and dental history checked?					
Routine medication taken?					
Last meal or drink checked?					
Fasting patient?					
If Yes – has glucose been given?					
Patient has consumed alcohol today?					
If Yes – advise to postpone session?					
Responsible escort present?					
Weight recorded?					
BP recorded?					
OPERATOR'S NAME IN CAPITALS:					

Figure 2.1 Checklist for operator before giving sedation (Courtesy of Miss A.M. Skelly)

DSA = Dental surgery assistant (dental nurse)

2. Not to attempt to drive a vehicle, ride a bicycle or pillion on a motorcycle, work with unguarded machinery, or make important decisions, until the day after having had a general anaesthetic.

3. Not to drink alcohol or take drugs, particularly sleeping tablets, the night before or until the day after having had a general anaesthetic.

Obviously it is impossible to control the behaviour of irresponsible patients, but it is essential to point out the dangers in the clearest possible terms. Patients may also fail to

Table 2.5 Deaths associated with dental treatment: England and Wales

Year	Total	Number of deaths (including GA)	Place of operation	
			Dental surgery	Hospital
1979	11	9	4	5
1980	5	4	1	2
1981	5	4	4	0
1982	8(1)	7(1)	3(1)	4(0)
1983	5(1)	5(1)	4(1)	1(0)
1984	3(1)	3(1)	2(1)	1(0)
1985	4(4)	4(4)	1(1)	3(3)
1986	4(2)	3(2)	3(2)	1(0)
1987	5(2)	4(2)	2(1)	3(1)
1988	3	1	0	1

Figures in brackets relate to children under the age of 16 years.

take in or forget verbal instructions, particularly after benzodiazepine sedation. To protect both the patient and operator the patient and escort should be given written instructions (Appendix 4 to this chapter), and every other item should be checked (*Fig. 2.1*).

Preoperative assessment for general anaesthesia

Deaths related to dental treatment are rare (*Table 2.5*), but most of them occur as a result of general anaesthesia.

Adequate preoperative assessment is crucial to the safety of the patient, and many diseases are relative or absolute contraindications to general anaesthesia in the dental surgery, as discussed in subsequent chapters. However, the first consideration is that a dentist should *never* act as both operator and anaesthetist (*see* Appendix 1 to this chapter). Quite apart from the risk to the patient, any accident involving an operator–anaesthetist in the UK is certain to provoke disciplinary action by the General Dental Council. If a death results, a charge of manslaughter may have to be faced. By contrast, local anaesthesia is remarkably safe and, in competent hands, even minor complications are uncommon. In those few cases where general anaesthesia is unavoidable, it is wiser to refer patients to hospital or a suitably equipped and staffed clinic for this purpose.

The following comments apply mainly to GA in the dental surgery, as inpatients should

be assessed by the anaesthetist who can also ensure that any supplementary investigations are carried out. The reader should also refer to the Poswillo Report, the Working Party report produced for the Standing Dental Advisory Committee (Department of Health, 1990) (*see* Appendix 2 to this chapter).

Though every precaution must be taken to assess fitness for anaesthesia, and especially to make sure that all details of a patient's medication are known, it must be accepted that diseases such as some congenital cardiac defects may cause no symptoms and remain completely unsuspected until complications develop. More common still is unsuspected hypertension or coronary artery disease, which is one of the main causes of death under anaesthesia. Under the circumstances, it is obviously essential that general anaesthesia should only be given in the dental surgery if absolutely essential. If, however, this has to be done, then it is the responsibility of the dentist to tell the anaesthetist all he knows about the patient's medical state, particularly about the presence of any of the following:

1. Respiratory disease.
2. Cardiovascular disease or hypertension.
3. Diabetes mellitus.
4. Neuromuscular disorders.
5. Medication and allergies, including details of smoking and alcohol intake.
6. Previous anaesthetic complications and any recent general anaesthetics (*see* halothane hepatitis, Chapter 10).
7. Pregnancy.
8. Symptoms or signs such as productive cough, dyspnoea, palpitations, chest pain, ankle oedema, raised blood pressure, dysrhythmias.
9. Any airway obstruction or threat to the airway or possible intubation difficulty.
10. Infections, particularly hepatitis or HIV.

Special investigations that may be needed preoperatively should be checked with the anaesthetist. The following may be required (*see* Appendix 1 to Chapter 1 for normal values and interpretation of abnormalities):

1. Haemoglobin estimation and blood picture.
2. Sickle test in Afro-Caribbeans, and Indians, Pakistanis, Bengalis and Chinese.
3. Blood pressure estimation.

4. Chest radiograph.
5. Electrocardiogram (ECG), particularly for patients over 60.
6. Urinalysis.
7. Urea and electrolytes if an intravenous infusion is to be used, or the patient is on diuretic therapy.
8. Liver function tests.

The question of routine screening has been discussed elsewhere, particularly in respect of the possible cost/benefit ratio. A suggested protocol for preoperative investigation is suggested in *Fig. 2.1*.

If there is any doubt about fitness for general anaesthesia a specialist medical opinion should be obtained; indeed the proper person to check the preoperative assessment is the anaesthetist.

The relative indications and contraindications for general and local anaesthesia and sedation are shown in *Table 2.1*.

In the case of general anaesthetics or, more frequently, sedation given in the dental surgery, it is also important to give the patient a questionnaire to make sure that nothing has been forgotten and, in the event of any mishap, to provide documentary evidence that this assessment has been carried out.

INTRAOPERATIVE CARE

An essential aspect of operative care is constant monitoring of the patient's state by:

1. Clinical observation of colour, respiration and pulse.
2. Where anything more than a local anaesthetic alone is used, use of:
   (a) blood pressure monitor;
   (b) pulse oximeter.

A stethoscope and suitable resuscitative equipment must always be available.

Ideally, there should also be an electrocardiograph monitor, but this is rarely practicable in the absence of expert interpretation of the tracing unless an automatic read-out of possible diagnoses is available. However, it is now regarded as essential to have an ECG and, in addition, a capnograph for measurement of end-tidal carbon dioxide when endotracheal anaesthesia is practised. Resuscitative equipment should include a defibrillator.

Nevertheless, a UK survey by postal questionnaire (Allen *et al.*, 1990) of 95 practitioners showed that though six of them were still using methohexitone and 11 were using methohexitone with halothane, none had a pulse oximeter. Fewer than 1 in 5 had a pulse monitor but variable numbers had other emergency equipment such as oral airways, endotracheal tubes or a laryngoscope and the majority had an emergency drug kit.

Pulse oximeters provide a measure of the degree of haemoglobin oxygen saturation by means of spectrophotometry. They are usually very accurate and are a valuable safety measure. However, they are expensive and under certain circumstances can give misleading readings.

COMMON POSTOPERATIVE LOCAL COMPLICATIONS

Operative care carried out expeditiously, with careful handling of tissues, asepsis, wound toilet and careful closure of the wound, will minimize local complications, as will the appropriate use of analgesics and antimicrobials. Nevertheless, some pain is to be expected after surgical procedures, and bleeding or wound infection is not always totally avoidable.

Pain

Pain after surgery usually starts after anaesthetic drugs have worn off, and may result from unavoidable operative trauma. Alternatively, it may result from a complication such as a fractured jaw.

Postoperatively, analgesics should be given as necessary, but if a general anaesthetic has

Table 2.6 Analgesics

Analgesic	Comments	Tablet contains	Route	Adult dose
NSAIDS[a]				
Aspirin	Mild analgesic. Causes gastric irritation. Interferes with haemostasis Contraindicated in bleeding disorders, children, asthma, late pregnancy, peptic ulcers, renal disease, allergy	300 or 325 mg	Oral	300–600 mg up to 6 times a day after meals (use soluble or dispersible or enteric-coated aspirin) (max 4 g daily)
Mefenamic acid	Mild analgesic. May be contraindicated in asthma, gastrointestinal, renal and liver disease, and pregnancy. May cause diarrhoea or haemolytic anaemia	250mg 500 mg	Oral	250–500 mg up to 3 times a day
Diflunisal	Analgesic for mild to moderate pain. Long action: twice a or day dose only. Effective against pain from bone and joint. Contraindicated in pregnancy, peptic ulcer, allergies, renal and liver disease	250 mg or 500 mg	Oral	250–500 mg twice a day
Non-NSAIDS				
Paracetamol/ Acetoaminophen	Mild analgesic. Hepatotoxic in overdose or prolonged use. Contraindicated in liver or renal disease, anorexia, or those on zidovudine. Available with methionine to prevent liver damage in overdose, as co-methiamol	500 mg	Oral	500–1000 mg up to 6 times a day (max 4 mg daily)
Nefopam	Moderate analgesic. Contraindicated in convulsive disorders. Caution in pregnancy, elderly, renal, liver disease. May cause nausea, dry mouth, sweating	30 mg	Oral *or* i.m.	30–60 mg up to 3 times daily
OPIOIDS				
Codeine phosphate	Analgesic for moderate pain. Contraindicated in late pregnancy and liver disease. Avoid alcohol. May cause sedation and constipation. Weakens cough reflex	15 mg	Oral	10–60 mg up to 6 times a day (or 30 mg i.m.)
Dextropro- poxyphene	Analgesic for moderate pain. Risk of respiratory depression in overdose, especially if taken with alcohol. May cause dependence. Occasional hepatotoxicity. No more effective as an analgesic than paracetamol/aceto- aminophen or aspirin alone. Available with paracetamol as co-proxamol	65 mg	Oral	65 mg up to 4 times a day
Dihydrocodeine tartrate	Analgesic for moderate pain. May cause nausea, drowsiness, constipation. Contraindicated in children, hypothyroidism, asthma, renal disease. May increase postop. dental pain. Reduce dose for elderly. Available with paracetamol as co-dydramol	30 mg	Oral	30 mg up to 4 times a day (or 50 mg i.m.)

continued

Table 2.6 *Continued*

Analgesic	Comments	Tablet contains	Route	Adult dose
Pentazocine	Analgesic for moderate pain. May produce dependence. May produce hallucinations. May provoke withdrawal symptoms in narcotic addicts. Contraindicated in pregnancy, children, hypertension, respiratory depression, head injuries or raised intracranial pressure. There is a low risk of dependence.	25 mg	Oral	50 mg up to 4 times a day (or 30 mg i.m. or i.v.)
Buprenorphine	Potent analgesic. More potent analgesic than pentazocine, longer action than morphine, no hallucinations, may cause salivation, sweating, dizziness and vomiting. Respiratory depression in overdose. Can cause dependence. Contraindicated in children, pregnancy, MAOI, liver disease and respiratory disease.	0.2 mg	Sublingual	0.2–0.4 mg up to 4 times a day (or 0.3 mg i.m.)
Meptazinol	Potent analgesic. Claimed to have a low incidence of respiratory depression. Side effects as buprenorphine.	No tablet	i.m. *or* i.v.	75–100 mg up to 6 times a day
Phenazocine	Analgesic for severe pain. May cause nausea	5 mg	Oral *or* sublingual	5 mg up to 4 times a day
Pethidine	Potent analgesic. Less potent than morphine. Contraindicated with MAOI. Risk of dependence.	No tablet available	s.c. *or* i.m.	25–100 mg up to 4 times a day
Morphine	Potent analgesic. Often causes nausea and vomiting. Reduces cough reflex, causes pupil constriction, risk of dependence	As required	s.c. *or* i.m. *or* oral *or* suppository	5–10 mg
Diamorphine	Potent analgesic. More potent than pethidine and morphine. Euphoria and dependence	10 mg	s.c., i.m. *or* oral	2–5 mg by injection, 5–10 mg orally

[a]There are many other NSAIDS.

been given, the anaesthetist should be consulted first (*Table 2.6*). Immediately postoperatively after oral surgery it may be necessary to use a long-acting local analgesic, or a strong analgesic such as pethidine or morphine. In some cases this is best controlled by the patient (patient-controlled analgesia: PCA). Patients on monoamine oxidase inhibitors must not be given pethidine or other opioids. Morphine is also contraindicated if there is allergy to it, or in patients with respiratory disease or head injury (*see also* Chapter 25).

However, after most dental procedures codeine (or co-proxamol or co-dydramol Table 2.6) will be effective and, if after a few hours analgesia is still required, it is better to use paracetamol.

Wound infection

Wound infection is uncommon after oral procedures unless there has been significant contamination, such as in a road traffic accident, foreign bodies are present, local vascularity is poor or the patient immunocompromised. Infection may present with pain, discharge or fever (or a combination) and is best managed by drainage, with wound toilet, antimicrobials and analgesics as indicated.

The diagnosis must first be made, and therapy guided by the likely pathogen. If staphylococci or streptococci are implicated, the first choice therapy in the absence of allergy is flucloxacillin; for Gram-negative organisms it is cefuroxime; for anaerobic infections it is metronidazole or clindamycin; and for enterococcal infection it is amoxycillin.

Bleeding

Postoperative haemorrhage usually is from damaged soft tissues and has a local cause (*see* Chapter 4) and responds to local pressure or suturing of the soft tissues. Patients should be given written as well as verbal guidance on how to care for their wounds (*see* Appendix 4 to this chapter).

CARE AFTER GENERAL ANAESTHESIA OR SEDATION

The immediate postoperative period is a particularly dangerous time and is mainly the responsibility of the anaesthetist. However, merely because the operative procedure has been completed, the dental surgeon must not neglect his or her patient. The patient must be closely supervised also with pulse oximetry, until conscious, by the dental surgeon and then by the nurse or other responsible adult, until the patient is alert and able to stand without dizziness or ataxia.

During recovery the patient should be laid in the semi-prone (tonsillar) position and the airway must be protected. Up to 20 per cent of patients may become hypoxic after intravenous sedation and therefore supplemental oxygen should be given during recovery.

Morbidity and mortality after general anaesthesia

Many patients have a relatively smooth postoperative recovery, especially after short procedures. However, drowsiness, headache (particularly with halothane), sore throat, muscle pains and vomiting are seen in over 60 per cent of patients after outpatient general anaesthesia.

Headache seems more common in women, especially if halothane has been used. Sore throat, if the patient was intubated, and muscle pains if suxamethonium has been given, are common.

More important complications include the following:

1. Collapse.
2. Cardiorespiratory complications.
3. Delayed recovery of consciousness.
4. Nausea and vomiting.
5. Fever.
6. Jaundice.
7. Behavioural problems.
8. Low urine output.
9. Thromboses.
10. Death.

Collapse
Postoperative collapse is shown by signs of shock, loss of consciousness, hypotension, weakness, sweating and rapid pulse with pallor. The causes can be difficult to find but include:

1. Haemorrhage.
2. Pulmonary embolism.
3. Cardiac arrest (usually myocardial infarction).
4. Adrenal insufficiency.
5. Adverse reactions to general anaesthetic agents.

These are outlined in Chapter 27.

Cardiorespiratory complications
After prolonged anaesthesia, especially in the elderly, there are dangers of postoperative complications such as atelectasis (Chapter 8). The patient should therefore be strongly encouraged to undertake breathing exercises and to cough up any sputum. Physiotherapy may be helpful. A transient rise in temperature is common after general anaesthesia and is usually caused by localized pulmonary infection which may not be clinically detectable.

In essence, many post-anaesthetic complications result from or lead to hypoxia and therefore include both impaired respiratory function and cardiac disease. Important causes therefore include the following.
Upper airway obstruction: This is particularly important in dental surgery because of operating around the airway and the risk of inhaling foreign material. Facilities such as

suction must always be immediately available for locating and clearing any blockage. The recovery period is the most dangerous time and great care must be taken to keep the airway clear.

Lower airways obstruction: Accumulation of secretions is a frequent cause and this can be particularly severe in patients with chronic bronchitis (Chapter 8). In dentistry, inhalation of a tooth or fragments of materials is another possible cause of collapse of a lobe or lobule (atelectasis) and subsequent lung abscess.

Occasionally, bronchospasm can result from a hypersensitivity reaction to an intravenous anaesthetic agent or other drug used during the operation.

Respiratory weakness: Reversal of the action of neuromuscular blocking drugs (muscle relaxants) depends on many factors, but if delayed, results in weak respiratory movements which cannot be made stronger by the patient's conscious efforts. Suxamethonium apnoea is discussed in Chapter 15.

Impaired chest movements: Damage to the chest is a common accompaniment of maxillofacial injuries, particularly when they result from road traffic accidents (Chapter 22). This may inhibit respiration and coughing.

Respiratory depression: This can result from the effects of the anaesthetic and ancillary drugs. Methohexitone and pentazocine, for example, form a potent combination of respiratory depressants, which can be aggravated by hypoxia, often from a similar cause, during the operation.

Cardiac complications: Myocardial infarction, cardiac failure or severe dysrhythmias can follow anaesthesia and are the chief risk in those with pre-existing cardiac disease (Chapter 3). Pre-existing cardiac disease may be aggravated or myocardial infarction can follow at an unpredictable interval after the anaesthetic, especially in those with ischaemic heart disease (Chapter 3). Myocardial infarction is one of the chief causes of deaths associated with anaesthesia.

Peripheral circulatory failure: Shock syndrome is more likely to be a complication of major surgery. Contributory factors are pre-existing heart disease, dehydration, haemorrhage, sepsis or anaphylactic reactions. However, neurogenic circulatory failure is a possible consequence of anaesthesia in a pathologically anxious patient (Chapter 18).

Delayed recovery of consciousness
Important causes are overdose of anaesthetic agents or the use of long-acting opioids for premedication, suxamethonium sensitivity, diabetic coma or hypoglycaemia, cardiac complications mentioned earlier, or cerebrovascular accidents. The last may be either in susceptible patients (elderly hypertensives) or as a result of emboli (Chapter 4). Occasionally hysterical patients may feign persistent unconsciousness.

Nausea and vomiting
Postoperative vomiting is both unpleasant for the patient and dangerous if protective laryngeal reflexes have not returned, allowing inhalation of vomit. Nausea and vomiting are usually the result of opioids used for premedication rather than modern anaesthetic agents and are less likely to follow oral surgery than some other types of operation unless a considerable amount of blood has been swallowed. In many cases the cause of postoperative nausea is unclear but some patients seem to be particularly susceptible. An anti-emetic such as metoclopramide, ondansetron, domperidone, cyclizine or prochlorperazine is usually effective (Chapter 25). Parenteral or rectal administration may be needed if vomiting is severe. Metoclopramide, and domperidone are best avoided in the young and elderly, as they can induce dystonic reactions.

Fever
A transient rise in temperature is common within a few hours of major operations and may be thought of as 'physiological'. Persistent fever for several days postoperatively, especially if spiking, may indicate haematoma, wound infection, deep vein thrombosis, urinary tract infection, infection of an intravenous line or more serious pulmonary infection. Occasionally pneumonia or a lung abscess can be precipitated, especially in those with chronic respiratory disease, if foreign material is inhaled or if an emergency operation has had to be carried out in spite of the presence of an acute upper respiratory tract infection (Chapter 8).

Jaundice

Postoperative jaundice can result from many causes, including the following:

1. Viral hepatitis (usually hepatitis C if blood has been given).
2. Halothane hepatitis and hepatotoxic effects of other drugs (Chapter 10).
3. Alcoholic hepatitis.
4. Aggravation of pre-existing liver disease.
5. Hepatic necrosis secondary to circulatory failure.
6. Transfusion reactions.

These conditions are discussed more fully in Chapter 10 and it is only necessary to emphasize here that liver damage should not be a consequence of anaesthesia for oral surgery if care is taken to exclude the high-risk groups listed above. However, it must be appreciated that anaesthesia for high-risk patients cannot be avoided for emergencies such as maxillofacial injuries, and this group of patients includes an unduly high proportion of alcoholics.

Halothane should be avoided if the patient has been exposed to it within the previous 6 months or has had a previous episode of halothane hepatitis. In a series of 300 patients who had been given halothane on more than one occasion within a month and who subsequently developed hepatitis, no fewer than 46 per cent died. Isoflurane, desflurane or sevoflurane are appropriate alternatives and in some hospitals have replaced halothane, though the cost is a concern.

Behavioural complications

Causes of confusion may include:

1. Drugs (anaesthetic, alcohol, others).
2. Hypoxia.
3. Infection (wound, lungs, urinary tract, abscess, septicaemia).
4. Urine retention or disturbed urea and electrolytes.

Amnesia that persists for at least 5 hours is common after sedation with diazepam or midazolam. As a result, patients are likely to forget post-sedation instructions, or worse, have an accident as a result of forgetting to take normal precautions when using power tools or other dangerous equipment. Bizarre behaviour has also been described even 24 hours after sedation.

It is also important to make sure that the patient is not anticipating going abroad immediately after the anaesthetic or sedation. Complications might develop on board an aircraft or at a destination where medical care is limited. That aside, it is difficult enough for most people to have to deal with the problems of getting through an airport without having their faculties blunted by the after-effects of a drug. As mentioned earlier, therefore, it is essential to give the patient written instructions to cover the necessary precautions of the post-anaesthetic or sedation period.

Low urine output

Low urine output is usually due to a reduced intake over the period but may be caused by urine retention. The patient should be examined for retention, and if it is present should be catheterized unless urine can be passed after a warm bath. If there is no retention, the patient should be given fluids orally if possible, and if there is no increase in output it may be necessary to try a diuretic such as frusemide.

Thromboses

Superficial vein thrombosis may follow injections that are irritant, or cannulae that have entered the tissues. Analgesics usually suffice, though antibiotics are occasionally indicated.

Deep vein thrombosis is mainly seen after prolonged major operations, and affects the calves. It may lead to pulmonary embolism (Chapter 4).

Deaths under general anaesthesia

The mortality rate for general anaesthetics carried out in the dental surgery is small, as mentioned earlier, but has been estimated (Lewis, 1983) as about 10 deaths for every million anaesthetics administered. Nevertheless, any deaths related to dental treatment are unacceptable. The true mortality rate cannot be determined since the total number of administrations is unknown. However, the number of deaths in dental practices has fallen from four in 1979 to zero in 1988, and deaths from general anaesthesia in dentistry have fallen from more than 10 each year in the 1950s to only one or two in the 1990s. This is probably as a result of the declining use of general anaesthesia in dentistry. Deaths under general anaesthesia for more major surgery have, also, incidentally, steadily declined in the same period, despite the great number of high-risk patients now undergoing surgery and the adventurous nature of modern operations, particularly cardiovascular surgery.

Of even more concern is the fact that, unlike deaths during major surgery, those who have died under dental anaesthesia have frequently been fit young people. Those who have died during conservative dentistry appear to have been between 8 and 28 years of age (average 17), and those who died during extractions were between 4 and 72 (average 26). It must not be assumed that all these deaths have been at the hands of dentists; specialist anaesthetists have been involved in some cases. In the period 1979 to 1988 there was a total of 40 deaths associated with dental treatment in dental practice and 20 deaths associated with dental treatment in hospitals in England and Wales. Between 1982 and 1987 in England and Wales, 15 died in dental practices and of these seven were under the age of 16.

The information about deaths under dental anaesthesia is of limited value since (a) the numbers are small, (b) information about factors relating to the causes of death is often scanty and (c) even when information is available, the causes of death sometimes remain obscure. Nevertheless, such information as there is strongly suggests that there is a highly unpredictable element involved in dental anaesthesia and, in view of the kind of patients who die under such circumstances, it must be assumed that unsuspected systemic disease has escaped recognition or that anaesthetic mishaps are more common than they should be. This excess of deaths of young, apparently fit patients during dental anaesthesia reinforces the need for taking a careful history and for referring patients with any suspicion of systemic disease to hospital. The last consideration is particularly important in view of the fact that many practitioners still do not possess resuscitation equipment adequate for use in an emergency. However the increased popularity of sedation as well as the restrictions imposed by some guidelines has greatly reduced the use of anaesthesia in the dental surgery and it is to be hoped that deaths under dental anaesthesia will cease to occur.

HAZARDS OF GASEOUS GENERAL ANAESTHESIA TO DENTAL PERSONNEL

Nitrous oxide and halothane can accumulate in appreciable concentrations in operating areas and particularly around the patient's face, close to where the operator is working. As a consequence, there has been much concern about the possible teratogenicity or carcinogenicity that might result from continual exposure to anaesthetic agents. The consensus of data from animal experiments at subanaesthetic concentrations has, however, not yielded convincing evidence of toxicity.

Epidemiological studies also suggest that there is no convincing evidence of any effect of chronic exposure to anaesthetic agents on mental performance, cancer, or fetal disorders such as low birth weight, stillbirth or malformation.

By contrast, megaloblastosis and a neurological disorder resembling subacute combined degeneration of the cord has been reported in dentists *abusing* nitrous oxide as a result of its interference, in the long term, with vitamin B_{12} metabolism (Chapter 24).

These considerations are discussed elsewhere (Scully *et al.*, 1990). Nevertheless, the following precautions should be taken where general anaesthesia or relative analgesia is used.

1. Every effort should be made to reduce contamination of the surgery atmosphere by anaesthetic gases by avoiding over-usage of general anaesthesia or relative analgesia, by careful use of the anaesthetic machine, adequate surgery ventilation and, most important, by using a scavenger system.
2. Pregnant staff, or staff likely to become pregnant, should not work in a contaminated environment unless there is an effective scavenging system.

BIBLIOGRAPHY

Allen N.A., Dinsdale R.C.W. and Reilly C.S. (1990) A survey of general anaesthesia and sedation in dental practice in two cities. *Br. Dent. J.* **169**, 168–72.

Applebaum P.S and Grisso T. (1988). Assessing patients' capacities to consent to treatment. *N. Engl. J. Med.* **319**, 1635–8.

Assem E.K. (1992) Highlights on controversial issues in anaesthetic reactions. In Assem E.K. (ed), *Allergic Reactions to Anaesthetics: Clinical and Basic Aspects.* Basle, Karger, pp. 1–14.

Bailey B.L. (1985) Informed consent in dentistry. *J. Am. Dent. Assoc.* **110**, 709.

Barker I., Butchart D.G.M., Gibson I. *et al.* (1986) Sedation for conservative dentistry. *Br. J. Anaesth.* **58**, 371–7.

Becker L.C. (1987) Is isofluorane dangerous for the patient with coronary artery disease? *Anesthesiology* **66**, 259–62.

Beeby C. and Thurlow A.C. (1986) Pulse oximetry during general anesthesia for dental extractions. *Br. Dent. J.* **160**, 123–5.

Bell C.J. (1995) Local anaesthetic solutions. *Postgrad. Dentist* **5**, 2–6.

Brahams D. (1989) Benzodiazepine sedation and allegations of sexual assault. *Lancet* **i**, 1339–40.

Brain A.I.J. (1983) The laryngeal mask – a new concept in airway management. *Br. J. Anaesthesiol.* **55**, 801–5.

Campling E.A., Devlin H.B., Hoile R.W. and Lunn J.N. (1996) *The Report of the National Confidential Enquiry into Perioperative Deaths, 1993/1994.* London, NCEPOD.

Cannell H. (1996) Evidence for safety margins of lignocaine local anaesthetics for peri-oral use. *Br. Dent. J.* **181**, 243–9.

Cattermole R.W., Verghese C., Blair I.J. *et al.* (1986) Isoflurane and halothane for outpatient dental anaesthesia in children. *Br. J. Anaesth.* **58**, 385–9.

Cawson R. A. (1969) The problem of the newer drugs in dentistry. *Br. Dent. J.* **120**, 109–10.

Cawson R.A., Curson I. and Whittington D.R. (1983) The hazards of dental local anaesthetics. *Br. Dent. J.* **154**, 253–7.

Cawson R.A., Spector R.G. and Skelly A.M. (1995) *Basic Pharmacology and Clinical Drug Use in Dentistry*, 6th edn. Edinburgh, Churchill Livingstone.

Clinical Standards Advisory Group (1995) *Dental General Anaesthesia.* London, HMSO.

Coplans M.P. and Curson I. (1993) Deaths associated with dentistry and dental disease. *Anaesthesia* **48**, 435–8.

Council on Scientific Affairs, American Medical Association (1993) The use of pulse oximetry during conscious sedation. *J. Am. Med. Assoc.* **270**, 1463–8.

Department of Health (1990) *General Anaesthesia, Sedation and Resuscitation in Dentistry.* Report of an Expert Working Party, Prepared for the Standing Dental Advisory Committee. London, DoH.

Department of Health (1993) *General Anaesthesia for Dentistry; Continuing Education and Training Courses for Non-Consultant Anaesthetists.* Royal College of Anaesthetists/Faculty of Dental Surgery/Faculty of General Dental Practitioners Working Party. London, DoH.

Dinsdale R.C.W. and Dixon R.A. (1976) Anaesthetic service to dental patients: England and Wales. *Br. Dent. J.* **144**, 271–9.

Doyal L. and Cannell H. (1995) Informed consent and the practice of good dentistry. *Br. Dent. J.* **178**, 454–60.

European Resuscitation Council (1992) *Guidelines for Advanced Life Support.* London, Hammersmith Hospital.

Fahy A. and Marshall M. (1969) Postanaesthetic morbidity in outpatients. *Br. J. Anaesth.* **41**, 433–8.

Fraser C.G. (1985) Urine analysis. *Br. Med. J.* **291**, 321–5.

Gall H., Kaufmann R. and Kalveram C.M. (1996) Adverse reactions to local anesthetics: analysis of 197 cases. *J. Allerg. Clin. Immunol.* **97**, 933–7.

Gandy S.R. (1995) The use of pulse oximetry in dentistry. *J. Am. Dent. Assoc.* **126**, 1274–8.

Gold B.D. and Wolfersberger W.H. (1980) Findings from routine urinalysis and hematocrit on ambulatory oral and maxillofacial surgery patients. *J. Oral Surg.* **38**, 677–8.

Greenblatt D.J., Ehrenberg B.L., Gunderman J. *et al.* (1989) Pharmokinetic and electroencephalographic study of intravenous diazepam, midazolam and placebo. *Clin. Pharmacol. Ther.* **45**, 356–65.

Gross J.B., Bailey P.L. and Cote C.J. (1996) Guidelines for sedation and analgesia by non-anesthesiologists. *Anesthesiology* **84**, 459–71.

Harrison G.G. (1978) Death attributable to anaesthesia: a 10-year survey (1967–76). *Br. J. Anaesth.* **50**, 1041–6.

Hersh E.V. (1996) Local anesthetics in dentistry; clinical considerations, drug interactions, and novel formulations. *Compend. Contin. Educ. Dent.* **14**, 1020–30.

Hiller A., Olkkola K.T., Isohanni P. and Saarnivaara L. (1990) Unconsciousness associated with midazolam and erythromycin. *Br. J. Anaesth.* **65**, 826–8.

Hodgson T.A., Shirlaw P.J. and Challacombe S.J. (1993) Skin testing after anaphylactoid reactions to dental local anesthetics. *Oral Surg.* **75**, 706–11.

Hunter J.M. (1996) Rocuronium; the newest aminosteroid neuromuscular blocking drug. *Br. J. Anaesth.* **76**, 481–3.

Joint Faculties Working Party on Sedation (1994) Report. Faculty of Dental Surgery/Faculty of General Dental Practitioners, Royal College of Surgeons of England. London.

Leading Article (1988) Midazolam – is antagonism justified? *Lancet* **ii**, 140–2.

Leading Article (1989) Nausea and vomiting after general anaesthesia. *Lancet* **i**, 651–2.

Lewis B. (1983) Deaths and dental anaesthetics. *Br. Med. J.* **286**, 3–4.

Lindsay S.J.E. and Yates J.A. (1985) The effectiveness of oral diazepam in anxious child dental patients. *Br. Dent. J.* **159**, 149–53.

Lu D.P. and Lu G.P. (1996) Hypnosis and pharmacological sedation for medically compromised patients. *Compend. Contin. Educ. Dent.* **17**, 32–40.

Lunn J.N. and Mushin W.W. (1982) *Mortality Associated with Anaesthesia.* London, Nuffield Provincial Hospitals Trust.

Matthews R., Malkawi Z., Griffiths M. and Scully C. (1992) Pulse oximetry in patients undergoing minor oral surgery with and without intravenous sedation. *Oral Surg., Oral Med. Oral Pathol.* **74**: 537–43.

Matthews R.W., Scully C. and Levers B.G.H. (1984) The

efficacy of diclofenac sodium with and without para-cetamol in the control of postsurgical dental pain. *Br. Dent. J.* **157**, 357–9.

McAteer P.M., Carter I.A., Cooper G.M. and Prys-Roberts C. (1986) Comparison of isoflurane and halothane in outpatient paediatric dental anaesthesia. *Br. J. Anaesth.* **58**, 390–3.

McGimpsey J.G., Kawar P., Gamble J.A., Browne E.S. and Dundee J.W. (1983) Midazolam in dentistry. *Br. Dent. J.* **155**, 47–50.

Norman J. (1980) Use of anaesthesia. Preoperative assessment of patients. *Br. Med. J.* **1**, 1507–8.

O'Boyle C.A., Harris D. and Barry H. (1986) Sedation in outpatient oral surgery. *Br. J. Anaesth.* **58**, 378–84.

Ogg T.W. (1976) Assessment of preoperative cases. *Br. Med. J.* **1**, 82–3.

Ogg T.W. (1980) Use of anaesthesia: implications of day-case surgery and anaesthesia. *Br. Med. J.* **2**, 212–13.

Ogg T.W., MacDonald I.A., Jennings R.A. *et al.* (1983) Day case dental anaesthesia. *Br. Dent. J.* **155**, 14–17.

Padfield A. (1989) The future of general anaesthesia in the dental surgery: a discussion paper. *J. R. Soc. Med.* **82**, 30–2.

Parbrook, G.D. (1986) Death from anaesthesia in the general and community dental services. *Br. J. Anaesth.* **58**, 369–70.

Porter S.R., Matthews R.W., Scully C., Midda M. and Bain S.E. (1992) Local analgesia infiltration. *Dent. Health* **31**, 4–6.

Porter S.R. and Scully C. (1996) *Innovations and Developments in Non-Invasive Oral Health Care.* Northwood, Science Reviews.

Richards A., Scully C. and Griffiths M.J. (1993). Wide variation in patient response to midazolam sedation for out-patient oral surgery. *Oral Surg. Oral Med. Oral Pathol.* **76**, 408–11.

Royal College of Surgeons of England (1993) *Guidelines for Sedation by Non-Anaesthetists.* Report of a Commission on the Provision of Surgical Services Working Party. London, Royal College of Surgeons.

Rule J. and Veatch R. (1993) *Ethical Questions in Dentistry.* Chicago, IL, Quintessence.

Scully C. (1988) *The Dental Patient.* Oxford, Heinemann.

Scully C. (1989) *The Mouth and Perioral Tissues.* Oxford, Heinemann.

Scully C. (1989) *Patient Care: a Dental Surgeon's Guide.* London, British Dental Association.

Scully C. and Griffiths M.J. (1990) Conscious sedation. In Bell C.J. (ed), *Heinemann Dental Handbook.* Oxford, Heinemann, pp. 374–84.

Scully C., Cawson R.A. and Griffiths M.J. (1990) *Occupational Hazards to Dental Staff.* London, British Dental Journal.

Seymour R.A. (1985) Prescribing analgesics. *Br. Dent. J.* **159**, 177–81.

Shirlaw P.J., Scully C., Griffiths M.J. *et al.* (1986) General anaesthesia, parenteral sedation and emergency drugs and equipment in general dental practice. *J. Dent.* **14**, 247–50.

Smiddy F.G. (1976) *The Medical Management of the Surgical Patient.* London, Arnold.

Smith B.L. and Young P.N. (1976) Day stay anaesthesia. *Anaesthesia* **31**, 181–9.

Stephens A.J., Sapsford D.J. and Curzon M.E.J. (1993) Intravenous sedation for handicapped dental patients: a clinical trial of midazolam and propofol. *Br. Dent. J.* **175**, 20–5.

Summers L. (1981) An investigation into the effects of surgical stress on the fit and poor-risk patient including the modifying effects of relative analgesia and B blockade. *Br. J. Oral Surg.* **19**, 3–12.

Sykes P. (1980) Should dental practitioners give anaesthetics? *SAAD Digest* **28**, 101–9.

Vessey M.P. and Nunn J.F. (1980) Occupational hazards of anaesthesia. *Br. Med. J.* **281**, 696–8.

Weinstein B. (ed) (1993) *Dental Ethics.* Philadelphia, Lea and Febiger.

Wilson I.H., Richmond M.N. and Strike P.W. (1986) Regional analgesia with bupivacaine in dental anaesthesia. *Br. J. Anaesth.* **58**, 401–5.

Wynn R.L. (1993) Erythromycin and ketoconazole (Nizoral) associated with terfenadine (Seldane) – induced ventricular arrhythmias. *Gen. Dent.* **41**, 27–9.

Young I.V.I. (1975) General anaesthesia for ambulant dental patients. *Br. J. Hosp. Med.* **13**, 441–8.

APPENDIX 1 TO CHAPTER 2

AMENDMENTS TO THE *PROFESSIONAL CONDUCT AND FITNESS TO PRACTISE* BOOKLET, APPROVED BY THE GENERAL DENTAL COUNCIL, MAY 1996

Consent

34. (iii)   Consent: dentists must obtain valid consent prior to carrying out treatment. For consent to be valid the dentist must himself or herself have explained to the patient and, if appropriate, his/her parent or guardian, the treatment proposed, the risks involved in the treatment and alternative treatments. If an anaesthetic or sedation is to be given, all the procedures to be undertaken must be explained to and discussed with the patient and, if appropriate, his/her parent or guardian. The onus is on the dentist to ensure that all necessary information and explanations have been given to the patient or parent/guardian by the dentist or by the anaesthetist. If a general anaesthetic or sedation is to be administered, consent must be obtained in writing.

General Anaesthesia, Sedation and Resuscitation

17.   General anaesthesia is a procedure which is never without risk. In assessing the needs of the individual patient due regard should be given to all aspects of behavioural management and anxiety control before deciding to proceed with general anaesthesia.

18.   Prior to the administration of general anaesthesia or sedation, a full medical history of the patient must be taken and patients must be given in advance clear and comprehensive pre- and post-treatment instructions in writing. Careful contemporaneous records of treatment and the procedures undertaken must be kept.

19.   Where a general anaesthetic is administered, the Council considers that it must be by a person other than the operating dentist treating the patient, and that person must remain responsible for the patient throughout the anaesthetic procedure until the patient's protective reflexes have returned and the patient has recovered control of his or her airway.

20.   This second person aforementioned must be a dental or medical practitioner with appropriate postgraduate training and evidence of relevant continuing clinical education.

21.   The anaesthetist should be supported by an assistant specifically trained and experienced in the necessary skills to assist in monitoring the patient's condition and in any emergency. Contemporary standards of monitoring should be adopted. Provision for Advanced Life Support must be immediately available within the operatory and in this connection the current Guidelines issued by the European Resuscitation Council would be appropriate. The dentist should also have the assistance of an appropriately trained dental nurse.

22.   Where conscious sedation techniques are employed a suitably experienced practitioner may assume the responsibility of sedating the patient as well as operating, provided that the practitioner has undertaken relevant postgraduate training. As a minimum requirement a second appropriate person who is capable of monitoring the clinical condition of the patient must be present throughout. Should the occasion arise he or she should also be capable of assisting the dentist in case of emergency.

23.   For these purposes, the following definition of conscious sedation should be understood to apply: 'A technique in which the use of a drug, or drugs, produces a state of depression of the central nervous system enabling treatment to be carried out, but during which communication can be maintained and the modification of the patient's state of mind is such that the patient will respond to command throughout the period of sedation. Techniques used should carry a margin of safety wide enough to render unintended loss of consciousness unlikely.'

24.   In all cases the technique chosen should be the most appropriate to enable successful treatment to be given and in the case of intravenous sedation this will normally be by the use of a single drug. Contemporary standards of monitoring should be adopted during conscious sedation and where more than one sedative drug is utilized the provision of Advanced Life Support must be immediately available. The current Guidelines issued by the European Resuscitation Council would also be appropriate in this connection.

24. (a)   Intravenous sedation is unpredictable in children. The therapeutic margin between sedation and anaesthesia may be very narrow, and there is always the possibility of a paradoxical reaction. In view of this, intravenous sedation in children should be administered only under very special circumstances.

continued

25. Patients who are recovering from general anaesthesia or sedation should be appropriately protected and monitored in adequate recovery facilities. When in the opinion of the anaesthetist or sedationist sufficiently recovered to leave the premises, the patient should be accompanied by a responsible adult. The only situation in which a dentist may exercise discretion as to whether an adult patient may be discharged unaccompanied is that in which nitrous oxide/oxygen sedation alone is the technique used. All patients must be specifically assessed for fitness for discharge.

26. Neither general anaesthesia nor sedation should be employed unless proper equipment for their administration is used and adequate facilities, including appropriate drugs, for the resuscitation of the patient are readily available, with both dentist and staff trained in the anaesthetic or sedation procedure and resuscitation techniques.

27. A patient could collapse in a dental practice at any time and the collapse may not be associated with the administration of general anaesthesia or sedation. Dentists should therefore ensure that all members of their staff are properly trained and prepared to deal with an emergency should one arise. The requirement to practise resuscitation routines frequently in a simulated emergency against the clock is not restricted to those dentists who provide general anaesthesia or sedation in their practices. The Council considers it essential that suction apparatus to clear the oropharynx, oral airways to maintain the natural airway, equipment with appropriate attachments to provide intermittent positive pressure to the lungs, and a portable source of oxygen, must be available in all dental practices. In this connection the current Guidelines issued by the European Resuscitation Council should be adopted.

28. A dentist who carried out treatment under general anaesthesia or sedation without ensuring that the conditions set out above were fulfilled would risk being considered to have acted in a manner which constituted serious professional misconduct.

APPENDIX 2 TO CHAPTER 2

RECOMMENDATIONS FROM THE POSWILLO REPORT (Department of Health, 1990)

(i) The use of general anaesthesia should be avoided wherever posssible.
(Para 3.8)

(ii) The same general standards in respect of personnel, premises and equipment must apply irrespective of where the general anaesthetic is administered.
(Para 3.11)

(iii) Dental anaesthesia must be regarded as a postgraduate subject.
(Para 3.13)

(iv) All anaesthetics should be administered by accredited anaesthetists who must recognize their responsibility for providing dental anaesthetic services.
(Para 3.14)

(v) Anaesthetic training should include specific experience in dental anaesthesia.
(Para 3.14)

(vi) Health authorities should review the provision of consultant dental anaesthetic sessions to ensure they are sufficient to meet local needs.
(Para 3.16)

(vii) Doctors and dentists with knowledge, experience and competence sufficient to satisfy the College of Anaesthetists and the Faculty of Dental Surgery to be under no detriment.
(Para 3.17)

(viii) The no detriment arrangements must have been implemented within two years of the publication of this report.
(Para 3.17)

(ix) The administration of general anaesthesia in dental surgeries and clinics equipped to the recommended standards of monitoring necessary for patient safety shall continue.
(Paras 3.16 and 3.19)

(x) An electrocardiogram, a pulse oximeter and a non-invasive blood pressure device are essential for the non-invasive monitoring of a patient under general anaesthesia.
(Para 3.20)

continued

(xi)   A capnograph to be used where tracheal anaesthesia is practised.
(Para 3.20)

(xii)   A defibrillator must be available.
(Para 3.21)

(xiii)   Equipment conforming to recognized standards should be purchased and installed, regularly serviced and maintained in accordance with manufacturer's instructions.
(Para 3.21)

(xiv)   General anaesthetic surgeries be subject to inspection and registration.
(Para 3.22)

(xv)   Intravenous agents should be administered via an indwelling needle or cannula which should not be removed until the patient has fully recovered.
(Paras 3.25 and 4.15)

(xvi)   Appropriate training must be provided for those assisting the anaesthetist and the dentist.
(Para 3.26)

(xvii)   At no time should the recovering patient be left unattended.
(Para 3.26)

(xviii)   Adequate recovery facilities should be available.
(Para 3.26)

(xix)   Good contemporaneous records of all treatments and procedures be kept.
(Para 3.30)

(xx)   Written consent be obtained on each occasion prior to the administration of a general anaesthetic.
(Para 3.31)

(xxi)   Consideration be given to developing a national general anaesthetic/sedation consent form for general dental practitioners.
(Para 3.31)

(xxii)   Patients be provided with comprehensive pre- and post-treatment instructions and advice.
(Para 3.31)

APPENDIX 3 TO CHAPTER 2

CLASSIFICATION OF OPERATIONS

Emergency
Immediate life-saving operation, resuscitation simultaneous with surgical treatment (e.g. trauma, ruptured aortic aneurysm). Operation usually within one hour.

Urgent
Operation as soon as possible after resuscitation (e.g. irreducible hernia, intussusception, oesophageal atresia, intestinal obstruction, major fractures). Operation within 24 hours.

Scheduled
An early operation but not immediately life-saving (e.g. malignancy). Operation usually within 3 weeks.

Elective
Operation at a time to suit both patient and surgeon (e.g. cholecystectomy, joint replacement).

Day case
A patient who is admitted for investigation or operation on a planned non-resident basis (i.e. no overnight stay).

continued

CLASSIFICATION OF ADMISSIONS

Elective

At a time agreed between the patient and the surgical service.

Urgent

Within 48 hours of referral/consultation.

Emergency

Immediately following referral/consultation, when admission is unpredictable and at short notice because of clinical need.

AMERICAN SOCIETY OF ANESTHESIOLOGISTS (ASA) CLASSIFICATION OF PHYSICAL STATUS

Class 1

The patient has no organic, physiological, biochemical or psychiatric disturbance. The pathological process for which operation is to be performed is localized and does not entail a systemic disturbance. Examples: a fit patient with impacted third molars.

Class 2

Mild to moderate systemic disturbance caused either by the condition to be treated surgically or by other pathophysiological processes. Examples: non- or only slightly limited organic heart disease, mild diabetes, essential hypertension, or anaemia. Some might choose to list the extremes of age here, either the neonate or the octogenarian, even though no discernible systemic disease is present. Extreme obesity and chronic bronchitis may be included in this category.

Class 3

Severe systemic disturbance or disease from whatever cause, even though it may not be possible to define the degree of disability with finality. Examples: severely limiting organic heart disease, severe diabetes with vascular complications, moderate to severe degrees of pulmonary insufficiency, angina pectoris or healed myocardial infarction.

Class 4

Severe systemic disorders that are already life-threatening, not always correctable by operation. Examples: patients with organic heart disease showing marked signs of cardiac insufficiency, persistent angina, or active myocarditis, advanced degrees of pulmonary, hepatic, renal or endocrine insufficiency.

Class 5

The moribund patient who has little chance of survival but is submitted to operation in desperation. Examples: major head injury with rapidly increasing intracranial pressure, massive pulmonary embolus. Most of these patients require operation as a resuscitative measure with little if any anaesthesia.

APPENDIX 4 TO CHAPTER 2

ROUTINE CHECKS BEFORE GENERAL ANAESTHESIA OR INTRAVENOUS SEDATION FOR DENTAL TREATMENT

Always check:
1. Patient's name (and hospital number).
2. Nature, side and site of operation.
3. Medical history, *particularly* of cardiorespiratory disease or bleeding tendency.
4. That consent has been obtained in writing from patient or, in a person under 16 years of age, from parent or guardian, and that patient adequately understands the nature of the operation and sequelae.
5. That necessary oral investigations, e.g. radiographs, are available.
6. That patient has had *nothing by mouth, including drugs* for *at least* the previous 4 hours.
7. That patient has emptied the bladder.
8. That patient's dentures have been removed and bridges, crowns and loose teeth have been noted by anaesthetist.
9. That any premedication (and, where indicated, regular medication such as the contraceptive pill, anticonvulsants or antidepressants) has been given but not usually within the previous 4 hours.
10. That anaesthetic and suction apparatus are working satisfactorily and that emergency drugs are available and not date-expired (see *Fig. 2.1*).
11. That patient is escorted by a responsible adult.
12. That patient has been warned not to drive, operate unguarded machinery, drink alcohol or make important decisions for 24 hours postoperatively.

INSTRUCTIONS TO PATIENTS BEFORE GENERAL ANAESTHETIC OR INTRAVENOUS SEDATION (PREFERABLY IN WRITING)

1. Do not take food or liquids after midnight before a morning appointment, or after a light breakfast at 8 a.m. before an afternoon appointment. In any event a general anaesthetic will *not* be given until at least 4 hours have elapsed since the taking of food or liquid.
2. You must be accompanied by a responsible adult, over the age of 18 years, who will undertake to escort you home and remain with you 24 hours after treatment. You must not be accompanied by children under 14 years of age.
3. Do not wear nail varnish or make-up.
4. After a general anaesthetic or sedation *you must not* on the same day:
   – drive a motor vehicle
   – ride a bicycle or motorcycle, even as passenger
   – cook or use unguarded machinery
   – take alcohol
   – take sedative drugs without medical advice
   – make important decisions or sign any documents
5. If you develop a cold before your appointment, please telephone the hospital or dental surgery for advice.
Patients who fail to comply with these simple safety precautions will not be given a general anaesthetic or sedation

INSTRUCTIONS TO PATIENTS AFTER TOOTH EXTRACTION (PREFERABLY IN WRITING)

After a tooth has been extracted the socket will usually bleed for a short time. This bleeding stops because a healthy blood clot forms in the tooth socket. These clots are easily disturbed and if this happens bleeding will recur. To avoid disturbance of the clot please follow these instructions:
1. After leaving the hospital or dental surgery do not rinse out your mouth for 24 hours, unless you have been told otherwise by the dentist.
2. Do not disturb the clot in the socket with your tongue or fingers.
3. For the rest of the day take only soft foods.
4. Try not to chew on the affected side for at least 3 days.
5. Avoid unnecessary talking, excitement or exercise for the rest of the day.

continued

6.   Do not take alcoholic or very hot drinks for the rest of the day.

If the tooth socket continues to bleed after you have left the surgery, do not be alarmed – much of the liquid which appears to be blood, is saliva. If bleeding persists make a small pad from a clean handkerchief or cotton wool, place over the socket and close the teeth firmly on it. Keep up the pressure for 15–30 minutes. If the bleeding still does not stop, seek dental or medical advice.

SUGGESTIONS FOR THE CARE OF THE MOUTH AFTER TOOTH EXTRACTION

Your tooth socket may heal more quickly if you keep it clean and use hot salt mouth baths, but not until 24 hours after the extraction. Dissolve a teaspoonful of table salt in a tumbler of hot water (about the same temperature as a hot cup of tea). Take a mouthful and tilt your head so that the hot salt water bathes the affected area. After about 15 seconds, spit out and repeat the bathing until you have used the whole tumblerful. If possible, the hot salt water mouth baths should be used three times daily for three days, after meals.

Brush your teeth in the normal way. The affected area can be cleaned by wiping with cotton wool moistened with the hot salt water if it is tender.

Discomfort or mild pain after tooth extraction may be relieved by the pain-killer you would normally use. Paracetamol tablets, one or two every 4 hours, are recommended for adults. Children may take paracetamol syrup, the dose depending on their age (follow instructions on the container).

You should seek the advice of your dentist if you have pain which is severe or persists for more than 24 hours.

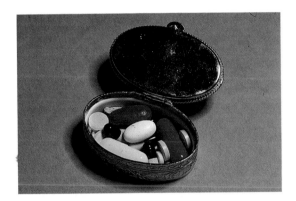

Plate 1 Pill box presented by an outpatient who proved
to be taking eight different medications, including a
corticosteroid, daily

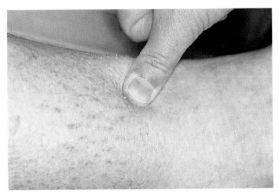

(a)   *(b)*

Plate 2(a,b) Pitting oedema

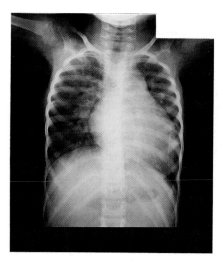

Plate 3 Chest radiograph of a child with congenital heart disease showing gross cardiac enlargement (the heart normally occupies less than half the width of the chest)

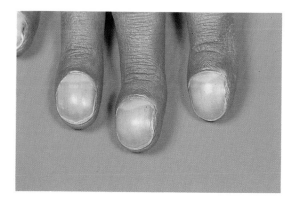

Plate 4 Finger clubbing in a patient with Fallot's tetralogy. Finger clubbing can be found in several different disorders, particularly cyanotic heart disease, chronic respiratory disease, lung cancer, Crohn's disease etc., but is sometimes benign and hereditary

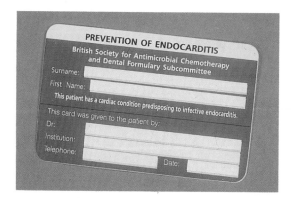

Plate 5 Endocarditis warning card

ADVANCE MEDICAL DIRECTIVE/RELEASE
(Child)

I the undersigned   , the
lawful parent of   , born
the   day of   19   , being one of
Jehovah's Witnesses with firm religious convictions have resolutely
decided to obey the Bible command "Keep abstaining . . . from
blood" (Acts 15:28, 29). With full realisation of the implications of
this position I HEREBY:

1.   *CONSENT* (subject to the *exclusion of the transfusing of blood
or blood components*) to all such necessary emergency treatment
including general anaesthesia and surgery as the doctors treating the
child may in their professional judgement deem appropriate to
maintain life.

2.   *DIRECT* (a) that such consent is temporary and only effective

until such time as I am contacted and am able to discuss further
proposed treatment and give informed consent;

       (b) that such consent and any subsequent consent that I may
give *EXCLUDES the transfusion of blood or blood components* but
includes the administration of non-blood volume expanders such as
saline, dextran, Haemaccel, hetastarch and Ringer's solution;

       (c) that my express refusal of blood is absolute and is not to be
overridden in ANY circumstances by a purported consent of a relative
or other person. Such refusal remains in force even though the
doctor(s) treating the child consider that such refusal may be life
threatening;

and   (d) that this Advance Directive shall remain in force and bind all
those treating the child unless and until I expressly revoke it in writing.

3.   *ACCEPT* full legal responsibility for this decision and *RE-
LEASE* all those treating the child from any liability for any
consequences resulting from such exclusion.

Dated the _____ day of _____ 19

Signed: _____

Witnesses to Signature:

Signature: _____ Relationship: _____

Signature: _____ Relationship: _____

                                        Printed in Britain

IDENTITY CARD

Child's Name _____

Parents: _____

_____

Address

_____
                                   Telephone

IMPORTANT MEDICAL INFORMATION
ON OTHER SIDE

As parents we are deeply interested in the welfare of
our child   . Because of
our family's convictions as Jehovah's Witnesses we *do
not accept blood transfusions*. We do accept non-blood
expanders and other medical treatment. In case of
accident, please contact us immediately. We likely can
provide information as to doctors who respect our
religious convictions and may already have provided
medical care for us.

SEE INSIDE

Allergies: _____

Current medication: _____

_____

Medical problems: _____

_____

_____

(a)   *(b)*

Plate 6(a,b) Jehovah's Witness refusal of blood transfusion

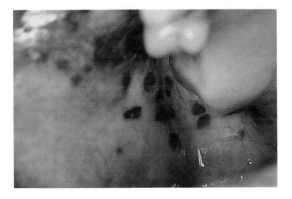

Plate 7 Oral purpura

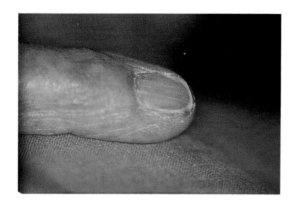

Plate 8 Koilonychia

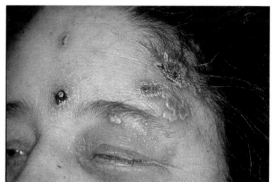

Plate 9 Zoster

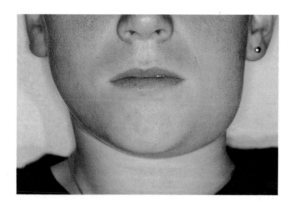

Plate 10 Cat scratch disease

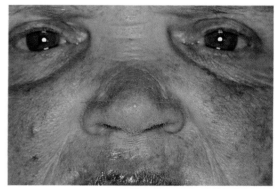

Plate 11 Saddle nose

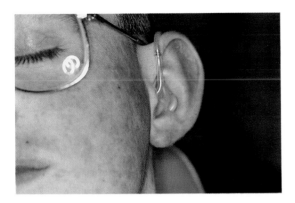

Plate 12 Toxoplasmosis: congenital infection can lead to deafness

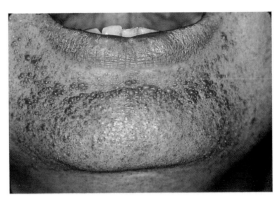

Plate 13 Tuberous sclerosis showing adenoma sebaceum

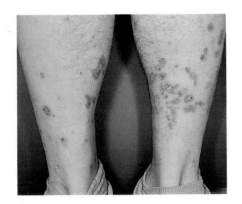

Plate 14 Lichen planus: skin lesions

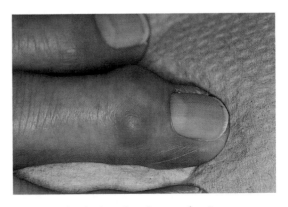

Plate 15 Heberden's nodes of osteoarthrosis

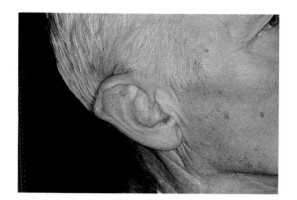

Plate 16 Gouty tophi

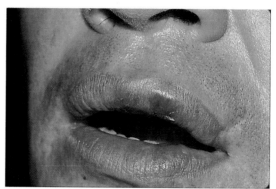

Plate 17 Kaposi's sarcoma in AIDS

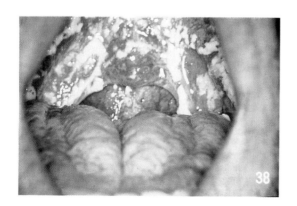

Plate 18 Candidosis in AIDS

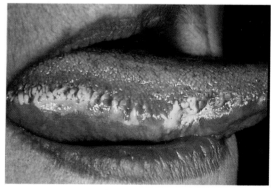

Plate 19 Hairy leukoplakia in AIDS

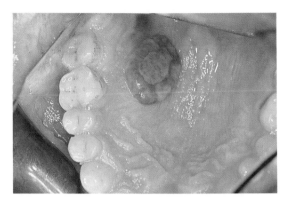

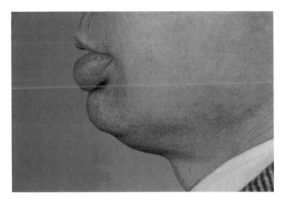

Plate 20 Kaposi's sarcoma in a diabetic following renal transplantation

Plate 21 Angio-oedema

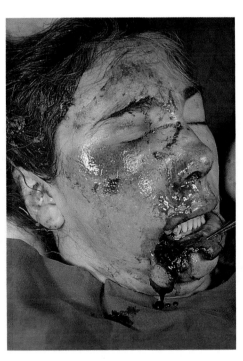

Plate 22 Maxillofacial injuries after a road traffic accident

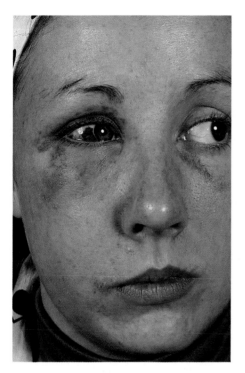

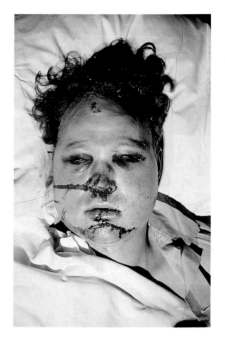

Plate 24 Victim of violence

Plate 23 Subconjunctival haemorrhage associated with zygomatic fracture

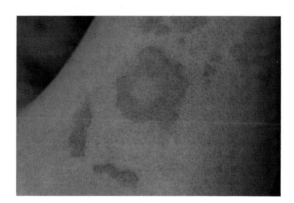

Plate 25 Urticaria

3

Cardiovascular disease

Key points

- Cardiac disease is common.
- Dyspnoea, chest pain, hypertension, central cyanosis, ankle oedema, abnormal pulse rate or rhythm, splinter haemorrhages and finger clubbing can all be features of cardiac disease.
- General anaesthesia (GA) constitutes a particular risk to cardiac patients.
- Patients with cardiac disease may become breathless if laid flat (as in the dental chair).
- The evidence that adrenaline in local anaesthetics used in sensible doses (up to 0.04 mg) is a hazard to cardiac patients is little more than theoretical.
- Local anaesthetics containing noradrenaline are totally contraindicated. Even in normal persons they have caused fatal hypertensive attacks.
- Anxiety and pain cause enhanced sympathetic activity. This increases the load on the heart and the risk of angina or dysrhythmias.
- A mild premedicant such as 5 mg diazepam orally can be valuable in cardiac patients before a dental appointment.
- Routine dentistry using short appointments is safe for most patients with heart disease unless they are over-anxious.
- Sedation with nitrous oxide is pleasant and usually acceptable and probably safer than intravenous sedation in cardiac patients.
- Extractions under local anaesthesia can usually be carried out one or two at a time but the trauma and blood loss of multiple extractions should be avoided.
- Patients on digoxin are at especial risk of electrocardiographic changes and dysrhythmias after tooth extractions.
- More major oral surgery for cardiac patients should only be carried out in hospital.
- GA is contraindicated within 3 months of a myocardial infarct.
- GA is also particularly hazardous for the following conditions:
  Angina pectoris, especially of recent origin or unstable.
  Severe hypertension.
  Intractable dysrhythmias (particularly digitalis toxicity).
  Some congenital heart diseases.
- Methohexitone should not be used even for so-called sedation in cardiac patients – it is a potent general anaesthetic agent which is a respiratory depressant with cardiovascular effects.
- Cardiac patients may have a bleeding tendency if on anticoagulants.
- Patients with cardiac valvular defects may be at risk for infective endocarditis if receiving dental treatment that produces a bacteraemia.
- Cardiac patients that may need antimicrobial cover to prevent endocarditis include those with:
  congenital cardiac defects
  rheumatic heart disease

> prosthetic cardiac valves
> previous history of endocarditis
> hypertrophic cardiomyopathy
> aortic valve disease (bicuspid valves).
> * Those with a prosthetic cardiac valve, or with a history of endocarditis are at special risk from infective endocarditis.
> * Prevention depends on giving prophylactic antimicrobials before dental extraction, surgery or scaling.
> * Antimicrobial prophylaxis should be started only a few hours preoperatively.
> * Equipment such as MRI, diathermy, electrosurgery, ultrasonic scalers and pulp testers can interfere with pacemakers.
> * Myocardial infarction can happen anywhere, including in the dental surgery. Dental treatment may possibly contribute to precipitating such an event – or be blamed for it.

Cardiovascular diseases, particularly hypertension and ischaemic heart disease, are still the most common causes of adult death in the developed world. There are some millions of ambulant patients with some form of heart disease, treated or untreated.

Dental procedures, or drugs used in dentistry, can aggravate heart disease, can precipitate angina, or possibly even provoke a heart attack. Changes in heart rate and blood pressure can be seen before the administration of a dental local anaesthetic injection, during tooth extraction and even when adrenaline-impregnated gingival retraction cords are used, but most of all when the patient experiences any pain. These changes appear to be *unrelated* to the administration of the local anaesthetic, and more related to anxiety or pain experienced. Interestingly, the blood pressure and pulse rate of dental staff are also raised when at work.

Moreover, a dental procedure can occasionally be the main factor precipitating a potentially lethal form of heart disease, namely infective endocarditis. Some patients require an antibiotic cover before dental treatment, in order to prevent infective endocarditis. It is also possible that periodontal disease is a risk factor for atherosclerosis and thromboembolism. Myocardial infarction is one of the most serious emergencies that can happen in the dental surgery and is one where the dental staff may be able to help save the patient's life.

Cardiac failure is present when the heart is unable to supply the circulatory demands of the body. Any increase in these demands as a result of tachycardia worsens the problem. At one extreme the person with a failing heart can manage fairly well if exertion is limited but, at the other extreme, established failure causes severe breathlessness even at rest. Failure is usually the result of disease of the heart, but an otherwise normal heart can fail as a consequence of overwork caused by hyperthyroidism or the attempt to oxygenate the tissues in severe anaemia.

Failure is usually progressive but, if adequately treated, may cause few symptoms. Activity is, however, always limited to some degree. Cyanosis and dependent oedema (usually swollen ankles) are prominent signs.

Cardiac arrest is a sudden event in which the heart stops beating. Immediate collapse and (if untreated) death follow within a few minutes. Arrest may follow ventricular fibrillation but the two conditions are not clinically distinguishable.

Patients with heart disease, particularly ischaemic heart disease, are at greatest risk from cardiac arrest. This is important to bear in mind, since awareness of the possibility of arrest may make it possible to start resuscitation immediately.

Shock (peripheral circulatory failure) is the clinical term for hypotension, coldness, pallor and sweating as a result of severe reduction in the circulating volume, because of haemorrhage or other causes. In severe shock, if the circulatory volume is not maintained by, for example, blood transfusion, the heart fails. Shock can also be caused by acute heart failure, typically the result of myocardial infarction, or can occasionally result from anaphylaxis

Ischaemia is a local interruption or reduction of blood supply to a single part. It is especially important when it affects the heart or brain. Ischaemic heart disease is due to occlusion of the coronary arteries (usually by atheroma) and leads to angina pectoris or myocardial infarction, which, if severe, causes acute failure of the whole circulation, loss of cerebral blood supply and often death.

Common signs and symptoms of cardiovascular disease

Serious heart disease is frequently asymptomatic and patients can die suddenly from myocardial infarction in particular, despite never having experienced chest pain or any other symptoms. Possibly 20 per cent of myocardial infarcts are silent (subclinical). However, in many cases signs and symptoms can be effectively controlled so that most patients with cardiac disease coming to the dental surgery appear well. Only the drug history may give a clue as to the nature of their illness.

Breathlessness (dyspnoea) is a typical symptom of left-sided heart failure. *Chest pain* is the typical symptom of ischaemic heart disease. *Palpitations* may be a symptom of dysrhythmia and *sudden loss of consciousness* can be a sign of a defect in cardiac conduction (heart block).

Cyanosis: central cyanosis (seen in the lips or within the mouth) is usually an indication either of cardiac failure or of respiratory disease, or both together in cor pulmonale. It is an indication of gross hypoxia and such patients must not therefore be given a general anaesthetic or sedation in the dental surgery, but should be treated in hospital.

Palpation of the pulse enables a clinician to assess the heart rate, force of contraction and rhythm, disturbances of which may signify cardiac disease and can be informative when, for example, a patient loses consciousness or appears to be having a heart attack.

The *blood pressure* measured on only a single occasion and showing *hypertension* can

be misleading, as it is frequently raised by anxiety. However, a check-up in the surgery may not raise the pressure and the finding of either normal levels (less than 160/95 for a male of 45 or over) or grossly raised levels is informative. In an injured patient a falling blood pressure is also a danger sign which must not be ignored, since it implies a serious complication such as haemorrhage or shock. Signs of cardiac disease may be seen on the hands, particularly *finger clubbing* (which can have many causes), and *splinter haemorrhages* beneath the nails in infective endocarditis.

The stethoscope is mainly of use to those with experience; even to the cardiologist the differentiation between functional (harmless) murmurs and those caused by cardiac disease may occasionally be difficult. However, absence of heart sounds, a cardinal feature of cardiac arrest, should be instantly detectable with a stethoscope, but absence of pulse is more quickly detected by palpation.

Enlargement of the heart, for example in cardiac failure or hypertension, can be reliably seen in a chest radiograph, while electrocardiography is invaluable for the diagnosis of dysrhythmias and of ischaemia or damage to the myocardium.

• Dental aspects of cardiovascular disease

The specific problems are detailed below but the most important aspect is to consider how well the patient is compensated, and the exact procedure which is contemplated. A well-compensated patient receiving atraumatic treatment under local anaesthesia is quite different from one who requires general anaesthesia and is poorly compensated with dyspnoea on minimal exertion, cyanosis, frequent angina or a recent infarct. The latter clearly requires treatment in hospital.

Types of cardiovascular disease

Organic disease can affect the myocardium, endocardium or pericardium in any combination. Myocardial disease secondary to hypertension or coronary artery disease is the most common and important cardiac disease. Functional disorders, where there is no organic disease of the heart itself, can also cause circulatory failure, as in shock (*Table 3.1*).

Table 3.1 Causes of heart disease

Organic disease of the heart

- Myocardial
  Myocardial overload secondary to hypertension or valve disease*
  Coronary (ischaemic) heart disease*
  Cardiomyopathies
- Endocardial
  Rheumatic heart disease
  Congenital anomalies*
  Infective endocarditis
- Pericardial
  Pericarditis
  Pericardial effusion

Functional disorders

- Hypertensive heart disease*
- Disorders of cardiac control
  Tachycardia
  Bradycardia
  Other dysrhythmias
- Changes in circulatory volume
  Hypovolaemia (shock syndrome)
  Hypervolaemia (circulatory overload)
  Others

*Common causes of heart failure.

A variety of common extracardiac diseases can aggravate heart disease, particularly if there is impaired oxygenation, as in severe anaemia.

HEART FAILURE

Heart failure is not a single disease but an effect of many disorders. Heart failure is a common cause of death and patients with failure are poor risks for general anaesthesia.

The heart fails either because it has excessive demands thrown upon it by, for example, arteriovenous shunts, anaemia or hyperthyroidism (high-output cardiac failure), or because the heart itself is damaged or restricted by, for example, myocardial disease (ischaemic heart disease, cardiomyopathy), excessive preload such as in mitral regurgitation, excessive afterload such as in hypertension or aortic stenosis, restricted activity as in pericarditis, or due to disease or drugs slowing the rate (heart block, β-blockers) (low-output failure). The common causes are ischaemic heart disease, hyper-

tension, valve disease and chronic obstructive pulmonary disease (*Table 3.1*). Failure can predominantly affect either the left or right side of the heart, but failure of one side usually leads to failure of the other.

Left-sided heart failure

Left-sided heart failure is more common than right-sided failure. Causes of left-sided heart failure include:

1. Ischaemic heart disease.
2. Aortic and mitral valvular disease (left-side valves).
3. Hypertension.

Clinically, left-sided failure presents mainly with pulmonary oedema. Failure causes congestion and oedema primarily of the lungs, but function of the brain and kidneys is also impaired. As the left ventricle fails, blood is dammed back in the pulmonary circulation where the venous pressure rises, causing oedema. Pulmonary oedema causes difficulty in breathing (dyspnoea), the most troublesome symptom of left-sided heart failure. Initially, dyspnoea mainly follows effort, but later is present at rest and persists or worsens when lying down (orthopnoea). Coughing is another typical consequence of pulmonary oedema. The sputum is frothy and, in severe cases, pink with blood. Paroxysmal nocturnal dyspnoea (cardiac asthma) is a sudden attack of severe dyspnoea due to pulmonary oedema which wakes the patient from sleep with a terrifying sensation of suffocation. Lying down increases pulmonary congestion and oedema and also makes respiration less efficient, because the abdominal viscera move the diaphragm higher and reduce the vital capacity of the lungs. It is obviously dangerous, therefore, to lay a patient with left-sided failure supine during dental treatment.

In the more advanced stages of left-sided heart failure there is inadequate cerebral oxygenation leading to symptoms such as loss of concentration, restlessness and irritability or, in the elderly, disorientation.

Right-sided heart failure

Right-sided failure presents mainly with peripheral oedema, fatigue and abdominal discomfort. Often a sequel to left-sided failure, particularly when there is mitral stenosis, the resulting condition is known as congestive cardiac failure. Failure of the right side of the heart alone is uncommon and most often secondary to chronic obstructive lung disease (cor pulmonale) or pulmonary embolism.

In contrast to left-sided failure, pulmonary congestion in right-sided failure is minimal, but congestion of the systemic and portal venous systems predominantly affects the liver, gastrointestinal tract, kidneys and subcutaneous tissues. The liver is usually enlarged due to passive congestion and, in severe cardiac failure, raised portal venous pressure also leads to escape of large amounts of fluid into the peritoneal cavity (ascites). Subcutaneous oedema gravitates to dependent parts; ankle oedema (*Plate 2*) is therefore seen in ambulant patients and sacral oedema in patients in bed.

Clinical aspects of heart failure

Obvious signs and symptoms of established cardiac failure include:

1. Breathlessness (dyspnoea).
2. Oedema.
3. Distension of neck veins.
4. Cyanosis.
5. Fatigue.

The pulse may be rapid and irregular, particularly if there is atrial fibrillation, and in extreme cases patients are cyanotic, polycythaemic, dyspnoeic at rest and oedematous as a result of advanced failure beyond the control of drugs.

• General management of heart failure

The medical treatment typically includes diuretics or drugs such as angiotensin-converting enzyme (ACE) inhibitors (captopril, cilazapril, enalapril, fosinopril, lisinopril, moexipril, perindopril, quinapril, ramipril or trandolapril). Digoxin or digitoxin are glycosides used to increase cardiac efficiency mainly when there are dysrhythmias. Phosphodiesterase inhibitors (enoximone or milrinone) may be useful in congestive cardiac failure.

• Dental aspects of heart failure

Elective surgery under general anaesthesia is contraindicated until cardiac failure is under control, but even then should be conducted in hospital. In uncontrolled cardiac failure, the patient should receive medical attention before dental treatment. In the patient with controlled cardiac failure, dental treatment under local anaesthesia can safely be carried out providing that consideration is given to the underlying cause of the cardiac failure (*Table 3.1*) and to the fact that those on digoxin are most at risk from electrocardiographic changes such as ST segment depression following tooth extraction (Blinder *et al.*, 1996). In these, cardiac monitoring would be wise, and bupivacaine should be avoided (Roitman *et al.*, 1993). Placing the patient supine may worsen dyspnoea and should therefore be avoided. Care should be taken after general anaesthesia especially, since there is a predisposition to venous thrombosis and pulmonary embolism. Some of the drugs that may complicate treatment include digitalis (vomiting), procainamide (leucopenia or a lupus-like reaction) or acetazolamide (facial paraesthesia). ACE inhibitors may cause erythema multiforme, angioedema or, sometimes, burning mouth. NSAIDs should be avoided in those patients taking ACE inhibitors since they increase the risk of renal damage.

HYPERTENSION

Hypertension is a persistently raised blood pressure resulting from increased peripheral arteriolar resistance. Dental management can be complicated, since any procedure causing stress can further raise the blood pressure and may precipitate acute complications such as a cardiac arrest or a cerebrovascular accident. Chronic complications of hypertension, especially impaired renal function, can affect dental management.

The blood pressure is easily measured (by convention in the right arm) with a sphygmomanometer (*Table 3.2*). Since the blood pressure rises with anxiety, measurements should be made with the patient relaxed and fully at rest. The blood pressure rises even before a visit for dental care. The diagnosis of what is hypertension is not absolutely clear. A

Table 3.2	Manual technique for recording the blood pressure

1. Allow the patient to sit at rest for as long as possible
2. Place sphygmomanometer cuff on right upper arm with about 3 cm of skin visible at the ante-cubital fossa
3. Palpate right radial pulse
4. Inflate cuff to about 200–250 mmHg, or until the radial pulse is no longer palpable
5. Deflate cuff slowly while listening with stethoscope over the brachial artery over skin on inside of arm below cuff
6. Record the systolic pressure as the pressure when the first tapping sounds appear
7. Deflate cuff further until the tapping sounds become muffled (diastolic pressure)
8. Repeat; record blood pressure as systolic/diastolic pressures

Table 3.3	Causes of hypertension

- Idiopathic (essential) hypertension
- Secondary hypertension
  - Renal disease
    - Renal artery disease
    - Pyelonephritis
    - Glomerulonephritis
    - Polycystic disease
    - Post-transplant
  - Endocrine disease
    - Cushing's syndrome, and corticosteroid therapy
    - Hyperaldosteronism
    - Phaeochromocytoma
    - Acromegaly
  - Cerebral disease
    - Cerebral oedema (mainly strokes, head injuries or tumours)
  - Coarctation of aorta (hypertension in upper half of body only)

blood pressure (BP) of systolic/diastolic of less than 130 mmHg/less than 85 is clearly normal for an adult. Above those values, hypertension is when either or both are persistently raised. In practice, the diagnosis of hypertension is made at an arbitrary point when the blood pressure at rest exceeds 160/95 mmHg (systolic/diastolic) and on remeasurement, and by this criterion probably over 10 per cent of the population are hypertensive.

Hypertension is secondary to defined diseases, particularly renal or endocrine disorders, in only about 10 per cent of cases (*Table 3.3*) and occasionally to pregnancy or an oral contraceptive.

The cause of hypertension is unknown in more than 90% of cases and the condition is then termed *essential hypertension* which becomes more frequent as age advances and appears related to genetic influences, obesity and a variety of other factors. About 40 per cent of hypertensive patients have raised levels of circulating catecholamines (adrenaline or noradrenaline) and may therefore have abnormal sympathetic activity. Acute emotion, particularly anger and anxiety, can cause great increases in catecholamine output and transient rises in blood pressure. Alcohol, caffeine and nicotine can also cause a rise in BP.

Uncomplicated hypertension causes no symptoms and is one of the few diseases in which the diagnosis can be entirely mechanical and quantitative, that is, by means of a sphygmomanometer. Some may live out their lives

with a persistently raised blood pressure which has no overt effects but common and important complications, particularly heart failure, stroke, retinal and renal disease – several of which are life-threatening – are as follows.

Heart failure: Persistent hypertension causes the heart to hypertrophy until it outgrows its blood supply and heart failure may thus result without any other significant complications. However, atheroma (atherosclerosis) of the coronary arteries frequently also develops and this reduces the heart's blood supply even further. A very common result is angina pectoris or myocardial infarction.

Brain damage: Hypertension, particularly when associated with atheroma, is a major cause of strokes, either as a result of haemorrhage into the brain from rupture of an artery or as a result of thrombosis complicating an atheromatous plaque.

Blood vessel disease: In addition to contributing to development of atherosclerosis, hypertension causes thickening of the walls of the arterioles of the kidney and this may lead ultimately to renal failure. Epistaxes may result from the combined effect of the raised blood pressure and weakening of the nasal vessel wall.

Malignant (accelerated) hypertension

Malignant hypertension is uncommon: it can have an acute onset or can develop in pre-existing essential hypertension.

Table 3.4   Important antihypertensive drugs (apart from diuretics)

	Possible oral effects	*Other comments and adverse effects*	*Examples*
Beta-adrenoreceptor blockers	Dry mouth Lichenoid lesions Paraesthesiae with labetalol	May cause bronchospasm Contraindicated in asthma Avoid in heart failure or heart block Muscle weakness Lassitude Disturbed sleep	Acebutolol Atenolol Bextaxolol Bisoprolol Metoprolol Nadolol Oxprenolol Pembutolol Pindolol Propranolol Sotalolol Timolol
Vasodilators	—	Headache May cause hypertrichosis Oedema	Hydralazine Minoxidil
Angiotensin-converting enzyme inhibitors	Sinusitis with quinapril Lichenoid reactions Loss of taste with enalapril Burning sensation or ulceration or loss of taste with captopril	First dose may cause sudden fall in blood pressure May impair renal function, especially if NSAIDs also given Cough Angioedema	Captopril Enalapril Lisinopril Perindopril Quinapril Ramipril
Calcium-channel blockers	Gingival hyperplasia Salivation with nicardipine	Headache and flushing Swollen legs	Amlodipine Diltiazem Felodipine Isradipine Lacidipine Nicardipine Nifedipine Nimodipine Verapamil

Malignant hypertension typically affects young adults, especially Afro-Caribbeans, and, like essential hypertension, causes no symptoms until complications develop. The chief complication is a severe form of nephrosclerosis with resulting ischaemic damage to the kidneys and renal failure. *Facial palsy is an occasional complication.*

Rapid deterioration in renal function was a common cause of death which, in the absence of treatment, often followed within a year of diagnosis. However, vigorous treatment, if started before renal damage is too far advanced, can greatly improve the expectation of life. About 50 per cent of such patients can now expect to live for at least 5 years.

Other causes of death are cardiac failure or cerebrovascular accidents.

• General management of hypertension

Lifelong treatment is usually necessary, even for mild hypertension, and significantly reduces the above complications. Weight loss, a reduction in salt intake and more exercise are beneficial. Smoking should be stopped as it increases the risks of ischaemic heart disease, and alcohol consumption should be restricted.

Specific antihypertensive therapy is indicated where the systolic pressure exceeds 200 mmHg, or the diastolic 110 mmHg, and may be indicated at lower levels, particularly if there are vascular complications, diabetes or end-organ damage such as renal impairment. The aim is to maintain the BP below 160/90. Antihypertensive agents currently used are shown in *Table 3.4*. Side-effects can sometimes be troublesome and antihypertensive treatment has to be tailored to each patient's response and the optimal result, in terms of lowering blood pressure with the least adverse effects, may require a combination of drugs. Diuretics are usually the first line of drug treatment, but may occasionally cause hypokalaemia in the elderly. Thiazide diuretics are mostly used (bendrofluazide, benzthiazide, chlorothiazide, chlorthalidone, clopamide, hydrochlorothiazide, indapamide, mefruside, metalazone, polythiazide or xipamide).

Adrenergic inhibitors, particularly beta-blockers are the usual first choice of additional drugs if these measures fail but not in patients with asthma or chronic obstructive pulmonary disease. Propranolol is the main beta-blocker used but a range of others is available (Table 3.4). Angiotensin-converting enzyme (ACE) inhibitors and calcium-channel blockers (Table 3.4) are now also commonly used.

• Dental aspects of hypertension

Blood pressure tends to rise during oral surgery under local anaesthesia, and adrenaline theoretically can contribute to this but this is usually of little practical importance. Alcohol, caffeine and nicotine can undoubtedly raise the blood pressure. Among the many other drugs that may induce or aggravate hypertension are corticosteroids, danazol, some antidepressant drugs, non-steroidal anti-inflammatory agents and ketamine. By contrast, dangerous *hypotension* can result from potentiation of hypotensive drugs by general anaesthetic agents. However, antihypertensive drugs should not be stopped, as rebound hypertension can result. The management of such patients should therefore be in the hands of specialist anaesthetists in hospital.

Postural hypotension: An important side-effect of some antihypertensive drugs such as thiazides, frusemide, methyl dopa and the calcium-channel blockers is a tendency to produce acute postural hypotension. Raising the patient suddenly from the supine position may therefore cause loss of consciousness.

General anaesthesia: All antihypertensive drugs are potentiated by general anaesthetic agents, especially barbiturates, and by opioids for premedication; severe hypotension can result. A severely reduced blood supply to vital organs can be dangerous even in a normal person, but in the chronically hypertensive patient the tissues have become adapted to the raised blood pressure which becomes essential (hence the term 'essential

hypertension') to overcome the resistance of the vessels and maintain adequate perfusion. A fall in blood pressure below the critical level needed for adequate perfusion of vital organs, particularly kidneys, can therefore be fatal.

Though mild hypertension is not a contraindication to general anaesthesia, the latter may be hazardous if there are any of the following:

1. Severe hypertension.
2. Cardiac failure.
3. Coronary or cerebral artery insufficiency.
4. Renal insufficiency.

When a general anaesthetic is given, the risks of cerebrovascular accidents and cardiovascular instability that result from withdrawal of antihypertensive medication and rebound hypertension outweigh the dangers of drug interactions which to some extent are predictable and manageable by an expert anaesthetist. Antihypertensive treatment is usually therefore maintained, but the management of such patients is a matter for the specialist anaesthetist.

Intravenous barbiturates in particular can be dangerous in patients on antihypertensive therapy, but halothane, enflurane and isoflurane may also cause hypotension in patients on beta-blockers. In practice, therefore, the severe (BP over 200/150) or elderly hypertensive, whether on hypotensive treatment or not, should not be given a general anaesthetic in the dental surgery. Patients with hypertension are best treated under local anaesthesia. Local anaesthetics with adrenaline (*see* Chapter 2) are safe and unlikely to cause trouble. No more than 4 ml of a solution containing 1 in 80 000 adrenaline should be used however.

Chronic administration of some diuretics such as frusemide may lead to potassium deficiency and thereby predispose to dysrhythmias and increased sensitivity to muscle relaxants such as curare, gallamine and pancuronium. Frusemide should therefore be discontinued a few days before a general anaesthetic is given.

Dental management: The anxiety associated with dental treatment typically causes a rise in blood pressure and may rarely precipitate cardiac arrest or a cerebrovascular accident. Preoperative reassurance is therefore important and sedation may be helpful. Patients are best treated in the morning with continuous BP monitoring, and given short appointments only.

The patient's blood pressure should be controlled before elective dental treatment or the opinion of a physician should be sought first. Since endogenous adrenaline released in response to pain or fear may induce dysrhythmias, it is important to avoid anxiety and pain. Adequate analgesia must be provided; NSAIDs are best avoided. Though its benefits are unproven, an aspirating syringe should be used to give a local anaesthetic, since adrenaline in the anaesthetic given intravenously may (theoretically) increase hypertension and precipitate dysrhythmias. Gingival retraction cords containing adrenaline should be avoided.

The management of hypertensive patients may also be complicated by the underlying disease (*Table 3.3*) or others such as cardiac or renal failure. Systemic corticosteroids may raise the blood pressure and antihypertensive treatment may have to be adjusted accordingly.

There are no recognized oral manifestations of hypertension but antihypertensive drugs can sometimes cause side-effects (*Table 3.4*), such as xerostomia, salivary gland swelling or pain, lichenoid reactions, erythema multiforme, angio-oedema, gingival hyperplasia, sore mouth or paraesthesiae.

CORONARY (ISCHAEMIC) HEART DISEASE

Ischaemic heart disease (IHD) is the result of progressive myocardial ischaemia due to persistently reduced coronary blood flow, usually because of atherosclerosis (atheroma). Hypertension is a major contributory factor.

Coronary heart disease affects at least 20 per cent of adult males under 60 years and increasingly thereafter. In Western populations, atheroma may affect up to 45 per cent of young adult males and ischaemic heart disease accounts for about 35 per cent of total mortality in Britain and the United States. It is a disease predominantly of males, particularly of affluent societies, linked to smoking, hypertension and high fat diets. There is a genetic component in some, but more commonly, smoking, hypertension, lack of exercise and hyperlipidaemia, possibly from the consumption of too much saturated (animal and dairy) fat, are contributory.

Hyperlipidaemia and hypertension seem to be linked. Nevertheless, immigrants from the Indian subcontinent have a higher than average morbidity and mortality from coronary heart disease despite a lower fat consumption than the rest of the population. There is a higher incidence of IHD in the hyperlipoproteinaemias, diabetes mellitus and hypothyroidism. Aspirin, beta-blockers and cholesterol-lowering appear to be the most effective way to treat patients with ischaemic heart disease. Lipid-lowering drugs include statins – inhibitors of 3-hydroxy-3-methylglutaryl coenzyme A (HMG CoA) reductase (simvastatin, fluvastatin and pravastatin) – nicotinic acid-related drugs (nicotinic acid and acipimox) and fibrates (clofibrate, bezafibrate, ciprofibrate, fenofibrate, and gemfibrozil). Cholesterol-lowering agents reduce both hypertension and risk of myocardial infarction; simvastatin reduces the risk of myocardial infarction and of premature death. There may also be benefit from beta-carotene and vitamins C and E and hormone replacement therapy.

IHD itself causes no symptoms but impaired coronary blood flow causes progressive damage to the heart, can go on to cardiac failure and can cause dysrhythmias. Usually the first signs of IHD are its dramatic complications, namely angina pectoris or myocardial infarction without warning or history of heart disease. Angina pectoris and myocardial infarction, the main acute manifestations of IHD, have many features in common but there are also important differences.

First, both diseases are the result of ischaemia and are common. The blood supply to the myocardium is chronically reduced but additional factors are involved in precipitating the acute attack. Second, chest pain is more severe and persistent in myocardial infarction. Third, angina (unlike myocardial infarction) is reversible and the pain is typically controlled by rest. Nevertheless, angina is typically followed sooner or later by myocardial infarction. Fourth, myocardial infarction leads to irreversible cardiac damage or sudden death.

Angina pectoris

Angina pectoris is the name given to paroxysms of severe ischaemic chest pain which are typically precipitated by effort and relieved by rest. The usual cause of angina is coronary atherosclerosis. Arterial spasm or reduced filling of the coronary arteries can contribute or, occasionally, be responsible alone.

Angina is termed *stable* if it occurs only on exertion and is relieved by rest, within 10 minutes, and there have been no changes in the frequency or duration of symptoms, or precipitating factors within the previous 60 days. *Unstable* angina is that in which there are changes in pattern, frequency or duration of precipitating factors; sudden onset angina is considered to be unstable. *Prinzmetal's* angina is angina at rest, commonly at night, and is caused by coronary artery spasm. *Syndrome X* describes patients with typical exertional chest pain simulating angina, but with arteriographically normal coronary arteries.

The most common precipitating cause of angina is physical exertion, particularly in cold weather. Emotion, especially anger or anxiety, can also induce attacks and some patients who can tolerate moderate exercise are vulnerable to angina when emotionally stressed.

The pain of angina is often unmistakable and described as a sense of strangling or choking. Tightness, heaviness, compression or constriction of the chest may be complaints but the pain is rarely of the unbearable, crushing and persistent nature of myocardial infarction. The typical site is behind the sternum radiating to the left particularly, sometimes to the left upper arm and occasionally to the left mandible or rarely to the teeth, tongue or palate. Patients who develop angina often have no history of heart disease. They may then have repeated attacks of angina over a long period or have a myocardial infarct soon after the first one or two attacks. The mortality rate in angina is about 4 per cent per year. The prognosis depends on the degree of coronary artery narrowing and is therefore highly variable and unpredictable.

Although the pain of angina can be relieved by rest it is more quickly relieved by giving nitrates, such as glyceryl trinitrate (nitroglycerin), which lowers peripheral vascular resistance and reduces the oxygen demands of the heart. Amyl nitrate, isosorbide dinitrite and erythrityl tetranitrate are also used. Calcium-channel blockers (occasionally also potassium-channel activators such as nicorandil) may be used, and aspirin is often prescribed for the anti-platelet activity.

Artery or vein coronary bypass grafts, or angioplasty, may be used to improve the coronary flow when angina fails to respond to drugs. Coronary artery bypass grafts (CABG) typically using saphenous vein, or percutaneous transluminal coronary angioplasty (PTCA), are commonly used, both resulting in a 5-year survival of over 85 per cent, though bypass is probably better than angioplasty in diabetics.

Although the typical picture of angina has been described, there are many patients who have painless acute myocardial ischaemia as shown by arteriography and the ECG changes in response to exercise.

In an experiment to assess whether those who had painless myocardial ischaemia were hyposensitive to pain, electrical pulp stimulation was used as an objective measure of response to pain. In a study on 108 patients with proven coronary artery disease, 71 per cent of those who had painless exercise-induced ischaemia had no discomfort from maximal pulpal stimulation. By contrast, over 80 per cent of patients who had exercise-induced angina had intense pain from maximal electrical pulp stimulation.

These findings suggest that the majority of those who suffer acute but painless myocardial ischaemia have hyposensitivity to pain.

• **Dental aspects of angina**

Dental care should be carried out with effective local analgesia, minimal anxiety, oxygen saturation and blood pressure and pulse monitoring, and at short appointments. Ready access to medical help, oxygen and nitroglycerin is crucial. Local analgesia should be given with an aspirating syringe. Adrenaline-containing LA solutions are satisfactory but a maximum of 4 ml solution containing 1 in 80 000 adrenaline should be used. Gingival retraction cords containing adrenaline should be avoided. Mepivacaine 3 per cent is preferable for use in patients taking beta-blockers. Preoperative glyceryl trinitrate and oral sedation, with intraoperative nasally delivered oxygen and ECG/BP monitoring, are advised.

Stable angina: Before dental treatment, patients with stable angina should be reassured and possibly sedated with oral diazepam, but prophylactic administration of glyceryl trinitrate may be more effective. If angina follows dental attention, the patient should be given their usual medication (usually glyceryl trinitrate). In any event the vasodilator should be readily available for use as required. Other medication, such as propranolol, should not be interfered with. For anything but minor treatment under local anaesthesia, the physician should be consulted and consideration should be given to any other complicating factors such as beta-blocker therapy, hypertension or cardiac failure.

Unstable angina: Elective dental care should be deferred until a physician has agreed to it, because of the risk of dysrhythmias or infarction. Emergency dental care should be the least invasive possible. Preoperative 0.5 mg glyceryl trinitrate sublingually or by inhalation (Matsura *et al.*, 1989), together with relative analgesia monitored by pulse oximetry and local analgesia, has been effectively used (Findler *et al.*, 1993) but such patients are best cared for in a hospital environment, as coronary vasodilators may be indicated intravenously.

Angina in the dental office: If a patient experiences chest pain, dental treatment must be stopped. If there is a history of angina, the patient should be given glyceryl trinitrate 0.5 mg sublingually and oxygen, and be kept sitting upright. Vital signs should be monitored. The pain should be relieved in 2–3 minutes; the patient should then rest and be accompanied home. If chest pain is not relieved within about 5 minutes, myocardial infarction is the probable cause (*see below*) and medical help should be summoned.

General anaesthesia should be deferred for at least 3 months in patients with recent onset angina, unstable angina or recent development of bundle branch block, and in any case, it should be given in hospital. Intravenous barbiturates are particularly dangerous. Tricyclic antidepressants are best avoided as they can disturb cardiac rhythm. Sumitriptan is contraindicated as it may cause coronary artery vasoconstriction.

Patients with bypass grafts do not require antibiotic cover against infective endocarditis.

Angina is a rare cause of pain in the mandible, teeth or other oral tissues, as mentioned earlier. On the other hand, untreated dental pain may precipitate angina in an affected individual. Patients with IHD appear to have more severe dental caries and periodontal disease than the general population, but whether these infections bear any causative relationship to the heart disease or whether they share some aetiological factor remains speculative.

Drugs used in the care of patients with angina may cause oral adverse effects such as lichenoid lesions (calcium channel blockers) or ulcers (nicorandil).

Myocardial infarction

Myocardial infarction (often called a coronary thrombosis or heart attack) is the most severe and lethal form of coronary heart disease. Between 30 and 50 per cent of patients die within the first hour after the attack and a further 10–20 per cent within the next few days.

Fewer than 50 per cent of patients have any premonitory symptoms, but some may have warnings, such as a change in the character of anginal pain or indigestion-like pain.

The pain may start either at rest or during activity, is typically unbearably severe and terrifying in character, is unrelieved by rest or nitrates, and can persist for hours if death does not supervene. Vomiting, facial pallor, sweating, restlessness and apprehension are common. Other features may include breathlessness, cough and loss of consciousness, but the clinical picture is variable.

The pain is felt in the chest but can radiate to the same sites as angina. On rare occasions pain is felt in the left mandible alone. A significant number of patients have silent (painless) infarctions and, as discussed earlier, this may be due to hyposensitivity to pain, including dental pain. In about 10 per cent of cases pain is slight or even absent and the first signs of a myocardial infarct may then be the sudden onset of left ventricular failure, shock, loss of consciousness, or death. Characteristic electrocardiographic (EGG) changes and the release of heart muscle enzymes into the blood confirm the diagnosis. Severe disorders of rhythm are common and may be fatal.

Sudden cardiac death

Death soon after the onset of chest pain is common: less often there is sudden cardiac death characterized by immediate collapse without premonitory symptoms, and loss of pulses. In such cases the precipitating event is a severe dysrhythmia such as ventricular fibrillation. Nevertheless, immediate cardiopulmonary resuscitation can be life-saving. The fact that at least 50 per cent of survivors of such attacks have no evidence (from the EGG or serum creatinine phosphokinase, lactic dehydrogenase and aspartate transaminase levels) of damage to the myocardium, suggests that sudden cardiac death is not the same as a myocardial infarct.

- **Diagnosis and management of myocardial infarction**

The onset of myocardial infarction is usually obvious from the clinical features (*Table 3.5*). Nausea and vomiting are common.

The patient should be kept at rest, reassured as well as possible and given oxygen by a face mask. Morphine, 10 mg, preferably by slow intravenous injection (2 mg/min) or up to 15 mg i.m. according to the size of the patient, plus cyclizine 50 mg, or alternatively, nitrous oxide with at least 28 per cent oxygen, should be given to relieve pain. Pentazocine is contraindicated as it can cause dysphoria and raises pulmonary arterial pressure. An ambulance should be called. Ventricular fibrillation is an important cause of death, but controllable by defibrillation. Nearly 50 per cent of deaths are in the first hour. If there is cardiac arrest the patient must be given external cardiac massage and oxygen or mouth-to-mouth ventilation (Chapter 27). Thrombolytic agents and aspirin may be indicated.

Prevention or reduction of the risks from myocardial infarction include stopping smoking, low fat intake, more exercise and aspirin 75 mg daily or 300 mg on alternate

---

Table 3.5   Myocardial infarction – diagnosis

- Changes in heart rate
- Dysrhythmias
- Hypotension
- Shock
- Fever and leucocytosis
- ECG changes
- Rise in serum enzymes

---

days. Such are the complexities of prostaglandin metabolism and the difficulties in interpreting clinical trials, that though the antiplatelet effect of aspirin is agreed to be valuable, there is, as yet, no consensus as to the optimal dose. Beta-blockers, particularly atenolol or metoprolol given intravenously in the acute phase, can lessen mortality and oral propranolol or timolol, in the convalescent stage, can reduce the risk of recurrence after a myocardial infarct, but such drugs are contraindicated for patients with asthma or in heart failure.

- **Dental aspects of myocardial infarction**

The severity of a myocardial infarct (MI) is suggested by the resulting disability, by the length of the acute illness and whether or not the patient was hospitalized. Nevertheless, it is important to consult the patient's physician before undertaking operative treatment. General anaesthesia is contraindicated after a recent myocardial infarct, though the risk declines with time. The incidence of myocardial infarction after general anaesthesia in patients with documented preoperative infarcts is up to eight times that of patients with no previous history. Nearly 30 per cent of patients having a general anaesthetic within 3 months of an infarct have another in the first postoperative week and at least 50 per cent die. The prognosis of recurrent infarction is also influenced by the time after the first attack; elective surgery under general anaesthesia should therefore be postponed for at least 3 months and preferably a year.

For patients with a history of MI, neither general anaesthesia nor advanced oral surgical procedures should be carried out in the general dental surgery; hospital care is more

Table 3.6 Main causes of acute chest pain*

Cause	Features	Predisposing factors
Myocardial infarction	Severe persistent crushing retrosternal pain possibly radiating to left arm. Unrelieved by glyceryl trinitrate. May be nausea or vomiting	Coronary heart disease Hypertension
Angina pectoris	Retrosternal pain possibly radiating to left arm. Often previously experienced. Relieved in 3 minutes by glyceryl trinitrate	Coronary heart disease Hypertension
Oesophagitis	Low retrosternal pain on lying down or stooping. Improved by antacids	Hiatus hernia
Anxiety (hyperventilation syndrome)	Anxious patients with precordial pain. Overbreathing, panic and precordial pain	Stress

*Other cardiovascular causes such as dissecting aneurysm, and conditions outside the chest (e.g. acute abdominal pain), may present with chest pain.

appropriate. Drugs such as sumitriptan are contraindicated. Anxiety and pain must be minimized and the physician may advocate preoperative use of glyceryl trinitrate. There must be ready access to oxygen and medical help. Local analgesia, possibly supplemented with relative analgesia, and monitoring of blood pressure, pulse and oxygen saturation are indicated.

Recent myocardial infarction: Patients within 3 months of an MI are at greatest risk of further MI or dysrhythmias or other complications and therefore the opinion of a physician should be sought before dental treatment. Elective dental care should be deferred. Simple emergency dental treatment under local anaesthesia may be given during the first 6 months after a myocardial infarct. Treatment under local anaesthesia should be carried out with care using an aspirating syringe to avoid excess dosage and intravenous injection, and anything that might cause undue anxiety. Prilocaine with felypressin is frequently advocated as the local analgesic but there is no evidence that it is safer than lignocaine with adrenaline which is a more effective local anaesthetic. Mepivacaine 3 per cent may be preferred for patients taking beta-blockers. Thrombolytic agents can produce a bleeding tendency (Chapter 4).

Symptomatic previous but older MI: The above considerations apply but elective dental procedures can normally be carried out.

Asymptomatic patients with previous older MI: Elective dental care can normally be carried out safely, but again it is wise to minimize pain and anxiety.

The management of myocardial infarction as an emergency in the dental surgery is along the lines mentioned in the previous section and summarized in Chapter 27. Pentazocine is less effective than morphine, even when given by injection but, worse, does not relieve or may even increase anxiety. Pentazocine can also increase the load on the heart to an undesirable degree: it is also now a Controlled Drug and is therefore no easier to obtain or store than morphine.

Heart block resulting from damage to the conduction tissues by an infarct may necessitate insertion of a cardiac pacemaker and result in other complications, as discussed later.

Other causes of chest pain

Angina or myocardial infarction are the main possible causes to bear in mind, but other causes are listed in *Table 3.6*.

KAWASAKI'S DISEASE

Kawasaki's disease (mucocutaneous lymph node syndrome; MLNS or MCLS) is an acute febrile illness with lymphadenopathy and desquamation of the lips, fingers and toes, simulating scarlet fever and erythema multiforme. It is now a considerably more common cause of severe childhood heart disease in many countries than rheumatic fever, and although considerably more prevalent in Japanese and Korean persons, cases have now been recognized in many other races. The most important complication is cardiac involvement with coronary arteritis leading to aneurysms that may thrombose with an overall mortality of 5–10 per cent.

The cause is unknown, and though an infection is likely, presumably in persons of certain genetic backgrounds, no agent has yet been consistently isolated. Some have suggested exposure to detergents, mites or mercury as causes, but again there is no real evidence for this. Superantigens (bacterial toxins that stimulate T lymphocytes) are another possible cause.

Children from 7 weeks to 8 years are mainly affected, with a male preponderance in a ratio of more than 2 to 1. The main clinical features are: (i) fever lasting at least 5 days; (ii) erythema and oedema of the extremities followed by desquamation; (iii) a polymorphous rash; (iv) oral mucosal erythema; (v) cervical lymphadenopathy; (vi) conjunctival infection; and (vii) mood changes (extreme misery). There are cardiac complications in approximately 25 per cent of cases.

Other less common complications include aseptic meningitis or encephalopathy, arthritis or arthralgia, abdominal pain, diarrhoea or vomiting, and hepatosplenomegaly. The majority have leukocytosis and thrombocytosis but a few have normochromic normocytic anaemia, leucopenia or thrombocytopenia.

- **Diagnosis and management of Kawasaki's disease**

Echocardiography should be carried out on suspicion and repeated at least at 14–21 days, 60 days and 12 months after the onset.

Intravenous gammaglobulin, in a single infusion of 2 g/kg, or as 400 mg/kg daily for 4 days, appears to reduce the cardiac involvement. Aspirin or systemic steroids may help.

- **Dental aspects of Kawasaki's disease**

Characteristic oral changes are a strawberry tongue, labial oedema, crusting or cracking of the lips, pharyngitis and oropharyngeal erythema. Cervical lymphadenopathy is also common and usually unilateral but occasionally massive. Facial palsy is sometimes seen; it is self-limiting but usually associated with cardiovascular involvement.

Any infant or young child with these features and particularly if there is also a desquamating rash on the extremities should be immediately referred to a paediatric cardiologist for investigation.

THE CARDIOMYOPATHIES

Cardiomyopathy is a disease of the myocardium other than that caused by hypertension, ischaemia, valve disease or cor pulmonale. There are many causes of cardiomyopathy, but all except alcoholic heart muscle disease are uncommon.

Alcoholic heart muscle disease

Chronic overindulgence in alcohol can damage both skeletal and cardiac muscle. The incidence of alcoholic heart disease appears to be higher still in those with sickle cell trait.

The clinical effects of alcoholism on the heart are variable but it may cause precordial pain and palpitations, dysrhythmias or pulmonary hypertension and right ventricular failure. Sudden unexpected death (probably caused by ventricular fibrillation) appears to be relatively common among young alcoholics.

Moderate social drinking (particularly one or two glasses of red wine a day), by contrast, may be associated with a lower than average mortality from myocardial infarction.

- **Dental aspects (*see* Chapter 24)**

Hypertrophic cardiomyopathy (idiopathic hypertrophic subaortic stenosis: IHSS)

This is regarded as a rare disease but may frequently pass unrecognized. Hypertrophic cardiomyopathy is characterized by hypertrophy of the septum and wall of the left ventricle causing progressive obstruction to its filling and outflow. Congestive cardiac failure with atrial fibrillation can result, or alternatively there may be mitral regurgitation, angina, sudden death or infective endocarditis.

Congestive cardiomyopathy

This is probably the most common form of idiopathic cardiomyopathy in Britain, but it is even more difficult to recognize than the hypertrophic type.

The essential features are weakening and distension of the left ventricle, valvular regurgitation and progress to failure of both ventricles.

• **Dental aspects of idiopathic cardiomyopathies**

Patients are at risk from infective endocarditis and are a poor risk for general anaesthesia because of dysrhythmias, cardiac failure, or myocardial ischaemia. Frequently, however, a patient is unaware of a cardiomyopathy until complications develop. Infantile supravalvular subaortic stenosis may be associated with hypercalcaemia and a characteristic elfin facies (William's syndrome: Chapter 15).

DYSRHYTHMIAS (ARRHYTHMIAS)

Disturbances of heart rhythm or gross disturbances of heart rate are usually caused by lesions of the sino-atrial or atrioventricular nodes, or of the cardiac conducting tissues, sometimes by drugs. Most dysrhythmias reduce cardiac efficiency and cardiac output.

Atrial fibrillation

Atrial fibrillation is the most common dysrhythmia. Atrial fibrillation is characterized by totally uncoordinated and ineffectual contractions. Common causes are congestive cardiac failure, ischaemic or rheumatic heart disease, or thyrotoxicosis. The effects of atrial fibrillation are impaired ventricular filling and an irregular, but usually rapid, ventricular rate. Thrombi may form in the atrium and can release emboli, for example to the brain. Anticoagulants may therefore be needed. Atrial fibrillation can also cause heart failure. Digoxin is the standard treatment.

Tachycardia

Tachycardia (abnormally rapid heart rate) increases the load on, and oxygen consumption of, the heart. It can cause serious complications, especially if associated with IHD, and can be fatal. Sinus tachycardia is a normal response to exercise or fear but can also result from diseases such as hyperthyroidism.

Atrial tachycardia is often paroxysmal, of unknown cause and produces no more than palpitations in a normal person. If severe, atrial tachycardia can impair ventricular filling and causes breathlessness or fainting. In the presence of heart disease, it can cause ischaemic pain or cardiac failure.

Ventricular tachycardia – a rate above about 140 per minute – is usually the result of IHD or digitalis overdosage. Myocardial pain or cardiac failure are typical consequences, but ventricular fibrillation may follow. Lignocaine is the usual treatment but bretyllium, mexilitine, moracizine, phenytoin or tocainide may be required. A particular form of ventricular tachycardia, known as *torsades de pointes* – because of peculiar ECG abnormalities – may be caused by interactions between terfenadine and ketoconazole or erythromycin (but not clarithyromycin).

Paroxysmal supraventricular tachycardia may remit spontaneously, but vagal pressure or intravenous adenosine are the standard measures to control it. Cardiac glycosides or verapamil may be needed.

Bradycardia

A slow heart rate may be unimportant in a young person and is often found in athletes. Bradycardia may follow myocardial infarction. A rate below about 60 per minute in an elderly person, especially when associated with heart disease, can cause sudden loss of consciousness (syncope). Atropine may be indicated.

In *sick sinus syndrome* the pacemaking function of the sino-atrial node becomes severely disturbed, with a variety of possible effects such as bradycardia, sino-atrial block, atrial tachycardia or atrial fibrillation. If there is sino-atrial block there is also dysrhythmia and, in severe cases, consciousness can be lost.

Disorders of conduction (heart block): These result from blocking of the cardiac impulse anywhere in the conduction system. Among the more common causes of conduction defects are IHD, drugs, especially digitalis and, in the past, rheumatic fever.

Mild heart block may only be detectable on an EGG. In complete heart block the ventricle contracts at its intrinsic rate of about 30–40 per minute. The result is severely reduced cardiac output with pallor or cyanosis and syncopal attacks (Stokes–Adams attacks). A pacemaker may be indicated.

Ventricular fibrillation

Ventricular fibrillation results in complete failure of cardiac output and is typically fatal within a few minutes. It is the most serious type of dysrhythmia and the most common cause of sudden death. Ventricular fibrillation is often a consequence of myocardial infarction or idiopathic fibrosis affecting the conduction mechanism, occasionally, thyrotoxicosis, halothane anaesthesia, or adrenaline or digitalis overdosage, and is a cause of sudden death in cocaine addicts.

Extrasystoles

These are the most common type of intermittent dysrhythmia and give rise to the well-known sensation of a missed heart beat. Extrasystoles are usually of no significance and are abolished by exercise in normal persons.

• Dental aspects of dysrhythmias

The probability of developing dangerous dysrhythmias with general anaesthesia is increased if there is a significant preoperative dysrhythmia.

Dysrhythmias can be induced by anaesthetic agents, especially halothane (isoflurane is safer); by manipulation of the neck, carotid sinus or eyes (vagal reflex); and by preoperative digitalization. The risk is greater in the elderly and those with coronary artery disease or aortic stenosis. Dysrhythmias can result if erythromycin or azole antifungal drugs are given to patients taking terfenadine, cisapride or astemizole.

Syncope may be the result of bradycardia, heart block or atrial tachycardia, and may be recognized by the slowness or irregularity of the pulse. It may need to be distinguished from a simple fainting attack by these means. Otherwise the initial treatment is the same.

Ventricular fibrillation is clinically indistinguishable from asystole and is one of the most serious emergencies that may have to be managed in the dental surgery (*see* Chapter 27).

Several anti-dysrhythmic drugs can cause oral lesions. Verapamil, enalapril and diltiazem may cause gingival hyperplasia, some beta-blockers may rarely cause lichenoid ulceration and procainamide can cause a lupus-like reaction.

Cardiac pacemakers

Pacemakers generate impulses to regulate the cardiac rhythm when there is absence of spontaneous cardiac rhythm. They can be temporary transvenous pacemakers, or permanent, and they operate either at a fixed rate (asynchronous mode) or, more commonly, only on demand (synchronous). Modern pacemakers are bipolar and typically located in the right ventricle, having been inserted via the subclavian or cephalic vein. They present few problems for dental treatment though high frequency, external electromagnetic radiation can interfere with the sensing function particularly of the monopolar type of pacemaker and may induce fibrillation in these patients. The chief hazards are magnetic resonance imaging, electrosurgery and diathermy. Ultrasonic scalers, pulp testers, dental induction casting machines, belt-driven motors in dental chairs, X-ray machines, microwave ovens and even television transmitters and faulty or badly earthed equipment *may* cause interference, but the risk is very small. Pulp testers are not a risk.

The only safe procedure under such circumstances is to avoid the use of all such equipment whenever a patient with a pacemaker is being treated, as it is difficult to assess the level of risk in any individual patient. Patients should be treated in the supine position; electrical equipment kept over 30 cm away; and repetitive switching of electrical instruments avoided.

If a pacemaker shuts off, all possible sources of interference should be switched off and the patient given cardiopulmonary resuscitation in the supine position. Artificial respiration should force the heart to resume its rhythm and the pacemaker to start up again.

Unless a cardiac valve lesion is also present, patients with permanent pacemakers do not need antibiotic cover to prevent endocarditis. If a temporary transvenous pacemaker is present, the physician should be consulted first. General anaesthesia if required should be given only in a hospital setting by a specialist.

It should be remembered, however, that despite the risks outlined above, the patient is generally at much greater risk from non-dental sources such as security systems in shops, airports etc.

THYROID-RELATED HEART DISEASE
(*see also* Chapter 14)

Hyperthyroidism raises the metabolic rate and activity of the heart, and sensitizes the myocardium to sympathetic activity. The heart has also to meet the increased demands resulting from the raised metabolic activity of the rest of the body.

Untreated thyrotoxicosis causes tachycardia and a tendency to dysrhythmias which can lead to cardiac failure or myocardial infarction, especially in the elderly. Beta-blockers are particularly useful.

Hypothyroidism slows the metabolic rate and activity of the heart and other tissues. In myxoedema, however, patients have hypercholesterolaemia associated with atherosclerosis. Ischaemic heart disease (angina or myocardial infarction) often develops but is unusual in that it predominantly affects women.

- ### Dental aspects of thyroid heart disease

The same reservations about general anaesthesia apply to patients with uncontrolled hyperthyroid heart disease as to those with other dangerous heart diseases, but sedation with diazepam should be beneficial. It has also been said that local anaesthetics containing adrenaline should be avoided because of the possible risk of dangerous dysrhythmias. There seems, however, scant confirmatory clinical evidence and the risk is probably only theoretical if overdose of local anaesthetics is avoided. Some prefer to use prilocaine with felypressin but there is no evidence that it is any safer.

Patients with uncontrolled hyperthyroidism can sometimes be difficult to manage, as a result of heightened anxiety, hyperexcitability and increased sympathetic activity. Sedation may therefore be particularly desirable.

Hypothyroid patients may be at risk in the dental surgery if they have IHD. Sjögren's syndrome is rarely associated with hypothy-roidism in spite of the fact that antithyroid autoantibodies are relatively commonly found in the former.

In severe myxoedema, diazepam and other CNS depressants can precipitate coma.

PULMONARY HEART DISEASE (COR PULMONALE)

Cor pulmonale is the term given to heart disease resulting from the excessive load imposed on the right ventricle by diseases of the lungs or pulmonary circulation, especially chronic obstructive airways disease (Chapter 8). The essential features are right ventricular hypertrophy leading to right-sided failure, systemic venous congestion and persistent hypoxia. In the early stages there is dyspnoea, a chronic cough, wheezing and often cyanosis. Right-sided cardiac failure, which may be precipitated by intercurrent respiratory infection, causes more severe dyspnoea and cyanosis, together with oedema of the ankles and ascites.

- ### Dental aspects of pulmonary heart disease

Under no circumstances should patients with cor pulmonale be given a general anaesthetic other than in hospital. Intravenous barbiturates are completely contraindicated and even diazepam may be dangerous because of its respiratory depressant effect in these hypoxic patients.

ACUTE RHEUMATIC FEVER

Rheumatic fever is a disease which sometimes follows a sore throat caused by certain strains of beta-haemolytic streptococci (*S. pyogenes*). The inflammatory changes appear to result from cross-reactivity with some of the streptococcal antigens and immunologically mediated tissue damage.

The chief importance of rheumatic fever was that, particularly in the past, it could lead, after the lapse of years, to chronic rheumatic heart disease as a result of fibrosis and distortion of the valves.

Rheumatic fever is now a very rare disease in the Western world and even among the

Table 3.7 Rheumatic fever – diagnostic criteria	
Major	*Minor*
Carditis	Pyrexia
Polyarthritis	Arthralgia
Chorea	Previous rheumatic fever
Erythema marginatum	ESR and C-reactive
Subcutaneous nodules	protein raised
	Characteristic ECG
	changes

few that are attacked, permanent cardiac damage hardly ever follows. In recent years, a few cases have appeared in the United States and Britain, but there appears to be no significant resurgence of the disease. It also appears to have changed in character. By contrast, in countries such as the Indian subcontinent, the Middle East and some of the Caribbean islands, rheumatic fever is common and is relatively quickly followed by permanent heart disease.

Children between 5 and 15 years are predominantly affected. In typical cases a sore throat is followed after about 3 weeks (2–26 weeks) by an acute febrile illness with pain flitting from one joint to another. The clinical manifestations are so variable, however, that the diagnosis should not be made unless at least two of the major criteria (*Table 3.7*) are fulfilled.

Preceding streptococcal infection is confirmed by a high or rising titre of antistreptolysin O (ASOT), and is suggestive, but not diagnostic, of rheumatic fever. However, a low ASOT virtually excludes the diagnosis.

The duration of the disease is usually from 6 to 12 weeks and in the great majority of cases there is resolution without apparent after-effects.

Any cardiac tissue can be affected but the most serious feature is subendocardial inflammation, particularly along the lines of closure of the valve cusps, resulting in the formation of minute fibrinous vegetations. The mitral and aortic valves are particularly affected. There is usually little detectable effect on cardiac function in the acute phase of the disease but, in unusually severe cases, myocarditis can cause death from cardiac failure.

Pain in the large joints (which gives rheumatic fever its name) is conspicuous, but heals

without permanent damage in about 3 weeks.

Other features are cerebral involvement causing spasmodic involuntary movements (Sydenham's chorea, St Vitus' dance), a characteristic rash (erythema marginatum), lung involvement and subcutaneous nodules, usually forming around the elbows.

- **General management of rheumatic fever**

Treatment consists principally of the use of salicylates for arthritis and penicillin if streptococcal infection is still active. Complications such as cardiac failure are treated along conventional lines.

Prompt antimicrobial treatment (within 24 hours of onset) of a streptococcal sore throat prevents the development of rheumatic fever in most cases. After an attack, there is a risk of recurrence and continuous antibiotic prophylaxis becomes necessary to lessen the risk of permanent cardiac damage. The drug of choice is usually oral phenoxymethyl penicillin (500 mg daily) until the age of 20. For those allergic to penicillin, sulphadimidine (500 mg daily) by mouth should be given. These doses are insufficient for prophylaxis against infective endocarditis and the oral bacteria are likely to be penicillin-resistant if long-term penicillin has been given. Chorea may recur during pregnancy or in patients taking the contraceptive pill, but does not indicate recurrent carditis.

- **Dental aspects of rheumatic fever**

Patients are unlikely to be seen during an attack but emergency dental treatment may be necessary, to relieve toothache for example. This can be done under local anaesthesia in consultation with the physician. General anaesthesia should be avoided because of the possibility of myocarditis but no other special precautions should be necessary as there appears to be little risk of infective endocarditis at this stage.

CHRONIC RHEUMATIC HEART DISEASE

In the past, approximately 60 per cent of children who survived acute rheumatic fever developed a cardiac lesion detectable after 10 years, but heart failure may take a further 10 or more years to develop. However, such complications have become increasingly rare and chronic rheumatic heart disease is only likely to be seen now in the middle-aged and some immigrants.

The essential features of rheumatic heart disease are fibrotic stiffening and distortion of the heart valves. The mitral valve is affected in most cases, either alone (60–70 per cent), or with the aortic valve in a further 20 per cent. The aortic valve alone is affected in only 10 per cent. Valve narrowing (stenosis) and regurgitation (incompetence) are associated in varying degrees.

Chronic rheumatic heart disease is essentially therefore a mechanical, haemodynamic disorder, in which the defective valves cause cardiac failure if function cannot be improved by surgery. Infective endocarditis may supervene at any time but is relatively rare.

The earliest sign of valve damage is a murmur. Later effects, particularly enlargement of the heart, may be detected clinically, radiographically and by ECG changes.

• Dental aspects of rheumatic carditis

The chief risk is of infective endocarditis which may follow dental surgery without antibiotic cover. Evaluation of a history of rheumatic fever is difficult. The only way to be certain is to refer the patient to a cardiologist to decide whether there has been any valve damage. The simpler alternative is to give antibiotic cover on the assumption that the history is valid, but this means that at least 70 per cent of such patients will receive the antibiotic unnecessarily (*see below*). It must be emphasized that all rheumatic heart lesions are at risk from infective endocarditis but the level of risk is not related to the severity of the defect. Asymptomatic lesions are often a greater risk than those which are severely disabling.

CONGENITAL HEART DISEASE

Congenital anomalies are now the most common type of heart disease among children and are now considerably more prevalent than rheumatic heart disease (*Plate 3*). Congenital heart disease is present in about 1 per cent of live births, and, in the absence of treatment, possibly 40 per cent of those affected would die within the first 5 years. The prognosis has been enormously improved by cardiac surgery.

Congenital defects can involve the heart or adjacent great vessels. Cardiac defects can be associated in different combinations and some 20 per cent have other congenital anomalies. Midline defects are often multiple: ventricular septal defect, for example, may be associated with cleft palate or imperforate anus.

The causes of congenital heart disease are unknown in most cases but the best known acquired causes are congenital rubella or cytomegalovirus infection (Chapter 11) and maternal drug misuse. The best known genetic cause is Down's syndrome (Chapter 23).

The most striking feature of some types of congenital heart disease is cyanosis (more than 5 g reduced haemoglobin per dl) caused by shunting deoxygenated blood from the right ventricle directly into the systemic circulation (right to left shunt). In severe cases, cyanosis is obvious at birth, particularly in Fallot's tetralogy. Chronic hypoxaemia causes severely impaired development and often gross finger and toe clubbing (*Plate 4*). Where the shunt is in the opposite direction (left to right) some of the output of the left ventricle is recirculated through the lungs. There is then pulmonary hypertension and, eventually, right ventricular hypertrophy. The direction of the shunt may then reverse and cyanosis develops later. Chronic hypoxaemia eventually results in polycythaemia which can cause haemorrhagic or thrombotic tendencies.

Dental management can be complicated by the hazard to some of these patients of general anaesthesia if the heart is failing, or of infective endocarditis. Congenital heart lesions are susceptible to infective endocarditis, *irrespective of the severity of the defect*. It is well recognized that congenital defects have occasionally been discovered only as a result of the development of infective endocarditis. Different types of congenital heart lesion vary in their vulnerability to infection, but this is only of statistical significance and antimicrobial prophylaxis is needed before dental surgery in all such patients (*see below*).

Only the main types of congenital heart disease can be briefly considered here.

Acyanotic congenital heart defects

Ventricular septal defect (VSD): This is a septal defect in the ventricular wall. These are one of the most common congenital defects and range from mere pinholes which are compatible with survival at least into middle age, to defects so large as to cause death in infancy if untreated. As described earlier, there may eventually be right ventricular hypertrophy, reversal of the shunt and late onset cyanosis. Right ventricular failure may develop.

Another effect of the left to right shunt is that the jet of blood hitting the endocardium of the right ventricle causes an area of endocardial thickening (jet lesion) to form. This lesion, or the margins of the defect, can later be the site of infective endocarditis. Ninety per cent of patients with VSD have an additional cardiac defect.

Atrial septal defect (ASD): This is a septal defect, often located near the foramen ovale. This has little effect on cardiac function and is initially acyanotic. Survival into middle age is usual, even in uncorrected cases. However, right ventricular failure usually develops eventually in the absence of surgical correction. Another complication of ASD is that an embolus from a vein can pass from the right ventricle into the left and therefore directly into the systemic circulation and can occasionally be fatal (paradoxical embolism).

The risk of infective endocarditis in ASD appears to be very small, but antibiotic cover should still be given for dental operations unless the defect has been repaired by direct suture more than 6 months previously.

Patent ductus arteriosus (PDA): PDA is a persistent opening (normally closed by the third month of life) between the aorta and pulmonary artery. This abnormal communication causes characteristically loud and continuous sawing, systolic and diastolic murmurs. Since the shunt is from left to right, it is initially acyanotic and the typical complication is right ventricular failure. Occasionally infective endocarditis supervenes. Antibiotic cover should therefore be given for dental operations unless the defect has been closed. If patency of the ductus is not necessary to maintain the systemic circulation, its closure

can be promoted in early infancy by giving intravenous indomethacin, a prostaglandin inhibitor. Alternatively, it is ligated.

Coarctation of the aorta: This is an aortic narrowing, usually sited beyond the origin of the subclavian arteries. The blood supply to the head, neck and upper body is not therefore obstructed and only the supply to the lower part of the body is restricted. The effect of the narrowing is to cause severe hypertension in the upper part of the body and a low blood pressure below. There are thus strong radial pulses at the wrists but weak or absent femoral pulses in the groins (radio-femoral delay).

Secondary changes are enlargement of collateral arteries (such as the intercostal) and degenerative changes in the aorta which can lead to a fatal aneurysm. A bicuspid aortic valve is associated in over 50 per cent of patients.

Infective endocarditis or left ventricular failure are other possible causes of death.

Pulmonary stenosis: This is narrowing of the pulmonary valve. The main symptoms are breathlessness and right ventricular failure, often in childhood.

Aortic stenosis: This is usually narrowing of the aortic valve.

Floppy mitral valve (mitral valve prolapse): This common condition is said to affect 4 per cent of the population. It is an autosomal dominant trait frequently present in otherwise normal persons, but is also a characteristic feature of Ehlers–Danlos and Marfan's syndromes (Chapter 16). Up to 50 per cent of patients with panic disorder have been reported to have mitral valve prolapse. The condition may also be seen in thyrotoxicosis, ischaemic heart disease and rheumatic heart disease.

A prolapsed mitral valve is typically asymptomatic, but if it causes a systolic murmur, can predispose to infective endocarditis, particularly in older persons.

Bicuspid aortic valve: This is usually asymptomatic, even in athletes, but is a high risk for infective endocarditis. The latter may be the first indication of the presence of the defect.

Cyanotic congenital heart defects

Transposition of the great vessels: Reversal of the origins of the pulmonary artery and aorta causes cyanosis and breathlessness from birth, and early congestive failure. Death in infancy is common unless there are associated defects such as a patent interventricular septum or patent ductus arteriosus, which provide sufficient collateral circulation for oxygenation of the blood to maintain life a little longer.

Tetralogy of Fallot: The four defects which give the condition its name comprise:

1. Ventricular septal defect.
2. Pulmonary stenosis.
3. Straddling of the interventricular septum by the aorta, into which blood flows from both ventricles – 'overriding aorta'. There is obstruction to the outflow from the right ventricle and thus also –
4. Compensatory right ventricular hypertrophy.

Among the most obvious clinical features are severe cyanosis and loud cardiac murmurs. Paroxysms of cyanosis and breathlessness, which typically cause cerebral anoxia and syncope, often supervene for no apparent reason. Another characteristic is that these children tend to squat, particularly after exertion, to get some relief from breathlessness.

The usual results of the persistent hypoxia are poor physical development, clubbing of the fingers and toes, and compensatory polycythaemia. In the absence of treatment there is typically heart failure, respiratory infection or, less often, infective endocarditis.

Eisenmenger's syndrome: This refers to cyanosis from any right-to-left shunt through a ventricular septal defect.

Tricuspid atresia: In this, there is absence of the tricuspid valve, right ventricle and pulmonary valve. The pulmonary circulation is maintained through a patent ductus arteriosus.

Pulmonary atresia: This is similar to tricuspid atresia. There is a three-chambered heart but the tricuspid valve is patent.

- **General management of congenital cardiac defects**

Many of the congenital cardiovascular defects can be improved by cardiac surgery. Medical treatment is needed for patients with cardiac failure, polycythaemia, infective complications or emotional disturbances.

- **Dental aspects of congenital cardiac disease**

Most important are the risks of general anaesthesia, infective endocarditis and bleeding tendencies. The last is caused by defective platelet function and increased fibrinolytic activity in cyanotic congenital heart disease. The dental management of these patients and prevention of infective endocarditis are discussed later, but general anaesthesia in the dental surgery is contraindicated and specialist referral is needed. A special hazard in some types of congenital heart disease is the development of cerebral abscess: this has very occasionally been reported as a consequence of dental sepsis or even to follow endodontic treatment.

Associated problems such as cleft palate, or syndromes such as Down's syndrome, Turner's syndrome, or idiopathic hypercalcaemia (William's syndrome) may also affect dental management (*see* Appendix to this chapter).

Oral abnormalities associated with cyanotic congenital heart disease include delayed eruption of both dentitions, with an increased frequency of positional anomalies and enamel hypoplasia. The teeth often have a bluish-white 'skimmed milk' appearance and there is gross vasodilatation in the pulps. There appears to be greater caries and periodontal disease activity, probably because of poor oral hygiene and lack of dental attention. After cardiotomy, transient small white, non-ulcerated mucosal lesions of unknown aetiology may be seen.

INFECTIVE (BACTERIAL) ENDOCARDITIS

Infective endocarditis is an uncommon but dangerous infection, predominantly affecting the heart valves but also capable of involving coarctation of the aorta or ductus arteriosus. The earlier name 'subacute bacterial endocarditis' is misleading – cases range from fulminatingly acute to chronic. Arteriovenous shunts for haemodialysis in chronic renal failure (Chapter 13) can also become infected and comparable diseases result.

The main effects of endocarditis are progressive cardiac damage and infection or embolic damage of many organs, especially the kidneys. Infective endocarditis may be fatal in about 30 per cent of patients overall, and there is also a high morbidity.

Predisposing factors to endocarditis

Infective endocarditis results from two main predisposing factors. First, a cardiac lesion such as congenital heart disease may allow endocardial infection to become established, and second, bacteraemia (caused by medical, surgical or dental procedures) may initiate the infection. Nevertheless, even an apparently normal heart can become infected and few cases can be reliably related to a preceding surgical procedure causing a bacteraemia. Many factors in the pathogenesis of the disease remain unidentified.

Invasive medical procedures, such as instrumentation of the urinary tract and the increasing prevalence of intravenous drug abuse, provide many portals of entry for microbes. Highly virulent bacteria such as staphylococci can be introduced into the bloodstream with the addict's needle or by open heart surgery and can cause particularly severe endocarditis. By contrast, micro-organisms which are harmless to the normal person can colonize the endocardium of a host with impaired defences.

The most common type of microbial isolate from patients with infective endocarditis are viridans streptococci, particularly *S. mutans* and *S. sanguis*. These account for nearly 40 per cent of the many different causative organisms. A possible reason for the importance of viridans streptococci in dentally related endocarditis is, first, that they are present in enormous numbers in the mouth, and second, are released into the bloodstream in large numbers during extractions in particular. They also have complex attachment mechanisms which may enable them to adhere to the endocardium. By comparison, other oral bacteria are only rarely incriminated.

The main local host factor is typically a ˙defective or damaged heart valve. Prosthetic valves also provide the site for a severe form of endocarditis, but this is infrequently due to oral bacteria. Surgical correction of some congenital heart defects has made some of these patients less susceptible to infection. By

Table 3.8	Aetiological factors for infective endocarditis

- *Bacterial factors*
Bacteraemia arising from
    Extractions and some other dental procedures
    Cardiac surgery, particularly insertion of prosthetic valves
    Intravenous medication
    Intracardiac or venous catheters
    Obstetric and gynaecological procedures
    Intravenous drug addiction
    Unknown sources
Number of bacteria entering the blood
Bacterial virulence
Ability of bacteria to adhere to endocardium

- *Host factors increasing susceptibility*
Local lesions
    Congenital
    Rheumatic and other acquired valvular disease
    Prosthetic heart valves
    Other cardiac disease
Drugs
Immunosuppressive treatment
    Cytotoxic drugs
    Underlying disease
    Alcoholism

- *Protective factors*
Antimicrobial chemotherapy

contrast, patients who have had a previous attack of infective endocarditis are particularly vulnerable.

Despite the varied factors affecting aetiology (*Table 3.8*), the peak prevalence of infective endocarditis is now in the sixth or seventh decade and the disease is very uncommon in children.

• Clinical features and mortality

The signs and symptoms are highly variable. In the previously healthy patient who acquires endocarditis due to viridans streptococci, the picture is likely to be that, 3 or 4 weeks after a dental operation, low fever and mild malaise develop and persist. Pallor (anaemia) or light (café-au-lait) pigmentation of the skin are typical. Later, increasing disability is associated with changing cardiac murmurs indicative of progressive heart damage, while release of emboli can have effects ranging from loss of a peripheral pulse to (rarely) sudden death from a stroke. Embolic phenomena include haematuria, which is common, cerebrovascular occlusion, petechiae or purpura of skin and mucous membranes, and splinter haemorrhages under the finger nails. Osler's nodes are small, tender vasculitic lesions in the skin.

Endocarditis, if not punctuated by some dramatic episode, can progress unsuspected for months and the mortality of approximately 30 per cent overall has not changed significantly since the introduction of penicillin. This results from the different risk factors that now operate. Thus, the increased age of the patients, the virulence of some infecting organisms and the presence of prosthetic heart valves or underlying disease all reduce the chances of survival. By contrast, the mortality from infective endocarditis caused by viridans streptococci (i.e. of oral origin) has fallen to between 5 and 15 per cent.

• Diagnosis and management of infective endocarditis

If a patient with known heart disease develops a febrile illness, especially with changing heart murmurs, after a surgical procedure, then there is little doubt as to the diagnosis. Echocardiography may be helpful in the diagnosis. Whether or not the diagnosis is obvious, blood culture is essential and must be carried out before antimicrobial treatment is started. At least three 20 ml samples of blood should be taken aseptically, at half-hourly intervals to increase the chances of obtaining a positive culture. The bacteriological findings determine the choice of antibiotics, but if viridans streptococci are the cause, then the usual treatment is with penicillin and gentamicin by injection for 2 weeks or more.

Early treatment is needed to minimize cardiac damage. In severe cases, such as prosthetic valve or candidal endocarditis, early removal of the infected valves and insertion of a sterile replacement can be highly effective.

The main cause of death is heart failure or, less frequently, uncontrollable infection. Cerebral or coronary embolism is relatively rare. The prognosis is poor in the elderly, the immunosuppressed, chronic alcoholics, in fungal or unusually virulent bacterial infections, or if the diagnosis is delayed. Further,

some 5 per cent of those who develop infective endocarditis have a further episode with increased heart damage or death.

• Dental disease and treatment as a cause of infective endocarditis

From the purely dental standpoint, it is obligatory to try to prevent the onset of infective endocarditis in view of the high morbidity and mortality. Although cardiologists sometimes state dogmatically that dental operations are the most common cause of infective endocarditis, this only illustrates outdated ideas. Indeed, cardiologists may be so vague about the dental history as to ascribe the disease to 'poor dental repair', 'gingivitis' or 'dental problems'. By contrast, large surveys have shown that dental treatment precedes only 5–10 per cent of cases. There has also been a steady decline in the frequency of a history of dentally related cases, since before the penicillin era. Moreover, the facts that (a) many of the patients are edentulous, that (b) the majority of patients are elderly and that (c) there is an increasing variety of non-dental causes of bacteraemia, indicate that few healthy ambulant patients acquire infective endocarditis as a result of dental treatment.

Experience in the pre-penicillin era showed that, even in patients with established rheumatic heart disease, infective endocarditis rarely followed dental extractions. Furthermore, it is clear that bacteria are released into the blood from the mouth (and other sites) on innumerable occasions unrelated to operative intervention, but cause no harm. The variables which determine whether micro-organisms will infect the heart are unclear, but the number released into the bloodstream is probably a deciding factor. Infective endocarditis can only be induced in animals under highly artificial conditions and with the use of huge inocula of bacteria.

The widespread but simplistic idea that bacteraemia is virtually synonymous with infective endocarditis is a gross misapprehension. If that were so, it would be necessary to give antibiotic cover even for brushing the teeth.

In simple terms, therefore, bacteria from the teeth and elsewhere can enter the bloodstream on many occasions, but only rarely infect the heart. In statistical terms, the chance of dental extractions causing infective endocarditis, even in a patient with valvular disease, may (it has been suggested) be as low as 1 in 3000. There is only one published study really supporting prophylaxis, that of a series of patients with cardiac valve prostheses, only about half of whom received an antimicrobial prophylaxis before subsequent surgical or dental procedures; there were no cases of endocarditis in those receiving prophylaxis, but a few cases occurred in the group receiving no antimicrobial (Horstkotte *et al.*, 1987). Nevertheless, antibiotic prophylaxis is still essential, where appropriate (*see below*).

- **Prevention of infective endocarditis in dental patients**

This depends in principle on:

1. Identification of patients at risk.
2. Planned preventive dental care.
3. Deciding which treatments require antimicrobial cover.
4. Giving the appropriate antibiotic(s) at the appropriate time.

Identification of patients at risk from infective endocarditis (Table 3.9)
Almost any type of heart lesion is susceptible to infection, but the most important lesions are where there is disturbed blood flow, such as:

- Prosthetic cardiac valves.
- Most congenital cardiac malformations.
- Surgically constructed systemic-pulmonary shunts.
- Rheumatic or other valvular disease.
- Idiopathic hypertrophic sub-aortic stenosis.
- Previous endocarditis.
- Mitral valve prolapse with insufficiency.

Identification of all patients at risk is not possible, but an attempt should be made to elicit a relevant history. Patients should therefore be asked if they have or have had:

- Valve defects, acquired (such as in some intravenous drug abusers) or congenital (mitral valve prolapse is common and usually asymptomatic; cover is required for it only when it gives rise to a murmur).

Table 3.9 Patients at risk from infective endocarditis

High risk
- Prosthetic valves
- Previous infective endocarditis

Variable risk
- Congenital heart disease
- Degenerative (calcific) aortic valve disease
- Hypertrophic cardiomyopathy
- Mitral valve prolapse with systolic murmur
- Rheumatic heart disease
- Surgically constructed systemic-pulmonary shunts
- Syphilitic heart disease
- Systemic lupus erythematosus
- Carcinoid syndrome
- Ankylosing spondylitis
- Marfan's syndrome
- Ehlers–Danlos syndrome
- Osteogenesis imperfecta
- Hurler's syndrome
- Kawasaki's disease

Note: The level of risk of infective endocarditis is very low in some of these diseases, such as isolated atrial secundum septal defects, those that have been repaired more than 6 months previously, and patent ductus arteriosus that has been ligated for more than 6 months.

- Heart surgery (and its nature).
- A heart murmur.
- A previous attack of infective endocarditis.
- Any other heart disease and its nature.

As mentioned earlier, the alternatives are to give antibiotic cover to all patients giving positive answers to any of these questions, or to refer the patient for a cardiologist's assessment of the need for prophylaxis. However, most patients will not need such cover and antibiotic treatment has its own risks.

On the other hand, patients do not always remember the advice to tell their dentist about heart disease. Some carry a warning card (*Plate 5*). There is also a large group who do not know that they have either a congenital defect or acquired valve disease, particularly calcific aortic degeneration. Overall, over 40 per cent of patients who suffer from infective endocarditis have a normal heart or an unsuspected defect.

Even the most careful dental surgeon has therefore to accept the possible embarrassment of a patient developing infective endocarditis in spite of a completely 'safe' history. This has happened in several dental practices in the writers' experience, as a result of totally unsuspected heart lesions. Nevertheless, the chances of this happening in any individual practice are very small.

At the other extreme, patients with Down's syndrome have a high frequency of congenital heart defects such as mitral valve prolapse, immunodeficiencies and also a tendency to gross plaque accumulation and periodontal disease, yet despite these three factors which should favour it, they do not appear to be particularly susceptible to infective endocarditis. Nevertheless, they should of course be given antibiotic cover.

There is a negligible risk of infective endocarditis after dental treatment in some cardiac conditions, and therefore antimicrobial prophylaxis is *not* considered essential:

- After myocardial infarction.
- After coronary artery bypass grafts.
- In isolated secundum atrial septal defects.
- Where a secundum atrial septal defect has been repaired more than 6 months previously.
- Where a patent ductus arteriosus has been repaired more than 6 months previously.
- After more than 6 months in a patient with a heart transplant.
- For implanted cardiac pacemakers or defibrillators.

Planned preventive care

All patients, particularly those with congenital or rheumatic heart disease, who have prosthetic heart valves or who have already had infective endocarditis, need meticulous preventive oral health care. The aim is to keep periodontal infection at its lowest possible level, to obviate the need for extractions or, if extractions are unavoidable, to lessen the severity of the bacteraemia by keeping the gingiva healthy. However, it must be appreciated that scaling also requires antibiotic cover. Unfortunately, this aspect of care is frequently neglected; a very high proportion of patients attending cardiology clinics have periodontal disease (Smith and Adams 1993).

Dental procedures for which prophylaxis should be given

Bacteraemia can follow virtually any dental procedure, even brushing teeth with clinically

---

Table 3.10 Procedures requiring antimicrobial prophylaxis in persons at risk from endocarditis

- Tooth extraction
- Oral surgery involving the periodontal tissues
- Periodontal surgery
- Subgingival procedures including scaling
- Intraligamentary injections
- Reimplantation of avulsed teeth

---

healthy gingivae, but mere bacteraemia should not be confused with infective endocarditis – many bacteraemias are so slight as to present no significant risk. However, there are such vast numbers of bacteria at the gingival margins and in the periodontal pockets that any operation disturbing these bacteria provides a good chance of precipitating infective endocarditis in a susceptible patient. In a survey of nearly 5000 cases of infective endocarditis attributable to dental treatment, it was found to have followed dental extractions in 95 per cent of cases. The current recommendations are therefore that antibiotic prophylaxis is mandatory only for the following types of dental treatment:

- Extractions.
- Scaling and subgingival procedures.
- Oral or periodontal surgery or raising mucogingival flaps for any other purpose.
- Reimplantation of avulsed teeth.
- Incision and drainage of infected tissue (*Table 3.10*), possibly.

Intraligamentary injections may also force large numbers of periodontal bacteria into the bloodstream. Though there appears to be no evidence as yet of these injections leading to infective endocarditis, they should be avoided in patients who are at risk. This is not to say that infective endocarditis *cannot* follow other forms of dental treatment but it does so so rarely as not to present a significant risk. The dentist who falls over backward in trying to give antibiotic protection against every kind of procedure, quickly runs out of antibiotics effective against the resistant bacteria that such measures produce. Any theoretical benefits are outweighed by the risks, as no antibiotic is without side-effects and the more frequently these drugs are used, the greater the risk of toxic effects and the greater the numbers of resistant bacteria that may need to be controlled.

There seems to be persistent anxiety about the need for antibiotic cover for endodontic treatment even though it is hard to find an authenticated case of it having caused endocarditis. It must be appreciated that in comparison with the gingival margins there are few bacteria in periapical lesions and that quite unusual violence is likely to be needed to send them into the bloodstream. If endocarditis follows root canal therapy it is likely therefore to be mere coincidence or incompetence on the part of the operator.

Dental procedures for which antimicrobial prophylaxis is not mandatory
Theoretically, antibiotics might be given for almost any other dental procedure but, since both the necessity and efficacy of prophylaxis is unproven, the stage can be reached when the side-effects from these drugs could outweigh any protection they might give. A study in the USA even suggests that the mortality from penicillin anaphylaxis far exceeds that of infective endocarditis. There is no evidence for the need for antibiotic prophylaxis for exfoliation of primary teeth, local anaesthetic injections (but intraligamentary injections may be a risk), non-surgical orthodontic, or prosthetic or restorative procedures which do not induce bleeding (*Table 3.11*). In these instances the risks from antibiotic prophylaxis are likely to far exceed any benefits.

- **Choice of prophylactic antibiotic regimen against infective endocarditis**

The recommendations are as follows:
1. *Patients not requiring a general anaesthetic and with no history of infective endocarditis:*
   (i) Not allergic to nor have received a penicillin more than once in the past month. Adults – 3 g amoxycillin orally 1 h before the operation, taken in the presence of the dentist or nurse. For children under 10, one-half the adult dose; for children under 5, a quarter of the adult dose.
   Note: Three grams of amoxycillin can be given on not more than two occasions in

Table 3.11   Procedures for which antimicrobial prophylaxis is not recommended in persons at risk for endocarditis

- Exfoliation of primary teeth
- Local anaesthetic injections, other than intraligamentary
- Non-surgical procedures that do not induce bleeding

a month as this dose is sufficient to destroy the relatively resistant streptococci that have emerged.
(ii) Patients allergic to or who have received a penicillin more than once in the previous month. Adults – a *single* oral dose of clindamycin – 600 mg for an adult, can be given one hour before the dental procedure. Children under 10 should have one-half the adult dose (300 mg) and children under 5 should have a quarter of the adult dose (150 mg). Clindamycin is now preferred to erythromycin as it is less likely to cause nausea and is better absorbed, as well as being marginally more effective in preventing post-extraction streptococcal bacteraemia. In a single dose it is not known to cause pseudomembranous colitis. If clindamycin is used, multistage procedures requiring antimicrobial prophylaxis should not be repeated at intervals of less than 2 weeks. Alternatively, 1.5 g erythromycin stearate can be given orally under supervision 1–2 h before the dental procedure, followed by a second dose of 0.5 g 6 h later. For children under 10, one-half the adult dose; for children under 5, a quarter of the adult dose.
   Patients who have had endocarditis should be managed as in (2) below.
2. *Treatment under general anaesthesia – patients with natural valve disease and no history of infective endocarditis, but not allergic to nor have had a penicillin more than once within the past month:* Amoxycillin 1 g intramuscularly or intravenously in 2.5 ml of 1 per cent lignocaine before induction plus 0.5 g of amoxycillin orally 6 h later. Alternatively, 3 g of amoxycillin may be given by mouth 4 hours before

induction and repeated as soon as possible after induction, if the anaesthetist agrees.

3. *Treatment under general anaesthesia – patients with prosthetic valves or previous endocarditis, not allergic to nor have had a penicillin more than once within the past month*: Amoxycillin 1 g intramuscularly in 2.5 ml of 1 per cent lignocaine or amoxycillin 1 g intravenously, plus gentamicin 120 mg intramuscularly or intravenously immediately before induction. A further 0.5 g of amoxycillin should be given orally 6 h later.

   If allergic to or have had a penicillin more than once in the past month: Vancomycin 1 g by intravenous infusion over 100 min followed by 120 mg of gentamicin intravenously before induction. Vancomycin, if given too rapidly, can cause facial or widespread erythema (red man syndrome) among other toxic effects. Alternatively, intravenous teicoplanin 400 mg plus gentamicin 120 mg may be given at induction, or intravenous clindamycin 300 mg may be given 10 minutes before induction followed by oral clindamycin 150 mg after 6 hours.

4. *Patients who have had a previous attack of infective endocarditis (irrespective of the type of anaesthetic) but are not allergic to the penicillins and have not had a penicillin more than once in the previous month*: Amoxycillin 1 g intramuscularly in 2.5 ml of 1 per cent lignocaine or amoxycillin 1 g intravenously plus gentamicin 120 mg intramuscularly or intravenously immediately before dental procedure. A further 0.5 g of amoxycillin should be given orally 6 h later.

   If allergic to or have had penicillin more than once in the past month: Vancomycin 1 g by intravenous infusion over 100 min followed by 120 mg of gentamicin intravenously, or the vancomycin may be replaced with teicoplanin 400 mg.

The reason different cover is given for those who are going to have a general anaesthetic is that (i) parenteral administration removes the risk of vomiting, (ii) it is not feasible to give such large doses (3 g) of amoxycillin (for example) by injection, hence it has to be supplemented with gentamicin.

- **Additional measures**

1. Application of an antiseptic such as 10 per cent povidone-iodine, 0.5 per cent chlorhexidine or tincture of iodine to the gingival crevice before the dental procedure may reduce the severity of any resulting bacteraemia and may usefully supplement antibiotic prophylaxis in those at risk. Chlorhexidine mouth rinses appear not to be helpful in this respect.
2. Good dental health should reduce the frequency and severity of any bacteraemias and also reduce the need for extractions.
3. It is **essential** that, even when antibiotic cover has been given, patients at risk should be instructed to report any unexplained illness. Infective endocarditis is often exceedingly insidious in origin and can develop 2 or more months after the operation which might have precipitated it. Late diagnosis considerably increases both the mortality or disability among survivors.
4. Patients at risk should carry a warning card to be shown to their dentist at each visit to indicate the danger of infective endocarditis and the need for antibiotic prophylaxis.

In summary therefore, it must be accepted that, although neither the need nor the efficacy of antibiotic prophylaxis can be established in any given case, antibiotics must be given before extractions, scaling and surgery involving the periodontal tissues to patients with a recognized predisposing cardiac disorder (*Tables 3.9, 3.10*). *In addition, it is essential to warn patients (whether or not antimicrobial prophylaxis has been given) to report back if even a minor febrile illness develops after dental treatment.*

It must be remembered that patients at risk from infective endocarditis may also have a heart lesion that makes them a poor risk for general anaesthesia and a few are on anticoagulant treatment or on other drugs.

VASCULAR SURGERY

Bypass grafts to the aorta and lower limb vasculature are often made of polytetrafluoroethylene, or of Dacron, and these remain non-endothelialized and liable to infection, typically with *Staphylococcus epidermidis*. Although there is no evidence for odontogenic infection of such grafts, the patients' periodontal health is not always good, and some have suggested the need for antimicrobial prophylaxis for dental procedures (Stansby *et al.* 1994) but there is no good evidence to support this. Magnetic resonance imaging is contraindicated where ferromagnetic vascular clips have been placed.

HEART SURGERY

Heart surgery is now frequently carried out for congenital cardiovascular disease, or some valve lesions. Correction of some congenital defects is only palliative but in many, such as patent ductus arteriosus, the results are excellent.

Heart valve defects may be corrected by valvotomy, grafts or prosthetic valves. The latter are particularly susceptible to infective endocarditis and there is then a high mortality. However, such infection is not usually of dental origin and replacement of the diseased valve while the infection is still active, together with vigorous antimicrobial treatment, frequently eradicates the disease.

- **Dental management of heart surgery patients**

Dental sepsis may be a threat to patients having cardiac surgery, as infective endocarditis can nullify any benefits from the operation and sometimes costs the patient's life. There may therefore be justification for preoperative clearance if the dental state is poor. However, the prospect of cardiac surgery is a great emotional stress and a source of severe anxiety to many patients. The idea of dental clearance at this time may therefore be too much for them to bear. It is desirable, however, if the opportunity is available, to reduce dental sepsis to the minimum before operation.

Candidal endocarditis is another threat and, though there is no evidence that these micro-organisms come from the patient's own mouth, it is an obvious precaution to eliminate any oral candidal infection before operation.

Management of patients after cardiac surgery may include attention to the following aspects:

1. Residual cardiovascular disease.
2. Regular dental care.
3. Infective endocarditis.
4. Anticoagulation (Chapter 4).
5. Immunosuppression (heart transplant patients) (Chapter 20).
6. Psychiatric or psychological disturbances.

CARDIAC TRANSPLANTATION

Heart transplantation is increasingly used to treat patients with otherwise uncontrollable cardiac disease, especially severe IHD and idiopathic cardiomyopathy. Although postoperative mortality and morbidity are falling, the one-year survival is variable (20–80 per cent). Heart–lung transplants are also increasingly used. After heart transplantation, patients are immunosuppressed, usually with cyclosporin or azathioprine, corticosteroids and antithymocyte globulin, or tacrolimus (*see* Chapter 20 for complications), and may be anticoagulated or taking aspirin and dipyridamole to reduce platelet adhesion and prolong the bleeding time. To minimize the development of atherosclerosis in the transplanted heart, patients are often placed on a low cholesterol diet and given simvastatin.

- **Dental aspects of cardiac transplants**

A meticulous pre-transplant oral assessment is required and dental treatment undertaken with particular attention to establishing optimal oral hygiene and eradicating sources of potential infection. Dental treatment should be completed before transplantation since there may be complications afterwards, related to:

1. Bleeding tendencies (Chapter 4).
2. Corticosteroid treatment (Chapter 14).
3. Immunosuppression (Chapter 20).
4. A risk of infective endocarditis in some cases during the first 6-month postoperative period.
5. There may rarely be viral hepatitis or HIV infection (Chapters 10 and 20).
6. Drug interactions.

Post-transplant patients may develop oral complications such as cyclosporin-induced gingival hyperplasia, or candidosis, herpetic or other infections or rarely hairy leukoplakia because of the immunosuppression (Chapter 20). Any invasive treatment should be carried out with considerable care in view of the bleeding tendency and immunosuppression; antimicrobial prophylaxis may be indicated.

Erythromycin, ketoconazole, itraconazole and possibly fluconazole may cause a rise in plasma cyclosporin levels. There may also be increased risk from nephrotoxicity with co-trimoxazole, aminoglycosides and quinolones.

Patients are also at risk from the oral complications of immunosuppression, notably viral and fungal infections, Kaposi's sarcoma and lymphomas, lip carcinoma and drug effects such as gingival hyperplasia (Chapter 20).

BIBLIOGRAPHY

Abraham-Inpijn L., Borgmeijer-Hoelen A. and Gortzak, R.A. (1988) Changes in blood pressure, heart rate and electrocardiogram during dental treatment with use of local anesthesia. *J. Am. Dent. Assoc.* **116**, 531–6.

Aitken C., Cannell H., Sefton A.M. *et al.* (1995) Comparative efficacy of oral doses of clindamycin and erythromycin in the prevention of bacteraemia. *Br. Dent. J.* **178**, 418–22.

Barnett M.L., Friedman D. and Kastner T. (1988) The prevalence of mitral valve prolapse in patients with Down's syndrome: implications for dental management. *Oral Surg. Oral Med. Oral Pathol.* **66**, 445–7.

Beck J., Garcia R., Heiss G., Vokonas P.S. and Offenbacher S. (1996) Periodontal disease and cardio-vascular disease. *J. Periodontol.* **67**, 1123–37.

Blinder D., Shemesh J. and Taicher S. (1996) Electrocardiographic changes in cardiac patients undergoing dental extractions under local anesthesia. *J. Oral. Maxillofac. Surg.* **54**, 162–5.

Bodenheimer M.M. (1996) Noncardiac surgery in the cardiac patient; what is the question? *Ann. Intern. Med.* **124**, 763–6.

Borea G., Montebugnoli L., Capuzzi P. and Vaccaro M.A. (1993) Circulatory dynamics during dental operations in patients with heart transplants. *Quintessence Int.* **24**, 749–51.

Brand H.S. and Abraham-Inpijn L. (1996) Cardiovascular responses induced by dental treatment. *Eur. J. Oral. Sci.* **104**, 245–52.

Campbell J.H., Huizinga P.J., Das S.K. *et al.* (1996) Incidence and significance of cardiac arrhythmia in geriatric oral surgery patients. *Oral Surg. Oral Med. Oral Pathol.* **82**, 42–6.

Cassidy J.P., Phero J.C. and Grau W.H. (1986) Epinephrine; systemic effects and varying concentrations in local anaesthetics. *Anesth. Prog.* Nov., pp. 289–97.

Cawson R.A. (1981) Infective endocarditis as a complication of dental treatment. *Br. Dent. J.* **151**, 409–14.

Cawson R.A. (1991) *Essentials of Dental Surgery and Pathology*, 5th edn. Edinburgh, Churchill Livingstone.

Cawson R.A. (1992) Antibiotic prophylaxis for dental treatment. *Br. Med. J.* **304**, 933–4.

Cawson R.A., Spector R.G. and Skelly A.M. (1995) *Basic Pharmacology and Clinical Drug Use in Dentistry*, 6th edn. Edinburgh, Churchill Livingstone.

Committee on Research, Science and Therapy, American Academy of Periodontology (1996) Periodontal management of patients with cardiovascular disease. *J. Periodontol.* **67**, 627–35.

Dajani A.S., Bisno, A.L., Chung, K.J. *et al.* (1990) Prevention of bacterial endocarditis. Recommendations by the American Heart Association. *J. Am. Med. Assoc.* **264**, 2919–22.

DeStefano F., Anda R.F., Kahn H.S. *et al.* (1993) Dental disease and risk of coronary heart disease and mortality. *Br. Med. J.* **306**, 688–91.

Duffin P.R., McGimpsey J.G., Pallister M.L. *et al.* (1992) Dental care of patients susceptible to infective endocarditis. *Br. Dent. J.* **173**, 169–72.

Durack D.T. (1995) Drug therapy; prevention of infective endocarditis. *N. Engl. J. Med.* **332**, 38–44.

Ehrmann E.H. (1986) Infective endocarditis and the dentist. *Aust. Dent. J.* **31**, 351–60.

Fairley J.W., Hunt B.J., Glover G.W. *et al.* (1990) Unusual lymphoproliferative oropharyngeal lesions in heart and heart–lung transplant recipients. *J. Laryngol. Otol.* **104**, 720–4.

Field E.A. and Martin M.V. (1990) Need for antibiotic prophylaxis for dental patients with a penile prosthesis. *Br. Dent. J.* **164**, 75.

Findler M., Galili D., Meidan Z. *et al.* (1993) Dental treatment in very high risk patients with active ischemic heart disease. *Oral Surg. Oral Med. Oral Pathol.* **76**, 298–300.

Friedlander A.H. and Gorelick D.A. (1987) Panic disorder: its association with mitral valve prolapse and appropriate dental management. *Oral Surg. Oral Med. Oral Pathol.* **63**, 309–12.

Furukawa F. (1995) Kawasaki disease. *Eur. J. Dermatol.* **5**, 549–57.

Glick M. (1995) Intravenous drug users: a consideration for infective endocarditis in dentistry? *Oral Surg. Oral Med. Oral Pathol.* **80**, 125.

Glueck C.J., McMahon R.E., Bouquot J., Stroop D., Tracy T., Wang P. and Rabinovich B. (1996) Thrombophilia, hypofibrinolysis, and alveolar osteonecrosis of the jaws. *Oral Surg. Oral Med. Oral Pathol.* **81**, 557–66.

Goode G.K. (1995) Hyperlipidaemia, hypertension, and coronary heart disease. *Lancet* **345**, 362–4.

Grace C.J., Levitz R.E., Katz-Pollak H. *et al.* (1988) *Actinobacillus actinomycetemcomitans* prosthetic valve endocarditis. *Rev. Infect. Dis.* **10**, 922–9.

Griffiths M.J. (1995) Artificial cardiac pacemakers. In Porter S.R. and Scully C. (eds), *Oral Health Care for Those with HIV Disease and Other Special Needs.* Northwood, Science Reviews, pp. 127–8.

Griffiths M.J. (1995) Heart and heart/lung transplantation. In Porter S.R. and Scully C. (eds), *Oral Health Care for Those with HIV Disease and Other Special Needs.* Northwood, Science Reviews, pp. 129–33.

Herman W.W. and Konzelman J.L. (1996) Angina: an update for dentistry. *J. Am. Dent. Assoc.* **127**, 98–104.

Hogevik H., Olaison L., Andersson R., Lindberg J. and Alestig K. (1995) Epidemiologic aspects of infective endocarditis in an urban population. *Medicine* **74**, 324–39.

Horstkotte D., Rosin H., Friedrichs W. *et al.* (1987) Contribution for choosing the optimal prophylaxis of bacterial endocarditis. *Eur Heart J.* **8** Suppl, 379–81.

Joshipura K.J., Rimm E.B., Douglass C.W. *et al.* (1996) Poor oral health and coronary heart disease. *J. Dent. Res.* **75**, 1631–6.

Larsson B., Johansson I., Hallmans G. and Ericson T. (1995) Relationship between dental caries and risk factors for atherosclerosis in Swedish adolescents? *Commun. Dent. Oral Epidemiol.* **23**, 205–10.

Lockhart P.B. (1996) An analysis of bacteremias during dental extractions. *Arch. Intern. Med.* **156**, 513–20.

Matsura H., Sugiyama K., Joh S. *et al.* (1989) Intravenous and sublingual nitroglycerin during dental treatment and minor oral surgery. *Anesth. Prog.* **36**, 169–77.

Mattila K.J., Nieminen M.S. and Valtonen V.V. (1989) Association between dental health and acute myocardial infarction. *Br. Med. J.* **298**, 779–81.

McGowan D.(1995) Infective endocarditis. In Porter S.R. and Scully C. (eds), *Oral Health Care for Those with HIV Disease and Other Special Needs.* Northwood, Science Reviews, pp. 117–25.

Michel M.F. (1986) Review of the guidelines of the Dutch Heart Foundation for the prevention of endocarditis. *Ned. Tijdschr. Geneeskd.* **130**, 2211–12.

Newburger J.W. (1996) Treatment of Kawasaki disease. *Lancet* **347**,1128.

Porter S.R. and Scully C. (1996) *Innovations and Developments in Non-invasive Oral Health Care.* Northwood, Science Reviews.

Rahn R., Schneider S., Diehl O. *et al.* (1995) Preventing post-treatment bacteremia. *J. Am. Dent. Assoc.* **126**, 1145–8.

Reichert S., Antuner A., Techot P. *et al.* (1997) Major aphthous stomatitis induced by nicorandil. *Eur. J. Dermatol.* **7**, 132–3.

Roitman K., Sprung J., Wallace M. *et al.* (1993) Enhancement of bupivacaine cardiotoxicity with cardiac glycosides and beta adrenergic blockers. *Anesth. Analg.* **76**, 658.

Sandre R.M. and Shafran S.D. (1996) Infective endocarditis: review of 135 cases over 9 years. *Clin. Infect. Dis.* **22**, 276–86.

Schweizerischen Arbeitsgruppe fur Endokarditis-prophylaxe (1984) Prophylaxe der bakteriellen Endokarditis. *Schweiz. Med. Wochenschr.* **114**, 1146–52.

Scully C. (1988) *The Dental Patient.* Oxford, Heinemann.

Scully C. (1989) *The Mouth and Perioral Tissues.* Oxford, Heinemann.

Scully C. (1989) *Patient Care: a Dental Surgeon's Guide.* London, British Dental Association.

Scully C. and Griffiths M.J. (1993) Antimicrobial prophylaxis and infective endocarditis. *Dent. Pract.* **31**, 3–4.

Scully C., Cawson R.A. and Griffiths M.J. (1990) *Occupational Hazards to Dental Staff.* London, British Dental Journal.

Scully C., Levers B.G.H., Griffiths M.J. *et al.* (1987) Antimicrobial prophylaxis of infective endocarditis: effect of BSAC recommendations on compliance in general practice. *J. Antimicrob. Chemother.* **19**, 521–6.

Smith A.J. and Adams D. (1993) The dental status and attitudes of patients at risk from infective endocarditis. *Br. Dent. J.* **174**, 59–64.

Stansby G., Byrne M. and Hamilton G. (1994) Dental infection in vascular surgical patients. *Br. J. Surg.* **81**, 1119–20.

Uyemura M.C. (1995) Antibiotic prophylaxis for medical and dental procedures. *Postgrad. Med.* **98**, 137–52.

Van der Meer J.T.M., van Wilk W., Thompson J. *et al.* (1992) Awareness of need and actual use of prophylaxis: lack of patient compliance in the prevention of bacterial endocarditis. *J. Antimicrob. Chemother.* **29**, 187–94.

Van Winkelhoff A.J., Overbeek B.P., Pavicic M.J. *et al.* (1993) Long-standing bacteremia caused by oral *Actinobacillus actinomycetemcomitans* in a patient with a pacemaker. *Clin. Infect. Dis.* **16**, 216–8.

Working Party of the British Society for Antimicrobial Chemotherapy (1982) The antibiotic prophylaxis of infective endocarditis. *Lancet* **ii**, 187–94.

Working Party of the British Society for Antimicrobial Chemotherapy (1986) Prophylaxis of endocarditis. *Lancet* **i**, 1267.

Working Party of the British Society for Antimicrobial Chemotherapy (1990) Antibiotic prophylaxis of infective endocarditis. *Lancet* **335**, 88–9.

Working Party of the British Society for Antimicrobial Chemotherapy (1992) Antibiotic prophylaxis of infective endocarditis. *Lancet* **339**, 1292–3.

Wynn R.E. (1993) Erythromycin and ketoconazole (Nizoral) associated with terfenadine (Seldane)-induced ventricular arrhythmias. *General Dentistry* February, pp. 27–9.

APPENDIX TO CHAPTER 3

GENETIC SYNDROMES WITH ASSOCIATED CARDIAC DEFECTS: MAIN FEATURES

Chromosomal disorders
Down's
Edward's
Patau's   Appendix to Chapter 5
Turner's
XXXY   Mental handicap: hypogonadism
XXXXX   Mental handicap: small hands

Hereditary disorders
Ehlers–Danlos'
Marfan's   Chapter 16
Osteogenesis imperfecta
The mucopolysaccharidoses (Hurler's   Appendix to Chapter 15
and related syndromes)
Ellis–van Creveld's   Appendix to Chapter 11
TAR   Thrombocytopenia: *Absent Radius*
Holt–Oram's   Hypoplastic clavicles: upper limb
                   defect

Multiple lentigenes   Basal cell naevi: rib defects
Rubenstein–Taybi's   Broad thumbs and toes: hypoplastic
                       maxilla

4

Disorders of haemostasis

Key points

- Disorders of haemostasis cause management problems mainly because of prolonged postoperative bleeding, but hypercoagulability and thromboses can be as, or more, life-threatening.
- About 90 per cent of post-extraction haemorrhage is from local causes:
    Excessive trauma (to soft tissue in particular).
    Inflamed mucosa at the extraction site.
    Poor compliance with postoperative instructions.
    Post-extraction interference with the socket, e.g. sucking and tongue pushing.
    Reactive hyperaemia.
- Consult the haematologist before undertaking investigations; bleeding and clotting times are unsatisfactory. Special assays, such as Factor VIII clotting activity, may well be required.
- Things to avoid in patients with bleeding tendencies:
    Trauma and surgery. Endodontics may be preferable to surgery.
    Regional local anaesthetic injections (may bleed into fascial spaces of neck and obstruct airway).
    Intramuscular injections.
    Drugs causing increased bleeding tendency (e.g. aspirin).
    Drugs causing gastric bleeding (e.g. aspirin and NSAIDs).
- Prothrombin times are reported as international normalized ratio (INR). The INR is the ratio of the patient's one-stage prothrombin time to that of controls. A normal healthy patient has an INR of 1.
- The relatively atraumatic removal of one or two teeth in patients on anticoagulants can be carried out using local measures to control bleeding, unless the INR is greater than about 3.5.
- Thrombocytopenia is significant if platelets are below 80–100 $\times 10^9$/l. Appropriate measures to raise the platelet count (platelet infusions) are required before surgery.
- Before surgery in patients with clotting defects, the bleeding tendency is corrected by giving an appropriate blood product rich in the deficient factor.
- Factor VIII or cryoprecipitate is used for haemophilia A and severe von Willebrand's disease, and Factor IX for Christmas disease
- Blood products may be used in lower doses if desmopressin and antifibrinolytic drugs are used.
- The possibility of viral hepatitis and HIV should be considered in persons with bleeding tendencies.

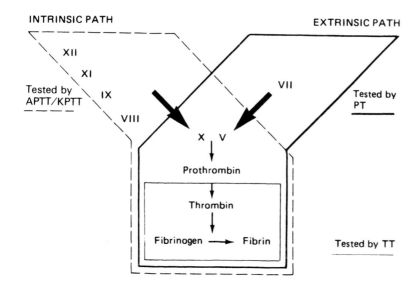

INTRINSIC PATH

EXTRINSIC PATH

Fig. 4.1 Blood clotting (*see* Table 4.3)

BLEEDING TENDENCIES

After injury to a blood vessel, primary haemostasis is by a platelet plug occluding the wound, mediated by interactions between platelets, coagulation factors and the vessel wall. There is also vasoconstriction. The injury also triggers the clotting cascade with the activation of thromboplastin, conversion of prothrombin to thrombin, and the ultimate end-point of the deposition of fibrin (*Fig. 4.1*).

Prolonged bleeding after dental extraction usually has a local cause, but is one of the most common signs of haemorrhagic disease and may amount to a haemorrhagic emergency. It is sometimes the way by which the disease is first recognized. Faced with a bleeding patient it is important to establish (1) if the situation is urgent and (2) if there could be a bleeding tendency.

1. *The situation is urgent if the patient is:*
   losing large quantities of blood;
   hypotensive (hypovolaemic); or
   bleeding internally.

   Under these circumstances an intravenous line must be established and plasma expanders or blood given. Blood transfusions are refused by Jehovah's Witnesses (*Plate 6*) and carry the risk of blood-borne viral infections (Chapters 10 and 20) and circulatory overload.

To stop bleeding, press firmly with a gauze pad over the socket for 10–15 minutes and consider suturing the socket under local anaesthesia

Significant histories suggesting a bleeding tendency include:

- a previous diagnosis of a bleeding tendency;
- bleeding for more than 36 hours or bleeding restarting more than 36 hours after operation;
- admission to hospital to arrest bleeding;
- blood transfusion for bleeding;
- spontaneous bleeding, e.g. haemarthrosis, deep bruising, or menorrhagia from little obvious cause;
- convincing family history of one of the above, combined with a degree of personal history;
- treatment with significant drugs (anticoagulants or, occasionally, aspirin).

Systemic causes include:

- acquired deficiencies of haemostasis, e.g. aspirin, anticoagulants, thrombocytopenia;
- hereditary deficiencies of clotting factors, e.g. von Willebrand's syndrome and haemophilia.

2. *There could be a bleeding tendency if:*
- the bleeding is unexplained by the degree of trauma;
- there is a previous, or family history of excessive bleeding.

Table 4.1   Platelet deficiency

Thrombocytopenia
Failed platelet production
Congenital disorders:
   Thrombocytopenia and absent radii (TAR),
   Wiskott–Aldrich syndrome, Bernard–Soulier
   syndrome, trisomy 13 or 18, thrombocytopenia with
   Robin syndrome, giant haemangiomas
   (Kasabach–Merritt syndrome), type IIb von
   Willebrand disease
Megakaryocyte depression:
   Drugs, viruses, chemicals
General marrow failure:
   Ethanol, cytotoxic drugs, irradiation, chemicals,
   drugs, viruses, aplastic anaemia, leukaemia,
   metastases, megaloblastic anaemia
Increased platelet destruction
Idiopathic thrombocytopenic purpura (ITP)
(autoimmune)
HIV-associated thrombocytopenic purpura
DIC, thrombotic thrombocytopenic purpura
SLE, chronic lymphocytic leukaemia, malaria
Drugs such as aspirin, cytotoxics, β-lactam antibiotics
and valproate
Abnormal platelet distribution
Splenomegaly
Dilutional loss (transfusion of stored blood)

Table 4.2   Coagulation defects

- Haemophilia
- Anticoagulants and thrombolytic agents
- Liver disease, including obstructive jaundice
- Von Willebrand's disease
- Others
     Chronic renal failure
     Dysproteinaemias, especially multiple myeloma
     Lupus erythematosus
     Bernard–Soulier syndrome
     Deficiencies of Factors XII and XIII and others
     Disseminated intravascular coagulation

Haemorrhagic disease can be caused by disorders of blood platelets, or of the clotting (coagulation) mechanism. The latter is most commonly caused by anticoagulant drugs sometimes by disorders such as von Willebrand's disease or by haemophilia (*Tables 4.1, 4.2*). Aspirin is one of the more common acquired causes of bleeding after a tooth extraction; one aspirin tablet impairs platelet function for almost one week. Warfarin is the most common anticoagulant

in use; von Willebrand's disease is the most common inherited bleeding disorder.

Platelet, or rarely, vascular defects give rise to purpura characterized by superficial (capillary) bleeding with the formation of petechiae or widespread ecchymoses into the skin or mucous membranes, and spontaneous gingival bleeding.

The coagulation disorders characteristically cause severe bleeding deep in the tissues and extensive haematoma formation after superficial injury, while bleeding after surgery or trauma can be so prolonged and severe as to be potentially lethal, if untreated.

INVESTIGATION OF THE PATIENT WITH HAEMORRHAGIC DISEASE

Haemorrhage is alarming to the patient and may be an emergency. An adequate history *is the single most important part of the evaluation*; physical examination is also necessary and laboratory tests are needed to confirm the diagnosis. The haematologist should be consulted about the most appropriate tests required. An accurate diagnosis is essential in order to provide replacement therapy where appropriate, and to enable other management procedures to be organized.

The history

Any suggestion of a haemorrhagic tendency *must* be taken seriously. Nevertheless, patients can be remarkably capricious as to the information they provide and, in any case, can hardly be expected to know when bleeding can legitimately be regarded as 'abnormal'. Previous dental extractions provide a useful guide, but prolonged bleeding (up to 24–48 hours) as an isolated episode is usually the result of local factors, especially excessive trauma, *which is the most common cause of excessive bleeding*. By contrast, even patients who know that they have a serious haemorrhagic tendency can keep the fact to themselves unless specifically asked. Special emphasis must therefore be placed on the following:

Features of previous episodes: Deep haemorrhage into muscles, joints or skin suggests a clotting defect. Bleeding from and into mucosae and skin ('bruising') suggests purpura (*Fig. 4.2*). Women with no bleeding

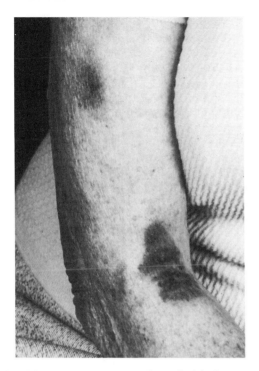

Fig. 4.2 Purpura in a patient with myeloid leukaemia

Relevant medical history: Many drugs such as anticoagulants, or corticosteroids, may cause bleeding tendencies, as may hepatic, renal, HIV and other disease. Patients may be aware of having haemorrhagic disease and carry an appropriate medical card. Patients who have received contaminated blood or blood products may be in high-risk groups for hepatitis B, D, C or G viruses, or HIV and other infections (Chapters 10 and 20).

Examination

Signs of purpura in the skin or mouth such as spontaneous gingival bleeding, petechiae or ecchymoses are seen mainly in platelet disorders (*Plate 7*).They include leukaemia and HIV disease. Alternatively, it may be localized to the mouth (sometimes grandiloquently termed 'angina bullosa haemorrhagica') and not associated with any abnormal bleeding tendencies. Joint deformities from haemarthroses, characteristic of haemophilia, should also be looked for but are infrequently seen now. Signs of underlying disease such as anaemia and lymphadenopathy in leukaemia, for example, must also be looked for.

Laboratory tests

It is important to consult the haematologist to ensure that appropriate blood samples are taken, but it is not necessary to specify individual tests on the request form. All that is needed is to say: 'History of prolonged bleeding. Would you please investigate haemostatic function?' and to give as much clinical detail as possible. A routine 'blood count' will not identify a clotting defect but may show platelet deficiency. The sample should be adequately labelled and sent immediately for testing together with relevant clinical information.

Essential tests include:

1. Full blood count, film, platelet count (EDTA sample).
2. Prothrombin time (PT), activated partial thromboplastin time (APTT) and thrombin time (TT) (citrated sample) (*see Tables 4.3, 4.4, Fig. 4.3*), but normal results do *not* rule out all mild bleeding disorders.
3. The bleeding time.
4. Serum for blood grouping and cross-matching (clotted sample).

disorder often state that they 'bruise easily', but any such bruises are usually insignificant and small. Excessive menstrual bleeding is rarely due to a bleeding disorder.

Past history: Most congenital bleeding disorders become apparent in childhood but mild haemophiliacs can escape recognition until adult life if they manage to avoid injury or surgery.

Surgery: Patients who have had tonsillectomy or dental extractions without trouble are most unlikely to have severe congenital bleeding disorders. By contrast, a mild haemophiliac can have oozing from an extraction socket for 2–3 weeks in spite of any local measures such as suturing.

Previous treatment: It is important to know how previous dental bleeding was controlled. If it responded to local measures then the patient is unlikely to have a serious haemorrhagic disease. On the other hand, admission to hospital and blood transfusion or comparable measures have obvious implications.

Family history: Haemorrhagic disease in a blood relative is strongly suggestive of a clotting defect.

Table 4.3 Laboratory findings in clotting disorders

Disorder	PT	APTT	TT	FL	FDP
Haemophilia A Haemophilia B von Willebrand's disease Deficiency of factors XI, XII	N	↑	N	N	N
Coumarin (warfarin) therapy Obstructive jaundice, or other causes of vitamin K deficiency Deficiency of factor V or X	↑	↑	N	N	N
Heparin therapy Disseminated intra-vascular coagulation	↑	↑	N	N	N
Parenchymal liver disease	↑	↑	↑	↓	↑
Deficiency of factor VII	↑	N	N	N	N

PT, Prothrombin time; APTT, activated partial thromboplastin time (or KPTT); TT, thrombin time; FL fibrinogen level; FDP, fibrin-degradation products.
Arrows indicate a value above ↑ or below ↓ normal (N).
Adapted from Nossel H. L. (1980) In Isselbacher K.J. et al. (ed.) *Harrison's Principles of Internal Medicine*. Tokyo, McGraw-Hill Kogakusha

Platelet defects: Platelet count and full blood examination are essential, and assays of platelet function may be indicated. Aspirin should be avoided for at least 7 days before assessing platelet function since even a single tablet can damage platelet function for up to a week.

In the Hess test (tourniquet test) more than a few petechiae appearing on the forearm when a sphygmomanometer cuff is inflated suggests a platelet or vascular defect but the test is not particularly sensitive and is not specific.

A valuable test of platelet function is the bleeding time but normal values range from 2 to 9 minutes so that it is not completely reliable. *In vitro* tests of platelet adhesion and aggregation may be required to demonstrate abnormal function. Platelet aggregation can also be measured using aggregating agents such as ristocetin. Unfortunately such tests are difficult to standardize and do not identify all platelet disorders; the clinical features are more important.

Table 4.5 shows comparative features of coagulation defects and platelet defects. It should be stressed again that a history of previous haemorrhagic episodes is the most important feature since screening tests of haemostasis do not always detect mild defects.

Coagulation defects: Precise characterization of a congenital clotting defect depends on assay of the individual factors and a wide range of other investigations may be indicated according to the type of case. For example, the assays usually used in diagnosis of haemophilia A are the APTT and the Factor VIII coagulant (FVIIIC) activity. The whole blood clotting time is uninformative and obsolete.

It is particularly important also to investigate patients for anaemia because: (a) anaemia is an expected consequence of repeated haemorrhages; (b) any further bleeding as a result of dental surgery will worsen the anaemia, or the anaemia may need to be treated before surgery can be carried out; and (c) anaemia may be an essential concomitant of the haemorrhagic tendency – as in acute leukaemia.

Table 4.4 Typical findings in platelet disorders

Disorder	Bleeding time	Platelets count	Clot retraction	Platelet aggregation	Platelet FIII activity
Thrombocytopenia	↑	↓	↓	—	—
Thrombasthenia	↑	N	↓	↓	↓
Storage pool deficiency	↑	N	N	N or ↓	↓
Aspirin: von Willebrand's disease	↑	N	N	↓ (only with ristocetin)	N
Thrombocythaemia	↑	↑	N or ↓	N or ↓	N or ↓

Arrows indicate a value above ↑ or below ↓ normal (N). FIII, Factor III.
Adapted from Nossel H. L. (1980) In Isselbacher K. J. et al. (ed) *Harrison's Principles of Internal Medicine*. Tokyo, McGraw-Hill Kogakusha

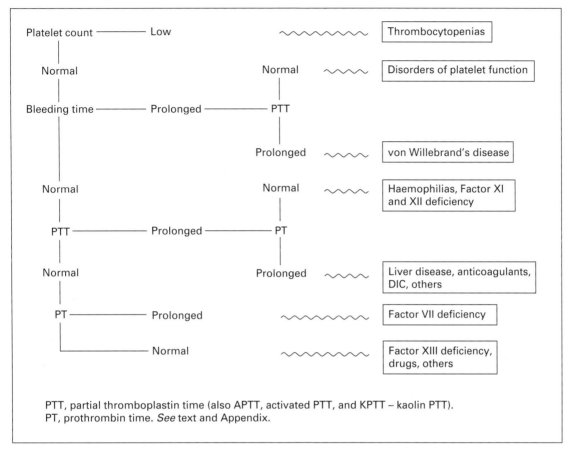

Fig. 4.3 Protocol for investigation of a bleeding disorder

Table 4.5 Features of bleeding disorders

Platelet defects	The purpuras*	Coagulation defects
Gender affected	Females more than males[†]	Males
Family history	Rarely	Positive
Nature of bleeding	Immediately after trauma	Delayed after trauma
	Relatively short-lived	Persistent
Effect of locally applied pressure	May cause bleeding to cease	Bleeding recurs when pressure removed
Spontaneous bleeding into skin or mucosa or from mucosa	Common	Uncommon
Bleeding from minor superficial injuries, e.g. needle prick	Common	Uncommon
Deep haemorrhages or haemarthroses	Rare	Common
Bleeding time	Prolonged	Normal
Tourniquet (Hess) test	Positive	Negative
Platelet count	Often reduced	Normal
Clotting function	Normal[‡]	Abnormal

*Purpura rarely vascular.
[†]Except in HIV disease and AIDS.
[‡]May be a prolonged prothrombin consumption test.

Patients may also need to be screened for infections, particularly HIV and hepatitis viruses, and for liver disease.

PLATELET DISORDERS

Platelet function may be impaired by many diseases or drugs (*Table 4.6*) but deficiencies of platelets (thrombocytopenias) are probably the most clinically important causes of purpura.

Thrombocytopenias

Thrombocytopenia exists when the platelet count falls below $100 \times 10^9/l$ and causes petechiae, ecchymoses and postoperative haemorrhage (*Table 4.7*). There are many causes of thrombocytopenia but idiopathic thrombocytopenic purpura (ITP), probably an autoimmune disorder, is one of the more common (*Table 4.1*). Corticosteroids, other immunosuppressive agents or sometimes splenectomy are needed to control it, and about 20 per cent of cases are resistant to treatment.

• Dental management in the thrombocytopenias

The main danger in dental treatment is haemorrhage. In patients with ITP, the bleeding tendency is sometimes effectively controlled by corticosteroids and should not therefore be a problem. However, if platelet levels are low, infusions may be indicated though these are not without risk – particularly from allergic reactions.

Local analgesia
Regional anaesthetic block injections are contraindicated if the platelet levels are below $30 \times 10^9/l$.

Minor surgery
Haemostasis after minor surgery is usually adequate if platelet levels are above $50 \times 10^9/l$. Platelets can be replaced or supplemented by platelet transfusions, but sequestration of platelets is very rapid. Platelet transfusions are therefore best used for controlling already established thrombo-

Table 4.6 Some drugs that may impair platelets or their function

* Non-steroidal anti-inflammatory drugs
  Aspirin
  Diclofenac
  Diflunisal
  Ibuprofen
  Mefenamic acid
* Beta-lactam antibiotics
  Ampicillin and derivatives
  Methicillin
  Penicillin G (benzyl penicillin)
  Cephalosporins (some)
  Gentamicin
  Rifampicin
  Sulphonamides
  Trimethoprim
* General anaesthetic agents
  Halothane
* Cytotoxic agents
  Asparaginase
  Carmustine
  Daunorubicin
  Vincristine
* Psychoactive agents
  Antihistamines (some)
  Diazepam
  Tricyclic antidepressants
  Chlorpromazine
  Haloperidol
  Valproate
* Diuretics
  Acetazolamide
  Chlorothiazide
  Frusemide
* Antidiabetics
  Chlorpropamide
  Tolbutamide
* Cardiovascular drugs
  Digitoxin
  Quinine
  Oxprenolol
  Heparin
  Methyldopa

Adapted from George and Shattil (1991).

cytopenic bleeding. When given prophylactically, platelets should be given half before surgery to control capillary bleeding and half at the end of the operation to facilitate the placement of adequate sutures. Platelets should be used within 6–24 hours after collection and suitable preparations include platelet-rich plasma (PRP), which contains about 90 per cent of the platelets from a unit of fresh blood in about half this volume, and platelet-rich concentrate (PRC), which contains about 50 per cent of the platelets from a unit of fresh whole blood in a volume

Table 4.7   Manifestations of thrombocytopenia and management of surgery

Platelet count ($\times 10^9/l$)	Severity of thrombocytopenia	Manifestations	Management in relation to type of oral surgery	
			Minor	Major
100–150	Mild	Mild purpura sometimes Slight increase in postoperative bleeding	No platelet transfusion Observe	Consider platelet transfusion Observe
50–100	Moderate	Purpura, postoperative bleeding	Platelets needed	Platelets needed
25–50	Severe	Purpura, postoperative bleeding, and even from venepuncture	Platelets needed	Platelets needed Avoid surgery where possible
<25	Life-threatening	Purpura, spontaneous bleeding	Platelets needed Avoid surgery where possible	Platelets needed Avoid surgery where possible

of only 25 ml. PRC is thus the best source of platelets. Platelet infusions carry the risk of iso-immunization, infection with blood-borne viruses and, rarely, graft-versus-host disease.

Where there is immune destruction of platelets (e.g. in ITP), platelet infusions are less effective. Long-term, corticosteroids can cause well-recognized problems (Chapter 14). Splenectomy predisposes to infections, typically with pneumococci, and especially within the first 2 years. Occasional reports of systemic infection post-splenectomy, involving oral streptococci, have prompted some to suggest that an antimicrobial prophylaxis should be given before invasive dental procedures (Chapter 20).

The need for platelet transfusions can be reduced by local haemostatic measures and the use of desmopressin or tranexamic acid or topical administration of platelet concentrates. Absorbable haemostatic agents such as oxidized regenerated cellulose (Surgicel), synthetic collagen (Instat) or microcrystalline collagen (Avitene) may be put in the socket to assist clotting.

Drugs that affect platelet function, particularly aspirin, should be avoided, as should other drugs rarely used in dentistry such as gentamicin, antihistamines, tricyclic antidepressants, phenothiazines and frusemide.

Major surgery
For major surgery, platelet levels over $75 \times 10^9/l$ are desirable.

Thrombasthenia (Glanzmann's syndrome)

Defective platelet aggregation is due to a defective membrane protein and causes a severe bleeding tendency. Platelet infusions are needed preoperatively.

Bernard–Soulier syndrome

Giant platelets characterize this heritable disorder, which in very many ways resembles von Willebrand's disease but is considerably more rare. The defect is in a platelet glycoprotein which acts as a receptor for von Willebrand factor.

Storage pool deficiency

Platelets may lack the capacity to store serotonin and adenine nucleotides and consequently fail to aggregate. Usually this is congenital with autosomal inheritance, and may be associated with albinism (Hermansky–Pudlak syndrome). Platelet infusion or cryoprecipitate corrects the bleeding tendency.

Purpura in HIV infection

Purpura is a relatively common feature of HIV infection. It may be autoimmune but there appears also to be a platelet defect resulting from the infection and drugs such as zidovudine or bone marrow disease may also contribute. Oral purpura in HIV infection may closely mimic oral lesions of Kaposi's sarcoma (Chapter 20).

Chronic renal failure (see Chapter 13)

Dysproteinaemias (see Chapter 6)

Myelodysplastic syndrome (see Chapter 6)

Drugs (heparin, dextrans).

Thrombocythaemia

In many conditions a raised platelet count (thrombocytosis) may be found and predisposes to arterial thrombosis. Thrombocythaemia, by contrast, is a myeloproliferative disease and may be an isolated disorder or associated with myelofibrosis, polycythaemia or chronic granulocytic leukaemia. Thrombocythaemia can give rise to both thromboses and bleeding tendencies as the main effects.

- ### Dental management in thrombocythaemia

Patients are sometimes treated with ^{32}P-labelled phosphorus but plateletphoresis, interferon, cytotoxic agents (chlorambucil or busulphan), corticosteroids or aspirin are increasingly used. Anticoagulants are sometimes employed.

The problems of dental management in thrombocythaemia can therefore be summarized as follows:

1. Haemorrhagic tendencies.

2. Thromboses.
3. Complications of cytotoxic agents or corticosteroids (Chapters 7 and 14).

VASCULAR PURPURA

Serious bleeding is caused rarely by vascular disorders. Bleeding into mucous membranes or skin starts immediately after trauma but stops within 24–48 hours.

Hereditary haemorrhagic telangiectasia (Osler–Rendu–Weber syndrome)

Hereditary haemorrhagic telangiectasia (HHT) is an autosomal dominant condition characterized by telangiectasia on the skin or any part of the oral, nasal, gastrointestinal or urogenital mucosa (*Fig. 4.4*). Fragility of the affected vessels leads to bleeding and consequently, sometimes, to iron deficiency anaemia or rarely even to cardiac failure. Cryosurgery is useful to treat oral telangiectases; small lesions may respond to argon laser treatment. Bleeding from oral surgery is unlikely to be troublesome but nasal intubation is clearly best avoided and close postoperative observation is advisable. There may be associated IgA deficiency or, rarely, von Willebrand's disease (*see below*). There have been occasional reports of brain abscesses or other infections following procedures that produce bacteraemias,

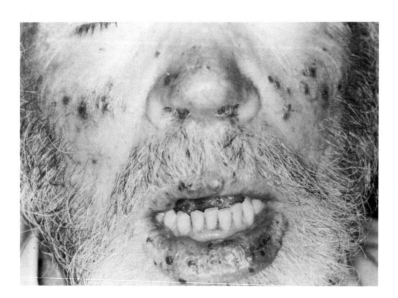

Fig. 4.4 Hereditary haemorrhagic telangiectasia

suggesting that antimicrobial cover may be indicated for dental treatment that might cause bacteraemia (Chapter 3).

Localized oral purpura

Causes of blood blisters in the mouth include:

1. Trauma.
2. Mucous membrane pemphigoid (Chapter 12).
3. Systemic causes such as platelet disorders, amyloidosis (causing Factor X deficiency, Chapter 6), leukaemia, infectious mononucleosis, HIV or rubella.
4. Localized oral purpura (angina bullosa haemorrhagica).

Blood blisters, especially in the soft palate, are occasionally seen in the absence of obvious trauma, generalized purpura, any other bleeding tendency or evidence of amyloidosis or autoimmune disease. However, a systemic cause of the blood blisters must be excluded before the diagnosis of localized oral purpura can be confidently made and the patient reassured.

These blood blisters may sometimes be a centimetre or more in diameter and after rupture may leave a sore area for a time. When a large blood blister of this type is in the pharynx it can cause an alarming choking sensation and was therefore originally termed 'angina bullosa haemorrhagica'. However, almost any site in the mouth can be affected.

CONGENITAL COAGULATION DEFECTS

The most important hereditary bleeding disorders in terms of prevalence and severity are haemophilia A and B (Christmas disease) and von Willebrand's disease. Less common disorders are summarized in the Appendix to this chapter. Many of the defects present a hazard to surgery and to local anaesthetic injections, but in general the teeth erupt and exfoliate without problems, and non-invasive dental care is safe.

Haemophilia A

Haemophilia A is the most common and best-known clotting defect, with a prevalence of about 5 per 100 000 of the population. It is about 10 times as common as haemophilia B except in some Asians, where frequencies are almost equal. Inherited as a sex-linked recessive trait, haemophilia affects males. A family history can, however, be obtained in only about 65 per cent of cases. All daughters of an affected male are carriers but sons are normal. Sons of carriers have a 50:50 chance of developing haemophilia while daughters of carriers have a 50:50 chance of also being carriers.

Haemophilia A is due to defective Factor VIII (antihaemophilia factor, AHF). This is a glycoprotein of several components, including Factor VIIIC (procoagulant that participates in the clotting cascade), VIIIR:Ag (von Willebrand factor, which binds to platelets and is the carrier for Factor VIIIC) and VIIIR:RCo (ristocetin cofactor, which supports platelet aggregation). In haemophilia A only Factor VIIIC is reduced.

Haemophilia typically becomes apparent in childhood when bleeding into muscles or joints (haemarthroses) follows injuries. Abdominal haemorrhage may simulate an acute abdomen. Haemarthroses can cause joint damage and cripple the patient, but bleeding after dental extractions is sometimes the first or only sign of mild disease. Bleeding into the cranium, bladder and other sites can cause severe or fatal complications. Haemorrhage in haemophiliacs is dangerous either because of loss of blood, or because there may be damage to joints, muscles and nerves, or pressure on vital organs if haemorrhage is internal. Thus compression of the larynx and pharynx following haematoma formation in the neck can be fatal. Dental extractions or deep lacerations are followed by persistent oozing for days or weeks and in the past have been fatal. The haemorrhage cannot be controlled by pressure and, although clots may form in the mouth, they fail to stop the bleeding. The characteristic feature of bleeding in haemophilia is that it seems to stop immediately after the injury (as a result of normal vascular and platelet response) but, after an hour or more, intractable oozing or rapid blood loss starts and persists.

The severity of bleeding is dependent on two main factors:

1. *The level of Factor VIIIC activity:* The severity of the disease is variable but corre-

Table 4.8 Severity of haemophilia

	% Factor VIII
Severe	<1
Moderate	1–5
Mild	>5–25
Normal	>25

lates well with the Factor VIII level of the plasma. Normal plasma contains 1 unit of Factor VIII per ml, a level defined as 100 per cent. If the Factor VIII level is above 5 per cent the disease is mild. Moderate haemophiliacs have a Factor VIII activity of less than 5 per cent (FVIIIC level less than 1 IU/dl) and severe haemophiliacs, less than 1 per cent.

In general, if the level of Factor VIII is above 25 per cent (FVIIIC over 5 IU/dl), the patient can lead a relatively normal life and may remain undiagnosed, although there can be prolonged bleeding after trauma or surgery (*Table 4.8*). In mild haemophilia, with Factor VIII levels of between 5 and 25 per cent (FVIIIC 1–5 IU/dl), comparatively minor trauma can lead to persistent bleeding. Between 1 and 5 per cent Factor VIII levels lead to moderate haemophilia and where levels are below 1 per cent bleeding is spontaneous.

2. *The severity of trauma:* Some very mild haemophiliacs may not bleed excessively even after a simple dental extraction, so that the absence of post-extraction haemorrhage cannot always be used to exclude haemophilia. Most will, however, bleed excessively after more traumatic surgery, such as tonsillectomy.

- **Diagnosis and management of haemophilia A**

The typical findings in haemophilia can be summarized as follows:

1. Prolonged activated partial thromboplastin time (APTT).
2. Normal prothrombin time (PT).
3. Normal bleeding time.
4. Low Factor VIIIC but normal VIIIR:Ag (von Willebrand factor) and R:RCo (ristocetin cofactor).

Factor VIII assay is required as even the APTT may be normal in mild haemophilia. If bleeding starts or is expected, treatment consists of replacement of the missing clotting factor, rest and often the use of antifibrinolytic agents.

Rarely, von Willebrand's disease may mimic haemophilia. The history may help to distinguish them (*Table 4.9*) but laboratory testing is essential (*see below*).

Factor VIII must be replaced to a level adequate to ensure haemostasis. Some years ago this was achieved with fresh plasma, or fresh frozen plasma, cryoprecipitate or fractionated human factor concentrates obtained from pooled blood sources, but these had, and may still occasionally have, the potential to carry blood-borne pathogens such as hepatitis viruses, HIV and various herpesviruses. Porcine Factor VIII and genet-

Table 4.9 Haemophilia A and von Willebrand's disease

	Haemophilia A	*von Willebrand's disease*
Inheritance	Sex-linked recessive	Dominant
Haemarthroses/deep haematomas	Common	Rare
Epistaxes	Uncommon	Common
Gastrointestinal bleeding	Uncommon	Common
Haematuria	Common	Uncommon
Menorrhagia	None (males)	Common
Post-extraction bleeding	Starts 1–24 hours after trauma, lasts 3–40 days	Starts immediately
	Not controlled by pressure	Lasts 24–48 hours and is often controlled by pressure
Bleeding time	Normal	Prolonged
Factor VIII coagulant activity	Reduced	Reduced
Factor VIIIR: RCo	Normal	Reduced

Note: von Willebrand's disease is occasionally identical to haemophilia.

ically engineered Factor VIII have been considerable advances. Regular prophylactic replacement of Factor VIII (antihaemophiliac globulin, AHF) is used when possible but necessitates daily injections. AHF is also in short supply and expensive, and its use may be complicated by antibody formation or viral infections (Chapters 2, 10 and 20), but heat treatment should inactivate HIV that might have been missed in the screening of donors. Increasing reliance is therefore placed on desmopressin and tranexamic acid.

Replacement therapy: Human freeze-dried Factor VIII concentrate (Factor VIII fraction, dried) is used when the deficiency is sufficiently severe. This preparation is stable for one year at 4 °C but once reconstituted should be used without delay. New recombinant Factor VIII is now available. In milder cases (Factor VIII levels within 5–25 per cent of normal) desmopressin and tranexamic acid may be satisfactory and are increasingly used.

- **Dental management in haemophilia A**

Difficulties in the management of haemophiliacs may include:

1. Dental neglect necessitating frequent dental extractions.
2. Trauma, surgery and subsequent haemorrhage.
3. Factor VIII inhibitors.
4. Hazards of anaesthesia, especially nasal intubation, and intramuscular injections.
5. Risks of hepatitis, and liver disease.
6. HIV infection.
7. Aggravation of bleeding by drugs.
8. Anxiety.
9. Drug dependence as a result of chronic pain.

Preventive dental care
Education of patient or parents, and preventive dentistry, should be started as early as possible. Dental neglect is common and can lead to serious consequences. Dental extractions are still a major problem for haemophiliacs

The use of fluorides, fissure sealants, dietary advice on the need for sugar restriction and regular dental inspections from an early age are crucial to the preservation of the teeth. Prevention of periodontal disease is also imperative. Comprehensive dental assessment is needed at the age of about

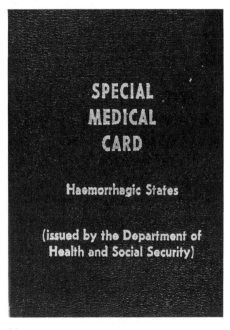

SPECIAL MEDICAL CARD

Haemorrhagic States

(issued by the Department of Health and Social Security)

IN CASE OF INJURY, BLEEDING, OR SERIOUS ILLNESS, THIS PERSON MAY HAVE URGENT NEED OF CARE AT A SPECIAL CENTRE.

IN EMERGENCY, TELEPHONE THE CENTRE NAMED OPPOSITE.

NEITHER INTRA-MUSCULAR INJECTIONS NOR ASPIRIN PREPARATIONS SHOULD BE GIVEN.

(a)   *(b)*

Fig. 4.5 (*a*) Special Medical Card that should be carried at all times by patients with haemorrhagic states; (*b*) special Medical Card showing warnings inside the cover

12–13, to plan for the future and to decide how best to forestall difficulties resulting from overcrowding or misplaced third molars or other teeth.

Surgery and postoperative haemorrhage
Dental extractions and surgery are dangerous for haemophiliacs. Surgery should therefore be carefully planned to avoid complications. All necessary surgery (and other dental treatment) should of course be performed at one operation. Haemophiliacs require the care of specialists of many disciplines and should therefore be treated in Haemophilia Reference Centres, or associated units (*see* Department of Health Memorandum FPN 105 HC (76)4). Haemophilia cards are issued to confirmed haemophiliacs and give details of the diagnosis and the Centre from which advice can be obtained (*Fig. 4.5*). Radiographs should be taken for any unsuspected disease and to assess whether further extractions might prevent future trouble.

Injections
Local anaesthesia should be avoided in the absence of Factor VIII replacement. Regional (inferior dental or posterior superior alveolar) blocks or injections in the floor of the mouth must not be used since they can cause haemorrhage which, by allowing blood to track down to cause airway obstruction, can be life-threatening. Rarely, even submucosal infiltrations have caused widespread haematoma formation, but intraligamentary injections may be safe. Infiltration anaesthesia may be used with caution and is adequate for conservative work in children, but lingual infiltration must be avoided.

If factor replacement therapy has been given, regional anaesthesia can be used, provided the Factor VIII level is maintained above 30 per cent, but infiltration is still preferable. Intravenous midazolam or relative analgesia can be used.

Intramuscular injections should be avoided unless replacement therapy is being given, as they can cause large haematomas. Oral alternatives are in any case satisfactory in most instances.

Conservative dentistry
Conservative treatment of the primary dentition and sometimes of the permanent denti-

tion may be carried out without anaesthesia. If conservative treatment is not tolerated without anaesthesia, papillary or intraligamentary infiltration may achieve sufficient analgesia and is unlikely to cause serious bleeding. Soft tissue trauma must be avoided and a matrix band may help prevent gingival laceration. However, care must be taken not to let the matrix band cut the periodontal tissues and start gingival bleeding. A rubber dam is also useful to protect the mucosa from trauma but the clamp must be carefully applied. High speed vacuum aspirators and saliva ejectors must be used with caution in order to avoid production of haematomas. Trauma from the saliva ejector can be minimized by resting it on a gauze swab placed in the floor of the mouth.

Endodontics: Root canal treatment may obviate the need for extractions and can usually be carried out without special precautions other than care to avoid reaming through the apex. Topical application of 10 per cent cocaine to the exposed pulp is the choice for vital pulp extirpation. However, in severe haemophilia, bleeding from the pulp and periapical tissues can be persistent and troublesome .

Periodontal treatment: In all but severe haemophiliacs scaling can be carried out under antifibrinolytic cover. Periodontal surgery necessitates factor replacement.

Orthodontics: There is no contraindication to the movement of teeth in haemophilia. However, there must be no sharp edges to appliances, wires etc., which might traumatize the mucosa.

Minor surgery
Endotracheal intubation for general anaesthesia may cause bleeding from nasal trauma and is dangerous in unprepared patients, but since replacement therapy has to be given for the surgical procedure, intubation can be carried out. An oral latex cuffed endotracheal tube is recommended to minimize trauma to the nasal and tracheal lining. The possibility of anaemia (Chapter 5) due to earlier blood loss must also be remembered if general anaesthesia is contemplated.

A Factor VIII level of between 50 and 75 per cent is required for dental extractions. AHF may also need to be given postoperatively but many patients can be managed with antifibrinolytic agents given during the subsequent 10 days. If oral bleeding recurs postoperatively, Factor VIII must be given. Some advise the administration of a further single dose of Factor VIII as a routine on the fourth or fifth postoperative day. However, this should be unnecessary if adequate Factor VIII has been given preoperatively.

Antifibrinolytics significantly reduce Factor VIII requirements. Tranexamic acid (Cyklokapron) is used in a dose of 1 g (30 mg/kg) orally, four times daily starting 24 hours preoperatively. Antifibrinolytics must not be used systemically where residual clots are present, for example in the urinary tract or intracranially. In haemophiliacs, the urine should therefore be examined preoperatively for haematuria.

Tranexamic acid used topically significantly reduces bleeding. Ten ml of a 5 per cent solution used as a mouth rinse for 2 minutes, four times daily for 7 days, is recommended. This solution can be made up by diluting 10 per cent tranexamic acid solution with sterile water.

Desmopressin (deamino-8-D arginine vasopressin: DDAVP) is a synthetic analogue of vasopressin which induces the release of Factor VIIIC, von Willebrand's factor (vWF) and tissue plasminogen activator (tPA) from storage sites in endothelium. Given as an intravenous infusion (0.3–0.5 µg/kg just before surgery, and repeated 12 hourly if necessary for up to 4 days), desmopressin can temporarily correct the haemostatic defect in mild haemophilia. Desmopressin may be useful for patients with Factor VIII inhibitors, and is also increasingly widely used, as mentioned earlier, for the management of mild haemophiliacs for such purposes as extractions. It is now available for subcutaneous or intranasal use when doses of 300 mg appear as effective as 0.2 mg/kg i.v. As desmopressin also causes release of plasminogen activator, tranexamic acid should also be given.

Desmopressin may cause facial flushing and slight tachycardia but the chief adverse effect is tachyphylaxis – declining response on repeated injection.

Local measures are also important to protect the operation area and minimize the risk of postoperative bleeding. Thus surgery should be carried out with minimal trauma to both bone and soft tissues, and careful mouth toilet postoperatively is also essential. Suturing (though theoretically unnecessary) is desirable to stabilize gum flaps and to prevent postoperative disturbance of wounds by eating. Non-resorbable sutures are preferred and should be removed at 4–7 days. Suturing carries with it the risk, if there is postoperative bleeding, of causing blood to track down towards the mediastinum with danger to the airway. However, such an eventuality is an indication of inadequate preoperative replacement therapy, although complications of this sort can result from the presence of Factor VIII inhibitors when postoperative haemostasis is less predictable.

In the case of difficult extractions, when mucoperiosteal flaps must be raised, the lingual tissues in the lower molar regions should preferably be left undisturbed since trauma may open up planes into which haemorrhage can track and endanger the airway. The buccal approach to lower third molars is therefore safer. Minimal bone should be removed and the teeth should be sectioned for removal where possible.

The packing of extraction sockets is unnecessary if replacement therapy has been adequate but some advise the packing of a small amount of oxidized cellulose soaked in tranexamic acid into the depths of the sockets. Acrylic protective splints are rarely used now, in view of their liability to cause mucosal trauma and to promote sepsis, but they may be needed in certain sites such as the palate. Local haemostasis can be aided by collagen, Gelfoam or Surgicel inserted into extraction sockets, and by cyanoacrylate or fibrin glues.

Prevention of infection: Antimicrobials such as oral penicillin V 250 mg four times daily should be given postoperatively for a full course of 7 days to reduce the risk of secondary haemorrhage. Infection also appears to induce fibrinolysis.

Postoperatively, a diet of cold liquid and minced solids should be taken for up to 10 days. Care should be taken to detect haematoma formation which may manifest itself by swelling, dysphagia or hoarseness. The patency of the airway must always be ensured.

Major surgery
Before major surgery the patient is assessed by haemostatic screening (APTT, PT, platelet

Table 4.10 Outline of management of haemophiliacs requiring surgery

Operation	Factor VIII level required	Preoperatively give	Postoperative schedule
Dental extraction, dentoalveolar or periodontal surgery	Minimum of 50% at operation	Factor VIII i.v.* Tranexamic acid 1 g i.v. (or by mouth starting 24 h preop.)	Rest as inpatient for 7 days unless resident close to Centre (then 3 days). Soft diet. For 10 days give tranexamic acid 1 g q.i.d. and pencillin V 250 mg q.i.d. If there is bleeding during this period give repeat dose of Factor VIII*
Maxillofacial surgery	100% at operation; 50% for 7 days postop.	Factor VIII i.v.†	Rest inpatient for 10 days. Soft diet. Twice daily i.v. Factor VIII* for 7–10 days

*Factor VIII dose in units = weight in kg × 25 given 1 h preoperatively.
†Factor VIII dose in units = weight in kg × 50 given 1 h preoperatively.

count), Factor VIII assay, specific antibody test, fibrinogen estimation, hepatitis B, C and HIV tests and liver function tests. The patient should be admitted to hospital and haemoglobin estimation carried out. Blood is also grouped and cross-matched for use in emergency. Surgery is best carried out on Thursdays and Fridays, since bleeding is most likely on the day of operation or from 4 to 10 days postoperatively. All surgical procedures must be covered with AHF which is given 1 hour preoperatively.

The dose of AHF given before operation depends both on the severity of haemophilia and the amount of trauma expected (*Table 4.10*). Factor VIII is effective only for about 12 hours and therefore must be given regularly at least twice-daily postoperatively for major surgery.

Trauma to the head and neck
Haemophiliacs with head and neck injuries are at risk from bleeding into the cranial cavity or into the fascial spaces of the neck. They should, therefore, be given factor replacement to a level of 100 per cent prophylactically after a head or facial trauma. If there are lacerations that need suturing, a minimum level of Factor VIII of 50 per cent is required at the time, with further cover for 3 days.

Other considerations
Haemophiliacs with inhibitors: Between 5 and 20 per cent of haemophiliacs who have had multiple infusions, and a few who have not,

develop inhibitory antibodies, which reduce the activity of Factor VIII. These problems are most common in severe haemophilia. Bleeding episodes are not more frequent when inhibitors are present but are more difficult to control. Two types of inhibitor are known – high and low titre inhibitors.

In general, those with low titre inhibitors can have dental treatment in the same way as those who have no antibodies. However, in those with high titre inhibitors surgery and other traumatic procedures must be avoided unless absolutely essential. If the concentration of inhibitors is low, Factor VIII may be effective for 4–5 days or longer if immunosuppressive therapy such as prednisolone or cyclophosphamide is given. In those with higher concentrations of inhibitors, monoclonal antibody-purified Factor VIII infusion or recombinant Factor VIII can often be effective. Human Factor VIII Inhibitor Bypassing Fractions (FEIBA) are also available; these are usually either non-activated prothrombin complex concentrates (PCC) or activated prothrombin complex concentrates (APCC) which act by activating Factor X directly bypassing the intrinsic pathway of blood clotting. The danger with these products is of uncontrolled coagulation with thromboses. In many cases, desmopressin is an effective alternative and antifibrinolytics may help, or immunosuppression may be required.

Hepatitis, infection with HIV and liver disease: Haemophiliacs are at risk from viral hepatitis and infection with HIV. Many patients treated before blood products were screened for hepatitis B or heat-treated against HIV are particularly at risk. Hepatitis C and D infection, however, are increasingly prevalent (Chapter 10).

Bleeding aggravated by drugs: Aspirin or other non-steroidal anti-inflammatory drugs such as indomethacin, should not be given to patients with haemophilia since they can cause gastric bleeding and worsen the haemorrhagic tendency by depressing platelet aggregation. Codeine and paracetamol are safer alternative analgesics.

Anxiety: Many haemophiliacs are acutely anxious about dental treatment. Emotional factors significantly increase fibrinolytic activity so that reassurance and use of sedatives may be helpful.

Drug dependence: The severe pain from haemarthroses may occasionally lead to drug dependence (Chapter 24), but this is uncommon.

Christmas disease (haemophilia B)

Christmas disease (Factor IX deficiency) is clinically identical to haemophilia A and inherited in the same way, but it is about one-tenth as common as haemophilia A. Female carriers often have a bleeding tendency.

• Dental management of haemophilia B

The earlier comments on dental management in haemophilia A apply equally to patients with haemophilia B, but Factor IX replacement is needed before surgery and desmopressin is not used. Human dried Factor IX concentrate is supplied as a powder to be reconstituted with sterile distilled water for intravenous administration. A dose of 20 units Factor IX per kg body weight is used intravenously 1 hour preoperatively. The standard preparation may also contain Factors II, VII and X. Factor IX is more stable than Factor VIII. Its half-life is often up to 2 days, so that replacement therapy can sometimes be given at longer intervals than in haemophilia A.

Factor XI deficiency (haemophilia C)

This is discussed below under 'Other congenital coagulation defects'.

Von Willebrand's disease

Von Willebrand's disease (pseudohaemophilia) is the most common inherited bleeding disorder and affects about 1% of the population. It is caused by a deficiency of, or defect in, von Willebrand factor (vWF). The vWF, synthesized in endothelium and megakaryocytes, normally acts as a carrier for Factor VIII protecting it from proteolytic degradation. A deficiency in vWF thus leads to a low Factor VIII concentration in the blood. vWF also bridges between platelets and damaged endothelium. Thus the bleeding tendency in von Willebrand's disease results both from a clotting defect and a defect in platelet function. Von Willebrand's disease not only affects females as well as males but the clinical presentation usually differs from haemophilia A (*Table 4.9*). The common pattern is bleeding from mucous membranes, with purpura of mucous membranes and the skin. Gingival haemorrhage is more common than in haemophilia. Excessive menstrual bleeding is a common presentation in females. Haemarthroses are rare. Although the disorder is usually less severe than haemophilia A, postoperative haemorrhage can be troublesome.

The low level of vWF results in poor platelet adhesion after trauma. Platelets usually fail to aggregate in the presence of ristocetin so that, unlike haemophilia, purpura is common and the bleeding time is prolonged but the best assay is the ristocetin cofactor assay. Von Willebrand's disease is thus characterized by a prolonged bleeding time, usually a prolonged APTT, low levels of von Willebrand's factor (Factor VIIIR:Ag), and low Factor VIIIC and VIIIR:RCo (ristocetin cofactor) levels.

There are various types of von Willebrand's disease and the severity varies from patient to patient and from time to time. Some patients have a clinically insignificant disorder, while others have Factor VIII levels low enough to cause severe clotting defects as well as a prolonged bleeding time. However, the severity does not correlate well with the Factor VIII level (*see* Appendix to this chapter). Pregnancy and the contraceptive pill may cause transient amelioration.

Von Willebrand's disease has over 20 variants but 80% have type I and nearly 20%

have type II disease. It is usually inherited as an autosomal dominant but a severe form of the disease may be inherited as a sex-linked recessive trait like true haemophilia. Rarely, von Willebrand's disease may be acquired, particularly in patients with autoimmune or lymphoproliferative diseases

- **Dental management in von Willebrand's disease**

Aspirin and NSAIDs should be avoided. In most patients with von Willebrand's disease, the haemostatic defect can be controlled with desmopressin, now mainly given via a nasal spray. The chief exceptions are, first, type IIB disease, in which desmopressin is contraindicated because it stimulates release of dysfunctional von Willebrand factor which leads, in turn, to platelet aggregation and severe but transient thrombocytopenia. Second, it is also contraindicated in type III disease, where so little von Willebrand factor is formed that essentially the same management is required as for haemophilia A. However, since Factor VIII has a prolonged half-life, less frequent infusions may be required.

Thus type I von Willebrand's disease can be treated with desmopressin but types II and III require clotting factor replacement.

Hereditary haemorrhagic telangiectasia, mitral valve prolapse, or Factor XII deficiency may be associated and may require to be considered in the management plan.

Other congenital coagulation defects

Factor XI deficiency (plasma thromboplastin antecedent deficiency) is one of the more common other congenital coagulation defects and is sometimes known as haemophilia C. Any of the other clotting factors can be deficient and all may be associated with a haemorrhagic tendency, except Factor XII deficiency (despite the prolonged clotting time and APTT in this defect there is actually a tendency to thromboses). Most are uncommon or rare defects.

Fresh frozen plasma will usually correct most of these coagulation defects, but local haemostatic measures should also be applied.

ACQUIRED COAGULATION DEFECTS

Acquired haemorrhagic disorders are much more prevalent than the congenital diseases but, except in anticoagulant therapy or liver disease, are usually less severe.

Important causes include:

1. Anticoagulant therapy.
2. Vitamin K deficiency or malabsorption.
3. Liver disease (deficiency of Factor XII).
4. Disseminated intravascular coagulation.
5. Fibrinolytic states.
6. Amyloidosis (deficiency of Factor X).
7. Autoimmune disorders (deficiency of Factor VIII).

Nevertheless, some of those with clinical bleeding tendencies do not have a defect detectable by current laboratory methods.

Anticoagulant treatment

The commonly used anticoagulants are coumarins, such as warfarin, for long-term, and heparin for short-term treatment. Anticoagulants are given for thromboembolic disease but their use varies widely (*Table 4.11*). Anticoagulants result in a bleeding tendency but, generally, postoperative haemorrhage will eventually subside spontaneously. Nevertheless, severe blood loss can occur.

Coumarins such as warfarin are given orally and antagonize the action of vitamin K so that the prothrombin and activated partial thromboplastin times are prolonged. The effects are delayed for 8–12 hours, are maximal at 36 hours, but persist for 72 hours. Nicoumalone and phenindione are seldom used. Oral anticoagulants are teratogenic. Coumarin anticoagulant therapy should maintain a prothrombin time of 2–2 1/2 times the control (control 11–15 seconds), or a thrombotest of 5–20 per cent. Prothrombin

Table 4.11	Important conditions for which anticoagulants may be used

- Atrial fibrillation
- Cerebral thrombosis
- Deep vein thrombosis
- Embolization secondary to myocardial infarction
- Heart valve replacements
- Renal dialysis

times are often now recorded as the international normalized ratio (INR), a ratio of 2–3 being the usual therapeutic range for deep vein thrombosis, and up to 4.5 being required for patients with prosthetic heart valves.

Heparin is not given orally but by injection and acts immediately, mainly by inhibiting the thrombin–fibrinogen reaction. The prothrombin, activated partial thromboplastin (APTT) and thrombin times are therefore prolonged. Most patients are monitored with the APTT. Platelet counts should also be monitored if heparin is used for more than 5 days, since thrombocytopenia can result. The anticoagulant effect of heparin is usually lost within less than 6 hours of stopping heparin. Low molecular weight heparins, which include dalteparin, enoxaparin and tinzaparin, have a longer duration of action. Related agents include danaparoid, ancrod and epoprostenol. There should be no interference with anticoagulant treatment without the agreement of the clinician in charge. Neglect of this important point has led to rebound thrombosis which has damaged prosthetic cardiac valves and even caused thrombotic deaths.

• Dental management of patients on oral (coumarin) anticoagulation

The prothrombin time (PT) is the standard laboratory test for monitoring oral anticoagulant activity. Blood (citrated) for the prothrombin time is tested as soon as possible (within a few hours of venepuncture) by adding calcium and tissue thromboplastin to activate the clotting cascade (*Table 4.12*). The prothrombin time is expressed as the ratio of the PT of the patient (in seconds) to that of a control value but because the thromboplastin and the control values vary between laboratories, leading to different meanings of PT, an INR has been devised, this being the PT ratio (patient's PT/control PT) that would have been obtained if an international reference thromboplastin type 67/40 had been used. In a person with a PT within the normal range, the INR is approximately 1. It is important to recognize that the INR is valid only for patients on stable anticoagulant therapy.

Patients on coumarin anticoagulants should not have their medication stopped or changed before dental treatment except under special supervision. Minor surgery (simple extrac-

Table 4.12	Assessment of oral anticoagulant therapy		
	Prothrombin time	*Thrombo-test*	*INR*
Normal level	<1.3	>70%	0.9–1.2
Therapeutic range	2–4.5	5–20%	2.0–4.5
Levels at which minor surgery can be carried out	<2.5	>15%	<3.5

tions of two or three teeth) may be carried out safely with *no* change in anticoagulant treatment if the prothrombin time is within 1.5–3 times normal (INR up to 3.5). Regional blocks should be avoided. Surgery should be as atraumatic as possible, and a little haemostatic material (e.g. oxidized cellulose or fibrin), but is not essential.

Patients requiring major oral surgery are best admitted to hospital 48 hours before the operation, as are patients with INR above 3.5 and, with the agreement of the clinician in charge, anticoagulation may need to be modified. If anticoagulants are to be continued, vitamin K should preferably be avoided as it makes subsequent anticoagulation difficult.

If postoperative bleeding occurs, vitamin K may be given to counteract the coumarins. If the use of vitamin K cannot be avoided, only 10 mg should be given. In an emergency an antifibrinolytic agent (tranexamic acid) can be used to control haemorrhage.

Patients on oral anticoagulants are especially at risk from haemorrhage under the following circumstances.

1. Irregular tablet taking.
2. Liver disease or obstructive jaundice, which impair vitamin K metabolism or absorption.
3. Prolonged antimicrobial therapy (azole antifungals, penicillins, metronidazole, erythromycin, cephalosporins).
4. Liquid paraffin which leads to loss of vitamin K (theoretically).
5. Use of protein-binding drugs which displace the anticoagulant from plasma proteins and enhance its effect, e.g. aspirin, azole antifungals and sulphonamides. Co-trimoxazole, which contains a sulphonamide, and azoles, even as oral gels, may therefore be contraindicated.

6. Use of aspirin and other non-steroidal anti-inflammatory agents which can cause gastric bleeding and also interfere with platelet function.
7. Withdrawal of barbiturates; this decreases the breakdown of anticoagulants.

Under such circumstances the thrombotest should be repeated within 24 hours of surgery.

- **Dental management of patients on heparin anticoagulation**

The effect of heparin is best assessed by the thrombin time, which is usually maintained at 3–4 times normal (control 10–12 seconds). Low dose heparin therapy such as 'Minihep' (used to reduce postoperative complication of deep vein thrombosis) may have little effect on the thrombin time, APTT or on postoperative bleeding.

Heparin is given intravenously and its use is therefore restricted to inpatients. It has an immediate effect on blood clotting but acts for only 4–6 hours, so that no specific treatment is needed to reverse its effect. This can be achieved immediately during an emergency by intravenous protamine sulphate given in a dose of 1 mg per 100 IU heparin. Usually there is no need to interfere with anticoagulant treatment for simple extractions.

Surgery can safely be carried out after 6–8 hours, when the effects of heparinization have ceased. Low molecular weight heparins act for up to 24 hours, however. In renal dialysis patients surgery is best carried out on the day after dialysis as the effects of heparinization have then ceased and there is maximum benefit from dialysis (Chapter 13). It should be remembered that the condition for which anticoagulant therapy is being given, especially prosthetic heart valves, may also affect dental management (*Table 4.11* and Chapter 3).

Vitamin K deficiency and malabsorption

Vitamin K is taken in with the diet and also synthesized by the gut flora. It is a fat-soluble vitamin and its absorption in the small gut depends on the presence of bile salts. After transport to the liver, vitamin K is used for

Table 4.13 Clotting defects involving vitamin K

- Lack of vitamin K synthesis in gut*
  Broad spectrum antibiotics used for prolonged periods or inpatients on parenteral feeding
- Poor absorption*
  Malabsorption syndromes
  Obstructive jaundice
- Failure of utilization
  Oral anticoagulant treatment
  Liver failure

*Responds to parenteral vitamin K.

the synthesis of Factors II (prothrombin), VII, IX and X.

Haemorrhagic disease may, therefore, result from too little vitamin K reaching the liver, particularly as a result of obstructive jaundice or malabsorption. Alternatively, vitamin K metabolism may be impaired by anticoagulants or severe liver disease. In the last, many haemostatic functions are severely impaired and vitamin K is of little or no value (*Table 4.13*).

- **Dental aspects of vitamin K deficiency**

Dental management in vitamin K deficiency may be complicated by (a) the clotting defect and (b) the underlying disorder, particularly obstructive jaundice (Chapter 10). The latter may be caused by gallstones, viral hepatitis or carcinoma of the head of the pancreas.

The underlying disorder should preferably be corrected, but vitamin K can be given if surgery is urgent. Phytomenadione (5–25 mg) is the most potent and rapidly acting form and should preferably be given intravenously to avoid intramuscular injection. The prothrombin time should be monitored after 48 hours, and, if the defect has not been corrected by then, this suggests parenchymal liver disease.

Liver disease

Liver disease is an important cause of bleeding disorders. The haemostatic defects in liver failure include (a) impaired vitamin K metabolism; (b) increased fibrinolysis; (c) failure of synthesis or increased consumption of normal clotting factors; (d) synthesis of abnormal clotting factors; and (e) thrombocytopenia.

Haemorrhage can be severe and difficult to manage because of the complexity of these defects. Antifibrinolytic treatment and fresh frozen plasma may sometimes be effective. If there is an obstructive element to the disease vitamin K may be effective, but only if parenchymal disease is mild (Chapter 10).

Fibrinolytic drugs and states

Fibrinolytics, such as streptokinase, alteplase, anistreplase and urokinase, and local activation of plasmin by infection for example, may cause abnormal bleeding. Dental surgery should be deferred where possible in patients on fibrinolytic therapy.

Acquired haemophilia

This rare disorder is due to circulating antibodies to Factor VIII which typically are of idiopathic origin but may rarely form in rheumatoid arthritis, other autoimmune disorders, drug therapy – especially with penicillin, pregnancy or the puerperium. Specialist haematological attention is required before any invasive dental treatment is considered.

Other disorders associated with bleeding tendencies

These include the following:

1. Polycythaemia vera (Chapter 6).
2. Myelofibrosis, leukaemia or lymphoma (Chapter 6).
3. Chronic renal failure (Chapter 13).
4. Cyanotic congenital heart disease (Chapter 3).
5. Gram-negative shock.
6. After massive transfusions.
7. Antibodies to clotting factors.
8. Head injuries (Chapter 22).

TENDENCY TO THROMBOSIS

Hypercoagulability is when there is a risk of thrombosis under circumstances that would not cause thrombosis in a normal person.

Thrombophilia

A hereditary tendency to thrombosis is termed thrombophilia and is due to decreased fibrinolysis, or disorders of antithrombin or protein C. Thrombophilia and hypofibrinolysis due to resistance to activated protein C, or low protein C levels, or low levels of stimulated tissue plasminogen activator appear to underlie rare cases of alveolar necrosis which often present with severe pain (neuralgia-inducing cavitational osteonecrosis).

Acquired hypercoagulability

Acquired hypercoagulability can be seen in prolonged immobilization, obesity, congestive cardiac failure, postoperatively, in malignant and myeloproliferative disease, with oestrogen use and in homocystinuria.

Venous thrombosis

Venous thrombosis and subsequent pulmonary embolism are important causes of death or significant morbidity, especially in elderly, bed-ridden and postoperative patients. Venous thrombosis usually affects the deep calf veins (deep vein thrombosis; DVT) as a consequence of immobility. Pressure on the calf (from lying in bed) and increased blood coagulability follow general anaesthesia and surgery. Several other factors contribute, including sometimes, oral contraceptives.

Deep vein thrombosis can occasionally lead to pulmonary embolism. Superficial vein thrombosis may complicate intravenous injections, particularly of diazepam, but does not lead to pulmonary embolism (PE).

- **Prevention of deep vein thrombosis**

Prophylaxis against venous thromboembolism is important but not reliably effective. The calves must not rest on hard objects during surgery and stasis may be eliminated by calf contractions stimulated electrically, or by pneumatic compression. Early mobilization and leg movements postoperatively must be encouraged.

Anticoagulant therapy with heparin is the most effective method of preventing thromboembolism but must be balanced against the risks of haemorrhage. Current recommendations are either low dose subcutaneous heparin 5000 units given 2 hours before operation, then every 8–12 hours until the patient is ambulant, or low molecular weight heparins such as dalteparin 2500 units subcutaneously 2 hours before operation then again at 12 hours postoperatively, and then 5000 units once daily until the patient is ambulant.

• Management of deep vein thrombosis

Treatment of DVT is by intravenous heparin, starting with at least 5000 units, then continuous infusion at 1000 units per hour or subcutaneous heparin 15 000 units each 24 hours, with laboratory monitoring of APTT .

Pulmonary embolism

Pulmonary embolism secondary to venous thrombosis may be fatal as a result of sudden circulatory collapse, may cause minor pulmonary infarcts with haemoptysis or pleurisy, or may gradually cause pulmonary hypertension and right-sided heart failure.

• Management of pulmonary embolism

In massive pulmonary embolism with collapse and cardiac arrest, external cardiac massage may break up the embolus. Oxygen and intravenous heparin should also be given or streptokinase or urokinase. Minor pulmonary embolism usually resolves spontaneously but anticoagulants are given.

Disseminated intravascular coagulation

Disseminated intravascular coagulation (DIC), also known as consumption coagulopathy or defibrination syndrome, is an uncommon, complex and not fully understood process in which the main effect is probably activation of the haemostasis-related mechanisms within the circulation. Precipitating causes include incompatible blood transfusions, severe sepsis, obstetric complications, severe trauma or burns and cancers in various sites. In one series of head injuries some degree of DIC was found in 57 per cent.

Possible effects of DIC include the following.

Haemorrhagic tendencies: These result from the consumption of platelets and clotting factors internally and from activation of the fibrinolytic system. Purpura and bleeding from sites such as the gastrointestinal tract can result. In the case of head injuries, DIC may lead to intracranial haemorrhage.

Thrombotic phenomena: Clotting in capillaries can damage any organ, but the kidneys, liver, adrenals and brain are particularly vulnerable. Brain ischaemia by vascular occlusion may therefore complicate head injury, as a result of DIC.

Haemolysis: Red cells become damaged as a result of the changes in the capillaries (microangiopathic haemolysis).

Shock: Shock may be caused by adrenal damage or obstruction of the pulmonary circulation by fibrin deposition and other factors.

• Management of DIC

The management of disseminated intravascular coagulation is controversial and must in any case depend on the cause and pathological changes taking place. In general, the underlying cause and any hypoxia or acidosis should be corrected. In addition, heparinization, replacement of clotting factors and platelets, or antifibrinolytic therapy may be given as appropriate. No single programme of treatment is effective for all cases.

DIC is an acute emergency and dental treatment is highly unlikely to be considered – except afterwards in survivors.

BIBLIOGRAPHY

Abubaker A.O., Bontempo F.A. and Braun T. (1987) Use of deamino-8-D arginine vasopressin in a patient with moderate von Willebrand's disease. *J. Oral Maxillofac. Surg.* **45**, 728.

Bailey B.M.W. and Fordyce A.M. (1983) Complications of dental extractions in patients receiving Warfarin anticoagulant therapy. *Br. Dent. J.* **155**, 308–10.

Barnard N. and Scully C. (1993) Epstein's syndrome; implications for the oral surgeon. *Oral Surg. Oral Med. Oral Pathol.* **76**, 32–4.

Barrett A.W., Griffiths M.J. and Scully C. (1993) The Cornelia de Lange syndrome in association with a bleeding tendency. *Int. J. Oral Maxillofac. Surg.* **22**, 171–2.

Benoliel R., Leviner E., Katz S. *et al.* (1986) Dental treatment for the patient on anticoagulant therapy. Prothrombin-time value: what difference does it make? *Oral Surg. Oral Med. Oral Pathol.* **62**, 149–51.

Cameron C.B. and Kobrinsky N. (1990) Perioperative management of patients with von Willebrand's disease. *Can. J. Anaesth.* **37**, 341–7.

Campbell H.D. and Payne R.W. (1977) Dental extractions in a family with von Willebrand's disease. *Br. Dent. J.* **142**, 402.

Capitano A.M., Sacco R. and Mannucci P.M. (1991). Pseudopathologies of hemostasis and dental surgery. *Oral Surg. Oral Med. Oral Pathol.* **71**, 184–6.

Castaldi P.A. (1980) The patient with easy bruising and bleeding. *Medicine (UK)* **28**, 1416–20.

Cawson R.A., Spector R.G. and Skelly A.M. (1995) *Basic Pharmacology and Clinical Drug Use in Dentistry*, 6th edn. Edinburgh, Churchill Livingstone.

Chadwick B. (1995) Congenital coagulopathies. In Porter S.R. and Scully C. (eds), *Oral Health Care for Those with HIV Infection and Other Special Needs*. Northwood, Science Reviews, pp. 85–92.

Colin W. and Needleman H.L. (1985) Medical and dental management of a patient with congenital Factor XIII deficiency. *Pediatr. Dent.* **7**, 227–30.

Colquhoum M.C., Daly M., Stewart P. and Beeley L. (1985) Interaction between warfarin and miconazole oral gel. *Lancet* **1**, 695–6.

Declerck D., Vinckier F. and Vermylen J. (1992) Influence of anticoagulation on blood loss following dental extractions. *J. Dent. Res.* **71**, 387–90.

Di Michele D. (1996) Hemophilia 1996. *Pediatr. Clin. North Am.* **43**, 709–36.

Durham T.M., Hodges E.D., Harper J. *et al.* (1993) Management of traumatic oral-facial injury in the hemophiliac patient with inhibitor. *Pediatr. Dent.* **15**, 282–7.

Editorial (1983) DDAVP in haemophilia and von Willebrand's disease. *Lancet* **ii**, 774–5.

Evans B.E. (1989) Dental management. In Hilgartner M.W. and Pochedly, C. (eds), *Hemophilia in the Child and Adult*, 3rd edn. New York, Raven Press, pp. 89–119.

Geffner I. and Porteous S.R. (1981) Haemorrhage and pain control in conservative dentistry for haemophiliacs. *Br. Dent. J.* **151**, 256–8.

George J.N. and Shattil S.J. (1991) The clinical importance of acquired abnormalities of platelet function. *N. Engl. J. Med.* **324**, 27–39.

Green D. (1980) Von Willebrand's disease. *Postgrad. Med. J.* **67**, 241–8.

Haska J. and Hehlmann R. (1993) Local treatment of thrombocytopenic mucosal haemorrhage. *Lancet* **342**, 55.

Hobson P. (1981) Dental care of children with haemophilia and related conditions. *Br. Dent. J.* **151**, 249–53.

Johnson W.T. and Leary J.M. (1988) Management of dental patients with bleeding disorders: review and update. *Oral Surg. Oral Med. Oral Pathol.* **66**, 297–303.

Kantarci A., Cebeci I., Firatli E., Atamer T. and Tuncer O. (1996) Periodontal management of Glanzmann's thrombasthenia: report of 3 cases. *J. Periodontol.* **61**, 816–20.

Katz J.O. and Terezhalmy G.T. (1988) Dental management of the patient with hemophilia. *Oral Surg. Oral Med. Oral Pathol.* **66**, 139–44.

Larson C.E., Chang J-L., Bleyaert A.L. *et al.* (1980) Anesthetic considerations for the oral surgery patient with hemophilia. *J. Oral Surg.* **38**, 516–19.

Leading Article (1983) DDAVP in haemophilia and von Willebrand's disease. *Lancet* **ii**, 774.

Lethagen S.R. (1995) Pathogenesis, clinical picture and treatment of von Willebrand's disease. *Ann. Med.* **27**, 641–51.

Levine P.H. (1985) The acquired immunodeficiency syndrome in persons with hemophilia. *Ann. Intern. Med.* **103**, 723–6.

Libre J.M., Cucurull J., Aloy A. *et al.* (1991) Antimicrobial prophylaxis for dental extractions after splenectomy. *Lancet* **337**, 1485–6.

Ludlam C.A. and Steel C.M. (1993) Haemostasis; von Willebrand's variants. *Lancet* **341**, 997.

Lusher J.M. and Warrier M.D. (1992) Hemophilia A. *Hematol. Oncol. Clin. North Am.* **6**, 1021–33.

Manabe M., Tsujimaki M., Kakuta S. *et al.* (1993) Acquired factor X deficiency. *J. Oral Maxillofac. Surg.* **51**, 922–4.

Mandalaki T. (1991) General principles of hemophilia care; retrospective review and perspectives. In Lushler J.M. and Kessler C.M. (eds), *Hemophilia and von Willebrand's Disease in the 1990s*. New York, Excerpta Medica, pp. 3–8.

McDonough R.J. and Nelson C.L. (1989) Clinical implications of factor XII deficiency. *Oral Surg. Oral Med. Oral Pathol.* **68**, 264–6.

Monsour P.A., Kruger B.J. and Harden P.A. (1986) Prevalence and detection of patients with bleeding disorders. *Aust. Dent. J.* **31**, 104–10.

Morrison A.E. and Ludlam C.A. (1995) Acquired haemophilia and its management. *Br. J. Haematol.* **89**, 231–6.

Mulligan R. and Weitzel K.G. (1988) Pretreatment management of the patient receiving anticoagulant drugs. *J. Am. Dent. Assoc.* **117**, 479–83.

O'Neil D.W. and Lowe J.W. (1989) Dentistry and the hemophiliac. *Compend. Contin. Educ. Dent.* **10**, 86–8, 156–60.

Peery W.H. (1987) Clinical spectrum of hereditary haemorrhagic telangiectasia. *Am. J. Med.* **82**, 989–97.

Poker I.D., Reade, P.C. and Cook R.M. (1990) Factor XI deficiency disclosed following haemorrhage related to a dental extraction. *Aust. Dent. J.* **35**, 258–60.

Porter S.R. and Scully C. (1996) *Innovations and Developments in Non-Invasive Oral Health Care*. Northwood, Science Reviews.

Porter S.R. and Singh N. (1995) Other bleeding disorders. In Porter S.R. and Scully C. (eds), *Oral Health Care for Those with HIV Infection and Other Special Needs*. Northwood, Science Reviews, pp. 93–110.

Rakocz M., Mazar A., Varon D. *et al.* (1993) Dental extractions in patients with bleeding disorders; the use of fibrin glue. *Oral Surg. Oral Med. Oral Pathol.* **75**, 280–2.

Redding S.W. and Stiegler K.E. (1983) Dental manage-
ment of the classic hemophiliac with inhibitors. *Oral Surg. Oral Med. Oral Pathol.* **56**, 145–8.

Richards A., Scully C., Eveson J. and Prime S.S. (1991) Epstein's syndrome: oral lesions in a patient with nephropathy, deafness and thrombocytopenia. *J. Oral Pathol. Med.* **20**, 512–13.

Rick, M. (1994) Diagnosis and management of von Willebrand's disease. *Med. Clin. North Am.* **78**, 609–23.

Royer J.W. and Bates W.S. (1988) Management of von Willebrand's disease with desmopressin. *J. Oral Maxillofac. Surg.* **46**, 313–4.

Saulnier J., Marey A., Horellou M-H. *et al.* (1994) Evaluation of desmopressin for dental extractions in patients with hemostatic disorders. *Oral Surg. Oral Med. Oral Pathol.* **77**, 6–12.

Schafer A.I. (1994) Hypercoagulable states: molecular genetics to clinical practice. *Lancet* **344**, 1739–42.

Sciubba J.R. and Parrado C. (1992) Parapharyngeal hemorrhage secondary to thrombolytic therapy for acute myocardial infarction. *J. Oral Maxillofac. Surg.* **50**, 413–5.

Scully C. (1988) *The Dental Patient.* Oxford, Heinemann.

Scully C. (1989) *The Mouth and Perioral Tissues.* Oxford, Heinemann.

Scully C. (1989) *Patient Care: a Dental Surgeon's Guide.* London, British Dental Association.

Scully C., Cawson R.A. and Griffiths M.J. (1990) *Occupational Hazards to Dental Staff.* London, British Dental Journal.

Sekine J., Tsuruda K., Matsunaga S-I. *et al.* (1994) Surgical management in the patient with congenital factor XII deficiency. *Oral Surg. Oral Med. Oral Pathol.* **77**, 13–15.

Sindet-Pedersen S. and Stenbjerg S. (1986) Effect of local antifibrinolytic treatment with tranexamic acid in hemophiliacs undergoing oral surgery. *J. Oral Maxillofac. Surg.* **44**, 703–7.

Sindet-Pedersen S., Ingerslev J., Ramstrom G. *et al.* (1988) Management of oral bleeding in haemophiliac patients. *Lancet* **ii**, 566.

Sindet-Pedersen S., Ramstrom G., Bernvil S. *et al.* (1989) Hemostatic effect of tranexamic acid mouthwash in anticoagulant-treated patients undergoing oral surgery. *N. Engl. J. Med.* **320**, 840–3.

Stephenson P., Lamey P.I., Scully C. *et al.* (1987) Angina bullosa haemorrhagica: clinical and laboratory features in 30 patients. *Oral Surg. Oral Med. Oral Pathol.* **36**, 25–9.

Stephenson P., Scully C., Prime S.S. *et al.* (1987) Angina bullosa haemorrhagica: lesional immunostaining and haematological findings. *Br. J. Oral Maxillofac. Surg.* **25**, 488–91.

Travis S., Wray R. and Harrison K. (1989) Perioperative anticoagulant control. *Br. J. Surg.* **76**, 1107–8.

Triplett D.A. (1993) Low molecular weight heparins. Is smaller better? *Arch. Intern. Med.* **153**, 1541–6.

Triplett D.A. and Brandt J. (1993) International normalized ratios, has their time come? *Arch. Pathol. Lab. Med.* **117**, 590–2.

Vinckier R. and Vermylen J. (1985) Dental extractions in hemophilia: reflections on ten years experience. *Oral Surg. Oral Med. Oral Pathol.* **59**, 6–9.

Werner E.J. (1996) Von Willebrand disease in children and adolescents. *Pediatr. Clin. North Am.* **43**, 683–707.

White G.C. and Lesesne H.R. (1983) Hemophilia, hepatitis and the acquired immunodeficiency syndrome. *Ann. Intern. Med.* **98**, 403–4.

Zakrzewska J. (1983) Gingival bleeding as a manifestation of von Willebrand's disease. *Br. Dent. J.* **155**, 157–60.

APPENDIX TO CHAPTER 4

RARE COAGULATION-RELATED FACTOR DEFECTS

Coagulation factor defect	Bleeding tendency	APTT	PT	Basic defect
V	+	–	–	Genetic: AR Streptomycin Liver disease, others
VII	+	–	–	Genetic: AR Liver disease; anti-coagulants, many others
X Stuart–Prower factor	+ usually	–	–	Genetic: AR Primary amyloid; others
XI Plasma thromboplastin antecedent	+	–	–	
XII Hageman factor	–	–	–	Genetic: AR Liver disease

continued

Coagulation factor defect	Bleeding tendency	APTT	PT	Basic defect
XIII fibrin stabilizing factor	+	–*	–*	Genetic: AR
α-Antiplasmin (Miyasato disease)	+	–†	–†	Genetic: AR many others
Fibrinogen	+	–	–	Genetic: AR
Prekallikrein (Fletcher factor)	–	–	–	Genetic: AR Nephrotic syndrome Liver disease

AR, autosomal recessive. *Assay by clot solubility. †Assay by α-antiplasmin function.

DISORDERS PREDISPOSING TO THROMBOSES

Factor involved	Aetiology	Management
Platelets (thrombocytosis and thrombocythaemia)	Exercise; pregnancy; trauma; post-splenectomy; chronic inflammatory disease; malignancy	Treat underlying cause Preoperative aspirin, dipyridamole or heparin
Antithrombin III deficiency	Genetic: AD Eclampsia, DIC Nephrotic syndrome	Superficial and deep vein thromboses with pulmonary embolism triggered by surgery, trauma, infection or pregnancy. Resistant to heparin anticoagulation – use oral anticoagulants ± fresh frozen plasma
Protein C deficiency or Protein S deficiency	Genetic: AD Liver disease DIC	Clinical features as for antithrombin III deficiency In addition, skin necroses if oral anticoagulants given

AD, autosomal dominant; DIC, disseminated intravascular coagulopathy.

SUB-TYPES OF VON WILLEBRAND'S DISEASE

	Type I	Type IIA	Type IIB	Type IIC	Type III
Inheritance	AD	AD	AD	AR	AR
Bleeding time	↑	↑	↑	↑	↑
Factor VIIIC	↓	↓ or N	↓ or N	N	↓↓
Factor VIIIR:Ag (von Willebrand factor)	↓	↓ or N	↓ or N	N	↓↓
Factor VIIIR:Rco (ristocetin cofactor	↓	↓↓	↓ or N	↓	↓↓
Platelet aggregation with ristocetin	↓ or N	↓	↑	↓	↓
Other comments	Mild bleeding tendency. Desmopressin restores haemostasis	↑	May have Thrombo-cytopenia	↑	May be severe bleeding tendency

AD, autosomal dominant; AR, autosomal recessive; N, normal; ↑ = increased; ↓ = decreased.

5

Anaemia

Key points

- Anaemia is a fall in haemoglobin level below the normal for age and sex.
- Anaemia can (a) be a contraindication to general anaesthesia and (b) cause oral complications, i.e. sore mouth, burning tongue, glossitis, ulcers, angular stomatitis.
- Anaemia is caused mainly by haemorrhage, depressed erythropoiesis, or haemolysis.
- The type of anaemia should be established, the cause found and remedied.
- The most usual cause of anaemia in most of the developed world is iron deficiency caused by chronic haemorrhage (commonly menorrhagia).
- In iron deficiency, if menorrhagia is not the cause, the site of blood loss should be sought, usually in the gastrointestinal tract.
- Folate deficiency is commonly dietary in origin.
- Vitamin B_{12} deficiency is rarely dietary in origin; more commonly it is caused by pernicious anaemia or a gastrointestinal lesion.
- Deficiencies of multiple haematinic factors, e.g. iron, folate and vitamin B_{12}, may be caused by disease of the small intestine.
- Sickle cell anaemia is a hereditary defect of haemoglobin structure, found mainly in patients of African ancestry and some from the Mediterranean countries and Asia.
- Screen all black patients for sickle cell anaemia. Do a full blood picture and a screening test, and record results.
- In sickle cell anaemia, at low oxygen tensions, the red cells sickle and cause infarcts or haemolyse.
- General anaesthesia may be dangerous to patients with sickle cell anaemia and should not be given in a dental practice.
- Even mild hypoxia can prove fatal in patients with sickle cell anaemia.
- Drugs may precipitate haemolysis in glucose-6-phosphate dehydrogenase deficiency. Aspirin and co-trimoxazole are contraindicated and prilocaine is best avoided.

Anaemia is not a disease in itself and may be a feature of many diseases (*Table 5.1*). The essential feature of anaemia is a haemoglobin level below the normal for the age and sex (Appendix 1 to Chapter 1). Up to puberty a haemoglobin level below 11.0 g/dl, and in adult females below 11.5 g/dl and adult males below 13.5 g/dl are the values regarded as indicative of anaemia.

The effect of anaemia is to reduce the oxygen-carrying capacity of the blood. Anaemia, particularly sickle cell disease, can thus make general

---

Table 5.1 Causes of anaemia

- Poor intake of haematinics (uncommon)
    Socioeconomic reasons
    Dietary fads
    Dysphagia
- Impaired absorption of haematinics
    Diseases of small intestine particularly
- Increased demands for haematinics
    Pregnancy and haemolysis, especially
- Impaired erythropoiesis
    Aplastic anaemia and leukaemia
    Drugs
    Chronic disease
    Viral infections
- Haemolytic anaemias
    Sickle cell and thalassaemia mainly
- Blood loss (most common cause)
    Menorrhagia
    Any gastrointestinal lesion (e.g. ulcers, carcinoma)
    Lesions of the urinary tract
    Trauma

Table 5.2 Clinical features of anaemia

- Sometimes none
- General lassitude
- Cardiorespiratory
    Dyspnoea
    Congestive cardiac failure
    Murmurs
    Angina pectoris
- Cutaneous
    Pallor
    Brittle nails
    Koilonychia (iron deficiency)
- Oral
    Sore mouth
    Oral ulceration
    Angular stomatitis
    Glossitis

---

anaesthesia hazardous. Some anaemias can also cause oral lesions such as ulcers, glossitis or angular stomatitis, or sometimes affect dental management in other ways.

In the early stages anaemia is frequently asymptomatic; skin colour is misleading but pallor of the oral mucosa, conjunctiva or palmar creases suggests severe anaemia. The different types of anaemia have many clinical features in common (*Table 5.2*). Anaemia also exacerbates or can cause heart failure and aggravate angina and the effects of pulmonary disease.

The most common cause of anaemia in Britain is chronic blood loss and consequent iron deficiency. Folate and vitamin B_{12} (cobalamin) deficiency are the next most common causes, but the precise nature of anaemia can only be established by clinical and laboratory investigation (*see* Appendix 1 to Chapter 1).

Classification of anaemias

Anaemia is classified on the basis of red cell (erythrocyte) size as *normocytic, microcytic* and *macrocytic*. Most common is microcytic anaemia, where the mean corpuscular (cell) volume (MCV) is below 78 fl; this is usually due to iron deficiency, occasionally to thalassaemia. Macrocytic anaemia (MCV more than 99 fl) is usually caused by vitamin B_{12} or folate deficiency (not infrequently in alcoholics), sometimes because folate and

vitamin B_{12} are used up in chronic haemolysis, pregnancy or malignancy. Macrocytic anaemia may also be seen in liver disease, myxoedema, or sometimes aplastic anaemia. Normocytic anaemia (MCV between 79 and 98 fl) may result from leukaemia, chronic disease, liver disorders, renal failure, infection, malignancy or other causes, particularly sickle cell disease, as discussed later.

Laboratory investigations

The most basic, and in many ways most useful, investigations are haemoglobin estimation and examination of a stained blood film. The terminology used in description of a blood film is shown in the Appendix to this chapter. Automated examination of blood provides a quick and reliable count of all the blood cells and important cytological features of red cells such as red cell distribution width (RDW), mean cell volume (MCV) and haemoglobin content. For this purpose a 4 ml sample of EDTA anticoagulated blood should be sent, with as much clinical information as possible, to the haematologist. A blood film may also be required, especially as a mixed macro- and microcytic picture may sometimes not be revealed by an automated counter and there may be other abnormalities seen. Special investigations are discussed with the specific diseases. The laboratory investigation of the common anaemias is summarized in *Fig. 5.1* (*see also* Appendix 1 to Chapter 1).

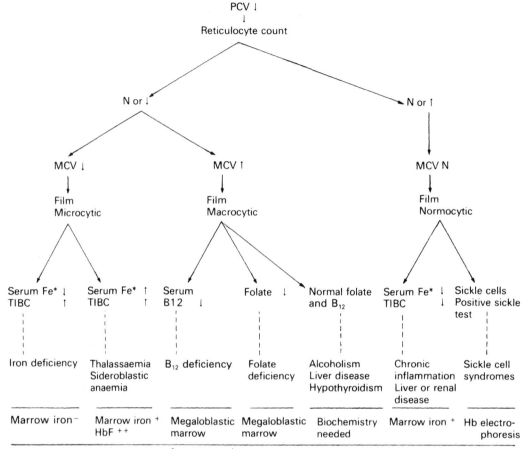

Fig. 5.1 Laboratory investigations for the cause of anaemia. PCV, packed cell volume; MCV, mean cell volume; TIBC, total iron binding capacity; HbF, fetal haemoglobin

Treatment

Blood transfusions should be used only when absolutely necessary, since they may carry the risk of infection, circulatory overload and allergic reactions. It is better to treat with haematinics such as iron or folic acid, or erythropoietin. Transfusions are usually indicated only when the haemoglobin concentration has fallen to below 7 g/dl.

• Dental aspects of anaemia: general considerations

Specific treatment of the different types of anaemia is considered later. The main danger is when a general anaesthetic is given, as it is vital to ensure full oxygenation. Nevertheless, the myocardium may be unable to respond to the demands of anaesthesia (Chapter 3). Whenever possible therefore, the cause of the anaemia should be corrected preoperatively, but at least the haemoglobin level must be raised, if necessary by transfusion.

Elective operations under general anaesthesia should not usually be carried out when the haemoglobin is less than 10 g/dl (male). In an emergency, anaemia can be corrected by whole blood transfusion, but this should only be given to a young and otherwise fit patient. Packed red cells avoid the risk of fluid overload and can be given in emergency to the elderly patient or those with incipient congestive cardiac failure. A diuretic given at the same time further reduces the risk of congestive cardiac failure. The patient should be stabilized at least 24 hours preoperatively and it should be noted that haemoglobin estimations are unreliable for 12 hours post-transfusion. Nitrous oxide is possibly contraindicated in vitamin B$_{12}$ deficiency (*see below*).

DEFICIENCY ANAEMIAS

Iron deficiency anaemia

The most common cause of anaemia worldwide is iron deficiency as a result of nutritional deficiencies in developing countries or chronic blood loss in the West. Women of child-bearing age and older are therefore mainly affected. In some studies, about 5 per cent of American women had mild iron deficiency anaemia and up to 25 per cent had low iron levels without anaemia. Excessive menstrual losses or gastrointestinal blood loss are the main causes. Very many children are mildly iron deficient because of the high demands for growth, especially during adolescence. By contrast, iron deficiency in an adult male almost invariably indicates blood loss, usually from the gastrointestinal or genitourinary tracts. The same holds true for post-menopausal women. Dietary iron is found mainly as iron salts partly as haem from the myoglobin and haemoglobin in meat. Gastric acid is required for the adequate conversion of iron salts for their absorption from the proximal small intestine. Some foods such as meat, poultry and fish and orange juice also promote the intestinal absorption of iron; others such as tannins in

Table 5.3	Causes of iron deficiency

- Blood loss
- Poor intake
- Poverty
- Ignorance
- Old age
- Malabsorption
- Achlorhydria

tea decrease absorption. Iron is stored in the bone marrow.

The important features of iron deficiency anaemia are summarized in *Fig. 5.1* and *Tables 5.2–5.4*. Impaired exercise capacity, koilonychia (*Plate 8*) and beeturia (urine appearing red after eating beetroot) may be seen. In childhood, iron deficiency may also predispose to developmental or behavioural disorders. However, symptoms ascribed to iron deficiency do not always respond to iron replacement.

Iron deficiency only manifests after iron stores are depleted. Thus in the early stages, iron is lost from the bone marrow (*Table 5.4*). Then there are erythrocyte size changes showing as an abnormal red cell distribution width (RDW) on automated red cell-sizing before the transport iron levels fall (with low serum iron and ferritin). A fall off in erythrocyte size (microcytosis and a low MCV) with increasing red cell protoporphyrin concentrations, follow. Falling serum ferritin levels are one of the most sensitive indices of iron deficiency but this test is not universally available. The serum iron binding capacity rises and transferrin saturation (serum iron/total iron binding capacity) falls: a value of less than 16 per cent indicates iron deficiency. Later there is a reduction in

	MCV	Hb	MCHC	Serum ferritin	Transferrin saturation*	Marrow iron stores
Normal	N	N	N	N	33%	N
Mild anaemia	↓	N or ↓	N	↓	>16%<33%	↓
Moderate anaemia	↓	↓	↓	↓	<16%	↓
Severe anaemia	↓↓	↓↓	↓↓	↓↓	<16%	↓↓

Table 5.4 Laboratory findings during the development of iron deficiency anaemia

Arrows indicate a value above or below normal (N).
*It is better to measure ferritin.

Table 5.5 Differential diagnosis of microcytosis*

Index	Iron deficiency	Heterozygous α- or β- thalassaemia trait	Lead poisoning
Haemoglobin	Reduced	Reduced	Normal[†]
MCV	Reduced	Reduced	Normal[†]
RDW	Increased	Normal	Normal
FEP	Increased	Normal	Increased
Serum iron	Reduced	Normal	Normal
TIBC	Increased	Normal	Normal
Ferritin	Reduced	Normal	Normal

*MCV, mean corpuscular volume; RDW, red cell distribution width; FEP, free erythrocyte protoporphyrin; TIBC, total iron-binding capacity.
[†]May be decreased if the blood lead concentration is in excess of 100 μg per decilitre.

Table 5.6 Causes of vitamin B_{12} deficiency

- Poor intake
  Poverty
  Ignorance
  Strict vegetarians (vegans, some Hindu Indians)
  Old age
- Malabsorption
  Defect in intrinsic factor production
  Congenital
  Autoimmune (pernicious anaemia)
  Gastrectomy
  Ileal disease
  Coeliac disease
  Tropical sprue
  Crohn's disease (more frequently folate deficiency)
  Blind loop syndrome
  Resections
  Fish tapeworm (Finland, Asia)
  Transcobalamin II deficiency
- Drugs
  Colchicine
  Neomycin
  Nitrous oxide (administration for more than 12 hours)

haemoglobin and a hypochromic microcytic anaemia.

Hypochromic microcytic anaemia with normal marrow iron stores is not caused directly by iron deficiency; it is uncommon but is a feature of thalassaemia and sideroblastic anaemia, as discussed later (*Table 5.5*).

The cause of the iron deficiency must be sought and treated. Then the best treatment of iron deficiency is an iron salt by mouth. Ferrous salts are the best absorbed, such as ferrous sulphate 200 mg twice daily. Ferrous gluconate 250 mg/day can be given if ferrous sulphate is not tolerated. Nausea or constipation are fairly common side-effects. Staining of the teeth by iron can be prevented in children by using sodium ironedetate as the iron source, as it is also sugar-free and more palatable than ferrous sulphate. Oral iron may need to be given for 3 months or more to replenish marrow iron stores. Parenteral iron does *not* increase the haemoglobin level more rapidly than oral iron, it must be given intramuscularly, and it may cause reactions including dysrhythmias. Parenteral iron has no advantages except, for example, when inflammatory bowel disease is aggravated by oral iron or the patient cannot take iron by mouth.

Vitamin B_{12} (cobalamin) deficiency

Vitamin B_{12} is found in the diet in meat (especially liver), is bound to gastric intrinsic factor, absorbed in the terminal ileum and stored in the liver. Deficiency is usually due to a defect in intrinsic factor, as a result of pernicious anaemia or gastrectomy, a vegan diet or occasionally ileal disease (*Table 5.6*). Deficiency of vitamin B_{12} develops slowly since stores last up to 3 years. Nitrous oxide can also interfere with vitamin B_{12} metabolism and interfere with neurological function if administration continues for 12 or more hours or if it is used as a drug of abuse.

Pernicious anaemia

Pernicious (Addisonian) anaemia is the most common type of macrocytic anaemia and typically affects women in middle age or over, particularly of Northern European descent. It is caused by a specific defect of absorption of vitamin B_{12}, not by malnutrition. Autoantibodies against gastric parietal cells (which produce intrinsic factor) and/or to the intrinsic factor or both are found and the disease is sometimes seen with other autoimmune diseases, especially hypothyroidism, or less often, diabetes mellitus, vitiligo, Addison's disease or hypoparathyroidism (Chapter 14).

The underlying lesion is an atrophic gastritis causing failure of production of intrinsic

---

Table 5.7   Schilling test for B$_{12}$ deficiency

Radiolabelled vitamin B$_{12}$ (small dose) given orally
Unlabelled vitamin B$_{12}$ (large dose) given i.m. 2 hours later
Collect urine over 24 hours (or whole body counting)
    Normal: excrete more than 15 per cent of radiolabelled B$_{12}$ in 24 hours
    B$_{12}$ deficiency: excrete less than 15 per cent of radiolabelled B$_{12}$ in 24 hours
Repeat with added intrinsic factor
    Pernicious anaemia: excretion of B$_{12}$ increases to normal
    Ileal disease: excretion of B$_{12}$ remains low

---

factor by parietal cells and of gastric acid (achlorhydria). There may be gastrointestinal symptoms in pernicious anaemia and also an increased risk of stomach cancer. Ultimately there is macrocytic (megaloblastic) anaemia with depressed production of all blood cells (*see Fig. 5.1*).

In addition to the usual signs and symptoms of anaemia, neurological symptoms, particularly paraesthesiae of the extremities, develop in about 10 per cent. Early signs include loss of toe positional sense and diminished perception of the vibration of a tuning fork. These early neurological changes are reversible with treatment but, in the past particularly, could lead to subacute combined degeneration of the spinal cord and, ultimately, paraplegia. Premature greying of the hair is another well-recognized feature.

The diagnosis of pernicious anaemia depends on the clinical findings and low serum B$_{12}$ levels together with the autoantibodies. Impairment of vitamin B$_{12}$ absorption is shown by the Schilling test, summarized in *Table 5.7*.

Serum vitamin B$_{12}$ levels may occasionally be low in the absence of an abnormal Schilling test, may be low even though there is no deficiency or may remain normal in patients who are deficient. Vitamin B$_{12}$ is a cofactor for biochemical reactions that become abrogated during vitamin B$_{12}$ deficiency, leading to the accumulation of methylmalonic acid and homocysteine in the serum and spillover into the urine. Measurement of these metabolites appears to be more sensitive and specific for deficiency than is assay of serum vitamin B$_{12}$ itself, though renal and other disorders may confuse the interpretation.

In a large study in the USA, 5 per cent of persons over 50 were found to have low serum vitamin B$_{12}$ levels. This was previously thought to be of no significance but the early finding that neurological damage could precede anaemia or even macrocytosis was confirmed. Absence of macrocytosis in some cases is due to concomitant iron deficiency, but in another study on 70 patients with very low (less than 100 ng/l) serum vitamin B$_{12}$ levels, anaemia was absent in 19 per cent and macrocytosis was absent in 33 per cent. In some of these cases vitamin B$_{12}$ deficiency was manifested first as cerebral abnormalities and what has been termed 'megaloblastic madness'.

Pernicious anaemia is treated with intramuscular hydroxycobalamin 1 mg five times at 3 day intervals to replete liver stores, and then at about 3 monthly intervals for the rest of the patient's life.

Other causes of B$_{12}$ deficiency are shown in *Table 5.6*.

Folate (folic acid) deficiency

Folic acid is found in fresh leafy and other vegetables (folate) and is absorbed from the proximal small intestine. There are virtually no body stores of folic acid. Most folic acid deficiency is caused by dietary deficiency; some is caused by disease of the small intestine, such as coeliac disease. The main causes of folic acid deficiency are summarized in *Table 5.8*, but occasionally no cause can be discovered.

The effects of folate and B$_{12}$ deficiency are very similar. Both cause megaloblastic changes in the marrow and macrocytic anaemia (*see Fig. 5.1*), defective DNA synthesis, impaired production of blood cells and, ultimately, of many other cells. Folic acid deficiency in pregnancy appears to predispose to neural tube defects or cleft lip-palate in the fetus and thus folic acid prophylaxis is recommended. However, deficiency in adults does not lead to subacute combined degeneration of the cord. It is also essential to distinguish it from pernicious anaemia, as treatment of the latter with folic acid will improve the haematological picture to some degree but aggravates the neurological damage.

Table 5.8   Causes of folate deficiency

- Poor intake
    - Poverty
    - **Ignorance**
    - **Old age**
    - Alcoholism
- Malabsorption
    - **Coeliac disease**
    - Crohn's disease
    - Other malabsorption states
- Increased demands
    - Infancy
    - Pregnancy
    - Chronic haemolysis
    - Malignant disease
    - Exfoliative skin lesions
    - Chronic dialysis
- Drugs
    - Alcohol
    - Barbiturates
    - Phenytoin
    - Primidone
    - Methotrexate
    - Pyrimethamine
    - Triamterene
    - Co-trimoxazole
    - Pentamidine
    - Oral contraceptives

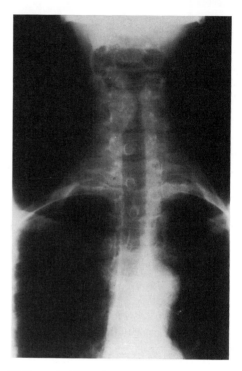

Fig. 5.2 Post-cricoid carcinoma in patient with Paterson–Kelly (Plummer–Vinson) syndrome

In folate deficiency the red cell folate levels are low, serum B_{12} normal, and the B_{12} absorption (Schilling) test is normal; these tests enable the important distinction to be made from B_{12} deficiency. Red cell folate levels, when low, are unequivocal evidence of folate deficiency but may remain normal for a time in a few folate deficient patients until older erythrocytes are replaced. Serum folate assays are considerably less reliable.

Once the cause has been found and rectified, treatment with folic acid (5 mg daily by mouth) rapidly restores the normal blood picture. Treatment is usually given for up to 4 months.

• Oral aspects of the deficiency anaemias

Oral mucosal lesions seem particularly frequent in the deficiency anaemias. For unknown reasons the tongue is especially affected, to the extent that soreness of the tongue can develop even before the haemoglobin falls below the lower limit of normal. Oral changes are of the following types.

The sore or burning, but otherwise normal tongue: Soreness of the tongue without depapillation or colour change can be caused by early deficiencies, often with normal haemoglobin levels. It is important to have haematological examination of these patients, especially as cobalamin deficiency can be the cause and, as discussed earlier, anaemia or macrocytosis may be absent at this stage. It can, also at this early stage, occasionally also be associated with neurological disorders. Though sore tongue is more frequently of psychogenic origin (Chapter 19), it is important not to make this assumption without full investigation.

Atrophic glossitis: The red, glossy smooth sore tongue is the best known effect of severe anaemia but is much less frequently seen than in the past.

Moeller's glossitis and other colour changes: In early B_{12} deficiency particularly, the tongue is sore and may also show a pattern of red lines without depapillation. In Moeller's glossitis a red line forms along the lateral margins and around the tip of the tongue, but this is rare. More commonly a less regular pattern of red lines forms on the dorsum. Alternatively, red sore patches may form. These may come and go but range from pin-head red spots to circular areas up to a centimetre across, which may resemble erythroplasia clinically and, though they resolve with treatment of the anaemia, may show dysplasia histologically.

Paterson–Kelly syndrome: The Paterson–Kelly (Plummer–Vinson) syndrome of glossitis and dysphagia with hypochromic (iron deficient) anaemia is uncommon. Women are mainly affected and the prevalence appears to be highest in Northern Europe. There is a substantial risk of carcinoma in the post-cricoid region or in the mouth (*Fig. 5.2*). Rarely this syndrome is associated with a macrocytic anaemia.

Candidosis: Candidosis can be aggravated or precipitated by anaemia and may be the presenting feature. In a few cases adequate treatment of anaemia alone, without antifungal treatment, relieves the infection. The majority of patients with chronic mucocutaneous candidosis, particularly the familial and diffuse types, are also iron deficient and treatment with iron appears to improve the response to antifungal treatment. On the other hand, very many patients with mild candidosis, particularly denture-induced stomatitis, appear not to have haematological disease (Chapter 20).

Angular stomatitis (cheilitis): Angular stomatitis is also a well-known sign, particularly of iron deficiency anaemia, but it affects only a minority of cases. Nowadays it is more frequently caused by infection, mainly by *Candida albicans* which may be promoted by the anaemia itself. Angular stomatitis is uncommon in pernicious anaemia.

Aphthous stomatitis: Aphthous stomatitis is sometimes associated with haematological deficiency, particularly of folate, which if remedied, can sometimes bring about a cure. Deficiencies should be suspected, especially in patients of middle age or over who develop aphthae.

ANAEMIA ASSOCIATED WITH SYSTEMIC DISEASE

Anaemia of various types may be associated with systemic disorders which include:

1. Chronic inflammation (infections or connective tissue disease).
2. Neoplasms including leukaemia (Chapter 6). Acute leukaemia is an important cause of anaemia and should always be considered when anaemia is seen in a child.
3. Liver disease (Chapter 10).

Or very rarely:
4. Hypothyroidism (Chapter 14).
5. Hypopituitarism (Chapter 14).
6. Hypoadrenocorticism (Chapter 14).
7. Uraemia (Chapter 13).
8. HIV infection (Chapter 20).

APLASTIC ANAEMIA

Aplastic anaemia is pancytopenia with a non-functioning bone marrow, a rare disease causing refractory normochromic, normocytic or macrocytic anaemia, leucopenia and thrombocytopenia. Chemicals such as benzene, and drugs are important causes (*Table 5.9*), but many cases are idiopathic, though probably viral or immunologically mediated and some are due to non-A, non-B, non-C hepatitis viruses. Irradiation or graft-versus-host disease may also cause bone marrow aplasia. The clinical manifestations are those of anaemia together with abnormal susceptibility to infection and a bleeding

Table 5.9 Causes of aplastic anaemia
• Genetic
Fanconi's anaemia
Dyskeratosis congenita
• Autoimmune (idiopathic)
• Drugs
NSAIDs
Anti-thyroids
Allopurinol
Phenylbutazone
Chloramphenicol
Sulphonamides
Gold
Penicillamine
Anticonvulsants
Cytotoxic agents
• Chemicals
Benzene
Toluene
Heavy metals
Glue-sniffing
• Viruses
Hepatitis

tendency. Purpura is often the first manifestation.

The prognosis is poor and 50 per cent of patients die within 6 months, usually from haemorrhage or infection. Iron overload may result from repeated blood transfusions.

The principles of management include the following:

1. Removal of the cause. Even when this is discoverable, as in the case of drugs such as chloramphenicol, marrow damage may still be irreversible.
2. Isolation and antibiotics to control infection.
3. Bone marrow transplantation after intense immunosuppression. This in turn may cause graft-versus-host disease (GVHD), which is often lethal (*see below*).
4. Androgenic steroids may be of some value (corticosteroids are of questionable benefit).
5. Blood transfusion – but this carries risks from iron overload or infection.

• **Dental aspects of aplastic anaemia**

Oral manifestations of aplastic anaemia, and management, are somewhat similar to those of leukaemia, namely:

1. Anaemia.
2. Haemorrhagic tendencies (Chapter 4).
3. Susceptibility to infections.
4. Effects of corticosteroid therapy (Chapter 14).
5. Hepatitis B and other viral infections (Chapter 10).

Oral lichenoid lesions, or a Sjögren-like syndrome, may develop if there is graft-versus-host disease if marrow transplantation has been carried out to relieve the anaemia (*see below* and Chapter 6). Gingival hyperplasia may develop if cyclosporin is used.

Fanconi's anaemia is a rare autosomal recessive syndrome characterized by skeletal defects, hyperpigmentation, pancytopenia and other congenital anomalies. It is associated with an increased susceptibility to oral or other head and neck carcinomas at an early age, as is dyskeratosis congenita.

Bone marrow transplantation

Bone marrow transplantation (BMT) is increasingly used, particularly in the treatment of aplastic anaemia, leukaemias and other haematological malignancies, and some genetic defects (Chapter 6). The transplant involves not only myeloid, erythroid and megakaryocyte but also lymphoid and macrophage cells. Most transplants are made between HLA-identical siblings, though other family members, or matched volunteers, may be used. Patients must first be prepared for transplant by suppressing their immune response, since that otherwise might reject the graft. In aplastic anaemia this is achieved with cyclophosphamide. In leukaemia, chemotherapy (often cyclophosphamide with busulphan) and total body irradiation are carried out to kill the malignant cells and achieve immunosuppression. The donor marrow is then mixed with heparin and infused intravenously, when it colonizes the marrow of the recipient and, over the next 2–4 weeks, starts to produce blood cells. Throughout this time and for the following 3 months or so, the patient is usually provided with an indwelling catheter (Hickman line) to facilitate therapy and intravenous feeding. The patient is essentially immuno-incompetent until the donor marrow is functioning fully, and must be isolated and protected from infections. Patients may require transfusions of granulocytes, platelets or red cells if problems arise. Granulocyte colony stimulating factors may be of some value. Recipients may then, after transplantation, be treated with methotrexate or more usually cyclosporin for 6 months or more to prevent or ameliorate graft-versus-host disease (Chapter 6).

Complications of BMT may include:

1. Graft rejection.
2. Infection: early on this is usually bacterial and must be treated vigorously. Later, opportunists such as cytomegalovirus may appear.
3. Bleeding tendency.
4. Veno-occlusive liver disease.
5. Graft-versus-host disease.
6. Complications of immunosuppression (Chapter 20).

• **Dental aspects of bone marrow transplantation**

Management problems can include:

1. Oral complications of cytotoxic treatment and radiotherapy (Chapter 7) and immunosuppression (Chapter 20), particularly oral bacterial, herpetic and fungal infections, which are the main causes of death. These develop usually within the first month of the transplant. Oral symptoms are the main complaint in patients after bone marrow transplantation and consist of mucositis, sinusitis, parotitis, pain or bleeding. Cyclosporin may induce gingival hyperplasia and this and other immunosuppressants have resulted in lip and occasionally oral carcinomas, Kaposi's sarcoma or lymphomas.
2. Immunosuppressive therapy (Chapter 20).
3. Bleeding tendencies.
4. Graft-versus-host disease with lichenoid reactions or xerostomia.

Pure red cell aplasia

Pure red cell aplasia is a rare disease which may be congenital or acquired – the latter is often associated with a thymoma and sometimes chronic mucocutaneous candidosis (Chapter 20). These patients need regular blood transfusions and are therefore at risk from hepatitis viruses and HIV infection.

Anaemia caused by marrow infiltration

Replacement of haemopoietic marrow by abnormal cells (metastases, leukaemias, myeloma or myelofibrosis) causes normocytic anaemia and often leucopenia or thrombocytopenia with a leucoerythroblastic peripheral blood picture. There may be extramedullary haemopoiesis in other organs.

Dental care may be complicated by susceptibility to infections, haemorrhage (as in aplastic anaemia) or the underlying disease.

HAEMOLYTIC ANAEMIA

Worldwide, malaria is the most common cause of haemolytic anaemia, but is rare in Britain. Haemolytic anaemia may also result from many other causes, including:

1. Inherited abnormal haemoglobin (the haemoglobinopathies).
2. Inherited abnormal structure or function of the erythrocyte (spherocytosis; G6PD deficiency).
3. Damage to erythrocytes (autoimmune, drug-induced or infective).

Accelerated erythrocyte destruction leads to bilirubin overproduction and sometimes jaundice. The spleen may enlarge and increased red cell turnover raises the reticulocyte count, plasma lactate dehydrogenase and uric acid levels. This increases the demand for folic acid and may in turn cause macrocytic changes.

Any of the haemolytic anaemias may be a contraindication to the use of general anaesthesia but, in practical terms, sickle cell disease is by far the most important cause of difficulties in dental management.

Haemoglobinopathies

The haemoglobinopathies are hereditary disorders characterized by abnormal haemoglobin production. Each of the haemoglobin peptide (globin) chains has a unique amino acid sequence which can be altered as a result of DNA mutations and lead to 'variant haemoglobins'. Quantitative rather than qualitative defects in the production of globins leads to the thalassaemias.

There is a spectrum of consequences from haemoglobinopathies. Some haemoglobinopathies, particularly sickle cell disease, cause significant morbidity and mortality, while others, such as haemoglobin E, have no significant clinical effect other than the need to be differentiated from iron deficiency anaemia. Patients may have combinations of more than one haemoglobinopathy.

The diagnosis of haemoglobinopathy rests on the history, examination and laboratory investigations. A family history is especially important as many of these disorders have a racial distribution. Afro-Caribbean, Mediterranean, Middle Eastern, Indian, Bangladeshi and Pakistani patients have a high prevalence of the sickling disorders, while Vietnamese, Cambodian, Laotian and Chinese are the ethnic groups most likely to have the thalassaemias and glucose-6-phosphate dehydrogenase deficiency. In the

Table 5.10 The sickling disorders

Disorder	Haemoglobin type	Origins of predominant ethnic groups affected	Clinical features
Sickle cell anaemia	SS	Africa, West Indies, Mediterranean, India	Severe anaemia
Sickle cell trait	SA	Africa, West Indies, Mediterranean, India	Usually asymptomatic
Sickle cell – HbC disease	SC	West Africa, South East Asia	Variable anaemia
Sickle cell – HbD disease	SD	Africa, India, Pakistan	Moderately severe anaemia
Sickle cell – HbE disease	SE	South East Asia	Moderately severe anaemia
Sickle cell – thalassaemia	SAF	Mediterranean, Africa, West Indies	Moderately severe anaemia

UK, about 1 in 10 Afro-Caribbeans carry the sickle cell trait and a similar proportion of Asians (from the Indian Sub-Continent) have thalassaemia. About 1 in 30 Chinese and 1 in 50 Afro-Caribbeans have thalassaemia, and 1 in 100 Cypriots and Asians have sickle cell trait.

Short stature, abnormal skeletal development and jaundice are often found, in addition to signs and symptoms of anaemia. A full blood picture and red cell indices should be obtained and blood should also be sent for electrophoresis (4 ml of EDTA anti-coagulated blood) and for assay of variant haemoglobins. Special tests such as the Sickledex may also be useful (*see below*).

The sickling disorders

Sickle cell disease can cause severe complications in general anaesthesia. Deoxygenation causes the erythrocytes to deform into sickle shapes which have a reduced survival and also form stacks which impede blood flow in small vessels.

The sickling disorders include (*Table 5.10*):

1. heterozygous sickle cell trait (HbAS), which is more common than
2. homozygous sickle cell anaemia or disease (HbSS);
3. heterozygous sickling trait associated with another haemoglobinopathy.

These diseases mainly affect Africans and Afro-Caribbeans but are also found in Asians and in those from the Mediterranean littoral. In West Africa some 2 per cent of the population have sickle cell disease and up to 30% have the trait.

Sickle cell trait is many times more common than sickle cell anaemia in Britain

Table 5.11 Features of sickle cell anaemia

- **Anaemia**
- **Haemolysis**
  - Jaundice
  - Gallstones
  - Reticulocytosis
- **Crises**
  - Painful crises
  - Aplastic crises
  - Dactylitis
  - Infarcts of CNS, lungs, kidney, spleen, bone
  - Skin ulcers
- **Impaired growth**
- **Skeletal deformities**
- **Susceptibility to infections**

and affects some 9 per cent of people of Afro-Caribbean descent, and 18 per cent of African descent.

Sickle cell trait (HbAS): The sickling trait is frequently asymptomatic, but sickle cell crises (*see below*) can be caused by low oxygen tension (general anaesthesia, high altitudes or unpressurized aircraft). At times such patients may have renal complications causing haematuria, or splenic infarcts (*Table 5.11*).

Sickle cell anaemia (HbSS): Sickle cell anaemia is usually a serious disease with widespread complications (*Table 5.11*). It frequently becomes apparent about the third month of life.

Sickle cell disease presents four main problems:

1. Crises.
2. Chronic anaemia.
3. Chronic hyperbilirubinaemia.
4. Predisposition to infections.

Crises of sickle cell disease are of two types, painful and haematological.

Painful crises: These are usually due to infarction as a result of sickling brought on by infection, dehydration, hypoxia, acidosis or cold and cause severe pain and pyrexia. Infarcts are seen mainly in the spleen (with eventual auto-splenectomy), bones and joints, brain, kidneys, lungs, retinae and skin. Infarcts in the jaws can cause pain which may be mistaken for toothache or osteomyelitis. Abdominal crises may mimic a surgical emergency. Pulmonary infarcts cause chest pain and eventually lead to pulmonary hypertension and right-sided cardiac failure. The kidneys may also be affected, with haematuria and a nephrotic syndrome. Ocular defects or a cerebrovascular accident – often with hemiplegia may arise.

Haematological crises: These are often caused by parvovirus infections and can be of three types, namely:

1. Haemolytic.
2. Aplastic.
3. Sequestration crises.

Anaemia with a haemoglobin level often as low as 5–9 g/dl and the results of infarctions may be incapacitating, but the main cause of death in sickle cell anaemia is infection, particularly by pneumococci, meningococci and salmonellae, because of an associated immune defect mainly as a result of splenic dysfunction subsequent to infarction (Chapter 20). Chronic haemolysis leads to hyperbilirubinaemia and predisposes to bile pigment gallstones.

The morbidity and early mortality rates are thus high in sickle cell disease; most succumb eventually to cardiac failure, renal failure or overwhelming infection.

- **Laboratory investigations in sickling disorders**

In sickle cell disease there is significant anaemia, with a haemoglobin level typically below 9 g/dl, target cells and reticulocytosis of from 5 to 25%. Sickled erythrocytes are sometimes seen in a stained blood film. By contrast, haematological findings are often normal in sickle cell trait. Sickling may be demonstrated in both sickle cell anaemia and

trait, by tests relying on the low solubility of HbS (Sickledex) or by the addition of a reducing agent (such as 10 per cent sodium metabisulphite or dithionite) to a blood sample. Haemoglobin electrophoresis shows HbS and up to 15 per cent HbF (fetal haemoglobin), but no HbA in sickle cell anaemia.

- **General management of the sickling disorders**

Patients with sickle cell anaemia need regular monitoring of their haematological state and a comprehensive care programme. Blood transfusions are needed for cerebrovascular symptoms in early childhood or recurrent pulmonary thromboses. Many patients, however, remain with moderate degrees of anaemia for most of their lives and transfusions can and should usually be avoided, especially because of the risk of hepatitis C and HIV infection. Folic acid needs to be given regularly, 5 mg per day, and infections must be treated early. Painful crises should be treated promptly with analgesics and hydration.

Nowadays an increasing number of patients with sickle cell disease survive into late middle age. Infections and thromboses are the main causes of death.

- **Dental aspects of the sickling disorders**

Sickling disorders should be suspected in those with a positive family history and in any patient of African, West Indian or (less frequently) Asian or Mediterranean descent. All those at risk should be investigated if general anaesthesia is to be given. If the sickle cell test is positive, haemoglobin electrophoresis is required to establish the diagnosis, but if the haemoglobin is less than 11 g/dl sickle cell anaemia is probable.

The main principles in the sickling disorders are to prevent trauma, infection, hypoxia, acidosis or dehydration, all of which can precipitate a crisis.

Sickle cell trait (HbAS): Patients with the common sickle cell trait present few problems in management but if general anaesthesia is necessary full oxygenation must be maintained throughout. Respiratory or other infections must be treated vigorously as they can cause a crisis.

Sickle cell anaemia (HbSS): Patients with sickle cell anaemia must be managed with the help of a haematologist and some are now treated with hydroxyurea, which increases the levels of HbF.

General anaesthesia is hazardous in sickle cell anaemia because of the severe anaemia and because a crisis may be precipitated. Wherever possible, therefore, disease should be prevented. Any dental treatment should be carried out under local anaesthesia though it is best to avoid prilocaine which may in overdose cause methaemoglobinaemia. Relative analgesia may be used together with pulse oximetry.

General anaesthesia should only be carried out in hospital with full anaesthetic facilities and blood available for transfusion. Drugs that can cause respiratory depression, including sedative agents, should not be given as they may lead to hypoxia; acidosis and hypotension must also be avoided. Some infuse sodium bicarbonate.

At least 30 per cent oxygen is needed and, provided that there is no respiratory depression or obstruction, normal anaesthetic procedures can be used. If a crisis develops, oxygen is given and bicarbonate infused. A packed red cell transfusion may be required if the haemoglobin falls below 50 per cent.

Elective surgery should be carried out in hospital in a phase when haemolysis is minimal. It is best if anaemia is corrected preoperatively and the haemoglobin brought up to at least 10 g/dl. Exchange transfusion is occasionally required for major surgery but only in selected patients and carries the risk of red cell alloimmunization in up to 20 per cent. Oral administration of folic acid may also be valuable in correcting the anaemia.

Prophylactic antimicrobials should be given for surgical procedures and infections must be treated vigorously, since the patient may be immunocompromised if the spleen is non-functional. Penicillin V or clindamycin are appropriate antimicrobials.

Some patients have such severe pain during crises that they abuse analgesics and become addicts (Chapter 24). As a consequence of this or of multiple transfusions some patients become infected with blood-borne viruses. Pain should be controlled with paracetamol or codeine rather than aspirin, which in large doses can upset the acid–base balance.

Infarction may cause pain and predispose to osteomyelitis, especially in the mandible, or to cranial neuropathies, including labial anaesthesia. Oral pain, if not of local dental origin, may be caused by infarction or osteomyelitis. On rare occasions severe bone pain can be felt in the mandible only and even the patient may not recognize it as a sickling crisis. Pulpal symptoms are common in the absence of any obvious dental disease and sometimes pulpal necrosis has resulted. Acute infections should be treated immediately, since they may precipitate a sickling crisis.

Hard tissue changes are conspicuous: hypercementosis may develop and there is bone-marrow hyperplasia with apparent osteoporosis of the jaw. Skeletal but not dental maturation is delayed. The lamina dura is distinct and dense and the permanent teeth may be hypomineralized, though neither caries nor periodontal disease is more severe. The skull is thickened but osteoporotic with a 'hair on end' pattern to the trabeculae. The diploe are thickened, especially in the parietal regions, giving a 'tower skull' form. Lesions suggestive of bone infarction – dense radio-opacities – may be seen in the skull and/or jaws. Bone scans using technetium diphosphonate show increased uptake in these areas.

The thalassaemias

The thalassaemias are characterized by depressed synthesis of one or more of the globin chains, leading to decreased haemoglobin production and hypochromic microcytic anaemia. The unaffected chains are, however, produced in excess and precipitate within the erythrocytes to cause increased erythrocyte fragility and haemolysis.

Thalassaemias are predominantly found in those of Mediterranean, Middle Eastern or Asian descent. Typical features in homozygotes are chronic anaemia, marrow hyperplasia and skeletal deformities, splenomegaly and gallstones. Heterozygotes for thalassaemia may be asymptomatic.

Alpha-thalassaemias are mainly found in Asians. There are four main subtypes, of varying degrees of severity.

Beta-thalassaemias (Mediterranean anaemia) mainly affect peoples from the Mediterranean littoral and Afro-Caribbeans. Heterozygous beta-thalassaemia (thalassaemia minor or thalassaemia trait) is common and usually asymptomatic, except for mild hypochromic anaemia which may be aggravated by pregnancy or intercurrent illness. Homozygous beta-thalassaemia (Cooley's anaemia: thalassaemia major) is the most serious type and is characterized by failure to thrive, increasingly severe anaemia, hepato-splenomegaly and skeletal abnormalities.

Affected children are susceptible to folate deficiency (as in other chronic haemolytic states) and also to infection. In spite of the anaemia, patients with homozygous beta-thalassaemia become overloaded with iron (haemosiderosis), which damages the heart, liver, pancreas, skin and sometimes salivary glands, causing a sicca syndrome. Most thalassaemic children develop cardiomyopathy and dysrhythmias and die in early adult life from cardiac haemosiderosis. Hepatic and pancreatic dysfunction are also common.

Although homozygous beta-thalassaemia is usually lethal in adolescence, some survive: these patients are thought to have a milder variant, such as beta-thalassaemia with high levels of HbF (*see Fig. 5.1*).

• General management of beta-thalassaemias

Diagnosis is confirmed by finding severe microcytic, hypochromic anaemia with gross aniso- and poikilocytosis, target cell formation and basophilic stippling of erythrocytes. In contrast to iron deficiency anaemia, serum iron and ferritin levels are normal or raised and total iron binding capacity (TIBC) is normal. There is a great increase in HbF (fetal haemoglobin) and some increase in HbA2.

The main measures in beta-thalassaemia are blood transfusions and folic acid supplements. Iron overload is common and requires treatment with iron chelating agents (desferrioxamine). Hydroxyurea is now being used but the side effects can be a significant disadvantage. Splenectomy may be required if there is hypersplenism causing increased blood destruction which leads to accumulation of iron elsewhere and other complications.

• Dental aspects of beta-thalassaemias

Homozygous thalassaemia has a poor prognosis; hospitalization is frequently needed and there may, as a consequence, be psychological problems. The major oral changes in thalassaemia are enlargement of the maxilla caused by bone marrow expansion (chipmunk facies) which may cause difficulties in intubation for the induction of general anaesthesia but the chronic severe anaemia, and often cardiomyopathy, are in any event contraindications to general anaesthesia. Hepatitis B or C, or HIV carriage, may be a complication in multiply transfused patients. Since splenectomy results in an immune defect, it may be prudent to cover surgical procedures with prophylactic antimicrobials.

Alveolar bone rarefaction produces a chicken-wire appearance on radiography. Pneumatization of the sinuses may be delayed. Expansion of the diploe of the skull causes a hair-on-end appearance that is frequently conspicuous on lateral skull radiographs. There is often spacing of the teeth and forward drift of the maxillary incisors, so that orthodontic treatment may be indicated. Less common oral complications include painful swelling of the parotids and xerostomia caused by iron deposition, and a sore or burning tongue related to the folate deficiency.

Sickle cell trait with another haemoglobinopathy

Double heterozygotes can have sickle cell trait accompanied by thalassaemia or have both sickle cell haemoglobin S and C (SC disease). These are usually milder than isolated sickle cell anaemia (*Table 5.10*). The degree of anaemia is variable but they are at about the same level of risk from general anaesthesia as are those with sickle cell disease. Patients with other combined defects should be managed in the same way as are those with sickle trait.

Other haemoglobin variants

There are over 60 haemoglobin variants in which changes in the peptide chain cause chronic haemolytic anaemia. Splenomegaly is common and splenectomy is necessary for severe disease. The diagnosis is made by determining the heat-stability of the haemoglobin. Various drugs may increase haemolysis and the physician must therefore be contacted.

Erythrocyte membrane defects

Hereditary spherocytosis (acholuric jaundice) is the main form of congenital haemolytic anaemia in Caucasians. It is an autosomal dominant trait characterized by haemolytic anaemia, jaundice, splenomegaly, gallstones, haemochromatosis and skin ulcers. Episodes of haemolysis may be precipitated by infections. Splenectomy and folic acid treatment are almost invariably required.

Hereditary elliptocytosis (ovalocytosis) and hereditary stomatocytosis are similar autosomal dominant disorders characterized by chronic haemolytic anaemia. Splenectomy is invariably needed.

• Dental aspects of erythrocyte membrane defects

Post-splenectomy there may be a case for antimicrobial prophylaxis before invasive dental procedures.

Erythrocyte metabolic defects

The most common disorder of this type is *glucose-6-phosphate-dehydrogenase (G6PD) deficiency*, seen mainly in those of Mediterranean, Middle Eastern or Asian descent.

The main problem in G6PD deficiency is that haemolysis can be precipitated by a number of factors. Haemolysis is caused by oxidant drugs (*Table 5.12*), eating fresh fava beans, by intercurrent infection or, occasionally, spontaneously. The diagnosis is confirmed by enzyme assays carried out in a specialist laboratory. Haemolysis in G6PD is self-limiting and splenectomy is usually not needed.

Table 5.12   Main drugs which may cause haemolysis in G6PD deficiency

- **Aspirin**
- Sulphonamides
- Ciprofloxacin and other 4-quinolones
- Antimalarials
- Dapsone
- Prilocaine

• Dental aspects of G6PD deficiency

Apart from the problems of anaemia, it is vital to avoid oxidant drugs such as the sulphonamides (including co-trimoxazole), dapsone, or ciprofloxacin, which can precipitate haemolysis. Metabolic acidosis also causes haemolysis and must be avoided during general anaesthesia. Aspirin may also precipitate haemolysis, but usually only when used in high dosage. Prilocaine may, in large doses, induce methaemoglobinaemia, and is therefore best avoided (*Table 5.12*).

Acquired haemolytic anaemia

Intravascular destruction of erythrocytes can be caused by factors such as gross trauma, complement-mediated lysis, toxins and malaria.

These diseases are rare, but may occasionally have dental relevance because of anaemia, corticosteroid treatment or haemorrhagic tendencies.

BIBLIOGRAPHY

Addy D.P. (1986) Happiness is iron. *Br. Med. J.* **292**, 969–70.

Banerjee A.K., Layton D.M., Rennie J.A. *et al.* (1991) Safe surgery in sickle cell disease. *Br. J. Surg.* **78**, 516

Barret A.P. (1986) Oral complications of bone marrow transplantation. *Aust. NZ J. Med.* **16**, 239–40.

Barthelemy H., Chouvet B., Cambazard F. (1986) Skin and mucosal manifestations in vitamin deficiency. *J. Am. Acad. Dermatol.* **15**, 1263–74.

Bishop K., Briggs P. and Kelleher M. (1995) Sickle cell disease; a diagnostic dilemma. *Int. Endodont. J.* **28**, 297–302.

Brain M.C. (1980) The clinical assessment of the anaemic patient. *Medicine (UK)* **27**, 1395–7.

Carmel R. (1988) Pernicious anemia: the expected findings of very low serum cobalamin levels, anemia, and macrocytosis are often lacking. *Arch. Intern. Med.* **148**, 1712–14.

Carmel, R., Sinow R.M., Siegel M.E. *et al.* (1988) Food cobalamin malabsorption occurs frequently in patients with unexplained low serum cobalamin levels. *Arch. Intern. Med.* **148**, 1715–19.

Cawson R.A., Spector R.G. and Skelly A.M. (1995) *Basic Pharmacology and Clinical Drug Use in Dentistry*, 6th edn. Edinburgh, Churchill Livingstone.

Challacombe S.J., Scully, C., Keevil B. *et al.* (1983) Serum ferritin in recurrent oral ulceration. *Oral Pathol.* **12**, 290–9.

Charache S., Terrin M.L., Moore D. *et al.* (1995) Effect of hydroxyurea on the frequency of painful crises in sickle cell anaemia. *N. Engl. J. Med.* **332**, 1317–22.

Crawford J.M. (1988) Periodontal disease in sickle cell disease subjects. *J. Periodontol.* **59**, 164–9.

Demas D.C., Cantin R.Y., Poole A. *et al.* (1988) Use of general anesthesia in dental care of the child with sickle cell anemia. *Oral Surg. Oral Med. Oral Pathol.* **66**, 190–3.

Duggal M.S., Bedi R., Kinsey S.E. and Williams S.A. (1996) The dental management of children with sickle cell disease and β thalassaemia: a review. *Int. J. Paediat. Dent.* **6**, 227–34.

Field E.A., Speechley J.A., Rugman F.R. *et al* (1995) Oral signs and symptoms in patients with undiagnosed vitamin B$_{12}$ deficiency. *J. Oral. Pathol. Med.* **24**, 468–70.

Goldfarb A., Nitzan D.W. and Marmary L. (1983) Changes in the parotid salivary gland of β-thalassemia patients due to hemosiderin deposits. *Int. J. Oral Surg.* **12**, 115–19.

Green R. (1996) Screening for vitamin B$_{12}$ deficiency: caveat emptor. *Ann. Intern. Med.* **124**, 509–10.

Gregory G. and Olujohungbe A. (1994) Mandibular nerve neuropathy in sickle cell disease. *Oral Surg. Oral Med. Oral Pathol* **77**, 66–9.

Griffiths M.J., Sherani M. and Scully C. (1992) Screening for anaemia in persons requiring in-patient dento-alveolar surgery. *Health Trends* **24**, 128–30.

Herbert V. (1988) Don't ignore low serum cobalamin (vitamin B$_{12}$) levels. *Arch. Intern. Med.* **148**, 1705–7.

Iwu C.O. (1989) Osteomyelitis of the mandible in sickle cell homozygous patients in Nigeria. *Br. J. Oral Maxillofac. Surg.* **27**, 429.

Jacobs A. and Bentley D.P. (1980) Clinical investigation and management of disorders of iron metabolism. *Medicine (UK)* **27**, 1398–405.

Lane P.A. (1996) Sickle cell disease. *Pediatr. Clin. North Am.* **43**, 639–64.

Leading Article (1980) Preventing iron deficiency. *Lancet* **i**, 1117–18.

Locksley R.M. (1985) Infection with varicella-zoster virus after marrow transplantation. *J. Infect. Dis.* **152**, 1172–81.

Luker J., Scully C. and Oakhill A. (1991) Gingival swelling as a manifestation of aplastic anaemia. *Oral Surg. Oral Med. Oral Pathol.* **70**, 55–6.

McClure S., Custer E. and Bessman D. (1985) Improved detection of early iron deficiency in nonanaemic subjects. *J. Am. Med. Assoc.* **253**, 1021–3.

O'Rourke C. and Mitropoulos C. (1990) Orofacial pain in patients with sickle cell disease. *Br. Dent. J.* **169**, 130–2.

Oski F.A. (1985) Iron deficiency – facts and fallacies. *Pediatr. Clin. North Am.* **32**, 493–7.

Oski F.A. (1993) Iron deficiency in infancy and childhood. *N. Engl. J. Med.* **329**, 190–3.

Patton L.L., Brahim J.S. and Travis W.D. (1990) Mandibular osteomyelitis in a patient with sickle cell anaemia. *J. Am. Dent. Assoc.* **121**, 602–4.

Peterson P.K. (1983) A prospective study of infectious diseases following bone marrow transplantation: emergence of aspergillus and cytomegalovirus as the major causes of mortality. *Infect. Control* **4**, 81–9.

Porter S.R. and Scully C. (1996) *Innovations and Developments in Non-Invasive Oral Health Care.* Northwood, IL, Science Reviews.

Sansevere J.J. and Miles M. (1993) Management of the oral and maxillofacial surgery patient with sickle cell disease and related hemoglobinopathies. *J. Oral Maxillofac. Surg.* **51**, 912–16.

Schilling R.F. (1986) Is nitrous oxide a dangerous anaesthetic for vitamin B$_{12}$ deficient subjects? *J. Am. Med. Assoc.* **255**, 1605–6.

Schubert M.M. (1986) Head and neck aspergillosis in patients undergoing bone-marrow transplantation. *Cancer* **57**, 1092–6.

Scully C. (1988) *The Dental Patient.* Oxford, Heinemann.

Scully C. (1989) *The Mouth and Perioral Tissues.* Oxford, Heinemann.

Scully C. (1986) Testing for sickle cell anaemia. *Br. Dent. J.* **160**, 40.

Scully C. (1989) *Patient Care: a Dental Surgeon's Guide.* London, British Dental Association.

Scully C., Cawson R.A. and Griffiths M.J. (1990) *Occupational Hazards to Dental Staff.* London, British Dental Journal.

Seto B.G. (1985) Oral mucositis in patients undergoing bone-marrow transplantation. *Oral Surg. Oral Med. Oral Pathol.* **60**, 493–7.

Smith D.B. and Gelbman J. (1986) Dental management of the sickle cell anaemia patient. *Clin. Prevent. Dent.* **8**, 21–3.

Smith H.B., McDonald D.K. and Miller R.I. (1987) Dental management of patients with sickle cell disorders. *J. Am. Dent. Assoc.* **114**, 85–7.

Stockman J.A. (1987) Iron deficiency anaemia: have we come far enough? *J. Am. Med. Assoc.* **258**, 1645–17.

Terezhalmy G.T. and Hall E.H. (1984) The asplenic patient: a consideration for antimicrobial prophylaxis. *Oral Surg. Oral Med. Oral Pathol.* **57**, 114–17.

Van Dis M.L. and Langlais R.P. (1986) The thalassemias: oral manifestations and complications. *Oral Surg. Oral Med. Oral Pathol.* **62**, 229–33.

Walters M.C. and Abelson H.T. (1996) Interpretation of the complete blood count. *Pediatr. Clin. North Am.* **43**, 599–622.

Young N.S. (1995) Aplastic anaemia. *Lancet* **346**, 228–32.

APPENDIX TO CHAPTER 5

TERMINOLOGY RELATED TO THE BLOOD FILM EXAMINATION

Features	Description	Significance
Acanthocytes	spiculated RBCs	a-betalipoproteinaemia
Anisocytosis	variably sized RBCs	iron deficiency, thalassaemia
Atypical mononuclear cells	large mononuclear cells	viral infections
Basophil stippling	bluish stippling of RBCs on H&E staining	lead poisoning, thalassaemia
Blasts	nucleated precursors	leukaemia, myelofibrosis
Burr cells	irregular RBCs	uraemia
Howell–Jolly bodies	RBCs containing nuclear fragments	after splenectomy
Hypochromia	pale RBCs	iron deficiency, thalassaemia
Left shift	immature WBCs	infections
Leptocytes	RBCs with dark periphery and centre	liver disease, thalassaemia
Leukoerythroblastic anaemia	immature cells	malignant disease in marrow
Metamyelocytes	immature cells	malignant disease in marrow
Myelocytes	immature cells	malignant disease in marrow
Normoblasts	immature cells	malignant disease in marrow
Pappenheimer bodies	granules of spherocytes	lead poisoning, tumours, after splenectomy
Poikilocytes	variably shaped RBCs	iron deficiency
Polychromasia	variably stained RBCs	new RBC after bleeding, haemolysis
Polymorphs	polymorphonuclear leucocytes	normal
Promyelocytes	immature cells	malignant disease in marrow
RBCs (red blood cells)	erythrocytes	normal
Reticulocytes	young RBCs	haemolysis
Right shift	hypersegmented post-mature WBCs	uraemia, liver disease, megaloblastic
Schistocytes	fragmented RBCs	haemolysis
Sickle cells	sickle-shaped RBCs	sickle cell anaemia
Spherocytes	spherical RBCs	hereditary spherocytosis, haemolysis
Target cells	*see* Leptocytes	
WBCs (white blood cells)	leucocytes	normal

RBC, red blood cell; H&E, haematoxylin and eosin; WBC, white blood cell

6

Malignant disease

Key points

- Malignant tumours in children are mostly leukaemias, lymphomas, CNS tumours, bone tumours, Wilms' tumours, neuroblastomas or retinoblastomas.
- Malignant tumours in adults are mostly carcinomas of the lung, breast, stomach or colon.
- Malignant tumours may arise in the mouth or upper aerodigestive tract, or lymph nodes, or may involve the region secondarily by metastasis to lymph nodes or bone mainly.
- Leukaemias and lymphomas may be complicated by septicaemias arising from oral sources.
- Leukaemias are neoplasms arising in white blood cells.
- Leukaemias often present with lymph node enlargement, splenomegaly, purpura and a bleeding tendency, liability to infections, and anaemia.
- Oral purpura, spontaneous gingival bleeding, herpetic infections, candidosis, mouth ulcers and cervical lymphadenopathy may be presentations of leukaemia.
- Cytotoxic chemotherapy is the main treatment for leukaemias, but radiotherapy and bone marrow transplantation may also be used.
- Strict attention to oral hygiene, asepsis, avoidance of aspirin, platelet infusions to cover surgery and avoidance of general anaesthesia are the main points in relation to oral health care in leukaemia.
- Myelodysplastic syndromes are a spectrum of pre-leukaemic states.
- Myeloproliferative disorders (polycythaemia rubra vera, thrombocythaemia, myeloid metaplasia) are a group of disorders with marrow cell proliferation which may be pre-leukaemic.
- Neoplasms of plasma cells (myelomatosis, Waldenstrom's macroglobulinaemia) give rise to hyperviscosity and often amyloid deposits, liability to infections and disordered haemostasis.
- Amyloidosis is a manifestation of a spectrum of diseases, with the common feature of deposits of hyaline material in tissues, and subsequent organ dysfunction, and a bleeding tendency.
- Lymphomas are solid tumours of lymphoid tissue, classified as Hodgkin's and non-Hodgkin's lymphomas.
- Lymphadenopathy, weight loss, fever and impaired immunity are features of lymphoma but widespread involvement may include the gastrointestinal tract and CNS.
- Chemotherapy and radiotherapy are the main treatments for lymphomas.
- Oral carcinoma in the developed world is mainly a disease of the elderly male who uses tobacco and alcohol. In developing countries it is seen mainly in younger persons using tobacco or betel.
- Oral carcinoma is treated mainly with surgery, sometimes with radiotherapy.
- Surgical treatment of malignant neoplasms in the head and neck is inevitably disfiguring to some degree, but cosmetic results are continually being improved and much can be offered.

LEUKAEMIAS

Leukaemias are potentially lethal diseases in which there is neoplastic proliferation of white blood cells associated with specific gene mutations, deletions or translocations. In acute leukaemias primitive blast leucocytes are released into the blood, whereas in chronic leukaemias the abnormal cells retain most of the morphological features of their normal counterparts. The neoplastic cells are usually lymphoid or myeloid stem cells and classification is essential since there are important differences in response to treatment of the various types of leukaemia.

Treatment of leukaemia is with cytotoxic drugs singly or in combination and some of these are used for other neoplasms (*Table 6.1*). These drugs kill malignant cells but are not totally selective and thus almost invariably damage proliferating cells of the epithelium, bone marrow, growth centres and gonads in particular. The drugs therefore typically cause severe nausea and vomiting and various other toxic effects, particularly impaired immunity, alopecia and sometimes mucositis, and are teratogenic (Chapter 7). Patients may need to be isolated during the induction of remission as they are highly susceptible to infection at this time. Granulocyte colony stimulating factors may be valuable in non-myeloid malignancies and newer treatments for leukaemias such as retinoids, monoclonal antibodies, cytokines, peptide vaccines and T-cell infusions are being introduced. Supportive care of patients on cytotoxic chemotherapy includes control of nausea, infections, haemorrhagic tendencies, anaemia, hyperuricaemia (gout) and renal malfunction. Nausea may be controllable with phenothiazines (prochlorperazine) or domperidone or, if severe, by 5HT antagonists (granisetron, ondansetron or tropisetron).

Cytotoxic drugs are also potentially hazardous to staff, who should only handle them wearing medical gloves and protective eyewear, should dispose of waste and sharps carefully, and should not handle them while pregnant.

Dental management in leukaemia can often be complicated by oral lesions (mucositis or ulcers especially), bleeding tendencies and susceptibility to infection. Septicaemias may arise from oral infections in these patients and in other immunocompromised persons (Chapter 20).

Acute leukaemias

The acute leukaemias account for less than 2 per cent of cancers overall, but in children represent nearly 50 per cent of all malignant disease and are the most common cause of non-accidental death. Acute lymphoblastic leukaemia (ALL) is the most common childhood leukaemia.

Acute lymphoblastic and non-lymphoblastic (myeloblastic) leukaemias are clinically indistinguishable (*Table 6.2*). Anaemia, lymphadenopathy, splenomegaly, infections, fever, bruising and bleeding tendencies are the main features. There is an excess of circulating white blood cells but there may be phases when they are few (aleukaemic leukaemia).

Diagnosis of leukaemia is confirmed by the blood picture and, in particular, a stained blood film and bone marrow biopsy. Cytochemistry, analysis of membrane markers and immunophenotyping are required for categorization of the cell type.

Table 6.1 Cytotoxic drugs (*see* Chapter 7)

- Alkylating drugs
- Cytotoxic antibiotics
- Antimetabolites
- Antimicrotubule assembly agents
- Others

Table 6.2 Acute leukaemia – typical features

General features	Features due to leukaemic infiltration of	
	Bone marrow	Lymphoreticular system
Weight loss	Anaemia (pallor)	Lymphadenopathy
Weakness	Bone pain	Splenomegaly
Anorexia	Ineffective leucocytes (Infections)	
	Thrombocytopenia (Purpura and bleeding from mucous membranes)	

Acute lymphoblastic leukaemia

Acute lymphoblastic leukaemia (ALL), the most common leukaemia of childhood, has a peak incidence at 3–5 years but can affect any age group.

Malignant lymphoblasts proliferate and infiltrate the bone marrow, viscera, skin and nervous system. Marrow infiltration causes granulocytopenia, anaemia and thrombocytopenia.

Common (non-B-cell, non-T-cell) ALL is the most frequent type affecting children; T-cell ALL affects males predominantly and has a poor prognosis, while B-cell ALL also has a poor prognosis and is refractory to chemotherapy.

• General management of acute lymphoblastic leukaemias

Treatment is with cytotoxic drugs such as doxorubicin or vincristine, crisantapase and prednisolone. Over 90 per cent of patients have a remission within 6 weeks and the 5-year survival rate in children is now over 50 per cent. The risk of relapse is greatest in the first 18 months and maintenance therapy is therefore usually continued for 3 years.

Relapse is higher in males, partly because of occult testicular or CNS disease. Craniospinal irradiation is no longer routine in low-risk ALL patients but intrathecal methotrexate may be given. Bone marrow transplantation may give better control if chemotherapy fails to prevent relapse, especially in adults, but there are usually difficulties in finding a compatible donor.

Adult acute lymphoblastic leukaemia

Adult ALL has a worse prognosis than childhood ALL, but treatment schedules are similar.

Acute non-lymphoblastic (myeloblastic) leukaemia

Acute non-lymphoblastic leukaemia is less common than ALL in children. About seven subtypes have been described. Acute myeloblastic leukaemia (AML) is the most common, and is the most common acute leukaemia of adults. The clinical features are similar to those of acute lymphoblastic leukaemia except that CNS involvement is rare, though the disease occasionally causes cranial nerve palsies.

• General management of acute myeloid leukaemia

Combination chemotherapy has greatly improved the prognosis in AML but is much less successful than in childhood ALL. Remission can be obtained in up to 85 per cent of patients but is rarely maintained, though high dose cytarabine is proving useful. Whenever possible, bone marrow transplantation is employed and 5-year survival rates of up to 60 per cent are then reported. Acute pro-myelocytic leukaemia is now successfully treated with a vitamin A analogue, trans-retinoic acid.

• Dental aspects of the acute leukaemias

The main dental management problems in acute leukaemia are as follows:

1. Oral infections and ulceration.
2. Bleeding (Chapter 4).
3. Anaemia (Chapter 5).
4. Hepatitis B or C (Chapter 10) and HIV infection (Chapter 20).
5. Corticosteroid treatment (Chapter 14).
6. Disseminated intravascular coagulopathy (Chapter 4).
7. Complications of bone marrow transplantation (Chapter 5).
8. Abnormal susceptibility to infection. Antimicrobial cover is needed for any surgery, particularly for those with indwelling atrial catheters.
9. Interaction between methotrexate and nitrous oxide (largely theoretical).

Dental treatment should only be carried out after consultation with the physician, as it may be affected by various aspects of management and the probable life expectation. Other preoperative precautions include screening for hepatitis B and HIV. The patient may be in isolation, such as in a laminar flow room, when strict asepsis is indicated.

Preventive oral health care is essential and, where indicated, conservative dental treatment may be possible, but surgery (except for

---

Table 6.3 Oral and perioral manifestations of leukaemia

- Lymph node enlargement
- Purpura, and bleeding from gingivae
- Infections
  Candidosis and other fungal infections
  Herpes virus infections
- Oral ulceration
  Caused by herpes viruses, drugs and other factors
- Gingival swelling
  Caused by leukaemic infiltrate
- Drug side-effects
  Oral ulceration (many of the cytotoxics)
  Dry mouth (adriamycin)
  Pigmentation (busulphan)
  Candidosis (antimicrobials)
  (*see also* Appendix to Chapter 25)

---

emergencies such as fractures, haemorrhage, potential airways obstruction or dangerous sepsis) should be deferred until a remission phase.

Regional local anaesthetic injections may be contraindicated if there is a severe haemorrhagic tendency. Extractions should be avoided because of the dangers of haemorrhage and infections such as osteomyelitis or septicaemia. Before surgery, desmopressin or platelet infusions or blood may be needed, and antibiotics given until the wound has healed. Penicillin is the antibiotic of choice; intramuscular injections should be avoided as a haematoma may result. Sockets should not be packed, as this appears to predispose to infection. Operative procedures must be performed with strict asepsis and as atraumatically as possible. Absorbable polyglycolic acid sutures (Dexon) or soft catgut are preferred. Aspirin should not be given, since it aggravates bleeding.

Anaemia may be a contraindication to general anaesthesia – intravenous sedation or relative analgesia may be used as alternatives. However, nitrous oxide, which interferes with vitamin B_{12} and hence folate metabolism, is possibly contraindicated if the patient is being treated with methotrexate since the toxic effects of the latter may be exacerbated.

Oral manifestations (*Table 6.3*): Oropharyngeal lesions can be the initial complaint in over 10 per cent of cases of acute leukaemia overall but develop in 65–90 per cent of cases of acute myelomonocytic leukaemia. They

result from the disease or treatment or both. Oral bleeding and petechiae are typical manifestations, together with mucosal pallor and sometimes gingival swelling (localized or generalized), mucosal or gingival ulceration, pericoronitis and cervical lymphadenopathy. Fungal and herpetic infections are common and may occasionally be fatal. Candidosis is particularly common in the oral cavity and the paranasal sinuses. Aspergillosis or mucormycosis can involve the maxillary antrum and be invasive. Herpetic oral and perioral infection is common. Pseudomonas and other Gram-negative species occasionally cause oral lesions. It is important to appreciate that the mouth is a major source of septicaemia or metastatic infections in leukaemic patients. Other oral findings include tonsillar swelling, paraesthesiae (particularly of the lower lip), extrusion of teeth, and painful swellings over the mandible and of the parotid (Mikulicz syndrome).

The different subtypes of acute leukaemia differ in their oral manifestations to some extent. Mucosal pallor, petechiae, tonsillar swelling and cervical lymphadenopathy are typical of acute lymphoblastic leukaemia but gingival swelling is uncommon. By contrast, acute myeloblastic leukaemia causes gingival swelling in 20–30 per cent of patients. Many of the drugs used in the treatment of leukaemia can also cause oral lesions, and patients may have complications from bone marrow transplantation (Chapter 5).

Radiographic findings may include destruction of the crypts of developing teeth, thinning or disappearance of the lamina dura, especially in the premolar and molar regions, and loss of the alveolar crestal bone. Bone destruction near the apices of mandibular posterior teeth may also be seen. These bone changes may be reversible with chemotherapy.

Many of the oral lesions are aggravated or caused by local infection and chemotherapy. Oral lesions are readily infected by opportunistic microbes and such infections may have serious or fatal consequences. Isolation to protect the patient may therefore be needed. Lesions tend to become infected with Gram-negative bacteria, including pseudomonas, serratia, klebsiella, enterobacter, proteus and escherichia, or with candida or aspergillus. In severely immunosuppressed patients over 50 per cent of systemic infections result from oropharyngeal micro-organisms. Microbiological investigations with care to obtain specimens for anaerobic culture are essential to enable appropriate antimicrobial therapy to be given. Meticulous oral hygiene should be carefully maintained, with regular frequent warm 0.2 per cent aqueous chlorhexidine mouth rinses and the use of a soft nylon toothbrush.

Candidosis is common in leukaemia. Prophylactic antifungal therapy, such as nystatin mouthwashes (10 ml of 100 000 units of nystatin per ml, four times daily) or pastilles, or amphotericin lozenges, is therefore indicated (*see* Appendix to Chapter 1).

Herpetic infections are also very common and a troublesome cause of oral ulceration, as are varicella-zoster infections. They should be treated vigorously with aciclovir. Varicella–zoster (VZV) and measles viruses can also cause encephalitis or pneumonia. Prophylactic aciclovir has greatly reduced the incidence, morbidity and mortality from VZV infections, including those secondary to bone marrow transplants. Such patients may need VZV immune globulin in the event of contact. They must not be given live vaccines and infected persons should be kept away.

Many of the cytotoxic drugs (*see* Chapter 7) can precipitate mucositis, sometimes with oral ulceration. Methotrexate is a major cause, but ulceration may be prevented or ameliorated by concomitant intravenous administration of folinic acid ('leucovorin rescue'). Topical folinic acid (1.5 mg in 15 ml of water) used three times daily may also be useful. Established oral ulcers may improve with chlorhexidine or povidone-iodine mouthwashes, or appropriate antibiotics for specific infections. All-trans retinoic acid (ATRA) used in the treatment of acute promyelocytic leukaemia, may produce gingival swelling.

Severe bleeding from the mouth, particularly from the gingival margin, may result from the thrombocytopenia, and needs treatment with desmopressin, or even platelet transfusion.

Chronic leukaemias

Chronic lymphocytic leukaemia

Chronic lymphocytic leukaemia (CLL) is the most common type of leukaemia (*Table 6.4*).

Table 6.4   Chronic lymphoid leukaemias*

Disorder	Particular features
Chronic lymphocytic leukaemia	Splenomegaly, skin lesions. Prolonged survival possible
Sézary syndrome	Generalized lymph node enlargement; pruritus; exfoliating erythroderma. Chemotherapy relatively ineffective
Hairy cell leukaemia	Splenomegaly; may be associated with HTLV-1 infection; predisposes to mycobacterial infection. Relatively long survival. Responds to alpha interferon
Prolymphocytic leukaemia	Splenomegaly; resistant to chemo- and radiotherapy
Adult T-cell leukaemia–lymphoma	Resembles lymphocytic leukaemia. Poor prognosis

*Except for T-cell leukaemia and Sézary syndrome, which involve T-cells, most involve B-cells.

Men are particularly affected and some 60 per cent of cases are now detected coincidentally during a blood screen for an unrelated reason. Some 15 per cent of patients are asymptomatic and life expectancy may not be affected. In others, the disease is insidiously progressive, with fatigue, fever, weight loss, anorexia, haemorrhage and infections. Lymph node enlargement is early, whereas the liver and spleen enlarge later. Other effects are anaemia and thrombocytopenia. Leukaemic infiltration of the skin is more common than in chronic myeloid leukaemia and may be a major manifestation. The 5-year survival is over 50 per cent.

• General management of CLL

Asymptomatic patients may not need treatment. Those that are symptomatic can be treated with radiotherapy, cytotoxic drugs and corticosteroids (*Table 6.5*). B-cell CLL responds better to treatment than T-cell CLL and chlorambucil is particularly effective, though it predisposes to epithelial cancers. Purine analogues (fludarabine; pentostatin) are effective but depress the CD4 count (Chapter 20), predisposing to infections

Table 6.5	Treatment of chronic lymphocytic leukaemia

- *Chemotherapy*
  Chlorambucil (Leukeran) usually ± mustine or cyclophosphamide (Endoxana)
  plus
  Corticosteroids if there is haemolytic anaemia, marrow failure or thrombocytopenia
  Interferon for hairy cell leukaemia
- *Radiotherapy*
  May be used for treating large lymph node masses
- *Supportive care* includes
  Antimicrobials
  Allopurinol

Treatment required only if there is progressive marrow failure or complications.

Chronic myeloid leukaemia

Chronic myeloid leukaemia (CML) is characterized by proliferation of myeloid cells in the bone marrow, peripheral blood and other tissues. Most patients with CML suffer from chronic granulocytic leukaemia (CGL), but there are several rare subgroups (*Table 6.6*).

Chronic granulocytic leukaemia (CGL) mainly affects those over 40 years of age. The clinical features are similar to those of other chronic leukaemias. Splenomegaly and hepatomegaly are common but lymphadenopathy is rare. Anaemia, weight loss and joint pains are not uncommon.

Table 6.6	Chronic myeloid leukaemia

Disorder	Particular features
Chronic granulocytic leukaemia	Splenomegaly Positive for Philadelphia chromosome Fairly responsive to chemotherapy
Atypical chronic granulocytic leukaemia	Negative for Philadelphia chromosome Less responsive to chemotherapy
Juvenile	Mainly young children; lymphadenopathy Poor response to chemotherapy
Chronic myelomono-cytic leukaemia	Little response to chemotherapy
Chronic neutrophilic leukaemia	Difficult to differentiate from a benign leucocytosis
Eosinophilic leukaemia	Eventual cardiac damage

Table 6.7	Treatment of chronic myeloid leukaemia

- *Chemotherapy*
  Busulphan (Myleran) ± 6-thioguanine
  In the proliferative phase it may be necessary to use hydroxyurea (Hydrea) or mitobronitol (Myelobromol) ± radiotherapy
- *Supportive care* may include
  Antimicrobials
  Allopurinol

The prognosis of CGL is variable, but sooner or later there is transformation to an acute phase similar to AML (blast crisis). Fever, haemorrhage or bone pain are then common.

• General management of CGL

Treatment has been by means of cytotoxic drugs, and remission for over 12 months may follow a single course of chemotherapy. Radiotherapy may be useful later (*Table 6.7*). Alpha interferon is now prolonging survival in CGL.

In blast transformation the same treatment is given as for AML, but the acute phase is usually refractory to treatment and the patient may die within a few months.

• Dental aspects of chronic leukaemias

The prognosis of most chronic leukaemias is better than for the acute leukaemias and routine dental treatment is more likely to be required. Close cooperation with the haematologist is needed since (as in all leukaemias) there may be:

1. Bleeding tendencies.
2. Liability to infection.
3. Anaemia.
4. Susceptibility to hepatitis B, C and HIV infection.
5. Side-effects of treatment, such as pulmonary fibrosis as a result of busulphan.

Ampicillin and amoxycillin may cause irritating rashes similar to those seen in infectious mononucleosis and are unrelated to penicillin allergy (*see* Appendix to Chapter 1).

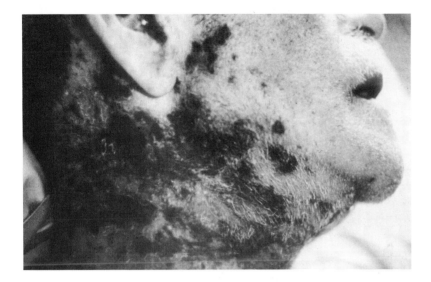

Fig. 6.1 Herpes zoster (shingles) of the upper cervical nerves in a patient dying from chronic leukaemia

Reports of oral manifestations relate mainly to CLL. Gingival swelling may be seen but less frequently than in the acute leukaemias. Palatal swelling (submucosal leukaemic nodules), gingival bleeding, oral petechiae or oral ulceration may also be features. Ulceration may be aggravated by cytotoxic therapy. Herpes simplex or zoster, and candidosis, are common (*Fig. 6.1*).

In CML oral haemorrhage may result from platelet deficiency. Leukaemic infiltration of lacrimal and salivary glands can cause Mikulicz syndrome. Granulocytic sarcoma is a rare tumour-like lesion which can affect the jaws or soft tissues and may rarely precede other manifestations or herald a blast crisis. Drug treatment of chronic leukaemia can also cause oral complications (Chapter 7).

MYELODYSPLASTIC (PRE-LEUKAEMIC) SYNDROMES

The myelodysplastic syndromes (MDS) are a group of stem cell disorders characterized by suppression of one or more cell lines in the bone marrow. Though the bone marrow is initially active, there is erythrodyspoiesis (*Table 6.8*). MDS affect mainly males over the age of 60 who present features of neutropenia, macrocytic anaemia and/or thrombocytopenia. Treatment includes erythrocyte and platelet transfusions, antibiotics, folic acid and vitamin B_6, and systemic corticos-

Table 6.8 The myelodysplastic syndromes	
• Refractory anaemia alone	RA
• Refractory anaemia with ring sideroblasts	RAS
• Refractory anaemia with excess blasts	RAEB
• Refractory anaemia with blasts in transformation	RABT
• Chronic myelomonocytic leukaemia	CML

teroids. Some patients succumb to marrow failure, others to acute leukaemia.

- ### Dental aspects of myelodysplastic syndromes

Dental management may be complicated by:

1. Bleeding tendencies due to thrombocytopenia (Chapter 4).
2. Anaemia (Chapter 5).
3. Neutropenia and a liability to infection, including HBV and HIV (Chapter 20).
4. Corticosteroids (Chapter 14).

Gingival infiltration and oral ulceration have been reported in chronic myelomonocytic leukaemia but not in the other myelodysplastic syndromes.

HYPEREOSINOPHILIC SYNDROME

Hypereosinophilic syndrome (HES) is an uncommon disorder in which there is hypereosinophilia in the absence of allergic disease, T-cell proliferation or parasitic infestation, together with disease of various organs, especially cardiomyopathy, and various rashes. Mucosal erosions may be an early feature.

HES is sometimes a pre-lymphomatous condition. Management is with systemic corticosteroids and usually hydroxyurea, or interferon.

MYELOPROLIFERATIVE DISORDERS

Proliferation of bone marrow cells, other than leucocyte stem cells, leads to myeloproliferative disorders (MPD). These are regarded as separate entities from leukaemias.

The main myeloproliferative disorders, which are all rare, are polycythaemia rubra vera, agnogenic myeloid metaplasia and essential thrombocythaemia. Chronic granulocytic leukaemia is sometimes also included in this group. Myeloproliferative disorders have several common features, transition between them is common, and any may progress to acute leukaemia (*Table 6.9*).

Polycythaemia rubra vera

Polycythaemia rubra vera is an expansion in the red cell population which may be primary and idiopathic (PRV) or, more commonly, secondary. PRV is uncommon, mainly a disease of the elderly and has a slight male predominance. The clinical features result from the essential disturbances, which are:

1. Proliferation of red cells.
2. Bone marrow replacement by erythropoietic tissue, and myeloid metaplasia in the liver and spleen.
3. Increased granulocyte and platelet production with platelet dysfunction.

The excessive red cell mass leads to *hyperviscosity syndrome* (*see below*) and the risk of thromboses, causing stroke, myocardial infarction or less serious consequences. Increased cell turnover may lead to hyperuricaemia, gout and renal damage. Bone marrow expansion causes bone pain and there may eventually be myelofibrosis. Haemostatic defects due to platelet dysfunction may cause bruising, bleeding or thromboses.

- **General management of PRV**

In the absence of treatment few patients with PRV survive more than 2 years. Repeated venesection reduces the red cell mass and extends survival to more than 10 years. Phosphorus-32 is also a simple and effective method of depressing erythropoiesis but may increase the risk of leukaemia. Cytotoxic agents (busulphan, chlorambucil or melphalan) may be given to suppress marrow activity, especially if there is thrombocytosis, but again they increase the risk of neoplasia. Cyproheptadine to control pruritus and allopurinol for gout may also be needed.

- **Dental aspects of PRV**

The main dental management problems are susceptibility to thrombosis and haemorrhage (Chapter 4). Venesection is especially important if surgery is indicated, since postoperative morbidity and mortality are greatly increased by thrombotic complications. There may also be oral complications from cytotoxic chemotherapy.

Table 6.9 Important findings in myeloproliferative diseases						
	RBC count	WBC count	Platelet count	Alkaline phosphatase	Marrow fibrosis	Spleno-megaly
Polycythaemia rubra vera	↑	↑	↑	↑	–	+
Agnogenic myeloid metaplasia	↓	↑	N or ↑	↑	+	++
Essential thrombocythaemia	N	N	↑↑↑	N	–	+

RBC, red blood cell; WBC, white blood cell.
Arrows indicate a value above ↑ or below ↓ normal (N).

Agnogenic myeloid metaplasia and myelofibrosis

Myelofibrosis may be primary (agnogenic myeloid metaplasia) or secondary (mainly to polycythaemia rubra vera, carcinomatosis or, rarely now, tuberculosis). Fibrosis of the bone marrow gradually depresses cell proliferation and extends throughout the reticuloendothelial system.

Most patients are elderly and suffer loss of weight, anaemia and thrombocytopenia. There may therefore be purpura and bleeding tendencies, weakness, bone pain, splenomegaly, hepatomegaly, gout and other features. The median survival time is about 5 years, but less in myelofibrosis secondary to carcinomatosis or polycythaemia.

• General management of myelofibrosis

Most patients need correction of anaemia and thrombocytopenia by transfusion. Bone pains and hyperuricaemia also need to be controlled. Corticosteroids are used occasionally.

• Dental aspects of myelofibrosis

Management problems may result from:

1. Anaemia.
2. Haemorrhage.
3. Possible hepatitis B, C or HIV carriage.
4. Corticosteroid treatment.

Essential thrombocythaemia

Thrombocythaemia may be an isolated abnormality, or associated with other myeloproliferative disorders. The common effects are thromboses or haemorrhages. There is usually gross thrombocytosis with functionally defective, giant platelets.

Radioactive phosphorus is the treatment of choice, but if this fails, cytotoxic drugs are used. Aspirin and dipyridamole are useful for preventing thrombosis, but heparin may be required. Surgery must be avoided until the disease is controlled, particularly because of the haemorrhagic tendencies.

CRYOGLOBULINAEMIA

Cryoglobulins are immunoglobulins which precipitate when cooled below the normal body temperature. Cryoglobulins are of three main types. Type I is monoclonal and a typical feature of lymphoproliferative and related diseases; types II and III are typically associated with the connective tissue diseases and some infections, where the effects may result from immune complex formation.

In most cases the underlying disease is more important and cryoglobulins are an incidental finding. However, cryoglobulins can occasionally cause effects as a result of their physical properties, particularly Raynaud's phenomenon, or occasionally, peripheral thromboses and obstruction of small vessels. Purpura or bleeding tendencies may also result. Plasmapheresis may be beneficial.

PLASMA CELL DISEASES

Plasma cell diseases are an uncommon group of B-lymphocyte disorders (*Table 6.10*), each characterized by overproduction of a specific immunoglobulin detectable, and often dominating other proteins, on electrophoresis. These homogeneous immunoglobulins (monoclonal immunoglobulins) are also

---

Table 6.10   Plasma cell diseases (dyscrasias)

- Multiple myeloma
- Solitary myeloma
- Waldenström's macroglobulinaemia
- Heavy chain disease
- Idiopathic monoclonal gammopathy

Table 6.11   Paraproteins found in the serum and urine in plasma cell diseases

	Serum	Bence-Jones proteinuria
Multiple myeloma	IgG (50%) IgA (25%) IgD or IgE rarely	+
Waldenström's macroglobulinaemia	IgM	Rarely
Heavy chain disease	Alpha chain (or gamma or μ)	–
Idiopathic monoclonal gammopathy	IgG (or IgA or IgM)	–

defective, and the rates of production of immunoglobulin light or heavy chains may be unbalanced, leading to overproduction of light chains (Bence-Jones protein) or heavy chains in the serum and urine (*Table 6.11*). Multiple myeloma, Waldenström's macroglobulinaemia, primary amyloidosis and the heavy chain diseases comprise this group, which are sometimes termed monoclonal gammopathies, or paraproteinaemias.

Multiple myeloma (myelomatosis)

Multiple myeloma is a disseminated plasma cell neoplasm that accounts for about 1 per cent of all malignant neoplasms. It is a disease mainly of the middle-aged and elderly, with a slight predilection for males, and is sometimes related to exposure to ionizing radiation or petroleum products.

The initial change is production of abnormal serum immunoglobulins, which are occasionally detectable by chance during routine haematological examination (by a raised ESR, rouleaux formation or high plasma viscosity) or serum protein investigations. Many years may elapse before symptoms appear. Neoplastic proliferation of plasma cells in the bone marrow and their release of cytokines such as interleukin-1, ultimately causes pain, osteoporosis and bone destruction, hypercalcaemia, renal failure, suppression of haemopoiesis, and many other secondary effects (*Table 6.12*). The abnormal immunoglobulins have defective antibody activity, and fail to protect against infections. There may also be plasma hyperviscosity with a clotting or bleeding tendency and neurological sequelae.

Findings leading to diagnosis (*Table 6.13*) include:

1. A monoclonal immunoglobulin peak (IgG in 55 per cent, IgA in 25 per cent and light chains only in 20 per cent) on electrophoresis of serum, or urine.
2. Plasma cell neoplasia on marrow biopsy.
3. Osteolytic lesions in skeletal radiographs or by bone scanning.

- **General management of multiple myeloma**

Anaemia, chronic renal failure, low serum albumin and high levels of serum β_2-

---

Table 6.12 Multiple myeloma: clinical findings

- Bone infiltration and destruction
- Bone pain (especially spinal)
  Pathological fractures
- Hyperviscosity syndrome
  Weakness
  Visual disturbances
  Bleeding tendencies
- Renal failure
- Anaemia
- Neurological lesions
  Paraesthesiae
  Weakness

Table 6.13 Multiple myeloma: investigational findings

- Radiological osteolytic lesions
- Biochemical
  Hypergammaglobulinaemia
  Bence-Jones proteinuria
  Monoclonal IgG (less often IgA, rarely IgD or IgE)
- Uraemia (in renal disease)
- Hypercalcaemia
- Hyperuricaemia (after treatment)
- Haematological
  Normochromic anaemia
  Leucopenia
  Thrombocytopenia
  ESR very high

---

microglobulin in the absence of renal disease, indicate a poor prognosis. Symptomatic patients, or those with progressive bone lesions or worsening paraproteinaemia, are treated by chemotherapy such as melphalan, cyclophosphamide or chlorambucil plus corticosteroids. The prognosis is variable, but the survival of treated patients averages 3 years. A few patients treated with cytotoxic chemotherapy develop acute myelomonocytic leukaemia.

More complicated chemotherapeutic regimens have not been shown to be consistently superior though relapses are probably best treated with vincristine, adriamycin (doxorubicin) and dexamethasone (VAD). New therapies include interferon, bone marrow transplantation and haematopoietic growth factors.

A growing number of asymptomatic patients are found to have myelomatosis by electrophoretic evidence of hypergammaglobulinaemia. Such patients must be followed and treatment started when appropriate.

• Dental aspects of multiple myeloma

Dental treatment may be complicated by:

1. Anaemia.
2. Infections.
3. Haemorrhagic tendencies.
4. Renal failure.
5. Corticosteroid therapy.

Oral manifestations: The skull, especially the calvarium, is ultimately affected in about 70 per cent of cases. Jaw lesions are seen less frequently. They mainly involve the posterior mandible but may be the first sign. Small, rounded, discrete (punched-out) osteolytic lesions are typical. Root resorption, loosening of teeth, mental anaesthesia and, rarely, pathological fractures are other possible effects. Rare complications are gingival bleeding, oral petechiae, cranial nerve palsies and herpes simplex or zoster infections. Amyloid may be deposited in the oral soft tissues causing local or more widespread swellings, such as macroglossia, the nature of which can be confirmed by biopsy.

Melphalan can cause severe mucositis. There is now some evidence that oral cooling with ice during the melphalan infusion can greatly reduce the mucositis.

Solitary plasmacytoma (localized myeloma)

A solitary plasmacytoma occasionally forms in the jaws or soft tissues nearby. There is usually no abnormal immunoglobulin production but, even when present, the levels are low.

Soft tissue plasmacytomas are more likely than bone lesions to remain localized. Local radiotherapy may be useful, but cytotoxic chemotherapy is contraindicated. Patients should be kept under observation as multiple myeloma develops in many, even after 20 years.

Waldenström's macroglobulinaemia (primary macroglobulinaemia)

Macroglobulinaemia is a rare disease in which B-lymphocytes produce excessive amounts of monoclonal IgM. These large globulin molecules make the blood abnormally viscous and cause hyperviscosity syndrome (*see below*). There is usually also anaemia, recurrent infections and haemorrhagic tendencies and a wide variety of other possible manifestations, particularly lymphadenopathy and splenomegaly.

Despite the analogous pathogenesis to multiple myeloma, foci of bone destruction and hypercalcaemia are not features of Waldenström's macroglobulinaemia, and renal involvement is uncommon. The prognosis of macroglobulinaemia is usually also slightly better than that of myeloma, but it may progress to lymphoma and a more rapid termination.

• General management of Waldenström's macroglobulinaemia

The clinical course is very variable but nearly 25 per cent of patients need no treatment for long periods and there is a median survival of over 3 years.

• Dental aspects of Waldenström's macroglobulinaemia

The major problems of dental treatment are:

1. Bleeding tendencies (Chapter 4).
2. Corticosteroid therapy (Chapter 14).
3. Anaemia (Chapter 5).

Oral manifestations: Haemorrhagic tendencies may cause spontaneous gingival bleeding or post-extraction haemorrhage. Deep punched-out ulcers of the tongue, buccal mucosa or palate have been reported, but are rare.

Heavy chain diseases

These are rare disorders in which gamma, alpha or mu immunoglobulin heavy chains appear in serum and urine. Gamma chain disease (Franklin's disease) may present with palatal swelling due to lymphoid swelling in Waldeyer's ring.

Benign monoclonal gammopathy and secondary macroglobulinaemia

Elderly patients who are otherwise healthy not infrequently produce excessive amounts of

Table 6.14   Diseases associated with amyloid formation

Disease	Amyloid fibril proteins
Idiopathic (primary) amyloidosis	AL proteins derived from immunoglobulin light chains
Myeloma-associated amyloidosis	AL proteins derived from immunoglobulin light chains
Secondary amyloidosis	AA protein derived from serum amyloid A (SAA) protein, an acute phase protein released by the liver under influence of chronic infections, chronic inflammatory states such as rheumatoid arthritis and ulcerative colitis via interleukin-1 from activated mononuclear phagocytes
Other forms of amyloidosis A heterogeneous group, some familial, others related to senility, medullary carcinoma of thyroid or calcifying epithelial odontogenic tumour and localized	A range of proteins, mainly like prealbumin

monoclonal immunoglobulin. It is essential not to interpret this finding as necessarily indicating myeloma. However, prolonged follow-up is essential to distinguish them from the 20 per cent who ultimately develop myeloma. Some others die from amyloid renal disease.

Many patients also produce large amounts of IgM secondary to connective tissue diseases, chronic liver disease or chronic lymphocytic leukaemia. This IgM is often polyclonal and not a precursor to myeloma or macroglobulinaemia.

Hyperviscosity syndrome

Hyperviscosity syndrome is characterized by slowing of the peripheral circulation caused by excessive amounts of high molecular weight plasma proteins. Polycythaemia, Waldenström's macroglobulinaemia or myeloma account for most cases.

The large protein molecules adsorb platelets and erythrocytes causing increased platelet adhesiveness and erythrocyte rouleaux formation. They also activate clotting factors and complement, causing local thrombosis and inflammation.

• General management of hyperviscosity syndrome

Venesection may be tried. Plasmapheresis reduces the viscosity, but treatment should be aimed at the primary condition. Penicillamine is useful for a short period only, since the side-effects can be severe.

• Dental aspects of hyperviscosity syndrome

Gingival haemorrhage or post-extraction haemorrhage, or taste loss or oral ulceration due to penicillamine, may be features.

AMYLOID DISEASE

Amyloid disease is the deposition in the tissues of an eosinophilic hyaline material with a characteristic fibrillar structure on electron microscopy. Amyloid disease can result mainly from deranged immunoglobulin synthesis, as in benign monoclonal gammopathy (primary amyloidosis) when the amyloid consists of AL protein, as does the amyloid associated with multiple myeloma, or more commonly from excessive stimulation of the reticuloendothelial system (secondary amyloidosis, *Table 6.14*). In the latter case the amyloid consists of AA proteins and is deposited mainly in and affects the function of the heart, skeletal muscle and gastrointestinal tract. Other secondary amyloid is of uncertain origin but affects mainly the spleen, liver, kidney and adrenals.

The widespread lesions in amyloid disease and the possible involvement of virtually any system, make this disorder protean in its manifestations including a bleeding tendency related to a Factor X defect.

• General management of amyloidosis

Amyloidosis is a manifestation of several diseases, not a disease in itself. An underlying cause must therefore be sought after the

Table 6.15 Simplified classification and main features of lymphomas	

Hodgkin's disease
Lymphocyte predominant
Nodular sclerotic
Mixed cellular
Lymphocyte depleted

Non-Hodgkin's lymphoma

Nodular	*Indolent course usually*
Poorly differentiated lymphocytic	Most frequent; disseminated
Mixed cellular (lymphocytic and histiocytic)	Good response to chemotherapy
Histiocytic	Aggressive; behaves like a diffuse lymphoma
Diffuse	*Aggressive course usually*
Lymphocytic	Chronic if well differentiated
	Others disseminated
Mixed cellular	Disseminated
Histiocytic	Formerly called reticulum cell sarcoma
Lymphoblastic	50 per cent develop acute lymphoblastic leukaemia
Burkitt's lymphoma	Good response to chemotherapy

Note: Many other classifications.

diagnosis is established by biopsy of lesional tissue, or by rectal or gingival biopsy examined with Congo red and polarized light. Combination therapy with corticosteroids, melphalan and fluoxymesterone may produce some improvement.

• Dental aspects of amyloidosis

Dental management may be influenced by the underlying disorder, or by cardiac, renal, adrenal, corticosteroid complications or a bleeding tendency. Macroglossia, gingival swellings, oral petechiae, bullae or, rarely, a sicca syndrome may result from amyloidosis, but virtually only in the primary type.

LYMPHOMAS

The lymphomas form a group of uncommon solid malignant tumours with a wide spectrum of clinical and pathological effects. Dental management may be complicated by anaemia, liability to infection and corticosteroid or cytotoxic therapy.

Lymphomas originate in lymph nodes or extranodal tissue in any part of the body, from any type of lymphocyte. They comprise Hodgkin's and non-Hodgkin's lymphomas. Immunological characterization of the cell lineage and the extent of the disease determine the treatment and prognosis (*Table 6.15*).

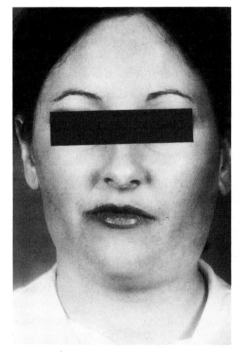

Fig. 6.2 Chronically enlarged cervical lymph nodes in a young patient raise the possibility of a lymphoma, tuberculosis or HIV infection

Hodgkin's disease

About 40 per cent of all lymphomas are Hodgkin's disease, which can affect any age group but particularly males in their thirties.

Table 6.16   Staging and treatment in Hodgkin's disease

Stage[a]	Definition	Treatment
I	Involvement of single lymph node or group of nodes	Radiotherapy
II	Involvement of two or more groups of lymph nodes on one side of diaphragm *or* Localized involvement of an extralymphatic organ or site and of one or more lymph nodes on the same side of diaphragm	Radiotherapy
III	Involvement of lymph nodes on both sides of diaphragm ± splenic or other sites	Radiotherapy (IIIA) *or* Quadruple therapy (IIIB)[b]
IV	Diffuse or disseminated disease of one or more extralymphatic organs or tissues ± associated lymph node involvement	Quadruple therapy[b]

[a]Stage is also qualified by a suffix A or B. B = presence of fever, night sweats or weight loss; A = absence of such systemic symptoms.
[b]Quadruple therapy is combined chemotherapy – either MOPP (Mustine, Oncovin, Prednisolone and Procarbazine) or ABVD (Adriamycin, Vincristine and Dimethyltriazenoimidazole-carboxamide).

Hodgkin's disease appears to originate in a cell of the monocyte–histiocyte series. There is progressive involvement of lymphoid tissue, often beginning in the neck (*Fig. 6.2*). The lymph nodes become enlarged, discrete and rubbery and can cause symptoms by pressure on other organs or ducts. Anaemia is common late in the disease.

Systemic symptoms including pain, remittent fever, night sweats, weight loss, malaise, bone pain and pruritus are common. Alcoholic drinks may cause pain in affected lymph nodes. Cellular immunity is impaired so that fungal and viral infections are common and may disseminate.

Treatment of Hodgkin's disease includes radiotherapy and chemotherapy (*Table 6.16*), depending on the staging of the disease. With such management the 5-year survival in the earlier stages is about 80 per cent and is over 60 per cent even in more advanced Hodgkin's disease. Those who relapse usually do so within the first 2 years.

Non-Hodgkin's lymphomas

Lymphomas other than Hodgkin's disease are increasing in frequency and have a variable but generally poor prognosis. Most non-Hodgkin's lymphomas (NHL) appear to be of B-cell origin and have a predilection for sites such as the gastrointestinal tract and CNS. They frequently involve the mesenteric lymph nodes and bone marrow but often enlargement of cervical lymph nodes is the first sign. NHL are being increasingly seen in persons infected with HIV and are second only to Kaposi's sarcoma in frequency in this group. They can also be a complication of the connective tissue diseases or cytotoxic chemotherapy.

In general, NHL are treated by multiple chemotherapy, since early dissemination is common, but radiotherapy may be useful in the initial stages.

• Dental aspects of the lymphomas

The main problems from lymphomas that may influence oral health care are:

1. Oral infections, especially with viruses and fungi.
2. Mucositis or oral ulceration caused by cytotoxic drugs.
3. Anaemia.
4. Corticosteroid therapy.
5. Bleeding tendencies.
6. Impaired respiratory function (pulmonary fibrosis due to irradiation).
7. Acute leukaemia (7 per cent of treated patients).

Oral manifestations: Painless enlarged cervical lymph nodes are the initial complaint in 50 per cent of cases. A lymphoma may form in the oral cavity or oropharynx but this is rare except in HIV infection.

Involvement of Waldeyer's ring is more common in NHL than in Hodgkin's disease. Lesions appear as erythematous swellings, often with surface ulceration as a result of trauma, and may involve the pharynx, palate, tongue, gingivae or lips, but lesions are frequently present systemically. The jaws may also rarely be involved. Herpes zoster, herpetic stomatitis and oral candidosis may be seen, especially in those on cytotoxic or radiation therapy. Zoster, secondary to immunodeficiency, may be the first sign of the disease. Though Hodgkin's disease frequently involves the cervical lymph nodes, it rarely affects the mouth, but when it does, is not clinically distinguishable from NHL.

Oral lesions are only rarely the initial manifestation of NHL but an oral lymphoma may be the first sign of HIV infection. A lymphoma in the mouth of a young male particularly should therefore lead to the suspicion of HIV infection.

In the perioral regions, NHL are one of the most common type of non-epithelial tumour of salivary glands in adults, but account for about 5 per cent of salivary gland tumours. Their diagnosis causes difficulties in this site because of possible confusion with benign lymphoepithelial lesion and Sjögren's syndrome, and the fact that either may progress to lymphoma in about 20 per cent of cases. By contrast, Hodgkin's disease of salivary glands is rare. The high frequency shown in some series is due to inclusion of disease of the cervical lymph nodes, but even these remain discrete and rarely involve the adjacent submandibular or parotid gland parenchyma.

Burkitt's lymphoma is often EBV-related and is seen particularly in Africa, in children, presenting mainly with jaw swellings but also frequently involving abdominal viscera. It responds well to chemotherapy.

A rare type of T-cell lymphoma is the cause of some cases of midline granuloma syndrome in which there may be oral complications (Chapter 21).

OTHER MALIGNANT DISEASE

Solid tumours in childhood

These are rare tumours most of which are treated with surgery plus radiotherapy and/or chemotherapy which can damage craniofacial and dental development (Chapter 7).

Brain tumours, especially gliomas, are the most frequent solid tumours in childhood. Most are low grade astrocytomas or medulloblastomas and are found in the posterior cranial fossa.

Wilms' tumour arises from the kidney but may metastasize to the lungs, liver or bone. It is often associated with aniridia.

Retinoblastomas have a strong hereditary basis, appear in pre-school children and cause blindness.

Neuroblastomas arise from neural crest cells, especially abdominally, and metastasize to lymph nodes, lungs, bone and liver.

Oral cancer

Oral cancer is usually squamous cell carcinoma; common sites are the lips, lateral border of the tongue and floor of mouth.

Oral cancer is mainly a disease of the elderly and there is a wide geographical variation in incidence, with very high rates particularly in India, Sri Lanka and Brazil.

Predisposing causes are obscure, though lip cancer is seen mainly on the sun-exposed lower lip, especially in white races, in sunny climates, and in persons frequently exposed to the sun. Alcohol and cigarette consumption is associated with mouth cancer. In some areas, betel and/or tobacco chewing, or the use of oral snuff, are responsible. A diet rich in fresh fruit and vegetables appears to have some protective effect.

Premalignant lesions include erythroplasia (erythroplakia) and particularly speckled leukoplakia or leukoplakias in the floor of the mouth. Syphilitic leukoplakia is now rare and the malignant potential of candidal leukoplakia is uncertain.

As a result of the HIV epidemic, oral lymphomas and Kaposi's sarcoma are now considerably more common. The hairy leukoplakia of HIV infection does not appear to be premalignant.

The majority of salivary gland tumours are pleomorphic adenomas but there is a higher proportion of malignant tumours in the sublingual and minor oral salivary glands than in the parotids. Though uncommon there is also a higher relative frequency of malignant salivary gland tumours in children.

Patients with any cancer may have severe psychological disturbances in view of the nature of the illness. These problems are compounded in oral cancer since there are additional disabilities, particularly interference with speech and swallowing, and disfigurement.

• General management of oral cancer

Any lesion of dubious nature should be biopsied and second primary tumours, usually in the upper aerodigestive tract, should be excluded by chest radiography and endoscopy. Patients with established oral cancer are best managed by a team of specialists, including the dental and maxillofacial surgeons, as well as the oncologist. Opinion varies as to the value of radiotherapy or surgery. Many early carcinomas can be treated by either method, while advanced cancer is, in general, incurable by any technique. Palliation is then the most that can be offered. Cytotoxic chemotherapy has not proved to offer any better prognosis and, indeed causes a greater morbidity and mortality.

Lingual and labial cancers are often managed with radiotherapy, which may also provide the best palliation in patients with advanced disease. Cancer of the floor of the mouth presents considerable problems in surgery and may necessitate partial mandibulectomy.

• Chemoprevention of oral cancer

Chemopreventive agents clearly show promise in the control of potentially malignant lesions such as leukoplakia. Retinoids (synthetic vitamin A derivatives) and carotenoids (vitamin A precursors) are used; their main drawback is that retinoids are often teratogenic and hepatotoxic. Isotretinoin is effective but at high doses is toxic. Beta-carotene is less toxic but less effective. Fenretinide may be better. Vitamin E may also be of benefit. The major drawback for most current chemopreventive agents, however, is recurrence when treatment is discontinued.

Antral carcinoma

Antral carcinoma is a rare neoplasm of unknown aetiology but woodworking is a known occupational hazard. It is a disease of the elderly.

Antral carcinoma causes maxillary pain or effects from expansion and infiltration of adjacent tissues. It may cause an intra-oral swelling or ulcer in the palate or upper vestibule; a swelling in the cheek; unilateral nasal obstruction or epistaxis; obstruction of the nasolacrimal duct with consequent epiphora; infraorbital anaesthesia if the nerve is involved; or proptosis and ophthalmoplegia if the orbit is invaded.

Further details can be found in standard texts of ENT and maxillofacial surgery: treatment is usually by surgery.

Nasopharyngeal carcinoma

Nasopharyngeal carcinoma (NPC) is a rare neoplasm which may be associated with Epstein–Barr virus and is especially common in Asia, particularly amongst the Southern Chinese, some Eskimo races and in parts of North Africa such as Tunisia. A similar tumour, *undifferentiated carcinoma with lymphoid stroma*, is one of the most common types of salivary gland cancer in Eskimos and Southern Chinese.

Often asymptomatic in itself, since the neoplasm does not obstruct the nasopharynx, NPC can present in a variety of ways.

1. Isolated cervical lymph node enlargement.
2. Unilateral conductive deafness (from obstruction of the Eustachian tube).
3. Elevation and immobility of the soft palate.
4. Pain, sometimes with anaesthesia, in the ipsilateral tongue, lower teeth and lower lip (invasion of the mandibular division of the trigeminal nerve).

A combination of the above is Trotter's syndrome. Treatment is usually by radiotherapy.

Cancer in other sites

Tumours involving other parts of the body are discussed in the appropriate chapters. Their most obvious oral importance is as a

Table 6.17 Oral manifestations of internal cancer

- Metastases in jaws or (rarely) oral soft tissues, especially from cancer of:
  Breast
  Lung
  Prostate
  Thyroid
  Kidney
  Stomach
  Colon
- Effects of tumour metabolites
  Facial flushing (carcinoid syndrome)
  Pigmentations (ectopic ACTH-secreting tumours)
  Amyloidosis (multiple myeloma)
  Oral erosions (glucagonoma)
- Changes caused by other functional disturbances
  Purpura, anaemia, infections (leukaemia)
  Infections (lymphoma)
  Bleeding (liver cancer)
  Anaemia (bleeding from gastrointestinal tumours)
- Mucocutaneous diseases
  Dermatomyositis (carcinoma)
  Acanthosis nigricans (gastric carcinoma)
  Erythema multiforme (lymphoma, leukaemia or carcinoma, especially after radiotherapy)
  Pemphigus vulgaris
  Paraneoplastic pemphigus
  Dermatitis herpetiformis
- Inherited disorders with predisposition to internal malignancy and oral lesions
  Cowden's syndrome
  Gardner's syndrome
  Multiple endocrine neoplasia type III
  Neurofibromatosis (von Recklinghausen's disease)
  Gorlin–Goltz syndrome
  Tylosis
  Tuberous sclerosis
  Maffuci syndrome

Table 6.18 Five-year survival (per cent) of cases of malignant disease[a]

Site	Sex	No. of registrations	5-year survival rate[b]
Lip	M	1 196	93.53
	F	194	84.01
Tongue	M	907	37.13
	F	628	45.93
Oesophagus	M	5 033	6.27
	F	3 983	7.88
Stomach	M	19 619	7.38
	F	12 938	7.25
Large intestine, except rectum	M	14 564	29.63
	F	19 703	29.35
Rectum and recto-sigmoid junction	M	13 003	30.79
	F	10 537	32.94
Pancreas	M	7 051	3.78
	F	6 071	3.12
Larynx	M	3 890	64.40
	F	725	56.85
Trachea, bronchus and lung	M	71 710	7.80
	F	16 461	7.02
Breast	M	472	59.57
	F	57 232	56.81
Cervix, uteri, excluding *in situ*	F	11 965	54.42
Prostate	M	17 943	35.93
Bladder	M	16 172	53.79
	F	5 629	47.35
Brain	M	3 717	14.81
	F	2 620	16.12
Hodgkin's disease	M	2 546	55.81
	F	1 581	57.28
Lymphatic leukaemia	M	2 560	30.41
	F	1 741	34.15
Myeloid leukaemia	M	2 314	7.60
	F	2 140	6.44
All leukaemias	M	5 555	18.17
	F	4 422	17.24

[a]1971–73 registrations: some may have improved recently.
[b]Corrected for age, etc.

source of metastases, which can form in the jaws or occasionally soft tissues and can mimic a simple epulis clinically. Histological examination of all such swellings is therefore essential. Studies of oral health in patients with advanced malignant disease have shown a high prevalence of oral symptoms, particularly xerostomia, which is seen in nearly three-quarters, but also soreness, taste disturbances and difficulties with wearing dentures. Candidosis is common.

Other oral manifestations of internal malignancy are summarized in *Table 6.17*.

Less obviously it must be borne in mind that any patient who has had cancer, even if treatment has apparently been successful, often has a limited expectation of life. If,

further, there are signs of spread of the tumour such as involvement of cervical or other lymph nodes, or the appearance of oral lesions, then the prognosis is very poor indeed. The dental care of such patients may therefore have to be modified accordingly. Though there is great individual variation, the overall 5-year survival rates are shown for important cancers in *Table 6.18*, as it is perhaps insufficiently widely appreciated how short survival may be in some cases. Thus in the case of carcinoma of the pancreas only 3–4 per cent survive for 5 or more years, but even the 1-year survival rate is only 10

Table 6.19   Langerhans cell histiocytoses

	Age of onset	Bone lesions	Skin or mucosal lesions	Visceral lesions	Pituitary lesions	Treatment	Prognosis
Solitary eosinophilic granuloma	>10 yr	+	±	–	–	Surgery Local radiotherapy	Good
Multifocal eosinophilic (Hand–Schüller–Christian disease)	<5 yr	+	+	±	+	Chemotherapy	Variable
Letterer–Siwe disease	Infancy	+	+	+	+	Chemotherapy Steroids	Often fatal

per cent. To put it another way, a patient who develops cancer of the pancreas has only a one in ten chance of surviving for more than a year.

LANGERHANS CELL HISTIOCYTOSIS (SOLITARY AND MULTIFOCAL EOSINOPHILIC GRANULOMA)

These diseases are tumours or tumour-like lesions of Langerhans cells – counterparts of macrophages which are antigen-presenting cells. This cell is recognizable by electron microscopy by the presence of rod-shaped Birbeck granules and by immunohistochemistry.

The three main types of disease are solitary eosinophilic granuloma, multifocal eosinophilic granuloma (Hand–Schüller–Christian disease) and Letterer–Siwe disease.

Both eosinophilic granuloma and Hand–Schüller–Christian disease are relatively benign. Letterer–Siwe disease is disseminated and malignant (*Table 6.19*).

Solitary eosinophilic granuloma

Eosinophilic granuloma is an osteolytic lesion of bone with a predilection for the mandible. Adults are mainly affected and typical symptoms are pain, tenderness, swelling or bone destruction. Radiographs show a tumour-like area of rarefaction. The diagnosis is by biopsy and typically shows foamy histiocytes and many eosinophils with ill-defined, somewhat fibrillar background and areas of necrosis. A bone scan should be carried out to ensure that the disease is not multifocal.

Eosinophilic granuloma is relatively benign and responds to curettage or, if recurrent, to modest doses of irradiation, or chemotherapy with vinblastine, prednisolone or cyclosphosphamide.

Eosinophilic granuloma can also affect the oral soft tissues, but less frequently than the mandible. However, a histologically somewhat similar lesion can be traumatic in origin or reactionary without any history of trauma and there must be some doubt about the nature of eosinophilic granulomas of soft tissues reported in the past.

Multifocal eosinophilic granuloma and Hand–Schüller–Christian syndrome

These lesions are the same histologically as the solitary eosinophilic granuloma and are sometimes referred to indifferently as Hand–Schüller–Christian disease. *Hand–Schüller–Christian syndrome*, strictly speaking, comprises osteolytic lesions of the skull, exophthalmos and diabetes insipidus and is a variant of multifocal eosinophilic granuloma. Multifocal eosinophilic granuloma most frequently develops before the age of 5 years.

Diagnosis is by biopsy which shows essentially the same features as solitary eosinophilic granuloma, and by skeletal radiography or bone scan to assess the extent of the disease.

Flat bones including the mandible are the main sites and soft tissues also become involved, but the classic Hand–Schüller–Christian triad develops in only 25 per cent. Lymphadenopathy and hepatosplenomegaly may develop in up to 50 per cent.

Malaise, fever and infections of the ear, mastoid and respiratory tract are common.

Nevertheless, in approximately 50 per cent of cases the lesions gradually resolve spontaneously over the course of years but can leave residual disabilities as a result of limb lesions or diabetes insipidus. To reduce such complications, or in refractory cases, chemotherapy in relatively modest doses may be used as for solitary lesions. The mortality may be 25–30 per cent. The younger the patient and the more widespread the disease, the worse the prognosis.

• Dental aspects of eosinophilic granuloma

Eosinophilic granuloma is an occasional cause of tumour-like swelling and radiolucent lesions of the mandible but the diagnosis can only be made by biopsy. Bone scans may show that the disease is (or becomes) multifocal, but the multifocal eosinophilic granuloma of childhood or Hand–Schüller–Christian syndrome rarely has initial manifestations in the jaws. However, either type of disease can produce a characteristic form of periodontal destruction with gross gingival recession and alveolar bone loss, typically involving a small group of teeth and often exposing the roots of the teeth, with a 'teeth floating in air' appearance on radiography.

Otherwise, complications can arise from treatment, either radiotherapy to the oral or para-oral regions, or chemotherapy with corticosteroids or cytotoxic agents.

In the case of solitary eosinophilic granuloma of soft tissues, care must be taken to distinguish the lesion from the traumatic eosinophilic granuloma. However, this depends upon the histopathologist. 'Traumatic' eosinophilic granuloma eventually resolves spontaneously, though it may need to be excised for cosmetic reasons. Alternatively, the lesion may be excised because of its clinical resemblance to a tumour.

Letterer–Siwe disease

Letterer–Siwe disease was previously thought to be a different disease from those just described. Nevertheless, the Langerhans cell can be identified in the lesions.

Clinically, Letterer–Siwe disease typically affects children between the ages of 2 and 3

years and may follow a rapidly fatal course. The main features are lymphadenopathy, hepatosplenomegaly, and bone and skin lesions. Fever, infections and bleeding tendencies are secondary to pancytopenia which results from marrow displacement by the histiocyte-like cells.

Diagnosis is by biopsy, showing infiltration of the tissues by proliferating histiocyte-like cells which, unlike those of eosinophilic granuloma, contain little or no lipid.

The disease is frequently rapidly fatal and occasionally death follows within a week of diagnosis. Treatment with radiotherapy, corticosteroids and cytotoxic drugs is rarely successful, but rarely, the course of the disease is less acute and recoveries have been reported.

• Dental aspects of Letterer–Siwe disease

In view of the age group mainly affected and the rapidity of the course, patients are unlikely to be seen by dentists. In the few older patients with a more chronic form of the disease, the features relevant to dentistry are essentially those of severe types of multifocal eosinophilic granuloma. Corticosteroid treatment may complicate dental management.

TERMINAL CARE

In any incurable disease, management must include particular attention to the psychological problems of the patient. Hope is all-important. Patients may or may not know, or may not want to know, that they have malignant disease, and even if they are aware of it may not appreciate, or be willing to accept, the prognosis. Many different persons are involved in the care of these individuals and it is most important that there is good communication so that all are aware of (a) the prognosis; (b) how much the patient understands about their disease; (c) their psychological reactions to cancer; and (d) the side-effects of treatment. The quality of life is as important as, or more important than, its duration.

The type of oral health care should to some extent be tailored to take account of the prognosis and must always be planned in relation to the interest that the patient has in their oral state. Just because patients are dying does not mean, however, that they should be allowed to suffer from pain, or that their appearance be neglected. Indeed, the provision of dental attention, for example the construction of a new denture, may help the patient's morale. Further details are given in Chapter 7.

Potent analgesics, such as narcotics, sedatives or antidepressants, may be needed in terminal cancer and can influence dental care. Morphine and diamorphine are the drugs of choice for severe pain. Phenazocine may be valuable in patients intolerant of, or allergic to, morphine. Pethidine has too short an action and the metabolite norpethidine can accumulate in renal failure and then cause convulsions. Buprenorphine is a partial agonist and should be avoided.

Dextromoramide is only very short-acting but can be useful to 'cover' painful procedures. NSAIDS may help ease bone pain, while dexamethasone helps headaches associated with raised intracranial pressure. Carbamazepine or tricyclic antidepressants may relieve pain due to tumour infiltrating nerves.

BIBLIOGRAPHY

Ali A. and Bennington I. (1995) Restorative care in oral malignancy. In Porter S.R. and Scully C. (eds), *Oral Health Care for Those with HIV Infection and Other Special Needs.* Northwood, Science Reviews, pp. 189–98.

Aractingi S., Janin A., Zini J.M. *et al.* (1996) Specific mucosal erosions in hypereosinophilic syndrome. *Arch Dermatol.* **132**, 535–41.

Armitage J.O. (1993) Treatment of non-Hodgkin's lymphomas. *N. Engl. J. Med.* **328**, 1023–30.

Barbas A.P. (1980) Surgical problems associated with polycythaemia. *Br. J. Hosp. Med.* **23**, 289–94.

Barnard N., Scully C., Eveson J.W., Cunningham S. and Porter S.R. (1993) Oral cancer development in oral lichen planus. *J. Oral Pathol. Med.* **22**: 421–4.

Bennett J.M. (1982) The French, American British (FAB) cooperative group proposals for the classification of myelodysplastic syndromes. *Br. J. Haematol.* **51**, 189–99.

Bloch S. (1980) Psychiatric management of the dying patient. *Medicine (UK)* **36**, 1837–41.

Bokkerink J.P.M. and de Vaan G.A.M. (1980) Histiocytosis X. *Eur. J. Pediatr.* **135**, 129–56.

Boyle P., MacFarlane G.J., Blot W.J., Chiesa F., Lefebvre J.L., Mano Azul A., Scully C. and de Vries N. (1995)

European School of Oncology Advisory Report to the European Commission for the 'Europe Against Cancer Programme'. *Oral Oncol: Eur. J. Cancer* **31B**, 75–85.

Boyle P., Macfarlane G.J., McGinn R., Zheng T., La Vecchia C., Maisonneuve P. and Scully C. (1990) International epidemiology of head and neck cancer. In: De Vries N. and Gluckman J. (eds), *Second Primary Cancers of Head and Neck,* Heidelberg, Springer-Verlag, pp. 80–138.

Boyle P., MacFarlane G.J., Maisonneuve P., Zheng T., Scully C. and Tedesco B. (1990) Epidemiology of mouth cancer in 1989. *J. R. Soc. Med.* **83**, 724–30.

Boyle P., MacFarlane G.J. and Zheng T. (1995) Recent advances in the epidemiology of head and neck cancer. *Curr. Opin. Oncol.* **4**, 471–7.

Boyle P., Veronesi Y., Tubiana M., Alexander F.E., Calais da Silva F. *et al.* (1995) European School of Oncology Advisory Report to the European Commission for the 'Europe Against Cancer Programme'. *European Code Against Cancer. Eur. J. Cancer.* **9**, 1395–405.

Boyle P., Zheng T., MacFarlane G.J., McGinn R., Maisonneuve P., La Vecchia C. and Scully C. (1990) Recent advances in etiology and epidemiology of head and neck cancer. *Curr. Opin. Oncol.* **2**, 539–45.

Carl W. (1980) Dental management and prosthetic rehabilitation of patients with head and neck cancer. *Head Neck Surg.* **3**, 27–42.

Cawson R.A., Spector R.G. and Skelly A.M. (1995) *Basic Pharmacology and Clinical Drug Use in Dentistry,* 6th edn. Edinburgh, Churchill Livingstone.

Coleman J.J. (1986) Complications in head and neck surgery. *Surg. Clin. North Am.* **66**, 149–69.

Cox M.F., Maitland N.J. and Scully C. (1993) Human herpes simplex-1 and papillomavirus type 16 homologous DNA sequences in normal, premalignant and malignant oral mucosa. *Oral Oncol.: Eur. J. Cancer* **29B**, 215–20.

Declerck D. and Vinckier F. (1988) Oral complications of leukemia. *Quintessence* **19**, 575–83.

Dreizen S., McCredie K.B., Bodey G.P. and Keating M.J. (1986) Quantitative analysis of the oral complications of anti-leukaemia chemotherapy. *Oral Surg. Oral Med. Oral Pathol.* **62**, 650–3.

Dunbar C.E. and Nienhuis A.W. (1993) Multiple myeloma; new approaches to therapy. *J Am. Med. Assoc.* **269**, 2412–16.

Dunn N.L., Russell E.C. and Maurer H.M. (1990) An update in pediatric oncology. *Pediatr. Dent.* **12**, 10–19.

Editorial (1980) Paraproteinaemia. *Br. Med. J.* **1**, 273–4.

Epstein J.B., Priddy R. W., Sparling T. *et al.* (1986) Oral manifestations in myelodysplastic syndrome. *Oral Surg. Oral Med. Oral Pathol.* **61**, 466–70.

Epstein J.B., Schubert M. and Scully C. (1991) Evaluation and treatment of pain in patients with orofacial cancer. *Pain Clinic.* **4**, 3–20.

Epstein J.B., Scully C. and Spinelli J.J. (1992) Toluidine blue and Lugol's iodine application in the assessment of oral malignant disease and lesions at risk of malignancy. *J. Oral Pathol. Med.* **21**, 160–3

Fayle S.A. and Curzon M.E.J. (1991) Oral complications in paediatric oncology patients. *Pediatr. Dent.* **13**, 289–95.

Fleming P. and Kinirons M.J. (1986) Dental health of children suffering from acute lymphoblastic leukaemia. *J. Paediatr. Dent.* **2**, 15.

Flint S.R., Sugerman P., Scully, C. *et al.* (1990) The myelodysplastic syndromes: a predisposing cause of oral ulceration and herpes labialis. *Oral Surg. Oral Med. Oral Pathol.* **70**, 450–3.

Gruppo Italiano Studio Policitemia (1995) Polycythemia vera; the natural history of 1213 patients followed for 20 years. *Ann. Intern. Med.* **123**, 656–64.

Hoagland H.C. (1995) Myelodysplastic (preleukaemia) syndromes; the bone marrow factory failure problem. *Mayo Clin. Proc.* **70**, 673–7.

Husby G. and Sletten K. (1986) Chemical and clinical classification of amyloidosis 1985. *Scand. J. Immunol.* **23**, 253–65.

Jobbins J., Bagg J., Finlay I.G. *et al.* (1992) Oral and dental disease in terminally ill cancer patients. *Br. Med. J.* **304**, 1612.

Kamp A.A. (1988) Neoplastic diseases in a pediatric population: a survey of the incidence of oral complications. *Paediatr. Dent.* **10**, 25–9.

Kuriakose M., Sankaranarayanan M., Nair M.K., Cherian T., Sugar A.W., Scully C. and Prime S.S. (1992) Comparison of oral squamous cell carcinoma in younger and old patients in India. *Oral Oncol.: Eur. J. Cancer* **28B**, 113–20.

Langdon J. (1995) The radiotherapeutic and surgical management of head and neck cancer. In Porter S.R. and Scully C. (eds), *Oral Health Care for Those with HIV Infection and Other Special Needs.* Northwood, Science Reviews, pp. 175–87.

Langdon J. and Henk J. (eds) (1995) *Malignant Tumours of the Mouth, Jaws and Salivary Glands.* London, Edward Arnold.

Leading Article (1980) Myelofibrosis. *Lancet* **i**, 127–9.

Leading Article (1989) Oral Cancer. *Lancet* **ii**, 311–12.

Lowe O. (1986) Oral concerns for the pediatric cancer patient. *J. Pedodont.* **11**, 35–46.

Luker J. (1995) Leukaemias. In Porter S.R. and Scully C. (eds), *Oral Health Care for Those with HIV Infection and Other Special Needs.* Northwood, Science Reviews, pp. 111–16.

MacFarlane G.J., Boyle P., Evstifeeva T. and Scully C. (1993) Epidemiological aspects of lip cancer in Scotland. *Commun. Dentistry Oral Epidemiol.* **21**, 279–82.

MacFarlane G.J., Boyle P., Evstifeeva T., Robertson C. and Scully C. (1994) Rising trends of oral cancer mortality in males worldwide: the return of an old public health problem. *Cancer Causes Control* **5**, 259–65.

Macfarlane G.J., Boyle P. and Scully C. (1992) Oral cancer in Scotland: changing incidence and mortality. *Br. Med. J.* **305**, 1121–3.

MacFarlane G.J., Evstifeeva T.V., Robertson C., Boyle P. and Scully C. (1994) Trends of oral cancer mortality among females worldwide. *Cancer Causes Control* **5**, 255–8.

Maitland N.J., Bromidge T., Cox M.F., Crane I.J., Prime S.S. and Scully C. (1987) Detection of human papillomavirus genes in human oral tissue biopsies and cultures by polymerase chain reaction. *Br. J. Cancer* **59**, 698–703.

Matthews J.B., Scully C., Jovanovich A., van der Waal I., Yeudall W.A. and Prime, S.S. (1993) The relationship of tobacco/alcohol use to p53 expression in patients with lingual squamous cell carcinomas. *Oral Oncol.: Eur. J. Cancer* **29B**, 285–90.

Peterson D.E., Elias E.G. and Sonis S.T. (1986). *Head and Neck Management of the Cancer Patient.* The Hague, Martinus Nijhoff, pp. 101–28.

Porter S.R. and Scully C. (1994) Gingival and oral mucosal ulceration associated with the myelodysplastic syndrome. *Oral Oncol.: Eur. J. Cancer* **30B**, 346–50.

Porter S.R. and Scully C. (eds) (1996) *Innovations and Developments in Non-Invasive Oral Health Care.* Northwood, Science Reviews.

Porter S.R., Luker J., Scully C. and Oakhill A. (1994) Oral features of a family with benign familial neutropenia. *J. Am. Acad. Dermatol.* **30**, 877–80.

Porter S.R., Matthews R.W. and Scully C. (1994) Chronic lymphocytic leukaemia with gingival and palatal deposits. *J. Clin. Periodontol.* **21**, 559–61.

Rodu B., Carpenter J.T. and Jones M.R. (1988) The pathogenesis and clinical significance of cytologically detectable oral candida in acute leukemia. *Cancer* **62**, 2042–6.

Rozman C. and Montserrat E. (1995) Chronic lymphocytic leukemia. *N. Engl. J. Med.* **333**, 1052–7.

Ruiz-Arguelles G.J., Garces-Eisele J. and Ruiz-Arguelles A. (1995) ATRA-induced gingival infiltration. *Am. J. Hematol.* **49**, 364–5.

Scheinberg D.A. (1995) Adult leukaemia in 1995; new directions. *Lancet* **346**, 455.

Scully C. (1983) An update on mouth ulcers. *Dent. Update* **10**, 141–52.

Scully C. (1983) Immunology and oral cancer. *Br. J. Oral Surg.* **21**, 136–46.

Scully C. (1983) Viruses and cancer: herpes viruses and tumours in the head and neck. *Oral Surg. Oral Med. Oral Pathol.* **56**, 285–92.

Scully C. (1985) Immunology and virology of oral cancer. In Henk J.M. and Langdon J. (eds), *Management of Malignant Tumours of the Oral Cavity.* London, Arnold, pp. 14–31.

Scully C. (1988) *The Dental Patient.* Oxford, Heinemann.

Scully C. (1989) *The Mouth and Perioral Tissues.* Oxford, Heinemann.

Scully C. (1989) *Patient Care; a Dental Surgeon's Guide.* London, British Dental Association.

Scully C. (1992) Viruses and oral squamous carcinoma. *Oral Oncol.: Eur. J. Cancer* **28B**, 57–9.

Scully C. (1993) Oral Cancer: new insights into pathogenesis. *Dent. Update* **20**, 95–100.

Scully C. (1993) Oncogenes, tumour suppressors and viruses in oral squamous carcinoma. *J Oral Pathol. Med.* **22**, 337–47.

Scully C. (1995) Carcinoma della lingua. In Boumassar E. and Costa A. (eds), *Oncologia*. Paris, Masson, pp. 31–6.

Scully C. (1995) Management of the sore mouth: other causes of oral soreness. *Eur. J. Palliative Care* **2** (Suppl 1), 13–15.

Scully C. (1995) Oral malignancy: diagnosis. In Porter S.R. and Scully C. (eds), *Oral Health Care for Those with HIV and Other Special Needs*. Northwood, Science Reviews, pp. 167–74.

Scully C. (1995) Oral precancer: preventive and medical approaches to management. *Oral Oncol.: Eur. J. Cancer* **31B**, 16–26.

Scully C. and Boyle P. (1992) Vitamin A and related compounds in chemo-prevention of potentially malignant oral lesions and carcinoma. *Oral Oncol.: Eur. J. Cancer* **28B**, 87–89.

Scully C. and Burkhardt A. (1993) Tissue markers of potentially malignant oral epithelial lesions. *J. Oral Pathol. Med.* **22**, 246–56.

Scully C. and Cawson R.A. (1996) Potentially malignant oral lesions. *J. Epidemiol. Biostat* **1**, 3–12.

Scully C. and Epstein J.B. (1996) Oral health care in cancer patients. *Oral Oncol.* **32B**, 281–92.

Scully C. and Field J. (1997) Genetic aberrations in squamous cell carcinoma of the head and neck (SCCHN) with reference to oral carcinoma. *Int. J. Oncol.* **10**, 5–21.

Scully C. and MacFarlane W.H. (1983) Orofacial manifestations in childhood malignancy: clinical and microbiological findings during remission. *J. Dent. Child.* **50**, 121–5.

Scully C. and Ward-Booth P. (1995) Detection and treatment of early cancers of the oral cavity. *Crit. Rev. Oncol./Haematol.* **21**, 63–75.

Scully C., Boyle P. and Tedesco B. (1992) The recognition and diagnosis of cancer arising in the mouth. *Postgrad. Doctor* **15**, 134–41; *Postgrad. Dentist* **5**, 42–7 (1995).

Scully C., Cawson R.A. and Griffiths M.J. (1990) *Occupational Hazards to Dental Staff*. London, British Dental Journal.

Scully C., Gill Y. and Gill Z. (1989) How pharmacists manage a patient with possible oral cancer. *Br. J. Oral Maxillofac. Surg* **27**, 16–21.

Scully C., Malamos D., Levers B.G.H., Porter S.R. and Prime S.S. (1986) Sources and patterns of referrals of oral cancer: the role of general practitioners. *Br. Med. J.* **293**, 599–601.

Singh N., Scully C. and Joyston-Bechal S. (1996) Oral complications of cancer therapies: prevention and management. *Clin. Oncol.* **8**, 15–24.

Stafford R., Sonis S., Lockhart P. *et al.* (1980) Oral pathoses as diagnostic indicators in leukaemia. *Oral Surg.* **50**, 134–9.

Ueland P.M., Refsum H. and Wesenberg F. (1986) Methotrexate therapy and nitrous oxide anaesthesia. *N. Engl. J. Med.* **300**, 1514.

Ward-Booth, P. and Scully, C. (1992) The management of mouth cancer. *Postgrad. Doctor* **15**, 166–75; *Postgrad Dentist* **5**, 65–71 (1995).

Whittaker J.A. (1980) Advances in the management of adult acute myelogenous leukaemia. *Br. Med. J.* **281**, 960–4.

Yeudall W.A., Torrance L.K., Elsegood K.A., Speight P., Scully C. and Prime S.S. (1993) Ras gene point mutation is a rare event in premalignant tissues and malignant cells and tissues from oral mucosal lesions. *Oral Oncol.: Eur. J. Cancer* **29B**, 63–7.

Zheng T., Boyle P., Hu H.F., Duan J., Jiang P.J. *et al.* (1990) Dentition, oral hygiene and risk of oral cancer: a case-control study in Beijing, People's Republic of China. *Cancer Causes Control* **1**: 235–42.

7

Cytotoxic chemotherapy and radiotherapy

Key points

- The main oral complications of cytotoxic chemotherapy are infections and ulceration.
- Lip cracking, gingival bleeding, xerostomia and delayed or abnormal dental development may also follow chemotherapy.
- Radiotherapy involving the oral tissues may give rise to a range of complications, especially mucositis, xerostomia, loss of taste, trismus and endarteritis obliterans and sequelae.
- Caries, candidosis, sialadenitis, osteoradionecrosis and dental and craniofacial maldevelopment are sequelae that may therefore follow radiotherapy that involves the salivary glands and jaws.
- In patients on cancer therapy, gentle reiteration of oral hygiene instruction and supervision, and scaling and polishing, will be not only valuable but will be appreciated.
- Treatment planning is essential to minimize trauma and infection, and to ensure any surgery is carried out at the optimum time in relation to cancer therapy.
- Tooth extraction, or other surgical procedures, should be done at least one week *before* radiotherapy is started, because of the risk of serious infection later.
- Haemorrhage needs the advice of a haematologist. If it is due to thrombocytopenia, a platelet transfusion, plus tranexamic acid, might be indicated.
- Corticosteroid mouthwashes may help ameliorate radiotherapy-induced mucositis and ice cubes may relieve chemotherapy-induced mucositis.
- Benzydamine rinses may ease discomfort of mucositis and ulceration.
- Salivary substitutes may help relieve xerostomia. Pilocarpine may help stimulate salivation.
- Dietary control and the use of fluorides are necessary to prevent caries.
- Prophylactic antimicrobials may help minimize herpetic and fungal infections.
- Infections with herpes viruses and candidosis may warrant systemic antimicrobials: aciclovir for herpes simplex infections, fluconazole for candidosis.

CYTOTOXIC CHEMOTHERAPY

Many of the cytotoxic agents used to treat malignant disease can cause complications, particularly if treatment is prolonged or in high dosage (*Table 7.1*). Furthermore, some 90 per cent of children and approximately 50 per cent of adults develop oral lesions (*Table 7.2*), particularly as, in many cases, radiotherapy is also given. When combined cytotoxic

Table 7.1a   Chemotherapeutic agents – main uses and toxicities: alkylating drugs

	Main uses	*Main toxicities*
Busulphan	CML	Myelosuppression Hyperpigmentation Pulmonary fibrosis
Carmustine	Multiple myeloma Lymphomas	Nephrotoxicity Pulmonary fibrosis
Chlorambucil	CLL	Myelosuppression Erythema multiforme
Cyclophosphamide	CLL Lymphomas	Cystitis (avoid with Mesna)
Estramustine	Prostatic carcinoma	Angina Gynaecomastia Liver dysfunction
Ifosfamide	CLL Lymphomas	Cystitis (avoid with Mesna)
Lomustine	Hodgkin's disease	Nausea and vomiting Delayed myelosuppression
Melphalan	Multiple myeloma	Delayed myelosuppression
Mustine	Hodgkin's disease	Severe vomiting
Thiotepa	Malignant effusions Bladder carcinoma	
Treosulfan	Ovarian carcinoma	

Note: All can interfere with gametogenesis, and predispose to acute leukaemias.

Table 7.1b   Chemotherapeutic agents – main uses and toxicities: cytotoxic antibiotics

	Main uses	*Main toxicities*
Aclarubicin	AML	
Bleomycin	Squamous carcinomas	
Dactinomycin	Paediatric tumours	Similar to doxorubicin but no cardiotoxicity
Daunorubicin	Kaposi's sarcoma	
Doxorubicin	Acute leukaemias Lymphomas	Mucositis Nausea and vomiting Cardiotoxicity Myelosuppression
Epirubicin	Breast carcinoma	
Mitomycin	Upper gastrointestinal and breast carcinomas	Myelosuppression Nephrotoxicity Lung fibrosis
Mitozantrone	Breast carcinoma	Myelosuppression Cardiotoxicity
Plicamycin (mithramycin)	Hypercalcaemic in malignancy	

Note: Should not be used with radiotherapy.

Table 7.1c   Chemotherapeutic agents – main uses and toxicities: antimetabolites

	Main uses	*Main toxicities*
Cladribine	Hairy cell leukaemia	Myelosuppression
Cytarabine	Acute leukaemias	Myelosuppression
Fludarabine	CLL	Myelosuppression Immunosuppression CNS and pulmonary toxicity

continued

Fluorouracil	Colon carcinoma	Mucositis
	Breast carcinoma	Myelosuppression
		Cerebellar syndrome
Gemcitabine	Non small-cell lung carcinoma	
Mercaptopurine	Acute leukaemias	
Methotrexate	ALL	Mucositis
	Rheumatoid arthritis	Myelosuppression (ameliorate with leucovorin)
	Psoriasis	
Thioguanine	Acute leukaemias	

Table 7.1d	Chemotherapeutic agents – main uses and toxicities: antimicrotubule assembly agents	
	Main uses	*Main toxicities*
Etoposide	Small cell carcinoma of lung lymphomas	Myelosuppression
		Nausea and vomiting
Vinblastine	Acute leukaemias	Myelosuppression
	Lymphomas	
Vincristine	Acute leukaemias	Neuropathies
	Lymphomas	Inappropriate ADH secretion
Vindesine	Acute leukaemias	Intermediate between vinblastine and vincristine
	Lymphomas	

Table 7.1e	Chemotherapeutic agents – main uses and toxicities: other antineoplastic drugs	
	Main uses	*Main toxicities*
Amsacrine	MAL	Mucositis
		Myelosuppression
		Dysrhythmias
Carboplatin	Small oat cell carcinoma of lung	Myelosuppression
		Others like cisplatin
Cisplatin	Ovarian carcinoma	Severe nausea and vomiting
	Testicular carcinoma	Ototoxicity
		Nephrotoxicity
Crisantapase	ALL	Anaphylaxis
		Glucose intolerance
		CNS changes
		Liver dysfunction
Dacarbazine	Hodgkin's lymphoma	Severe nausea and vomiting
		Myelosuppression
Hydroxyurea	CML	Nausea
		Rashes
		Myelosuppression
Paclitaxel	Ovarian cancer	Hypersensitivity
	Breast cancer metasatases	Myelosuppression
		Dysrhythmias
Pentostatin	Hairy cell leukaemia	Myelosuppression
		Immunosuppression
Procarbazine	Hodgkin's lymphoma	Myelosuppression
		Hypersensitivity
		Disulfiram reaction with alcohol
Interferon alpha	Kaposi's sarcoma	Flu-like symptoms
	Hairy cell leukaemia	Cardiotoxicity
	Non-Hodgkin's lymphoma	Hepatotoxicity
		Depression

Table 7.2 Drugs used in cancer chemotherapy that frequently cause mouth ulcers and may cause management difficulties

Group	Drug	Possible management problems
Antibiotics	Bleomycin	Lung fibrosis
	Dactinomycin	Vomiting
	Daunorubicin	Cardiac damage
	Doxorubicin	Cardiac damage
	Mitozantrone	Cardiac damage
Antimetabolites	Cytosine arabinoside	
	5-fluorouracil	
	Methotrexate	Liver and renal damage
Miscellaneous	Carboplatin	Neuropathy and renal damage
	Etoposide	Vomiting

Note: Most of these agents can depress the bone-marrow leading to a tendency to infection and a bleeding state: particular complications are noted here.
Oral ulceration can be a complication of virtually any cancer chemotherapeutic agent but is most common in these groups.

chemotherapy and radiotherapy are given, the most common complications are infections (23 per cent), mucositis (6 per cent) and bleeding (5 per cent).

Infections

Cytotoxic agents predispose to infections with fungi, viruses, toxoplasma or bacteria. Oral candidosis is common and is usually caused by *Candida albicans* or, less often, other candida species. Candidosis is promoted especially by severe leukopenia and the use of antibiotics (Chapter 20). Oral mucormycosis (phycomycosis) or aspergillosis are rare. Herpetic infections (*herpes simplex* or *herpes zoster*) are common and may cause chronic oral ulcers. Gram-positive bacterial infections (staphylococci) are less common as patients usually receive antibiotics prophylactically. Hospitalized patients on cytotoxic chemotherapy may, however, develop Gram-negative oral infections (with pseudomonas, klebsiella, escherichia, enterobacter, serratia or proteus) and dental infections may spread rapidly (*Fig. 7.1*).

Ulcers and mucositis

Oral ulceration is a particularly common complication in patients treated with antimetabolites and cytotoxic antibiotics (*see Table 7.1*), and may be severe enough to preclude further chemotherapy. Ulceration often begins shortly after chemotherapy is started and may resolve within a few weeks of

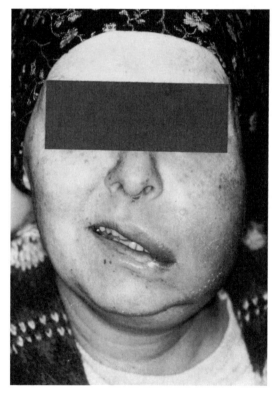

Fig. 7.1 Leukaemic with a dental abscess and spreading infection

completion of treatment. The ulcers are shallow and painful, affecting particularly the labial and faucial mucosa, but usually heal within 2–3 weeks of cessation of cytotoxic therapy.

Oral ulceration most often complicates treatment with methotrexate, 5-fluorouracil, doxorubicin, melphalan, mercaptopurine or bleomycin. Over 50 per cent of patients on methotrexate or 5-fluorouracil and 30 per cent of those on daunorubicin and 25 per cent of those on 6-mercaptopurine suffer from drug-induced oral ulceration. It is often the first sign of methotrexate toxicity and can follow within 24 hours of a single dose.

Lip cracking

Lip cracking is common when there are febrile episodes.

Bleeding

Drug-induced thrombocytopenia may cause gingival bleeding, mucosal petechiae or ecchymoses.

Xerostomia

Cytotoxic agents (especially doxorubicin) may cause xerostomia, similar to that resulting from radiation therapy, and can lead to caries and other oral infections.

Delayed and abnormal development

Prolonged chemotherapy can damage the developing dentition and jaws.

• Dental management of patients on cytotoxic chemotherapy

Before chemotherapy
A careful oral assessment should be carried out to enable extractions and any other surgery to be completed before cytotoxic treatment, as the latter can cause abnormal bleeding and susceptibility to infection (*Table 7.3*). Oral hygiene should be improved as far as possible.

During chemotherapy
It may be possible to avoid or reduce oral ulceration caused by methotrexate using systemic or topical folinic acid (leucovorin). Oral cooling with ice cold water or sucking ice during the infusion of the agent may lessen the stomatitis induced by 5-fluorouracil and melphalan.

Table 7.3 Dental treatment for patients on cytotoxic chemotherapy

Blood cell type	Peripheral blood count	Precautions
Platelets	$>50 \times 10^9/l$	Routine management though desmopressin or platelets are needed to cover surgery
	$<50 \times 10^9/l$	Platelets needed for any invasive procedure[a]
Granulocytes	$>2 \times 10^9/l$	Routine management
	$<2 \times 10^9/l$	Prophylactic antimicrobials for surgery
Erythrocytes	$>5 \times 10^{12}/l$	Routine management
	$<5 \times 10^{12}/l$	Special care with general anaesthesia

[a]Any procedure where bleeding is possible.

Established mucositis or oral ulceration is managed by maintaining good oral hygiene with twice-daily 0.2 per cent aqueous chlorhexidine mouth rinses. Viscous 2 per cent lignocaine or benzydamine rinse or spray can be used to help lessen discomfort.

Many patients develop oral candidosis and this usually also implies oesophageal candidosis which may be a portal for haematogenous dissemination. Nystatin suspension (100 000 U/ml) as a mouthwash or pastilles four to six times daily, may be given prophylactically. Some workers now recommend fluconazole for patients with candidosis who develop fever. Dentures should be carefully cleaned and stored overnight in 1 per cent hypochlorite to reduce candidal carriage.

Oral herpetic infections should be treated with aciclovir suspension or systemic aciclovir (tablets or infusion). Prophylactic aciclovir is used in some centres and has lowered the incidence of and mortality from zoster. Zoster immune globulin may help ameliorate varicella or zoster.

Although patients are frequently already on several antibiotics, Gram-negative infections may need treatment with gentamicin or carbenicillin as the oral lesions can be portals for systemic spread.

Aspirin should not be given to patients on methotrexate as it may enhance the toxicity of the latter (*see* Appendix to Chapter 25). Some cytotoxic drugs enhance the effects of suxamethonium (Chapter 15); others cause more serious complications that can influence dental management (*Table 7.2*).

After chemotherapy

Most acute oral complications develop during chemotherapy but even afterwards there should still be close attention to oral hygiene and preventive dentistry, as many patients continue to have anaemia, bleeding tendencies and be susceptible to infection (*see Table 6.17*).

RADIOTHERAPY INVOLVING THE ORAL CAVITY OR SALIVARY GLANDS

A range of oral complications can follow radiotherapy, but the most common is mucositis (*Table 7.4*).

Table 7.4   Oral complications of radiotherapy involving the salivary glands

- Mucositis
- Ulceration
- Candidosis
- Xerostomia
- Radiation caries
- Dental hypersensitivity
- Periodontal disease
- Loss of taste
- Trismus
- Osteoradionecrosis and irradiation-associated osteomyelitis
- Craniofacial defects

Mucositis

This is almost inevitable during radiotherapy where the field involves the oral mucosa. The degree of mucositis depends on the type of radiotherapy, dose and duration of treatment. The initial reaction is mucosal erythema followed by sloughing, ulceration and considerable discomfort. Dysphagia and oral soreness become maximal 2–4 weeks after radiotherapy but usually subside in a further 2–3 weeks.

Xerostomia and infections

The fields of radiotherapy to cancers of the head and neck often involve the major salivary glands. Radiotherapy of tumours of the naso- and oropharynx is especially liable to damage the salivary glands. Irradiation depresses salivary secretion and the saliva has a higher viscosity but lower pH. Salivary secretion diminishes within a week of radiotherapy in virtually all patients and the saliva becomes thick and tenacious. Some salivary function may return after many months.

Xerostomia predisposes to infections, particularly caries, oral candidosis and acute ascending sialadenitis.

Radiation caries and dental hypersensitivity

Patients frequently take a softer, more cariogenic diet because of dryness and soreness of the mouth and loss of taste. There is a change to a more cariogenic oral flora. Irradiation may also directly damage the teeth, which become hypersensitive, thus making oral hygiene difficult. These factors combine to cause rampant dental caries, including areas such as incisal edges and cervical margins which are normally free from caries. Caries begins at any time between 2 and 10 months after radiotherapy, and may eventually result in the crown breaking off from the root. A complete dentition may be destroyed within a year of irradiation.

Loss of taste

Hypoguesia follows radiation damage to the taste buds but xerostomia alone can disturb taste sensation. Taste may start to recover within 2–4 months but, if more than 6000 CGy have been given, loss of taste is usually permanent.

Trismus

Progressive endarteritis of affected tissues, with reduction in their blood supply, follows radiotherapy. The results may be replacement fibrosis of the masticatory muscles. Fibrosis becomes apparent 3–6 months after radiotherapy and can cause permanent limitation of opening.

Osteoradionecrosis and osteomyelitis

Death of bone of the jaw, particularly the mandible, is a potentially serious complication of irradiation endarteritis. If the soft tissues covering the bone are healthy and undisturbed, there may be no obvious consequences, but infection, often resulting from dental extractions carried out after radiotherapy, can lead to intractable osteomyelitis. In severe cases the whole of the body of the mandible may become infected, both the overlying mucosa and skin may be destroyed and the bone may become exposed internally and externally.

Irradiation-associated osteomyelitis may occasionally be precipitated by mucosal ulceration caused by a denture. As a consequence, some specialists refuse to permit patients to wear dentures, especially a full lower denture, after irradiation of the oral mucosa.

Osteoradionecrosis is, however, a less frequent problem now, as megavoltage radiotherapy has less effect on bone than did orthovoltage therapy. Osteoradionecrosis appears to develop mainly in patients receiving more than 6000 CGy, particularly to the floor of the mouth and mandible. Osteomyelitis may follow months or years after radiotherapy but about 30 per cent of cases develop within 6 months. Osteomyelitis is heralded by pain and swelling. The area of involved bone is often small (less than 2 cm diameter) and with antibiotics the signs and symptoms of inflammation may clear within a few weeks. Complete resolution can, however, take 2 or more years in spite of intensive treatment with antimicrobials. Hyperbaric oxygen may be required.

Craniofacial defects

Irradiation of developing teeth can cause hypoplasia and retarded eruption. Irradiation of growth centres in children can cause craniofacial maldevelopment.

• Dental management of patients receiving radiotherapy to the head and neck

Treatment planning
The complications of dental treatment after radiotherapy are such that planned treatment should be carried out before irradiation. Oral hygiene should be meticulous, preventive dental care instituted, and restorative procedures carried out at this stage. These measures can significantly reduce the caries incidence.

Most cancer patients are of middle age or over and many have neglected dentitions. In such patients, teeth in the radiation path should be extracted or, if the patient has no objection, a total clearance may be preferable. The latter is essential where the teeth have been consistently neglected. Alternatively, the patient may have so healthy a dentition and such good oral hygiene that dental complications after radiotherapy are unlikely.

The time interval permitted between extractions and radiotherapy is invariably a compromise because of the need to start radiotherapy as soon as possible. No bone should be left exposed in the mouth when radiotherapy begins since, once the blood supply is damaged by radiotherapy, wound healing is jeopardized. Many advise an interval of at least 2 weeks between extracting the teeth and starting radiotherapy but this is not always essential.

However, it is not always necessary to extract all the teeth before radiotherapy. In any case, clearance before irradiation may not be practicable, because the patient is too old or ill, or the prognosis is too poor. Some patients may even refuse radiotherapy rather than lose their teeth. Furthermore, it is not easy to construct dentures if there is mucosal soreness, and dentures cannot always be worn after radiotherapy.

During radiotherapy
Elimination of Gram-negative bacteria by using a polymyxin and tobramycin lozenge four times a day may result in a significant reduction in mucositis. Smoking and alcohol should be discouraged.

Mucositis may be relieved by using warm normal saline mouthwashes and a benzydamine oral rinse, lignocaine viscous 2 per cent, or sucralfate. A 0.2 per cent chlorhexidine mouthwash maintains oral hygiene. Antifungal drugs such as nystatin suspension, 100 000 units/ml, as a mouthwash or pastilles used four times daily, may be required.

A saliva substitute such as carboxymethylcellulose may provide some symptomatic relief. Trismus may be improved by jaw-opening exercises with tongue spatulas or wedges used three times a day.

After radiotherapy

Oral hygiene and preventive dental care should be continued and mucositis managed as outlined above.

Dental extractions may precipitate osteomyelitis in the irradiated jaw but, if extractions are unavoidable, trauma should be kept to a minimum, raising the periosteum as little as possible and ensuring that sharp bone edges are removed. Careful suturing is needed and prophylactic antibiotics should be given in adequate doses and continued for 4 weeks at least.

However, some specialists may refuse to carry out extractions in the irradiated area because of the severity of radiation-associated osteomyelitis which can develop in spite of all precautions. Under these circumstances, dental infections are controlled with antimicrobials.

Radiation caries and dental hypersensitivity can be controlled with daily topical fluoride applications (sodium fluoride mouthwash, stannous fluoride gel or acidulated fluoride phosphate gel). Occasionally full cover acrylic splints are used to protect the teeth (Coffin's caps). Unfortunately, only too many patients are told by their doctors to 'suck a sweet' to relieve the discomfort of their dry mouth. Clearly these patients must be disabused of such ideas and given practical guidance about diet. In essence all that should be necessary is avoidance of sweets and sweet confectionery and use of sugar substitutes such as saccharin or aspartame, wherever possible. Mouthwashes of sodium bicarbonate may help dissolve the stringy saliva that forms.

Mucosal trauma from dentures may predispose to osteomyelitis and some specialists therefore insist that dentures be abandoned. If dentures are required, they should be fitted at about 4–6 weeks after radiotherapy, when initial mucositis subsides and there is only early fibrosis.

The dryness of the mouth is managed as for Sjögren's syndrome (Chapter 9) but palliation with liberal use of artificial saliva is usually the best that can be achieved.

BIBLIOGRAPHY

Azul A.M. (1995) Oral complications of the non-surgical management of malignant disease. In Porter S.R. and Scully C. (eds), *Oral Health Care for Those with HIV Infection and Other Special Needs*. Northwood, Science Reviews, pp. 183–7.

Barrett A.P. (1987) A long-term prospective clinical study of oral complications during conventional chemotherapy for acute leukemia. *Oral Surg. Oral Med. Oral Pathol.* **63**, 313–16.

Bergmann O.J. (1989) Oral infections and fever in immunocompromised patients with haematologic malignancies. *Eur. J. Clin. Microbiol. Infect. Dis.* **8**, 207–13.

Beumer J., Harrison R., Sanders B. and Kurrasch M. (1983) Preradiation dental extractions and the incidence of bone necrosis. *Head Neck Surg.* **5**, 514–21.

Bochud P-Y., Calandra T. and Francioli P. (1994) Bacteremia due to viridans streptococci in neutropenic patients: a review. *Am. J. Med.* **97**, 256–64.

Charak B.S., Parikh P.M., Banavali S.D. *et al.* (1988) Comparison of clotrimazole with nystatin in preventing oral candidiasis in neutropenic patients. *Indian J. Med. Res.* **88**, 416–20.

Childers N.K., Shennett E.A., Wheeler P. *et al.* (1993) Oral complications in children with cancer. *Oral Surg. Oral Med. Oral Pathol.* **75**, 41–7.

Degregorio M.W., Lee W.M.F. and Ries C.A. (1982) Candida infections in patients with acute leukaemia: ineffectiveness of nystatin prophylaxis and relationship between oropharyngeal and systemic candidiasis. *Cancer* **50**, 2780–4.

Fortenja S.W., Newman M.G., Lipsey A.I. *et al.* (1980) Capnocytophaga sepsis: a newly recognised clinical entity in granulocytopenic patients. *Lancet* **i**, 567–8.

Goho C. (1993) Chemoradiation therapy: effect on dental development. *Pediatr. Dent.* **15**, 6–12.

Jones L.R., Toth B.B. and Keene H.J. (1992) Effects of total body irradiation on salivary gland function and caries-associated microflora in bone marrow transplant patients. *Oral Surg. Oral Med. Oral Pathol.* **73**, 670–6.

Kuhrer, I., Kuzmits R., Linkesch W. *et al.* (1986) Topical PGE2 enhances healing of chemotherapy associated mucosal lesions. *Lancet* **i**, 622.

Larson D.L. (1986) Management of complications of radiotherapy of the head and neck. *Surg. Clin. North Am.* **66**, 169–83.

Levendag P.C., Vikram B., Wright R. *et al.* (1989) Dental problems following surgery and external radiation therapy in patients with advanced carcinomas of the oral cavity and oropharynx. *Acta Oncol.* **28**, 550–5.

Loprinzi C.L., Cianflane S.G., Dose A.M. *et al.* (1990) A controlled evaluation of an allopurinol mouthwash as prophylaxis against 5-fluorouracil-induced stomatitis. *Cancer* **65**, 1879–82.

McElroy T.N. (1984) Infection in the patient receiving chemotherapy for cancer: oral considerations. *J. Am. Dent. Assoc.* **109**, 454–6.

Murray C.G., Daly T.E. and Zimmerman S.O. (1980) The relationship between dental disease and radiation necrosis of the mandible. *Oral Surg. Oral Med. Oral Pathol.* **49**, 99–104.

Peterson D. and Sonis S. (1983) *Oral Complications of Cancer Chemotherapy*. Boston, Nijhoff.

Peterson D.E., Elias E.G. and Sonis S.T. (1986) *Head and Neck Management of the Cancer Patient*. The Hague, Nijhoff.

Porter S.R. and Scully C. (1996) *Innovations and Developments in Non-Invasive Oral Health Care*. Northwood, Science Reviews.

Rand K.H., Kramer B. and Johnson A.C. (1982) Cancer chemotherapy associated symptomatic stomatitis. *Cancer* **50**, 1262–5.

Scully C. (1988) *The Dental Patient*. Oxford, Heinemann.

Scully C. (1989) *The Mouth and Perioral Tissues*. Oxford, Heinemann.

Scully C. (1992) Oral infections in the immunocompromised patient. *Br. Dent. J.* **172**, 401–7.

Scully C. (1995) Management of the sore mouth. *Eur. J Palliative Care* Suppl 1, 13–15.

Scully C. and Epstein J.B. (1996) Oral health care for cancer patients. *Oral Oncol.* **32**, 281–92.

Scully C. (1989) *Patient Care: a Dental Surgeon's Guide*. London, British Dental Association.

Scully C. and Gilmour G. (1986) Neutropenia and dental patients. *Br. Dent. J.* **160**, 436.

Scully C., Cawson R.A. and Griffiths M.J. (1990) *Occupational Hazards to Dental Staff*. London, British Dental Journal.

Scully C., MacFadyen E.E. and Campbell A. (1982) Orofacial manifestations in cyclic neutropenia. *Br. J. Oral Surg.* **20**, 96–101.

Seto B.G. (1985) Oral mucositis in patients undergoing bone marrow transplantation. *Oral Surg. Oral Med. Oral Pathol.* **60**, 493–7.

Singh N., Scully C. and Joyston-Bechal S (1996) Oral complications of cancer therapies: prevention and management. *Clin. Oncol.* **8**, 15–24.

Sinzinger H., Porteder H., Matjka M. *et al.* (1989) Prostaglandins in irradiation-induced mucositis. *Lancet* **i**, 556.

Tsavaris N., Caragiauris P. and Kosmidis P. (1988) Reduction of oral toxicity of 5-fluorouracil by allopurinol mouthwashes. *Eur. J. Surg. Oncol.* **14**, 405–6.

Wahhin Y.B. and Matsson L. (1988) Oral mucosal lesions in patients with acute leukemia and related disorders during cytotoxic therapy. *Scand. J. Dent. Res.* **96**, 128–36.

Williford S.K., Salisbury P.L., Peacock J.E. *et al.* (1989) The safety of dental extractions in patients with hematologic malignancies. *J. Clin. Oncol.* **7**, 798–802.

Wright W.E. (1985) An oral disease prevention program for patients receiving radiation and chemotherapy. *J. Am. Dent. Assoc.* **110**, 43–7.

8

Respiratory disorders

Key points

- Respiratory disease is common and relevant mainly because it influences choice of anaesthesia.
- General anaesthesia is potentially hazardous, because respiratory failure may be precipitated.
- Upper respiratory tract infections are a contraindication to non-urgent general anaesthesia, because the infection may be spread to the lower respiratory tract.
- Lower respiratory tract infections are a contraindication to general anaesthesia.
- Reduce or avoid sedatives and analgesics in patients with respiratory disease.
- Respiratory disease may present with dyspnoea, central cyanosis, or clubbing, as can cardiac disease.
- Wheeze, cough, production of sputum and haemoptysis are other features.
- Upper respiratory tract infections (URTI) are usually viral but may be secondarily infected with bacteria.
- Sinusitis may complicate URTI, and usually involves *Streptococcus pneumoniae* and *Haemophilus influenzae*. In chronic sinusitis, anaerobes are common.
- Sinusitis is treated, if necessary, with analgesics and inhalations or nose drops to help provide relief. Amoxycillin (with metronidazole in chronic sinusitis) or erythromycin may be needed.
- Fungal infections of the sinuses may be harmless aspergillomas or, in immunocompromised patients, potentially lethal aspergillosis, phycomycosis, or other mycoses.
- Lower respiratory infections often follow URTI and are bacterial, or may be bacterial or mycoplasmal or rarely fungal pneumonias *ab initio*. General anaesthesia is contraindicated.
- Tuberculosis affects one-third of the world population, is increasing and, in immunocompromised persons particularly, is becoming multi-drug resistant.
- Tuberculosis can be an occupational hazard to those working with high-risk groups such as people who are socially deprived, injecting drug users, HIV-infected, or from the developing world.
- *Mycobacterium tuberculosis* is the usual cause but non-tuberculous mycobacteria such as *M. avium-intracellulare* can also cause pulmonary or lymph node lesions in particular.
- Legionnaire's disease is a pneumonia with a high mortality, seen mainly in elderly patients infected with *Legionella pneumophila* emanating from infected aerosols, for example air from conditioning systems.
- Lung infection with abscess formation and sometimes septicaemia may result from inhalation of infected material from the mouth.
- Asthma, bronchitis and emphysema are the most common serious respiratory disorders. In these, as well as bronchiectasis and cystic fibrosis, dental treatment is best carried out under local anaesthesia.

- Lung cancer is most common in older males who smoke tobacco. It appears to be particularly common in dental technicians, and has also been related to dust inhalation.
- Lung cancer may be a second primary neoplasm in patients with oral cancer, but lung cancer may also metastasize to the jaws.
- Sarcoidosis is a chronic granulomatous multi-system disorder with protean manifestations but frequently hilar lymphadenopathy, respiratory lesions, and salivary or other oral disease.

Respiratory disorders are common and may significantly affect dental treatment, especially general anaesthesia. In particular, respiratory diseases are often also a contraindication to opioids, benzodiazepines and other respiratory depressants.

Cough – the most common symptom – is a reflex which helps defend the respiratory tract but it is abnormal to produce sputum for long periods. Mucoid sputum is often a feature of chronic bronchitis, whereas purulent sputum is produced in acute bronchitis, bronchiectasis or lung abscess. The coughing of blood (haemoptysis) may be a serious event and due to a carcinoma or tuberculosis for example. It is also common in bronchitis, bronchiectasis and acute infections.

Breathlessness (dyspnoea) is particularly ominous if it persists at rest. *Wheezing* is caused by airways obstruction and is typically a sign of asthma or bronchitis.

Other important signs of respiratory disease include chest pain, cyanosis, finger clubbing, use of accessory muscles of respiration with indrawing of the intercostal spaces (hyperinflation) and abnormalities in chest shape, movements and breath sounds. The most useful investigations are chest radiography and spirometric tests. The latter are used to estimate functional capacity of the lungs, and overall the most useful, especially for the assessment of obstructive airways disease such as asthma, is the peak expiratory flow rate (PEFR). Spirometry and carbon monoxide perfusion can be used to assess impaired lung ventilation or gaseous exchange. Radionuclide lung scanning, blood gas analysis and sputum cytology or culture are sometimes needed.

RESPIRATORY INFECTIONS

The most common respiratory infections are viral and seen in otherwise healthy persons. Tuberculosis is probably the most serious respiratory infection and is a particular problem in the developing world, where many are malnourished or immunocompromised.

Patients with HIV infection, other immunodeficient persons, and those with bronchiectasis or cystic fibrosis are susceptible to respiratory infections by a great variety of microbes. The otherwise harmless organism *Pneumocystis carinii* is a common cause of fatal pneumonia in immunocompromised patients, especially those with AIDS. Various mycoses may affect the paranasal sinuses in immunocompromised persons.

Upper respiratory tract viral infections

Most respiratory infections begin as viral infections of the upper respiratory tract. The incubation periods are frequently short and rarely exceed 14 days and these infections are highly infectious in the early stages.

Three main clinical patterns are seen:

1. The common cold syndrome (coryza).
2. Pharyngitis and tonsillitis.
3. Laryngotracheitis.

The common cold syndrome
The common cold syndrome can be caused by many different viruses, but usually rhinoviruses (*Table 8.1*). Nasal discharge and obstruction, with nasopharyngeal soreness, are only too well known. There is only mild systemic upset and serious complications are

<table>
<tr><td colspan="2">

Table 8.1 Main causes of upper respiratory tract infection

</td></tr>
</table>

Rhinoviruses Respiratory syncytial viruses Para-influenza virus Coxsackie viruses	Common cold
Echoviruses Adenoviruses Influenza viruses Epstein–Barr virus Beta-haemolytic streptococci	Pharyngitis and tonsillitis

rare in otherwise fit patients. However, sinusitis may develop and cause facial pain and tenderness. Earache may result from obstruction of the pharyngotympanic tube by oedema or more seriously by bacterial infection of the middle ear (otitis media).

Symptoms resembling the common cold can also precede other infections, such as measles or influenza.

Pharyngitis and tonsillitis
Most cases of pharyngitis and tonsillitis are caused by viruses (*Table 8.1*) but other agents, especially *Streptococcus pyogenes*, *Mycoplasma pneumoniae*, pneumococci or rarely *Corynebacterium diphtheriae* may need to be considered in the differential diagnosis.

The throat is sore with pain on swallowing (dysphagia) and sometimes fever and conjunctivitis. Complications, which are rare, include peritonsillar abscess (quinsy) and sometimes otitis media. Streptococcal sore throats may be associated with scarlet fever; acute glomerulonephritis or rheumatic fever may occasionally follow but the latter is now very rare. Nevertheless streptococcal throat infections should be treated with penicillin if the patient is not allergic, or erythromycin. Ampicillin and amoxycillin should be avoided as they tend to cause rashes, especially if the sore throat in glandular fever is misdiagnosed as a streptococcal sore throat.

Herpangina, glandular fever and diphtheria are discussed in Chapter 11.

Laryngotracheitis
Hoarseness, loss of voice and persistent cough are common in laryngotracheitis. In children, partial laryngeal obstruction may cause noisy inspiration (stridor or croup) and

is potentially dangerous. Various microbes may be involved, such as respiratory syncytial virus in children particularly.

- **Dental aspects of upper respiratory tract infections**

Dental treatment is best deferred until after recovery. General anaesthesia should be avoided since there is often some respiratory obstruction and infection can also be spread down to the lungs. If a general anaesthetic is unavoidable it is best to carry out intubation with a cuffed tube and the patient supine, so that nasal secretions do not enter the larynx. Antimicrobials may be indicated for prophylaxis.

Most upper respiratory tract infections are innocuous and have no oral manifestations. Oropharyngeal lesions are, however, prominent in herpangina, glandular fever and diphtheria (Chapter 11). The use of xylitol chewing gum has been shown to reduce otitis media, presumably by inhibiting pneumococci.

Sinusitis

Infection of the paranasal air sinuses (maxillary, ethmoidal, sphenoidal and frontal) is usually bacterial and commonly follows a viral upper respiratory tract infection. Maxillary sinusitis may also rarely follow periapical infection of upper posterior teeth or an oro-antral fistula. Sinusitis may also complicate prolonged endotracheal intubation and mechanical ventilation in critically ill patients, especially when nasotracheal intubation is used. The sinusitis predisposes to nosocomial pneumonia.

The bacteria most commonly incriminated in acute sinusitis are *Streptococcus pneumoniae* and *Haemophilus influenzae*, but *Moraxella catarrhalis*, *Staphylococcus aureus* and alpha haemolytic streptococci may also be found. Increasingly, *S. pneumoniae* is penicillin resistant. In chronic sinusitis anaerobes predominate; half are beta-lactamase producers. Bacteroides predominate. In patients on prolonged endotracheal intubation, Gram-negative bacilli, predominantly *Pseudomonas aeruginosa*, *Acinetobacter baumannii* and Enterobacteriaceae are common. In immunocompromised persons, other organisms may be involved, including mucor, aspergillus or other fungal species.

Features of maxillary sinusitis are pain in the cheek and/or upper teeth, worsened by tilting the head or lying down, and nasal obstruction with mucopurulent nasal discharge. There is tenderness over the maxilla, dullness on antral transillumination, and antral radio-opacity or a fluid level on occipitomental radiography.

Sinus opacity is difficult to evaluate. Some studies have shown sinus opacities in up to 50 per cent of children under the age of 6 years. Sinus opacity is sometimes due only to mucosal thickening rather than infection, but a fluid level is highly suggestive of sinusitis. Ultrasonography, CT or MRI may be helpful but the diagnosis can only be confirmed by sinus puncture and aspiration. Nevertheless the history, clinical examination and radiographs are usually sufficiently reliable.

Acute sinusitis resolves spontaneously in about 50 per cent of cases. Analgesics are often indicated. Antibiotics may sometimes be required. Treatment is then a two-week course of amoxycillin, erythromycin (or clindamycin or azithromycin or clarithromycin), or a tetracycline such as doxycycline. Drainage is aided by vasoconstrictors such as ephedrine or xylometazoline nasal drops, which improve the patency of the maxillary ostium. Inhalations of warm, moist air, possibly with benzoin, menthol or eucalyptus, may give some symptomatic relief.

Chronic sinusitis responds better to drainage, plus metronidazole with amoxycillin or erythromycin (alternative – clindamycin).

Oro-antral fistula is discussed in surgical textbooks, and *fungal infections* are discussed below (*see* Chapter 26).

Lower respiratory tract infections

Lower respiratory tract infections are frequently viral, although often complicated by bacterial infection, but may be mycoplasmal (atypical pneumonia).

Clinical features vary according to the part of the respiratory tract mainly affected. Bronchitis causes cough, wheezing and sometimes dyspnoea. Bronchiolitis, which is restricted mainly to infants, causes rapid respiration, wheezing, fever and dyspnoea.

Table 8.2   Factors predisposing to pneumonia

- Viral respiratory infections, including colds
- Old age
- Immobility
- Respiratory depression or chest injury
- Alcoholism
- Immune deficiency (especially HIV infection)
- Neurological disorders permitting aspiration of foreign material
- Underlying pulmonary disease such as carcinoma or emphysema

---

Pneumonia causes cough, fever, rapid respiration, breathlessness, chest pain, dyspnoea and shivering. Pneumonia in a previously healthy individual is classed as primary and is usually lobar. Pneumonia may be secondary to some other disorder and is usually bronchopneumonia.

Previous viral respiratory infections, aspiration of foreign material, pre-existent lung disease (for example bronchiectasis or carcinoma), or depressed immunity, as a result, for example, of alcoholism or immunosuppression, or oral micro-organisms, may contribute (*Table 8.2*). Poor oral hygiene and periodontal disease may promote oropharyngeal colonization with Enterobacteriaceae such as *Klebsiella pneumoniae*, enterobacter species, and *Escherichia coli*, and with *Staphylococcus aureus* and *Pseudomonas aeruginosa*. This is especially likely in the very aged and infirm, and in those mechanically ventilated in intensive care units. Bacterial pneumonia may result.

Pneumocystis carinii pneumonia is discussed in Chapter 20.

• Dental aspects of lower respiratory tract infections

Attention to oral hygiene is important in persons who are unable to maintain oral hygiene, as discussed above. Once established, however, the majority of lower respiratory tract infections are severe illnesses and are contraindications to all but emergency dental treatment. General anaesthesia is hazardous and is absolutely contraindicated. Dental treatment should therefore then be deferred until recovery or be limited to relief of pain.

Pulmonary tuberculosis

Tuberculosis (TB) is caused mainly by infection with *Mycobacterium tuberculosis*. Tuberculosis from *M. bovis* in milk has been virtually eliminated by the tuberculin testing of cattle, and pasteurization of milk. However, tuberculosis is a major global problem. One-third of the world's population is infected and it is particularly widespread in developing countries. Highest increases in incidence are in South East Asia, Sub-Saharan Africa and Eastern Europe.

In developed countries, the incidence is also rising, probably because of increases in social deprivation, homelessness, immigration, HIV infection and intravenous drug abuse. Between 1985 and 1991, the incidence doubled in some cities in the USA, and in many developed countries increased by up to 30 per cent. In the USA, TB is seen especially in Afro-American and Hispanic young males, in New York, Miami and San Francisco. In other developed countries, TB is seen mainly in the elderly who are homeless, in prisons, or in institutions. Tuberculosis has also been a problem especially of immigrants, such as those from the Indian sub-continent and Vietnam.

Diabetics, alcoholics, severely immunodeficient patients, such as those with HIV infection, vagrants and institutionalized patients are now mainly at risk. Tuberculosis is increasingly common in the HIV-infected population, especially in the USA. Intravenous drug abusers and those in penal care, who are often poorly compliant with treatment, are particularly affected. The organism is then frequently multi-drug resistant (MDR) and the presentation may be atypical, and the infection disseminated. It then presents a risk to health care workers. One recent outbreak of highly drug-resistant TB in the USA was in New York and involved at least 357 patients, most of whom contracted the infection in one of 11 hospitals. Nearly 90 per cent were HIV-positive persons, mostly young male blacks or hispanics.

Pulmonary tuberculosis is usually contracted by the inhalation of infected sputum. TB is transmitted by coughing infected sputum and has been transmitted to close contacts such as family members, but transmission is not invariable. Tuberculosis has been transmitted between patients and health care workers, including dental staff, and has even been transmitted between passengers during long-haul air flights.

Most primary infections are subclinical. Inhaled mycobacteria may cause subpleural lesions and in the regional lymph nodes (primary complex). Haematogenous dissemination can lead to genitourinary, bone or joint lesions. The pulmonary lesions may extend and result in a pleural effusion. Because it frequently passes unrecognized for so long, the mortality from pulmonary tuberculosis is high. Lymph node tuberculosis may lead to caseation of the nodes and pressure symptoms, for example on the bronchi. Miliary tuberculosis is characterized by widely disseminated lesions recognizable especially in the lungs but can be seen in the choroid of the eyes on ophthalmoscopy.

Post-primary tuberculosis follows reactivation of an old primary pulmonary lesion and results in lesions ranging from a chronic fibrotic lesion to fulminating tuberculous pneumonia.

The diagnosis of tuberculosis is suggested by a chronic cough, haemoptysis, loss of weight, night sweats and fever. Erythema nodosum may be associated. It is confirmed by physical examination, chest radiography, sputum smears and culture, and tuberculin testing (Mantoux or Heaf test). These are skin tests, looking for a delayed hypersensitivity reaction to protein from *M. tuberculosis* (purified protein derivative: PPD). Polymerase chain reaction techniques have greatly accelerated the diagnosis and speciation of mycobacteria and enabled treatment to be started earlier.

Other non-tuberculous (atypical) mycobacteria (NTM) frequently nowadays cause tuberculosis. *Mycobacterium avium-intracellulare* (MAI) can cause pulmonary tuberculosis while *M. scrofulaceum* is a rare cause of tuberculous cervical lymphadenitis, for example (*see also* p. 226).

Patients with HIV infection frequently develop tuberculosis due to NTM as well as *M. tuberculosis* and antimicrobial resistance is spreading.

• General management of TB

Chemoprophylaxis with isoniazid ± rifampicin is indicated when:

1. there has been close contact with a person actively infected with TB;
2. there is conversion of the tuberculin test within the past 2 years;
3. there is a positive tuberculin test in an immunocompromised person (such as diabetes, renal failure, cancer, HIV infection);
4. a person under 35 years, or an intravenous drug user, has a positive tuberculin test;
5. a foreign-born person has a positive tuberculin test and has migrated from a region of high prevalence within the previous 2 years;
6. there has been previous inadequate treatment of TB.

The efficacy of immunisation using BCG (bacille Calmette–Guerin) is controversial.

The first priority of tuberculosis control programmes is to identify and completely treat all patients with active tuberculosis. Treatment is started with three drugs in combination in order to avoid the emergence of bacterial resistance, given as a single daily dose with food (*Table 8.3*). Rifampicin plus isoniazid and pyrazinamide are used for the first 2 months, followed by the first two drugs only for a further 4 months. Chemotherapy must be given for at least 6 months (9 months in the immunocompromised) to be effective.

Patients are infectious until the sputum is negative to culture but the infectivity is greatly reduced by 2 weeks after the start of chemotherapy.

Pyridoxine is given to prevent isoniazid-induced peripheral neuropathy. Rifampicin interferes with the contraceptive pill. Alcoholics, drug-abusers, vagrants, the mentally handicapped or those with psychiatric disorders frequently default from treatment and, if chemotherapy is less than adequate, bacterial resistance readily develops.

Many patients with HIV disease now have multidrug-resistant TB. Capreomycin has been effectively used in some.

• Dental aspects of TB

The high infectivity of pulmonary tuberculosis is shown by cases of tuberculous infection of extraction sockets and cervical lymphadenitis in 15 patients treated by an infected member of a dental clinic staff. Tuberculosis is unlikely to be transmitted to staff during oral health care unless the person being treated has active pulmonary TB or the dental staff immunocompromised. Mortalities have been recorded in dental staff who themselves were HIV-positive, working in a dental clinic for HIV-infected persons in New York.

Patients with open pulmonary tuberculosis are thus clearly contagious and dental treatment is thus best deferred until the TB has been treated. If this is not possible, patients should be treated with special precautions to protect the respiratory tract against cross-

Table 8.3	Anti-tubercular therapy	
Drug	*Use*	*Main side-effects*
Rifampicin	Initial therapy[a]	Urine and saliva turn red
		Bullous lesions
	Continuation therapy[b]	Enhanced liver drug-metabolizing enzymes
		Hepatotoxicity
		Nephrotoxicity
Isoniazid	Initial therapy	Peripheral neuropathy
	Continuation therapy	Hepatotoxicity
Pyrazinamide	Initial therapy	Hepatotoxicity
Streptomycin*	Initial therapy	Vestibular nerve damage
		Circumoral paraesthesiae
Ethambutol*	Initial therapy	Ocular damage

[a]Initial therapy = rifampicin + isoniazid + streptomycin or ethambutol for 2 months.
[b]Continuation therapy = rifampicin + isoniazid for 9 months.
*Increasing resistance

infection. The aims are to prevent the release of mycobacteria into the air, to remove any that are present, and to stop the inhalation by other persons. Reduction of splatter and aerosols, by minimizing coughing and avoiding ultrasonic instruments, and use of rubber dam, are important. Improved ventilation, ultraviolet light, new masks and personal respirators are indicated. Mycobacteria are very resistant to disinfectants, so that heat sterilization should be used wherever possible. General anaesthesia is contraindicated for dental treatment, because of the risk of contamination of the anaesthetic apparatus or because of impaired pulmonary function. This could result from pleurocentesis, thoracoplasty or resection which were used before the introduction of chemotherapy.

Aminoglycosides such as streptomycin enhance the activity of some neuromuscular blocking drugs and in large doses may alone cause a myasthenic syndrome during general anaesthesia. The clearance of diazepam and the hepatotoxicity of paracetamol are enhanced by rifampicin. Isoniazid may also have the latter effect.

Other factors such as alcoholism or intravenous drug use (Chapter 24), hepatitis (Chapter 10) or HIV disease (Chapter 20) may also influence dental management.

Oral lesions can develop in pulmonary tuberculosis and in HIV-infected persons with tuberculosis, but are rare. Chronic ulcers, usually of the dorsum of the tongue, are the main manifestation. Occasionally the diagnosis of pulmonary tuberculosis is made as the result of biopsy of an oral ulcer. Such cases (usually middle-aged males) may result from neglect of symptoms or default from treatment. Unfixed material should also be sent for culture if possible. However the diagnosis is usually confirmed by sputum culture and chest radiographs after granulomas are seen microscopically. Acid-fast bacilli are rarely seen in oral biopsies even with the help of special stains.

Tuberculous cervical lymphadenopathy is the next most common form of the infection to pulmonary disease and is particularly common among those from the Indian Sub-Continent. NTM is a relatively common cause of cervical lymphadenitis in children under 12 years, and in HIV disease. In others, TB is the usual cause of mycobacterial lymphadeni-

tis. Most TB lymphadenitis is painless, with several enlarged rubbery nodes, and systemic symptoms only in a minority. Only about 15 per cent have pulmonary manifestations on radiography. Diagnosis relies on tuberculin testing but this can be positive both in tuberculous and NTM cervical lymphadenitis. Any person with a recent conversion from negative to positive tuberculin test should be suspected to have mycobacterial infection and should prompt biopsy, such as fine needle aspiration biopsy, for culture or histological confirmation. The polymerase chain reaction may improve diagnosis, as culture must wait 4–8 weeks for a result.

Oral complications of anti-tubercular therapy are rare but rifabutin and rifampicin may cause red saliva (*Table 8.3*).

Legionnaire's disease (legionellosis)

The term *Legionnaire's disease* was coined as a result of an outbreak of a previously unrecognized respiratory disease in an American Legion meeting in Philadelphia in 1976. Legionellosis is infection with one of the family Legionellaceae, a group of over 30 fastidious Gram-negative aerobic bacilli, ubiquitous in aquatic environments, and liable to infect especially persons who are immunocompromised. Most infections have involved *Legionella pneumophila*, and small epidemics have now been reported from many countries, since the first recognized outbreak. *L. bozemanii* and *L. micdadei* are occasionally implicated. The infection spreads mainly through aerosolization of infected water – especially from humidifiers in air-conditioning plants, and typically causes a lobular type of pneumonia. The latter ranges from discrete patches of inflammmation and consolidation to involvement of whole lobes.

Males over 45, smokers, the elderly and the immunocompromised are particularly at risk. The overall mortality may be as high as 10 per cent, but over 25 per cent in the elderly and up to 80 per cent in the immunocompromised. By contrast, many younger persons have been exposed to the infections and are seropositive but have remained healthy. However, in an outbreak due to the effluent from the air-conditioning system of Broadcasting House in London, young adults among passers-by in the street developed legionellosis.

A non-pneumonic form of the infection known as *Pontiac fever* manifests as a mild flu-like illness. Erythromycin is the standard therapy.

There is no evidence of person-to-person transmission and most infections have been traced to aerosol transmission involving warm water sources, such as air-conditioning systems, showers, nebulizers and the like. Many infections are contracted during travel abroad, particularly to Spain, Turkey and some other Mediterranean areas. Nearly 46 per cent of cases originate in this way.

• Dental aspects of legionellosis

Legionellae have been isolated from the stagnant water within dental units and could be disseminated in the dental surgery during aerosolization of water from dental equipment such as air-turbine sprays. Serological studies of dental school personnel have shown antibodies to Legionella species to rise with duration of work in the school. This suggests the bacteria could be spread in this way, but it has not been confirmed that the sources were dental equipment. Nevertheless, when dental units have to stand idle for long periods, over holidays or weekends for example, the system should be flushed through before treating patients.

Lung abscess

Lung abscess is a localized infection leading to cavitation and necrosis. The clinical features may be very ill-defined and diagnosis rests mainly on the chest radiograph. There is a risk of infection spreading locally or leading to a brain abscess.

Most cases result from pneumonia associated with infection by *Staphylococcus aureus* or *Klebsiella pneumoniae*. Bronchial obstruction by carcinoma or aspiration of foreign bodies are other important causes.

• Dental aspects of lung abscess

When undertaking endodontics or cementing restorations such as inlays or crowns, a rubber dam or other protective device should *always* be used to avoid the danger of inhalation of these foreign bodies. The main dangers in dentistry are with general anaesthesia, particularly if an inadequate throat pack has been used. A well-known cause of lung abscess is inhalation of a tooth or fragment, or rarely, endodontic instruments, but lung abscesses more often result from aspiration of oral bacteria, particularly anaerobes, even in the absence of dental intervention.

• General management of lung abscess

Patients who inhale tooth fragments or dental instruments must have chest radiographs (lateral and postero-anterior) and, if necessary, bronchoscopy.

Lung abscesses are usually treated by postural drainage or relief of the obstruction by bronchoscopy and antimicrobial chemotherapy.

Bronchiectasis

Bronchiectasis is dilatation and distortion of bronchi with excess sputum production and poor drainage causing recurrent lower respiratory tract infections. Bronchiectasis is often the result of respiratory damage as a result of measles, whooping cough, bronchiolitis or adenovirus infections in childhood. Some cases follow bronchial obstruction and cystic fibrosis or immunodeficiencies, but in many cases, no cause can be found. The damaged and dilated bronchi lose their ciliated epithelium, and mucus therefore tends to pool. Infection with *S. pneumoniae*, *H. influenzae* or *P. aeruginosa* is common.

Clinical features of bronchiectasis include overproduction of sputum, which is purulent during exacerbations, a cough (especially during exercise or when lying down) and finger clubbing. There are recurrent episodes of bronchitis, pneumonia and pleurisy. Haemoptysis is not uncommon and, in advanced bronchiectasis, pain, dyspnoea, cyanosis and respiratory failure may develop. Complications include cerebral abscess but amyloid disease is now rare since sepsis can usually be controlled.

• General management of bronchiectasis

Chest radiography and pulmonary function tests are required to establish the severity of bronchiectasis. Postural drainage is important and antimicrobials such as tetracycline, co-trimoxazole or amoxycillin are given for acute exacerbations and for long-term maintenance treatment.

- ### Dental aspects of bronchiectasis

General anaesthesia is contraindicated in the acute phases and should be avoided in the chronic phase. If a general anaesthetic must be given, safeguards should be taken as for patients with chronic obstructive airways disease and antibiotic cover should be given to prevent dissemination of infection.

OTHER RESPIRATORY DISORDERS

Cystic fibrosis

Cystic fibrosis (fibrocystic disease: mucoviscidosis) is an inherited disorder of the exocrine glands. It is inherited as an autosomal recessive trait and, with an incidence of about 1 in 2000 births, is the most common inherited error of metabolism in the UK and the USA and one of the most common, lethal hereditary disorders.

The essential feature of cystic fibrosis is increased viscosity of mucus. Obstruction of pancreatic ducts by mucus leads to pancreatic insufficiency in childhood with malabsorption and bulky, frequent, foul-smelling fatty stools and growth is frequently stunted (Chapter 9). Diabetes mellitus may be a complication, and some have cirrhosis.

Recurrent respiratory infections may result in bronchiectasis and usually a persistent productive cough. Most patients have recurrent sinusitis and nasal polyps. Viral infections such as measles can have severe sequelae. Cystic fibrosis also affects sweat and salivary glands. Most patients have a sweat sodium concentration in excess of 70 mmol/l (a change also reflected in the saliva) and these changes are used in diagnosis.

- ### General management of cystic fibrosis

Pancreatic replacement therapy (oral pancreatin) is given with each meal. A low fat intake and adequate vitamins in the diet are also necessary. Clearance of sputum is helped by regular physiotherapy, water aerosols and bronchodilators (terbutaline or salbutamol). Mucolytics such as carbocisteine, methyl cysteine and dornase alpha may be used but their effectiveness is questionable. Vaccination against measles, whooping cough and influenza are important preventive measures while amoxycillin or flucloxacillin are effective prophylactic antimicrobials. These may be given in an aerosol.

- ### Dental aspects of cystic fibrosis

General anaesthesia is contraindicated if respiratory function is poor, and liver disease and diabetes may also complicate treatment (Chapter 14).The major salivary glands may become enlarged. Tetracycline staining of the teeth was common, but should rarely be seen now. Enamel hypoplasia may be seen and both dental development and eruption are delayed. Pancreatin may cause oral ulceration if held in the mouth. The low fat, high carbohydrate diet predisposes to caries.

Chronic obstructive airways disease

Chronic obstructive airways disease (COAD: chronic obstructive pulmonary disease, COPD) is most frequently caused by chronic bronchitis and emphysema. Chronic bronchitis is defined as the excessive production of mucus and persistent cough with sputum production for more than 3 months in a year over 3 consecutive years. Emphysema is dilatation of air spaces distal to the terminal bronchioles with destruction of alveoli and a reduction in the alveolar surface area available for respiratory exchange.

Chronic bronchitis and emphysema are usually seen together in Britain, and are exceedingly common, especially among cigarette smokers living in cities. Deficiency of the anti-proteolytic enzyme α_1-antitrypsin is a rare cause of emphysema.

Chronic bronchitis leads to production of excessive, viscous mucus, which is ineffectively cleared from the airway, stagnates and becomes infected with *S. pneumoniae* and *H. influenzae*. Patchy areas of alveolar collapse may result. Both chronic bronchitis and emphysema cause cough, sputum and dyspnoea. There is initially an early morning mucoid cough which becomes mucopurulent during exacerbations. Dyspnoea on effort is mild at first, but deteriorates to leave a respiratory cripple ultimately dyspnoeic at rest and especially when recumbent (orthopnoea).

Chronic obstructive airways disease is complicated by chronic hypoxaemia. Eventually the sequence of pulmonary hypertension, right ventricular hypertrophy and cardiac failure (cor pulmonale) develops (Chapter 3). Chronic hypoxaemia leads to central cyanosis which, in association with ankle oedema and raised jugular venous pressure of cor pulmonale, gives rise to a 'blue bloated' appearance. At the other end of the spectrum, chronic obstructive airways disease may produce a 'pink panter' who is severely breathless and pink from vasodilatation caused by CO_2 retention. The reasons for these distinct clinical pictures are unclear.

The diagnosis is made clinically and supported by chest radiography, respiratory function tests and occasionally arterial blood gas estimations.

• General management of COAD

Patients with chronic bronchitis and emphysema must stop smoking. Immunization against influenza is recommended. Exacerbations of bronchitis are managed with amoxycillin, trimethoprim or tetracycline. Ipratropium bromide, other antimuscarinics (oxitropium) or other bronchodilators such as beta-agonists, or occasionally low dose systemic corticosteroids or theophylline, may be beneficial. Respiratory failure and cor pulmonale may also need to be treated. Severe cases are occasionally treated with bullectomy, or by lung transplantation.

• Dental aspects of COAD

The high prevalence of chronic bronchitis and emphysema means that all dental surgeons will have to treat these patients.

Wherever possible, dental treatment should be carried out under local anaesthesia. Patients are best treated in the upright position as they may become increasingly breathless if laid flat. It may also be difficult to use a rubber dam as patients may not tolerate the additional obstruction to breathing.

Patients with COAD should be given a general anaesthetic only if absolutely necessary, and only in hospital after full preoperative assessment. Secretions reduce airway patency, and if lightly anaesthetized the patient may cough and contaminate other areas of the lung. Intravenous barbiturates are totally contraindicated. Diazepam and midazolam are also mild respiratory depressants and should not be used for intravenous sedation by the dentist.

Patients taking corticosteroids should be treated with appropriate precautions (Chapter 14). Interactions of theophylline with drugs such as erythromycin, clindamycin or ciprofloxacin may result in dangerously high levels of theophylline. Those taking ipratropium may have a dry mouth.

• Pre-anaesthetic assessment

Postoperative respiratory complications are more prevalent in patients with pre-existing lung diseases, especially after prolonged operations and if there has been no preoperative preparation. Most patients with pre-existing respiratory disease present no problem if the assessment and anaesthesia have been managed appropriately. Spirometry and carbon monoxide perfusion are essential to assess respiratory function.

The most important single factor in preoperative care is cessation of smoking for at least 1 week preoperatively. Respiratory infections must also be eradicated. Sputum should first be sent for culture and sensitivity, but antimicrobials such as co-trimoxazole or amoxycillin should be started without awaiting results. Treatment can later be altered if necessary. Bronchodilator drugs are useful for bronchospasm. Thorough and frequent chest physiotherapy is important preoperatively and, if there is congestive cardiac failure, diuretics are indicated.

Many anaesthetists suggest that it is safest to avoid premedication. Morphine is certainly contraindicated since it can impair the cough reflex or precipitate bronchospasm. Pethidine can be used if the patient is in pain. Atropine and related antimuscarinics are also best avoided since they dry up the airways and increase the risk of postoperative pulmonary complications.

• **Postoperative care**

Postoperatively there should be close continuous assessment as it is difficult to detect hypoventilation. Arterial blood gases need to be monitored if any problems are anticipated and, rarely, if hypoventilation or excess secretions cannot be controlled by simple means, tracheostomy may be necessary. The 'blue-bloated' type of patient has a high arterial partial pressure of CO_2 ($PaCO_2$) and a low PaO_2. The main stimulus to respiration in these patients is hypoxia and there is little response to raised levels of CO_2. Such patients may hypoventilate postoperatively, especially if the respiratory drive of hypoxia is abolished by giving oxygen.

Bedridden patients with chronic obstructive airways disease may have added complications if given a general anaesthetic. Impaired cardiovascular responses may lead to profound hypotension if barbiturates are used. Cor pulmonale may be aggravated by the cardiodepressant activity of drugs used in anaesthesia or by the water retention that follows surgery or anaesthesia.

Secondary polycythaemia may predispose to thromboses postoperatively.

Asthma

Bronchial asthma is a state of bronchial hyper-reactivity characterized by paroxysmal expiratory wheezing and dyspnoea. Generalized reversible bronchial narrowing is caused by increased bronchial smooth muscle tone, mucosal oedema and congestion, and mucus hypersecretion. Precipitants can include non-allergens or allergens, especially aero-allergens.

Asthma is common, affects more than 2 per cent of the population and usually begins in childhood or early adult life. Asthma in children is typically allergic (extrinsic asthma) and, although such children are frequently asymptomatic between attacks, they often have had or develop other allergic diseases such as eczema, hay fever and drug sensitivities. This type of asthma, which tends to resolve by adult life, is associated with increased production of IgE on exposure to allergens, and the release of mast cell products which cause bronchospasm and oedema. Extrinsic asthmatic attacks may be precipitated by allergens in house dust,

animal dander, feathers, animal hairs, moulds, milk, eggs, fish, fruit, nuts, non-steroidal anti-inflammatory agents and some antibiotics. Intrinsic asthma, on the other hand, is not allergic in nature and appears to be related to mast cell instability and hyper-responsive airways. Factors that can initiate an episode of either type of asthma include infections (especially viral), irritating fumes including cigarette smoke, exercise, weather changes and emotional stress. Some drugs, particularly beta-blockers such as propranolol and non-steroidal anti-inflammatory drugs, are dangerous in either type of asthma and are absolutely contraindicated.

Children with asthma initially suffer from repeated 'colds' with cough, malaise and fever. Wheeziness with laboured expiration is prominent. The frequency and severity of attacks vary widely between individuals but symptoms are usually worse at night. Deaths from asthma are usually a result of failure to recognize deterioration, or inadequate treatment.

• **General management of asthma**

Investigations include blood examination for total IgE (usually raised and specific IgE antibody concentrations), skin tests which may help to identify any allergens and chest radiographs. Objective measurement of airways obstruction by a peak flow meter is important and treatment should be based on the amount by which peak flow is reduced.

Management of asthma includes the avoidance of identifiable irritants and allergens, and drug therapy. Sodium cromoglycate is used as an inhalant for prophylaxis, particularly in children, but some fail to respond. Selective beta$_2$-adrenoreceptor agonists or stimulants (salbutamol, terbutaline, fenoterol, rimiterol, bambuterol, pirbuterol, reproterol, tulobuterol, salmeterol or eformoterol) are the safest and most effective bronchodilators for the routine control of asthma. Ipratropium bromide is useful for some patients but particularly those with asthma associated with bronchitis. An alternative is oral sustained release theophylline preparations which have a prolonged action and are useful for controlling nocturnal asthma. If both of these fail, corticosteroid (beclomethasone, betamethasone valerate, budesonide or fluticasone) aerosol inhalations may be more effective and taken in conjunction with a bronchodilator, but must be taken regularly. High dose corticosteroid inhalants can cause some degree of adrenal suppression. If these also fail, oral corticosteroid treatment becomes necessary in addition.

Home use of peak flow meters allows patients to monitor progress of their disease and to detect any deterioration, which may require urgent modification of treatment.

• Dental aspects of asthma

Anxiety may occasionally precipitate asthmatic attacks and it is important to attempt to lessen fear of dental treatment by gentle handling and reassurance. Asthmatic patients should be asked to bring their usual medication with them when coming for dental treatment.

Dental treatment is best carried out under local anaesthesia. Occasional patients with asthma may react to sulphites present as preservatives in vasoconstrictor-containing local anaesthetics. It may be better, therefore, to avoid solutions containing vasoconstrictors. If adrenaline-containing local analgesics are indicated, they should be given with an aspirating syringe since adrenaline may theoretically enhance the risk of dysrhythmias with beta-agonists.

Relative analgesia with nitrous oxide and oxygen is preferable to intravenous sedation and gives more immediate control of the patient. Sedatives in general are better avoided as, in an acute asthmatic attack, even benzodiazepines can precipitate respiratory failure.

General anaesthesia may be complicated by hypoxia and hypercapnia, which can cause pulmonary oedema even if cardiac function is normal, and cardiac failure if there is cardiac disease. The risk of postoperative collapse of the lung or pneumothorax is also increased. General anaesthesia is therefore best avoided and in any event should only be given by a specialist anaesthetist in hospital. Halothane, or better, enflurane, isoflurane, desflurane or sevoflurane, are the preferred anaesthetics, but ketamine may be useful in children.

Drugs may also be liable to precipitate an asthmatic attack or anaphylaxis. Beta-blocker agents such as propranolol can precipitate severe or life-threatening bronchospasm, and are completely contraindicated. Aspirin and other NSAIDs, mefenamic acid, paracetamol and pentazocine are occasionally responsible and should be avoided. A few patients have *triad asthma* with nasal polyps, asthma and aspirin sensitivity. An asthmatic attack may also be precipitated by drugs causing histamine release directly: morphine and some other opioids, methohexitone, thiopentone, suxamethonium, tubocurarine and pancuronium should also therefore be avoided. Acrylic monomer and cyanoacrylates may occasionally precipitate an attack.

Allergy to penicillin may be more frequent in asthmatic patients. However, erythromycin, clindamycin and ciprofloxacin are also best avoided, since they may slow the metabolism of theophylline and cause toxicity.

Systemic corticosteroid treatment brings with it the risks from steroid complications and operations are dangerous on such patients without adequate preparation (Chapter 14). Acute asthmatic attacks are usually self-limiting or respond to the patient's usual medication such as a beta-agonist inhaler (salbutamol 5 mg). If severe, hydrocortisone 200 mg intravenously plus prednisolone 20 mg orally should also be given but asthma can occasionally persist despite these measures and continue for hours or days (status asthmaticus). This potentially lethal complication needs emergency treatment. Intravenous salbutamol or terbutaline, or aminophylline slowly, or subcutaneous adrenaline may be needed. Rapid injection of aminophylline or overdose can cause sudden severe dysrhythmias and death. This risk is increased in patients taking oral theophylline preparations. Oxygen should be given early and continued during the journey to hospital, if necessary by assisted positive pressure ventilation. Respiratory infections should also be treated.

Although there are no specific oral complications of asthma, the use of corticosteroid inhalers occasionally causes oral or pharyngeal thrush, while beta$_2$-agonists and ipratropium bromide (isopropyl atropine, Atrovent) can cause a dry mouth.

BRONCHOGENIC CARCINOMA (LUNG CANCER)

Bronchogenic carcinoma accounts for 95 per cent of all *primary* lung tumours, but lung tumours are frequently metastases. Bronchogenic carcinoma is the most common cancer in developed countries in males, and is the cause of death in some 10 per cent of them. Bronchogenic carcinoma most frequently affects urban, adult cigarette smokers, and it has become increasingly common in women to the extent that the mortality rate for the two sexes has become almost equal in the USA, where it is one of the most common types of cancer. Lung cancer is a fairly common cause of death in dental technicians but it is unknown whether this is due to smoking alone or to dust inhalation.

Recurrent cough, haemoptysis, dyspnoea, chest pain and recurrent chest infections are the predominant features. Cerebral metastases are common and can cause headache, epilepsy, hemiplegia or visual disturbances. Hepatic metastases may cause hepatomegaly, jaundice or ascites. Metastases can cause enlargement of the lower cervical lymph nodes. Bone metastases may cause pain, swelling or pathological fracture. Local infiltration may cause pleural effusion, or lesions of the cervical sympathetic chain (Horner's syndrome), brachial neuritis, or recurrent laryngeal nerve palsy. Obstruction of the superior vena cava may cause facial cyanosis and oedema (superior vena cava syndrome).

There are many non-metastatic extrapulmonary effects of bronchogenic or other carcinomas. Loss of weight and anorexia are common. Ectopic hormone production, neuromyopathies, thromboses (thrombophlebitis migrans), finger clubbing, muscle weakness and various skin manifestations may also be seen (Chapter 6) and are sometimes the first manifestations.

The diagnosis of bronchogenic carcinoma is based on history and physical examination supported by radiography (including CT), sputum cytology, bronchoscopy and biopsy.

- **General management of lung cancer**

About 25 per cent of patients are suitable for surgery but the 5-year survival is only about 25 per cent. Radiotherapy is frequently used but chemotherapy has, in general, given disappointing results except in small cell carcinomas. The overall 5-year survival rate is only 8 per cent.

- **Dental aspects of lung cancer**

Dental treatment under local anaesthesia should be uncomplicated. However, patients with bronchogenic carcinoma often have impaired respiratory function, especially after lobectomy or pneumonectomy and this, with any muscle weakness (myasthenic syndrome, Eaton–Lambert syndrome) which may make the patient unduly sensitive to the action of muscle relaxants, make general anaesthesia hazardous. General anaesthesia, if needed, should therefore be carried out by a specialist anaesthetist in hospital.

Metastases in the jaw are only rarely early or initial manifestations of a carcinoma of the lung. Even more rarely metastases can form epulis-like soft tissue swellings. Pigmentation of the soft palate is another rare early oral manifestation. Lung cancer may also be present in patients with oral cancer, and vice versa, or develop at a later stage (Chapter 5). Such synchronous or metachronous primary tumours must always be ruled out.

OCCUPATIONAL LUNG DISEASE

Workers in many industries are exposed to a variety of airborne particles that may cause lung disease. Pulmonary disorders related to the inhalation of dust particles are sometimes grouped as the pneumoconioses.

The clinical significance of these disorders varies widely (Appendix to this chapter). Some, such as siderosis, are benign, while others, such as asbestosis, can cause significant incapacity or cause lethal malignant complications. Berylliosis may be a hazard in some dental technical laboratories and lung cancer is increased. The major complication affecting dental treatment is that of respiratory impairment, and for this reason, general anaesthesia may be contraindicated. The physician should be contacted before treatment.

SARCOIDOSIS

Sarcoidosis is a multi-system granulomatous disorder of unknown aetiology. It most commonly affects young adults and typically causes bilateral hilar lymphadenopathy,

Table 8.4 Sarcoidosis – clinical findings	
Systemic symptoms	Fever, weight loss, fatigue
Pulmonary	Hilar lymphadenopathy; widespread infiltration
Ocular	Acute uveitis, cataracts, glaucoma
Lymph nodes	Lymphadenopathy (rarely lymphoma)
Dermatological	Erythema nodosum, infiltrates (lupus pernio) around eyes and nose
Hepatic	Asymptomatic hepatomegaly, sarcoid liver disease
Spleen	Splenomegaly
Renal	Nephrocalcinosis, renal calculi
Joints	Arthralgia, effusion
Neurological	Cranial or peripheral neuropathies
Skeletal	Cyst-like radiolucent areas
Oral/para-oral	Salivary gland swellings, gingival swelling

Table 8.5 Sarcoidosis – laboratory findings	
Histological findings	Non-caseating tubercle-like granulomas
Immunological findings	Anergy (partial) Negative response to tuberculin and some other common antigens on skin testing but positive response to Kveim antigen in about 80% Lymphopenia; reduced numbers of T-cells Raised serum levels of immunoglobulins
Biochemical findings	Hypercalcaemia. Raised serum levels of lysozyme, serum angiotensin converting enzyme (SACE) and adenosine deaminase

pulmonary infiltration and skin or eye lesions. It is twice as frequent in females as males and is seen especially in Afro-Caribbean populations.

The aetiology of sarcoidosis is unclear but is associated with limited impairment of cell-mediated immune responses (partial anergy) but no special susceptibility to infection. Sarcoidosis is protean in its manifestations and can involve virtually any tissue (*Table 8.4*). Pulmonary involvement is the most common and important, and causes impaired respiratory efficiency with cough and dyspnoea. Radiological changes such as enlarged hilar lymph nodes, may be more severe than suggested by the symptoms. Acute uveitis can progress to blindness. Hypercalcaemia is common and can result in renal damage. An increased susceptibility to lymphomas has been suggested.

• **General management of sarcoidosis**

Because of its vague and protean manifestations, sarcoidosis appears to be under-diagnosed. In the presence of suggestive clinical features, chest radiography, laboratory investigations such as raised levels of serum angiotensin-converting enzyme (SACE) (*Table 8.5*), a gallium scan of lachrymal and salivary glands, and labial gland biopsy may be indicated.

Mild anaemia, leucopenia and eosinophilia are common. Hypergammaglobulinaemia and a raised ESR are usual; serum albumin levels are low. Serum calcium levels are raised because of sensitivity to vitamin D, as are alkaline phosphatase in hepatic sarcoidosis, and lysozyme, adenosine deaminase and serum angiotensin-converting enzyme (SACE) in active cases.

Histological evidence of non-caseating epithelioid cell granulomas, and impaired delayed hypersensitivity reactions to some antigens may be useful. The Kveim test was carried out by intracutaneous injection of a heat-sterilized suspension of human spleen or lymph nodes affected with sarcoidosis. After 4–6 weeks the area was biopsied and, if positive, showed well-formed epithelioid granulomas. The test is positive in about 80 per cent of patients but is rarely used.

Patients with only minor symptoms often require no treatment. Corticosteroids are used especially if there is active ocular disease, progressive lung disease, hypercalcaemia, cerebral involvement or other serious complications.

• **Dental aspects of sarcoidosis**

Management problems of patients with systematic sarcoidosis may include:

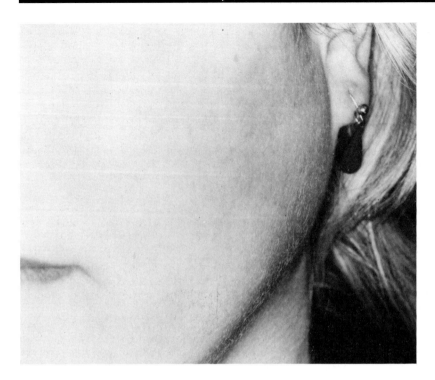

Fig. 8.1 Sarcoidosis presenting with parotid gland swelling

1. Respiratory impairment.
2. Uveitis and visual impairment.
3. Renal disease.
4. Jaundice.
5. Corticosteroid treatment (Chapter 14).

Sarcoidosis can involve any of the oral tissues but has a predilection for salivary glands. There is asymptomatic enlargement of the major salivary glands in about 6 per cent of cases (*Fig. 8.1*) and some have xerostomia. There is also an association of sarcoidosis with Sjögren's syndrome, when SS-A and SS-B serum autoantibodies are found. The association of salivary and lachrymal gland enlargement with fever and uveitis is known as uveoparotid fever (Heerfordt's syndrome). The salivary gland swellings usually resolve on treatment of sarcoidosis but this may take up to 3 years. Biopsy of minor salivary glands may confirm the diagnosis when other signs of the disease such as a suggestive chest film are present, and avoid the need for more invasive procedures.

Gingival enlargement can be an early or late feature and biopsy shows the typical sarcoid follicles. However, there is a group of patients who have histological features of sarcoid in one or more sites in the mouth, such as the gingivae, but no systemic manifestations and a negative Kveim test. A few of these patients may ultimately develop other more or less systematized disease but probably the majority have isolated lesions. Such cases, where no exogenous cause for the granulomatous reaction can be found, are regarded as having 'sarcoid-like' reactions and treatment is unnecessary. However, patients should be kept under observation for as long as possible.

There may be associated cranial neuropathies, especially facial palsy and rarely an association of thyroiditis, with Addison's disease and sarcoidosis (TASS syndrome).

Other causes of granulomatous reactions

If sarcoid-like follicles are found on biopsy of oral tissues, the differential diagnosis includes sarcoid and the following:

1. Tuberculosis and NTM.
2. Orofacial granulomatosis, Crohn's disease and Melkersson–Rosenthal syndrome.

3. As a reaction to some carcinomas.
4. Leprosy.
5. Zirconium.
6. Berylliosis.
7. Brucellosis.
8. Other foreign bodies.
9. Wegener's granulomatosis. However, it should be noted that midline granulomas (Chapter 21) are frequently not characterized by epithelioid granulomas histologically.
10. Other infections: syphilis, deep mycoses, cat-scratch disease, toxoplasmosis

POSTOPERATIVE RESPIRATORY COMPLICATIONS

Segmental or lobar pulmonary collapse and infection are the most common respiratory complications following surgical operations under general anaesthesia. These complications are more common after abdominal surgery or if there is pre-existent respiratory disease, smoking or occupational respiratory disorders (*see also* Chapter 2).

Postoperative respiratory complications can be significantly reduced by starting physiotherapy preoperatively in patients with respiratory disorders who require prolonged general anaesthesia.

Bronchodilators such as salbutamol may also be of value in preventing complications, especially if there is a strong element of bronchospasm.

If postoperative pulmonary infection develops, physiotherapy and antibiotics should be given and sputum sent for culture. The common microbial causes are *S. pneumoniae* and *H. influenzae*; suitable antibiotics include amoxycillin, erythromycin or co-trimoxazole. Hospital infections may include other micro-organisms such as staphylococci, klebsiella, pseudomonas and other Gram-negative bacteria. Microbiological examination of the sputum and antibiotic sensitivities are therefore essential.

Aspiration of gastric contents (Mendelson's syndrome)

Inhalation of gastric contents, such as alcoholic vomiting, may cause asphyxia and death. Aspiration of gastric contents into the lower respiratory tract causes pulmonary oedema and can be fatal (Mendelson's syndrome). Aspiration is most likely if a general anaesthetic is given to a patient whose stomach is not empty because, for example, food or drink has been taken or stomach emptying is delayed. Hiatus hernia may predispose to regurgitation.Vomiting during anaesthesia, and hence aspiration, is more likely in the last trimester of pregnancy.

The best treatment is prevention, by ensuring that the stomach is empty and by passing an endotracheal tube if not. The endotracheal tube must be passed by a skilled anaesthetist with the patient's head at a lower level than the stomach. Antacids or an H_2 receptor blocker, such as cimetidine or ranitidine, may be given by mouth before the anaesthetic to reduce gastric acidity in the event of aspiration.

If gastric contents are aspirated, the pharynx and larynx must be carefully sucked out. Systemic corticosteroids have been recommended, but recent reports have not confirmed any reduction in the mortality.

OBSTRUCTIVE SLEEP APNOEA SYNDROME

Obstructive sleep apnoea syndrome (OSAS) is when there are periods of apnoea during sleep because of airways obstruction in the region of the soft palate and tongue. Partial upper airways obstruction during sleep can cause snoring and there is an association between obstructive sleep apnoea, daytime sleepiness and cardiopulmonary complications, particularly in obese middle-aged men. Reduced activity of muscles in the tongue, palate and pharynx appears to contribute. Because of the apnoea, arterial oxygen saturation falls, and cardiac dysrhythmias may develop. In more severe cases pulmonary hypertension and right ventricular failure result. There is a raised mortality rate, not least from road traffic accidents since affected patients are constantly drowsy. Measures devised to overcome these problems include orthognathic surgery, uvulopalatopharyngoplasty (UPPP), nasal continuous airway pressure or even tracheostomy. Only the last two have been shown convincingly to reduce the mortality.

• Dental aspects of OSAS

Uvulopalatopharyngoplasty has been the standard treatment for OSAS but the efficacy is currently under review. Recent work suggests that where the obstruction is predominantly hypopharyngeal, surgical advancement of the facial skeleton and hyoid may effectively expand the airway. When there is both oro- and hypopharyngeal obstruction UPPP may need to be combined with mandibulo-maxillary and hyoid advancement. Nasal obstruction may also have to be relieved, but maxillofacial surgery carried out in stages to assess the degree of improvement, may relieve nocturnal hypoxia, snoring and daytime sleepiness.

Oronasal obstruction in weak senile patients: A dangerous degree of dyspnoea and cyanosis has been noted in some weak senile patients, even when awake. The oronasal obstruction results from blockage of the nose and lack of teeth or dentures causing the mouth to become over-closed.

Hypoxia, thus caused, may contribute to the death of these vulnerable patients. Provision of dentures may alleviate this hazard, but a nasal catheter provides a more rapid and simple solution.

RESPIRATORY DISTRESS SYNDROMES (RDS)

Respiratory distress in premature infants may be caused by bronchopulmonary dysplasia and necessitates endotracheal intubation for many weeks. This may in turn result in midface hypoplasia, palatal grooving or cleft-ing, or defects in the primary dentition. The same oral effects may be seen with prolonged use of orogastric feeding tubes. The degree to which subsequent growth corrects these deformations is currently unknown though the palatal grooves typically regress by the age of 2 years. Unfortunately, using soft endotracheal tubes does not obviate this problem and at present the best means of avoiding palatal grooving appears to be the use of an intraoral acrylic plate to stabilize the tube and protect the palate.

Adult respiratory distress syndrome (ARDS) is a sequel to several types of pulmonary injury and some infections, including with oral viridans streptococci.

BIBLIOGRAPHY

Almeida O.P. and Scully C. (1991) Oral lesions in the systemic mycoses. *Curr. Opin Dent.* **1**, 423–8.

Bagg J. (1996) Tuberculosis; a re-emerging problem for health care workers. *Br. Dent. J.* **180**, 376–81.

Bartlett J.G. (1996) Antibiotic selection in sinusitis. *Arch. Otolaryngol. Head Neck Surg.* **122**, 422–3.

Bert F. and Lambert-Zechovsky N. (1996) Sinusitis in mechanically ventilated patients and its role in the pathogenesis of nosocomial pneumonia. *Eur. J. Clin. Microbiol. Infect. Dis.* **15**, 533–44.

Brinker H. (1986) The sarcoidosis-lymphoma syndrome. *Br. J. Cancer* **54**, 467–73.

Brook M.G., Lucas R.E. and Pain A.K. (1988) Clinical features and management of two cases of Streptococcus milleri chest infection. *Scand. J. Infect. Dis.* **20**, 345–6.

Cawson R.A. Spector R.G. and Skelly A.M. (1995) *Basic Pharmacology and Clinical Drug Use in Dentistry*, 6th edn. Edinburgh, Churchill Livingstone.

Cleveland J.L., Gooch B.F., Bolyard E.A. *et al.* (1995) TB infection control recommendations from the CDC, 1994: considerations for dentistry. *J. Am. Dent. Assoc.* **126**, 593–600.

Cox N.H. and McCrea J.D. (1996) A case of Sjögren's syndrome, sarcoidosis, previous ulcerative colitis and gastric autoantibodies. *Br. J. Dermatol.* **134**, 1138–40.

Erkan M., Ozcan M., Arslan S. *et al.* (1996) Bacteriology of antrum in children with chronic maxillary sinusitis. *Scand. J. Infect. Dis.* **28**, 283–5.

Ferguson G.T. and Cherniack R.M. (1993) Management of chronic obstructive pulmonary disease. *N. Engl. J. Med.* **328**, 1017–22.

Fernald G.W., Roberts M.W. and Boat T.F. (1990) Cystic fibrosis: a current review. *Pediatr. Dent.* **12**, 72–8.

Fotos P.G., Westfall H.N., Synder I.S. *et al.* (1985) Prevalence of Legionella-specific IgG and IgM antibody in a dental clinic population. *J. Dent. Res.* **64**, 1382–5.

Goldsmith D. and Trieger N. (1980) Pulmonary assessment in the ambulatory patient. *J. Oral Surg.* **38**, 771–3.

Hagan J.L. and Hardy J.D. (1983) Lung abscesses revisited. *Ann. Surg.* **197**, 755–62.

Kauffman C.A. (1996) Quandary about treatment of aspergilloma persists. *Lancet* **347**, 1640.

Kenyon T.A., Valway S.E., Ihle W.W. *et al.* (1996) Transmission of multi-drug resistant *Mycobacterium tuberculosis* during a long airplane flight. *N. Engl. J. Med.* **334**, 933–8.

Kinirons M.J. (1989) Dental health of patients suffering from cystic fibrosis in Northern Ireland. *Commun. Dent. Hlth* **6**, 113–20.

Kuhn J.P. (1986) Imaging of the paranasal sinuses: current status. *J. Allerg. Clin. Immunol.* **77**, 6–9.

Larsen G.L.(1992) Asthma in children. *N. Engl. J. Med.* **326**, 1540–5.

Lee K.C. and Schecter G. (1995) Tuberculous infections of the head and neck. *ENT J.* **74**, 395–9.

Levin J.A. and Glick M. (1996) Dental management of patients with asthma. *Compend. Contin. Educ. Dent.* **17**, 284–92.

Lindemann R.A., Newman M.G., Kaufman A.K. *et al.* (1985) Oral colonisation and susceptibility testing of *Pseudomonas aeruginosa* oral isolates from cystic fibrosis patients. *J. Dent. Res.* **64**, 54–7.

Lowe A.A. (1990) The tongue and airway. *Otolaryngol. Clin. North Am.* **23**, 677–98.

Lu S-J., Chang S-Y. and Shiao G-M. (1995) Comparison between short-term and long-term post-operative evaluation of sleep apnoea after uvulopalatopharyngoplasty. *J. Laryngol. Otol.* **109**, 308–12.

Mahaney M.C. (1986) Delayed dental development and pulmonary disease in children with cystic fibrosis. *Arch. Oral Biol.* **31**, 363–7.

McCarthy F.M. (1984) Safe treatment of the emphysema patient. *J. Am. Dent. Assoc.* **106**, 761–6.

Menzies D., Fanning A., Yuan L. and Fitzgerald M. (1995) Tuberculosis among health care workers. *N. Engl. J. Med.* **332**, 92–8.

Molinari J.A. (1995) Tuberculosis infection control; a reasonable approach for dentistry. *Compend. Contin. Educ. Dent.* **16**, 1080–6.

Newton L.H., Joseph C.A., Hutchinson E.J. *et al.* (1996) Legionnaire's disease surveillance: England and Wales, 1995. *CDR* **6**, R151–155.

Porter S.R. and Scully C. (1996) *Innovations and Developments in Non-Invasive Oral Health Care.* Northwood, Science Reviews.

Primosch R.E. (1980) Tetracycline discoloration, enamel defects and dental caries in patients with cystic fibrosis. *Oral Surg. Oral Med. Oral Pathol.* **50**, 303–8.

Riben P.D., Epstein J.B. and Mathias R.G. (1995) Dentistry and tuberculosis in the 1990s. *J. Canad. Dent. Assoc.* **61**, 492–8.

Rotschild A., Dison P.J., Chitayat D. *et al.* (1990) Midfacial hypoplasia associated with long-term intubation for bronchopulmonary dysplasia. *Am. J. Dis. Childh.* **144**, 1302–6.

Ryberg M., Moller C. and Ericson T. (1991) Saliva composition and caries development in asthmatic patients treated with β2 adrenoceptor agonists; a 4 year follow-up study. *Scand. J. Dent. Res.* **99**, 1404–6.

Salzman G.A. and Pyszczynski R. (1988) Oropharyngeal candidiasis in patients treated with beclomethasone dipropionate delivered by metered-dose inhaler alone and with aerochamber. *J Allerg. Clin. Immunol.* **81**, 424–8.

Scannapieco F.A. and Mylotte J.M. (1996) Relationships between periodontal disease and bacterial pneumonia. *J. Periodontol.* **67**, 1114–22.

Scully C. (1988) *The Dental Patient.* Heinemann, Oxford.

Scully C. (1989) *The Mouth and Perioral Tissues.* Heinemann, Oxford.

Scully C. (1989) *Patient Care: a Dental Surgeon's Guide.* London, British Dental Association.

Scully C. (1995) The mycobacterioses. In Millard H.D. and Mason D.K. (eds), *1993 World Workshop on Oral Medicine.* Ann Arbor, University of Michigan Press, pp. 57–61.

Scully C., Cawson R.A. and Griffiths M.J. (1990) *Occupational Hazards to Dental Staff.* London, British Dental Journal.

Seinfeld E.D. and Sharma O.P. (1983) TASS syndrome; unusual association of thyroiditis, Addison's disease and sarcoidosis. *J. Roy. Soc. Med.* **76**, 883–5.

Shapiro G.G., Furukawa C.T. and Pierson W.E. (1986) Blinded comparison of maxillary sinus radiography and ultrasound for diagnosis of sinusitis. *J. Allerg. Clin. Immunol.* **77**, 59–62.

Skogberg K., Ruutu P., Tukiainen P. and Valtonen V. (1993) Effect of immunosuppressive therapy on the clinical presentation and outcome of tuberculosis. *Clin. Infect. Dis.* **17**, 1012–17.

Smith W.H.R. (1982) Intraoral and pulmonary tuberculosis following dental treatment. *Lancet* **i**, 842–4.

Strull G.E. and Dym H. (1995) Tuberculosis: diagnosis and treatment of resurgent disease. *J. Oral Maxillofac. Surg.* **53**, 1334–40.

Thompson P.J. *et al.* (1986) Assessment of oral candidiasis in patients with respiratory disease and efficacy of a new nystatin formulation. *Br. Med. J.* **292**, 699–700.

Tynan J.J. and Kamiyama K. (1984) Cystic fibrosis and oral health. *J. Canad. Dent. Assoc.* **50**, 833–5.

Uhari M., Kontiokari T., Koskela M. and Niemela M. (1996) Xylitol chewing gum in prevention of otitis media – double blind randomised trial. *Br. Med. J.* **313**, 1180–3.

Von Gonten A.S., Meyer J.B. and Kim A.K. (1995) Dental management of neonates requiring prolonged oral intubation. *J. Prosthodont.* **4**, 222–5.

APPENDIX TO CHAPTER 8

OCCUPATIONAL LUNG DISEASES

Disorder	Source of causal agent	Group at risk	Clinical significance
Anthracosis	Soot Carbon smoke	Urban dwellers	Benign
Asbestosis	Asbestos	Asbestos workers (crocidolite or amosite predispose to mesothelioma) Insulation Fertilizers Explosives	Pulmonary fibrosis leading to cor pulmonale Bronchial carcinoma Mesothelioma
Bagassosis	Mouldy sugar cane fibre	Farmers	Acute pneumonia or bronchiolitis
Bariliosis	Barium	Barium miners	Benign
Berylliosis	Beryllium Various alloys	Fluorescent lamps	Chronic respiratory disease leading to cor pulmonale
Byssinosis	Cotton, flax or hemp	Cotton workers	Periodic bronchospasm leading to obstructive airways disease
Coal miner's pneumoconiosis	Coal dust	Coal miners	Largely asymptomatic but may cause fibrosis and emphysema
Kaolin pneumoconiosis	China clay	China clay workers	Resembles silicosis (q.v.)
Siderosis	Iron dust	Welders Grinders	Benign
Silicosis	Silica (quartz) dust	Miners Sandblasting Potters	Pulmonary fibrosis leading to cor pulmonale Tuberculosis
Stannosis	Tin dust	Tin refining	Benign

9

Gastrointestinal disorders

Key points

- Disorders affecting the teeth are commonly of local origin but systemic disease may affect tooth development, structure and eruption.
- Oral ulcers are the common mucosal lesions and may have local causes, or be aphthae, carcinoma or other neoplasms, or be related to systemic diseases – notably infections, or blood, intestinal or skin diseases, or to drugs.
- Recurrent aphthae are uncommonly associated with systemic disease but similar lesions may be seen in Behçet's syndrome, vitamin deficiencies and immunodeficiencies, notably HIV disease.
- Salivary disorders are often of local cause but may be iatrogenic, or associated with connective tissue disease, liver disease, infections, endocrine or metabolic disease, or tumours.
- Dry mouth is often iatrogenic, due to drugs or irradiation of the glands, but may be caused by dehydration as in diabetes, or autoimmune exocrinopathy (Sjögren's syndrome).
- Sjögren's syndrome (SS) affects the salivary and lachrymal glands; if there is a connective tissue disease it is termed secondary, while alone it is termed primary.
- Complications of SS include caries, candidosis and sialadenitis. Salivary gland swelling may be due to the primary disease process, sialadenitis, or lymphoma. HIV can produce a similar picture.
- Cervical lymph node enlargement is usually caused by infection in the head and neck. Systemic infections, local or systemic neoplasms, and a miscellany of other disorders must be considered.
- Halitosis is usually caused by smoking, food or drugs, or periodontal or other infection in the mouth or upper airway. Respiratory, renal, hepatic, endocrine, gastrointestinal and psychiatric conditions should be excluded.
- Peptic ulceration is related to infection with *Helicobacter pylori*. Oral sources of this are thought not to be significant.
- Peptic ulceration is a contraindication to aspirin and other non-steroidal anti-inflammatory drugs. Acid regurgitation may cause dental erosion.
- Gastric disorders may increase the risk of vomiting after general anaesthesia.
- Coeliac disease is an inherited hypersensitivity to gluten, which presents with jejunal disease in particular, and consequent malabsorption.
- Crohn's disease is a chronic granulomatous disorder causing ulceration and mucosal tags, seen particularly in the ileum, but can affect any part of the gastrointestinal tract, including the mouth.
- Anaemia resulting from gastric conditions (ulceration, surgery, pernicious anaemia), coeliac or Crohn's disease may predispose to oral disease, especially ulcers, candidosis, glossitis and dysaesthesia.

ORAL DISEASE

Orofacial pain is discussed in Chapter 19. This chapter discusses many of the other oral complaints where there may be important medical implications.

DISORDERS AFFECTING THE TEETH

Teething

Teething is traditionally blamed for a variety of signs and symptoms in infancy. Restlessness, finger-sucking, gum-rubbing and drooling may be associated with the eruption of deciduous teeth. However, teething is not responsible for diarrhoea, fever, convulsions or other systemic disorders; these have systemic causes, usually infections.

Discoloration of teeth

Causes are outlined in *Table 9.1*. Most are extrinsic or related to caries or trauma but biliary atresia may cause green, and erythropoietic porphyria, red, teeth.

Odontogenic infections

Odontogenic infections arise mainly as a consequence of caries leading to pulpitis then periapical infection. Most respond to drainage, either by endodontic treatment, by incision, or by tooth extraction. Analgesics may be required.

Most odontogenic and orofacial infections contain a mixed flora, with a substantial proportion of anaerobes and, although most respond to drainage, antimicrobials may sometimes be indicated, particularly in the following circumstances.

1. Infections:
    of fascial spaces of the neck;
    necrotizing fasciitis;
    osteomyelitis;
    odontogenic infections in ill or immuno-compromised persons;
    acute ulcerative gingivitis;
    acute sinusitis.
2. Prophylaxis of:
    infective endocarditis;
    meningitis where there is cerebrospinal fluid leak or compound skull fracture after head injury;
    infection after facial fractures;
    infection in major maxillofacial surgery;
    infection after surgery in immunocompromised persons or after jaw irradiation;
    infection in ventriculoatrial or other shunts, penile prostheses, and sometimes joint prostheses.
3. Some cases of:
    dental abscess;
    pericoronitis;
    dry socket;
    minor oral surgery.

Most odontogenic infections respond well to phenoxymethyl penicillin or metronidazole. Amoxycillin, ampicillin, doxycycline or erythromycin are also usually effective. Co-trimoxazole is best now reserved mainly for treatment of *Pneumocystis carinii* pneumonia.

Fascial space infections

Fascial space infections are usually polymicrobial, involve predominantly anaerobes, and arise from the oral flora. They are dangerous since they may cause swelling and thus embarrass the airway, may erode the carotid vessels, may cause toxicity, and rarely spread to the mediastinum or intracranially. Patients with these infections should thus usually be admitted for hospital care, which may involve drainage and usually high dose antibiotics.

Table 9.1	Causes of discoloured teeth	
	Extrinsic	*Intrinsic*
Most teeth affected	Smoking	Tetracycline
	Beverages, e.g. tea	Fluorosis
	Drugs	Amelogenesis imperfecta
	e.g. iron,	
	chlorhexidine	Dentinogenesis imperfecta
	minocycline	
	Poor oral hygiene	Kernicterus
	Betel chewing	Porphyria
One or a few teeth affected	As above	Trauma
		Caries
		Internal resorption

Necrotizing fasciitis

Necrotizing fasciitis is an uncommon, potentially lethal infection of the subcutaneous tissues and deep fascia, with necrosis of the overlying skin due to thrombosis of blood vessels. It can arise from a dental source and may threaten the airway. The mortality has reached 30 per cent in some series.

A variety of micro-organisms have been implicated including beta-haemolytic streptococci, anaerobes such as porphyromonas and prevotella species, and others. Most patients are middle-aged or older, but few have detectable underlying predisposing factors though an immunodeficiency such as diabetes may be present.

Clinically there is pain disproportionate to the clinical appearance. Initially there is no fever, but within 24–48 hours there is rapidly spreading tissue necrosis. The skin is initially red, painful and oedematous but rapidly turns purplish, dusky and then black, and there is gas and exudate. Thoracic CT may be required to detect mediastinal spread.

Early aggressive therapy is indicated. The airway should be protected by intubation, and the area opened surgically to drain and excise the necrotic tissue. Penicillin or a cephalosporin plus metronidazole are indicated and hyperbaric oxygen if available.

DISORDERS AFFECTING THE ORAL MUCOSA

Oral ulcers

Oral ulcers are very common. Most are traumatic or recurrent aphthae; they are usually of little consequence, but more serious causes must always be excluded (*Table 9.2*). Particular care must be taken to exclude cancer, blood dyscrasias, mucocutaneous or gastrointestinal disease and HIV or other infections.

The clinical history is of great value in the differential diagnosis but if there is any doubt investigations, perhaps including biopsy, are essential. The history should establish any contributing factor such as drug use, or systemic disease such as anaemia or other blood dyscrasia, immunodeficiency, infections, skin, gastrointestinal, eye or genital

Table 9.2   Causes of oral ulceration

- Local causes
  Trauma
  Chemical irritation
  Burns
  Irradiation
- Recurrent aphthae
- Neoplasms
  Squamous cell carcinoma
  Others (Chapter 6)
- Systemic causes
  Mucocutaneous diseases (Chapter 17)
    Lichen planus
    Chronic ulcerative stomatitis
    Pemphigus
    Pemphigoid
    Localized oral purpura
    Erythema multiforme
    Epidermolysis bullosa
    Dermatitis herpetiformis
    Linear IgA disease
    Behçet's and Sweet's syndromes
  Connective tissue and other diseases (Chapter 16)
    Lupus erythematosus
    Reiter's syndrome
    Vasculitides
    Giant cell arteritis
    Wegener's granulomatosis
    Periarteritis nodosa
  Blood diseases (Chapters 4 and 5)
    Leucopenias including HIV disease
    Leukaemias and myelodysplastic syndrome
    Deficiency states or anaemia
    Hypereosinophilic syndrome
  Gastrointestinal disease
    Coeliac disease
    Crohn's disease
    Ulcerative colitis
  Drugs (*see* Chapter 25)
  Infections
  Viral mainly (Chapter 11)
    Herpes viruses
    Coxsackie viruses
    ECHO viruses
  Bacterial
  Acute necrotizing gingivitis
  Syphilis
  Tuberculosis
  Epithelioid angiomatosis
  Fungal
    Cryptococcosis
    Histoplasmosis
    Paracoccidioidomycosis
    Blastomycosis
    Zygomycosis
    Aspergillosis
  Protozoal
    Leishmaniasis

Table 9.3 Features of recurrent aphthae
• Onset usually in childhood or adolescence • Typically round or ovoid ulcers • Recurrences at intervals • Usually self-limiting. Ulceration typically ceases before middle age

Table 9.4 Different types of aphthae

• Minor aphthae
  Common
  Usually round or ovoid discrete ulcers
  Not on attached gingiva or hard palate and rarely on dorsum of tongue
  Most are 2–4 mm in diameter
  Most heal within 10 days without scarring
• Major aphthae
  Uncommon
  Usually round or ovoid discrete ulcers
  Ulcers may be one to several centimetres in diameter
  Persist for months before healing with scarring
• Herpetiform aphthae
  Uncommon
  Ulcers initially 1–3 mm across but later coalesce to form ragged ulcers
  Ulcers form in crops of 10–100 with widespread erythema

disease. The typical features of aphthae are summarized in *Table 9.3*.

Recurrent aphthae (recurrent aphthous stomatitis, RAS)

Recurrent aphthae are recurring mouth ulcers that typically start in childhood. They are common and may affect up to 25 per cent of the population at some time. Some groups, for example students, have a higher incidence, but only a minority of patients have ulcers so frequently or severely as to cause them to seek dental or medical advice.

Aphthae typically start in childhood or adolescence and become progressively more troublesome until, when patients reach their twenties or thirties, help is sought. Most patients are non-smokers. The disease is usually self-limiting and after a variable number of years the ulcers become less frequent or cease altogether. During the course of the disease spontaneous remissions of a month or two are common and this makes evaluation of treatment difficult. Several different clinical patterns are recognized (*Table 9.4*).

There appears to be a familial basis to the ulceration in some patients. A few show a clear relationship of ulcers with the luteal phase of menstruation. A few patients associate the ulcers with stress, particular foods or trauma and similar ulcers can be a troublesome feature of HIV infection.

Most patients are otherwise healthy. Deficiency states, particularly of iron, folate or vitamin B_{12}, however, are found in 10–20 per cent of patients, and aphthae may also be associated with some intestinal diseases, notably coeliac or Crohn's disease, or ulcerative colitis, or Behçet's syndrome (Chapter 21), when there may be genital ulceration, uveitis and other lesions.

Exceedingly rare causes of ulcers, clinically indistinguishable from RAS, are HIV infection, cyclic neutropenia and other immunodeficiencies. Major aphthae may be the presenting feature of HIV infection. They typically affect the palate and may be associated with pharyngeal or oesophageal ulceration.

Cyclic neutropenia typically causes recurrent infections, fever, malaise and enlarged cervical lymph nodes. Oral ulceration typically appears at 21-day intervals, coincident with the falls in circulating neutrophils, and may be the main manifestation of the disease. In others, severe periodontal disease may develop.

In vitro immunological abnormalities have been reported in RAS but there is scant evidence for an autoimmune basis, no association with typical autoimmune diseases and none of the common autoantibodies are found. There is also little evidence for an association with atopic disease.

• General management

In addition to a careful history, patients with aphthae should be screened haematologically, particularly if the history suggests a systemic disorder or if the ulcers develop or worsen in middle age or later. A full screen includes haemoglobin and blood indices. Serum ferritin (or iron and iron-binding capacity), vitamin B_{12} levels and corrected whole blood or red cell folate levels may sometimes be required (Appendix to Chapter 1). Systemic conditions such as Behçet's disease and HIV infection should be excluded if the history is suggestive of these.

There is no specific or reliably effective treatment for aphthae. Patients vary widely in their response to various medications and their assessment is complicated by spontaneous remissions or by placebo effects.

A mouthwash of chlorhexidine gluconate (0.2 per cent aqueous solution) is useful to maintain oral hygiene and mitigates ulcers in some patients. Others seem to respond to tetracycline mouth rinses. Topical corticosteroids may sometimes be effective. Hydrocortisone hemisuccinate pellets 2.5 mg dissolved in the mouth up to four times daily should be used continuously, whether ulcers are present or not, unless attacks are infrequent. This regimen should be continued for 2 months then stopped for a month to assess progress. Triamcinolone acetonide in Orabase paste can be used, but patients may find it difficult to apply. Topical betamethasone, beclomethasone, clobetasol or fluocinonide preparations are sometimes required. Systemic corticosteroids or other immunosuppressants are occasionally indicated.

Major aphthae remain a serious problem. Pain may be controlled with the use, topically, of lignocaine gels or viscous solutions. Experimentally, corticosteroids, thalidomide and azathioprine may be effective but such treatment is a matter for specialists. Pentoxyfilline appears promising. In patients with HIV infection major aphthae may respond to zidovudine or thalidomide.

White and red lesions

Most white lesions are of local aetiology, such as keratoses caused by irritation. White sponge naevus is a rare congenital disorder that can involve the vagina and anus. Lichen planus and lupus erythematosus are discussed in Chapter 12. Candidosis may cause white or red lesions (Chapter 20). Other red lesions are inflammatory (sarcoid, Crohn's disease) or atrophic (desquamative gingivitis, erythroplasia or due to a deficiency state) or sometimes due to Kaposi's sarcoma, or Wegener's granulomatosis.

Desquamative gingivitis

Desquamative gingivitis may be caused by lichen planus, pemphigoid, pemphigus, linear IgA disease or dermatitis herpetiformis (*see* p. 253).

Oral hyperpigmentation

Most oral pigmentation is racial in origin or a local lesion such as an amalgam tattoo. Though they are rare, the most important systemic causes to be excluded are drugs such as minocycline (Chapter 25), heavy metal poisoning, Addison's disease, Nelson's syndrome, melanoma and HIV disease. In the last case the pigmentation may be due to treatment with zidovudine or drugs such as clofazimine, occasionally to Addison's disease secondary to fungal infection or of unknown cause. Pigmentation of the soft palate is a rare manifestation of bronchogenic carcinoma (*Table 9.5*).

A number of rare congenital disorders have oral hyperpigmentation as a manifestation. Peutz–Jeghers syndrome (*Table 9.5*) includes oral and perioral hyperpigmentation with small intestine polyps. Carney complex includes lentiginosis due to adrenal disease and multiple neoplasia such as myxomas of the skin, heart and breast, schwannomas, pituitary adenomas, testicular tumours and thyroid tumours. Syndromes such as NAME (naevi, atrial myxoma, myxoid neurofibromata and ephelides) and LAMB (lentigines, atrial myxoma, mucocutaneous myxoma, blue naevi) fall into this category. Lentigenes may also be seen with hypertrophic cardiomyopathy in the LEOPARD syndrome, or occasionally with arterial dissections.

DRY MOUTH

Dry mouth (xerostomia) has many causes (*Table 9.6*). It may be a complaint even when salivary flow is normal but this is psychogenic. Important causes are drugs (*see* Appendix to Chapter 25), irradiation of the major salivary glands, Sjögren's syndrome and HIV infection.

Table 9.5   Oral hyperpigmentation

- Congenital
  Racial (even in some Caucasians)
  Naevi
  Syndromes
  Peutz–Jeghers syndrome (*Table 9.13*)
  Carney complex
  Laugier–Hunziker syndrome
- Acquired
  Endocrine or metabolic
  Addison's disease
  ACTH therapy
  ACTH-producing tumours (lung cancer)
  Haemochromatosis
  Nelson's syndrome
  Neoplastic
  Melanoma
  Kaposi's sarcoma
  Metals
  Amalgam tattoo
  Bismuth, mercury, lead, silver
  Drugs
  Smoking
  Antimalarials
  Cytotoxics (busulphan particularly)
  Oral contraceptives
  Phenothiazines
  Minocycline
  Zidovudine
  Clofazimine
  Others
  HIV infection and AIDS

Table 9.6   Causes of dry mouth

- Iatrogenic
  Drugs (antimuscarinics; sympathominetics)
  Cancer therapy (irradiation of salivary glands, radioactive iodine, cytotoxic drugs)
  Graft-versus-host disease
- Salivary gland disease
  Aplasia
  Sjögren's syndrome
  Sarcoidosis
  HIV disease
  Infiltrates (amyloidosis; haemochromatosis)
  Cystic fibrosis
  Others
- Dehydration
  Diabetes mellitus
  Diabetes insipidus
  Renal failure
  Haemorrhage
  Other causes of fluid loss or deprivation

Drugs

Smoking and alcohol use aggravate xerostomia. Any drugs with an antimuscarinic or sympathomimetic effect may cause a dry mouth (Appendix to Chapter 25) and these are especially drugs used in the treatment of psychiatric diseases. Tricyclic antidepressants, lithium and phenothiazine neuroleptics are some of the most potent causes of xerostomia. However, despite statements to the contrary, neither the commonly used 'tranquillizers', the benzodiazepines nor beta-blockers cause xerostomia. Indeed the latter may be used to relieve dry mouth secondary to anxiety in actors for example, for whom anxiety-induced dry mouth is an occupational hazard.

Irradiation

Ionizing irradiation affecting the major salivary glands, usually during treatment of a malignant neoplasm in the head and neck, regularly produces severe xerostomia (Chapter 6). Occasionally, the salivary glands are similarly affected by the use of ^{131}iodine in the treatment of hyperthyroidism, since the radionuclide is also taken up by salivary glands.

Sjögren's syndrome

Sjögren's syndrome is an autoimmune exocrinopathy, often with multi-system disease (*Table 9.7*).

The association of dry mouth (xerostomia) with dry eyes (keratoconjunctivitis sicca) in the absence of rheumatoid arthritis (the features originally observed by Sjögren) is sometimes referred to as 'sicca syndrome' (primary Sjögren's syndrome) and the term 'Sjögren's syndrome' (secondary Sjögren's syndrome) is reserved for the association of these features with rheumatoid arthritis, or less frequently with primary biliary cirrhosis, systemic lupus erythematosus, progressive systemic sclerosis, polymyositis, or other connective tissue diseases. Indeed the association with Sjögren's syndrome is a common feature which the connective tissue (collagen vascular) diseases share.

It has been estimated that probably 15 per cent of patients with rheumatoid arthritis develop Sjögren's syndrome and, since the same salivary gland changes can be associ-

Table 9.7 Sjögren's syndrome – features and systemic components

- Ocular
  Keratoconjunctivitis sicca
- Oral
  Xerostomia
  Lobulated tongue
  Infections
- Respiratory tract
  Dryness
- Gastrointestinal
  Dysphagia
- Pancreas
  Subclinical dysfunction
- Cutaneous
  Xeroderma
  Vaginal dryness
  Raynaud's phenomenon
- Haematological disorders
  Anaemia
  Leucopenia
- Associated autoimmune disorders
- Drug allergies

Table 9.8 Sjögren's syndrome – comparison of sub-types

Feature	Primary	Secondary
Other connective tissue disease	–	+
Oral involvement	More severe	Less severe
Recurrent sialadenitis	More common	Less common
Ocular involvement	More severe	Less severe
Extraglandular manifestations	More common	Less common
Lymphocyte-aggressive manifestations	More common	Less common
HLA associations	HLA-DR3 HLA-B8	HLA-DR4
Rheumatoid factor	50%	90%
Anti-SS-A (Ro)	5–10%	50–80%
Anti-SS-B (La)	54–73%	2–6%
Rheumatoid arthritis precipitin (RAP)[a]	5%	76%
Salivary duct antibody	10–36%	67–70%

[a]Also known as SS-C.

ated with other connective tissue diseases or can develop in apparent isolation, it is clear that Sjögren's syndrome is relatively common.

Sjögren's syndrome is an autoimmune exocrinopathy which mainly affects middle-aged or older women. The essential changes of Sjögren's syndrome are infiltration of the lachrymal, salivary and other exocrine glands by lymphocytes and plasma cells, with progressive acinar destruction. The parotid glands are chiefly affected but the changes are also detectable in the other major glands, and the minor labial glands (such as in the lower lip) in most patients. Sicca syndrome shares most of the serological abnormalities of rheumatoid disease, with autoantibodies (especially antinuclear antibodies SS-A or Ro, and SS-B or La), although overt rheumatoid arthritis is not present and there are other differences, as shown in *Table 9.8*.

Clinically, these syndromes are characterized by dryness of all mucosae. Despite the often troublesome nature of the oral symptoms, the most important effects of Sjögren's syndrome are on the eyes, where drying causes keratoconjunctivitis sicca. This can lead ultimately to impairment or loss of sight. Patients with dry eyes may have no symptoms or may complain of grittiness,

burning, soreness, itching, or inability to cry. They may wake in the morning with a pustular exudate in the eyes, crusting at the canthuses or have infections of the lids. It is essential for the patient to have an ophthalmological examination. A Schirmer test shows impaired lacrimation.

Bronchial involvement may lead to recurrent respiratory infections and this disease may also involve vaginal glands, pancreas or other organs (*Table 9.7*). Patients with Sjögren's syndrome may develop other autoimmune manifestations such as Raynaud's phenomenon.

Oral involvement results in discomfort caused by the reduced salivary flow, obvious dryness of the mucosa in severe cases and, erythema and lobulation of the tongue. Swelling of the parotids is seen in a minority and, rarely, these glands can also be persistently painful. Late onset of salivary gland swelling may indicate development of a lymphoma which is an uncommon but well-recognized and lethal complication of Sjögren's and, especially, sicca syndrome.

Apart from its dryness, the oral mucosa appears normal but the supervention of candidal infection causes redness and soreness. The main effects of persistent xerostomia are:

1. Discomfort and, in severe cases, difficulty in speaking, swallowing or managing dentures.
2. Disturbed taste sensation.
3. Accelerated caries.
4. Susceptibility to oral candidosis.
5. Susceptibility to ascending (bacterial) sialadenitis.

Surprisingly, perhaps, some patients can manage dentures in spite of virtual or complete absence of saliva and many such patients do not complain of dry mouth *per se*.

HIV infection

Parotitis can be seen in HIV infection and is a common feature in children. The infection can also cause salivary gland swellings due to lymphocytic infiltration, and dry mouth. Though the salivary gland changes in HIV infection are mainly due to lymphocytic infiltration, autoantibody findings typical of Sjögren's syndrome are lacking, and the age and sex distribution are also usually different.

• Management of dry mouth

The history should be directed particularly to discover any drugs likely to cause dry mouth and any symptoms suggestive of connective tissue disease, particularly rheumatoid arthritis, or of diabetes or HIV infection. Dryness of other mucous membranes, particularly of the conjunctivae, should be excluded. A Schirmer test shows decreased lacrimation.

Examination should include palpation of the major salivary glands for swelling. Oral examination may reveal obvious xerostomia with lack of salivary pooling and flow from the duct orifices, frothy saliva, debris on the dorsum of the tongue, or infections (candidosis or sialadenitis) or rampant dental caries. In Sjögren's syndrome the tongue typically becomes lobulated and red.

Since no single investigation will reliably establish the diagnosis of Sjögren's syndrome, a variety of tests *may* have to be carried out. These include the following.

1. *Immunological studies* are useful. Typical findings in Sjögren's syndrome are shown in *Table 9.8*, but the main abnormalities are hypergammaglobulinaemia mainly as a result of the presence of rheumatoid factor, and, frequently, other autoantibodies – particularly SS-A (Ro: Robair) and SS-B (La: Lattimer).

2. *Salivary flow rates.* These will confirm the presence and degree of xerostomia but are non-specific. Whole saliva collected without stimulation by allowing the patient to dribble into a sterile container over a measured period is now regarded as the best form of sialometry. Parotid output after stimulation with 10 per cent citric acid can also be objectively determined using a suction (Lashley or Carlsson–Crittenden) cup over the parotid duct orifice or by cannulation of the duct.

3. Labial gland biopsy is one of the most specific investigations. Biopsy of the parotid is theoretically preferable but labial gland biopsy is easier, safer and reflects the parotid changes in the majority of cases. This is probably the most useful single investigation.

Other investigations that may be useful include the following.

• *Sialography* is non-specific and time-consuming. Hydrostatic instillation of contrast medium typically shows a snow-storm appearance (punctate sialectasis) in well-established cases. Sialography is of course contraindicated if there is acute parotitis.
• *Radioactive pertechnetate uptake and concentration* in the major glands can be measured by scintigraphy which is sometimes useful, but involves the use of radio-isotopes and depends on the availability of specialized equipment.
• *Haematological examination.* The ESR is typically raised and anaemia may be associated with rheumatoid disease.

Having said all that, it must be accepted that, since no specific treatment is available, it is arguable whether intensive investigation is always justifiable. Certainly in a patient with known collagen disease, particularly rheumatoid arthritis, a dry mouth is virtually diagnostic of Sjögren's syndrome. It is, however, essential, as mentioned earlier, to arrange for ophthalmological investigation to exclude or treat early keratoconjunctivitis.

Dry mouth may be helped by frequently sipping water or drinks, sucking ice, chewing gum, or using frequent, liberal rinses of a salivary substitute containing carboxymethyl cellulose or mucin. Pilocarpine 5 mg three times daily with meals, or other anti-cholinesterase inhibitors such as pyridostigmine may increase salivation if any functional tissue remains, but systemic effects such as diarrhoea and blurred vision may be troublesome and there may be dysrhythmias. Malic acid stimulation may help salivation.

Preventive dental care is important. Patients have a tendency to consume a cariogenic diet because of the impaired sense of taste: this must be avoided, and caries should also be controlled by fluoride applications. Improved oral hygiene and the use of a 0.2 per cent chlorhexidine mouthwash will help to control periodontal disease and other infections.

Denture hygiene is important because of susceptibility to candidosis and antifungal treatment is often needed (Appendix to Chapter 1).

Generalized soreness and redness of a dry oral mucosa is typically caused by *Candida albicans* and often associated with angular stomatitis. Antifungal treatment is given as rinses of nystatin or amphotericin mixture.

Acute complications such as ascending parotitis should be treated with antibiotics. Pus should be sent for culture and antibiotic sensitivities but, in the interim, a penicillinase-resistant penicillin such as flucloxacillin in combination with metronidazole, because of the possible presence of anaerobes, should be started.

Patients with Sjögren's syndrome who need dental treatment may not be a good risk for general anaesthesia because of the tendency to respiratory infections. There may also be problems in management related to the associated connective tissue disease and complicating factors such as anaemia (Chapter 5).

SIALORRHOEA (HYPERSALIVATION)

A clear distinction should be made between hypersalivation and drooling. Normally, any excess of saliva is swallowed and causes no symptoms. Drooling is common in infants, and in patients who have poor neuromuscular coordination or are mentally handicapped, without any over-production of saliva. Drooling may be controllable with antimus-carinic agents such as propantheline bromide. If drooling is severe, transplantation of the parotid duct such that it discharges into the pharynx may be effective and the submandibular duct can be moved. True hypersalivation is very rare, although it may be induced by lesions or foreign bodies in the mouth, by rabies or by drugs such as anticholinesterases or clozapine (Chapter 25). However, often there is no objective evidence for the complaint and it has a psychogenic basis.

SALIVARY GLAND SWELLINGS

The most common cause of salivary swelling is mumps (Chapter 11), which usually affects children and causes bilateral painful swellings, but mumps is now less common since children are immunized at an early age. Other causes include sialadenitis, Sjögren's syndrome, sarcoidosis, some drugs (*Table 9.9*), HIV infection, neoplasms and sialosis.

Neoplasms (usually pleomorphic adenoma) must be considered, particularly when there is a persistent unilateral swelling

---

Table 9.9   Causes of salivary gland swelling

- Inflammatory
    Mumps
    Bacterial ascending sialadenitis
    Obstructive sialadenitis
    Sjögren's syndrome
    Sarcoidosis
    HIV infection
    Angiolymphoid hyperplasia
    Kimura's disease
- Neoplastic
    Pleomorphic adenoma and others
- Endocrine and metabolic
    Alcoholic cirrhosis
    Diabetes mellitus
    Acromegaly
    Malnutrition or bulimia
    Cystic fibrosis
    Chronic renal failure
    Amyloidosis
    Haemochromatosis
- Drugs (rarely)
    Isoprenaline
    Phenylbutazone
    Iodides
    Chlorhexidine

Table 9.10   Causes of neck lumps

- Cervical lymph node pathology (*Table 9.11*)
- Infections
    Abscess
    Actinomycosis
- Cysts
    Thyroglossal
    Branchial
    Cystic hygroma
- Hamartomas
    Haemangiomas
- Thyroid
    Goitre
    Nodules (and carcinoma)
- Carotid
    Aneurysm
    Body tumour
- Skin
    Sebaceous cyst
    Dermoid cyst
    Lipoma
    Carcinoma

Table 9.11   Swellings of the cervical lymph nodes

- Infections
    Viral
        Viral respiratory infections
        Herpetic stomatitis
        Infectious mononucleosis
        HIV infection
        Others such as rubella, Coxsackie, Echovirus
    Bacterial
        Dental, tonsil, nose, sinuses, face or scalp
        infections
        Tuberculosis
        Atypical mycobacterioses
        Syphilis
        Cat scratch disease
        Staphylococci
        Lyme disease
        Brucellosis
        Rickettsial
    Parasitic
        Toxoplasmosis
- Neoplasms
    Primary
        Hodgkin's disease and non-Hodgkin's lymphoma
        Leukaemia, especially lymphocytic
    Secondary
        Carcinoma – oral, cutaneous, salivary gland or
        nasopharyngeal
        Others – malignant melanoma and Ewing's
        sarcoma
- Miscellaneous
    Sarcoidosis
    Sinus histiocytosis
    Mucocutaneous lymph node syndrome
    (Kawasaki's disease)
    Kikuchi–Fujimoto's disease
    Kimura's disease
    Castleman's disease
    Angiolymphoid hyperplasia
    Phenytoin and other drug reactions
    Connective tissue diseases
    Some immunodeficiency diseases

in older patients. Painless salivary swelling (sialosis or sialadenosis) appears related to autonomic dysfunction and is thus a rare feature of alcoholic cirrhosis (Chapter 10), diabetes mellitus, acromegaly (Chapter 14), starvation or bulimia (Chapter 18), or it may be idiopathic.

FREY'S SYNDROME

Parotidectomy or trauma to the parotid region is sometimes followed by sweating and flushing of the preauricular skin on that side, in response to stimulation of salivation (Frey's syndrome or gustatory sweating). Similar conditions may follow surgery to other salivary glands. Antiperspirants such as 20 per cent aluminium chloride hexahydrate may be effective in controlling the sweating.

LUMPS IN THE NECK

The lumps in the neck of most significance to dentistry are enlarged cervical lymph nodes, but lumps may also be due to other pathology (*Table 9.10*)

CERVICAL LYMPH NODE ENLARGEMENT

Causes of cervical lymphadenopathy are shown in *Table 9.11*. Most of the conditions associated with cervical lymphadenopathy are discussed in other chapters.

Kikuchi–Fujimoto disease

Kikuchi–Fujimoto disease is a benign, self-limiting lymphadenopathy that is easily confused clinically with a lymphoma or systemic lupus erythematosus, presenting mainly in young adults with lymphadenopathy in cervical and sometimes axillary or other regions, and flu-like symptoms, also with mild fever. Many have a lymphocytosis and raised ESR, suggestive of a viral aetiology but the precise cause is unknown. Lymph node biopsy may be indicated but care must then be taken to differentiate from lymphoma.

Angiolymphoid hyperplasia with eosinophilia

Angiolymphoid hyperplasia with eosinophilia (ALHE) is a vascular lesion with eosinophilic infiltration and lymphoid hyperplasia, that produces cutaneous and mucosal nodules in the head and neck region in particular, and is seen mainly in young patients and in the West. It is regarded as an epithelioid haemangioma and responds to local excision.

Angiofollicular lymphoid hyperplasia (Castleman's disease)

Castleman's disease is characterized by a cervical mass resembling a lymphoma, but is benign, and consists of lymphoid and endothelial hyperplasia. It is usually excised as it may give rise to malignant blood vessel tumours.

Kimura's disease

Kimura's disease (eosinophilic lymphogranuloma) is an idiopathic chronic inflammatory disease which resembles, but is distinct from, angiolymphoid hyperplasia with eosinophilia. It presents mainly in oriental males, as subcutaneous nodules in the head and neck region particularly, often with cervical lymphadenopathy and salivary gland involvement. It is occasionally associated with nephrotic syndrome. The lesions are characterized by lymphoid hyperplasia, capillary proliferation and eosinophilic infiltration. Corticosteroids and even local irradiation have been used as treatment.

HALITOSIS

Family and friends are usually considerably more aware of halitosis than the patient. Most halitosis is due to habits such as cigarette smoking, or to oral infection. One of the most common and manageable causes of halitosis is periodontal disease, in which anaerobes are numerous and frequently produce foul-smelling metabolic products such as sulphides. Tonsillar, nasal, antral or pharyngeal infections are also important causes. In such cases also patients are usually unaware of the displeasure that they cause to others. Causes of halitosis are outlined in *Table 9.12*.

By contrast, when the patient is concerned about halitosis, in the majority of cases this is delusional and the breath does not smell unpleasant. Such patients should be firmly reassured, as they may be depressed. Some may have other psychiatric disorders; in a study of 137 patients troubled by halitosis, 50 were depressed, 36 seemed to be hypochondriacal and most of the remainder had schizophrenia or temporal lobe epilepsy.

DISTURBED TASTE SENSATION

The pathways of taste perception are outlined in Chapter 17. Taste buds are found on the tongue mainly but also on the soft palate, uvula, epiglottis, pharynx, larynx and oesophagus. Taste perception can be tested with salt

---

Table 9.12 Causes of halitosis

- Oral infections (especially periodontal)
- Dry mouth
- Foods, or smoking
- Drugs
  - Solvent abuse
  - Alcohol
  - Chloral hydrate
  - DMSO (dimethyl sulphoxide)
- Systemic disease
  - Respiratory tract tumours and infections (nose, sinuses, pharynx, larynx, bronchi, lungs)
  - Cirrhosis and liver failure
  - Renal failure
  - Diabetic ketosis
  - Gastrointestinal disease
  - Psychogenic disorders

(NaCl), sweet (saccharin), acidic (citrus) and bitter (quinine), or by electrogustometry.

Similar conditions to those that cause halitosis can cause a bad taste in the mouth (dysguesia (*see* Appendix to Chapter 17)). The sense of taste can also be temporarily disturbed by the use of chemicals such as chlorhexidine. Gymnemic acid abolishes the perception of sweet tastes while amiloride abolishes salt perception. Loss of taste can be due to medical conditions, or anaesthesia of the nerves involved, damage to the chorda tympani (herpes zoster oticus; otitis media; mastoiditis; cholesteatoma).

CONGENITAL DISORDERS

Some of those which involve the oral cavity and other parts of the gastrointestinal tract are shown in *Table 9.13*.

Table 9.13 Congenital intestinal disorders

Syndrome	Extra-intestinal features	Gastrointestinal lesions
Familial colonic polyposis	—	Colon polyps, adenocarcinoma
Peutz–Jeghers syndrome	Pigmented macules of mouth lips and digits Risk of neoplasia	Small intestine polyps and carcinoma rarely
Gardner's syndrome (familial adenomatous polyposis coli)	Osteomas of jaws (especially mandible), epidermal cysts, sebaceous cysts, lipomas, fibroma, dental anomalies	Colon polyps, adenocarcinomas, biliary neoplasia
Juvenile polyposis	—	Inflammatory polyps in small or large intestine
Tylosis (palmar–plantar hyperkeratosis)	Hyperkeratosis of palms and soles	Oral leucoplakia and oesophageal carcinoma
Multiple endocrine adenomatosis, type III	(*see* Chapter 10)	Mucosal neuromas

OESOPHAGEAL DISEASE

DYSPHAGIA

Dysphagia (difficulty in swallowing) is the common symptom of oesophageal disease. It has many possible causes, including disease in the mouth and elsewhere outside the oesophagus (*Table 9.14*), and is sometimes neurotic ('globus hystericus').

• General management

Dysphagia is a symptom that must never be dismissed lightly. The history is often the most important contribution to diagnosis but most patients, unless there are obvious oral causes, should be referred for medical investigation. Chest radiography and a barium swallow examination are usually required unless there are signs of neuromuscular disease. Oesophagoscopy may be needed if there is any suggestion of an organic lesion.

Treatment can be difficult. Surgery is required, particularly for impacted foreign bodies, strictures, pouches, achalasia or carcinoma. The last has an appallingly poor prognosis (Chapter 6).

Table 9.14   Causes of dysphagia

- Psychogenic
    Globus hystericus
- Organic
    Mouth
        Xerostomia
        Inflammatory or neoplastic lesions
    Pharynx
        Inflammatory or neoplastic lesions
        Foreign bodies
        Sideropenic dysphagia (Paterson–Kelly syndrome)
        Pouch
    Oesophagus
        Benign stricture
        Carcinoma
- Scleroderma
- External pressure from mediastinal lymph nodes
- Neurological and neuromuscular causes
        Achalasia
        Syringobulbia
        Cerebrovascular accidents
        Cerebrovascular disease (pseudobulbar palsy)
        Motor neurone disease
        Guillain–Barré syndrome
        Poliomyelitis
        Diphtheria
        Cerebellar disease
        Myopathies
        Myasthenia gravis
        Muscular dystrophies
        Dermatomyositis

- **Dental aspects**

Tonsillitis and pharyngitis are the most common causes of dysphagia, but oral causes include infections or ulcers of the palate, fauces, tongue or floor of the mouth. Almost any infection can cause dysphagia but particularly important are viral infections (herpetic stomatitis, herpangina and glandular fever) and bacterial infections such as pericoronitis. Rarely, pain–dysfunction syndrome, by making contraction of the jaw muscles painful, causes difficulty in the initiation of the swallowing process.

Infections involving the fascial spaces of the neck, particularly those tracking to the parapharyngeal space, peritonsillar infections and Ludwig's angina (bilateral sublingual and submandibular cellulitis) cause dysphagia which is, nevertheless, a minor feature of these serious diseases.

Oral ulcers can occasionally cause dysphagia. Severe recurrent aphthae are most often responsible, but other causes (*see Table 9.2*), particularly carcinoma, must be excluded. Carcinoma of the posterior lateral border of the tongue is an important cause and can be missed unless examination is thorough.

Dry mouth is an uncommon cause of dysphagia. Dysphagia may be particularly important in disorders of the medulla, since there may be defects of cranial nerves V, VII, IX, X, XI or XII (Appendix to Chapter 17).

REFLUX OESOPHAGITIS

Reflux oesophagitis is one of the most common kinds of dyspepsia and, although at one time considered to be a result of hiatus hernia, the relationship between the symptoms and appearances on barium swallow is inconsistent. Oesophageal spasm can complicate the picture.

Symptoms can be effectively relieved by taking frequent small meals, antacids, cimetidine or other H_2-blocker during the day, or using a proton-pump inhibitor such as omeprazole. Losing weight and raising the head of the bed by at least 4 inches are also helpful.

The gastric contents can have a pH as low as 1 and regurgitation if chronic can thus cause dental erosion, especially if there is impaired salivation for any reason. Some patients are convinced that oral symptoms or disease are caused by 'acid' but, apart from the few genuine cases with persistent regurgitation of gastric contents, which may lead to dental erosion, this is no more than a folk myth, probably fostered by advertisements for antacids (*see also* Anorexia nervosa and bulimia, Chapter 18).

THE STOMACH

Normal function

Gastric secretions include hydrochloric acid (secreted by parietal cells), pepsin (secreted by chief or peptic cells) and intrinsic factor (secreted by parietal cells). Gastric mucus contains several glycoproteins which help to protect the mucosa against erosion.

Gastrin stimulates gastric acid secretion and secretion of gastrin is controlled by the inhibitory effects of acid in the antrum or duodenum, decrease in gastric distension and release of the pancreatic hormones, cholecystokinin-pancreozymin and secretin. Gastrin acts by inducing local release of histamine which acts on specific (H_2) receptors on the parietal cells which then secrete acid. Acid secretion is also stimulated by synthetic analogues of gastrin (pentagastrin), by histamine and its analogues, and by hypoglycaemia.

Gastric function tests

Gastric acid secretion in response to various stimuli can be assessed by passing a nasogastric tube and measuring the volume, pH and acid concentration of the aspirate.

PEPTIC ULCER

Peptic ulcer develops in or close to acid-secreting areas, usually in the stomach (gastric ulcer) or proximal duodenum (duodenal ulcer). *Helicobacter pylori* is the most common contributory cause, though most infected individuals have no disease. The use of NSAIDs is the second most common contributor. Acid production is typically normal in those with a gastric ulcer, although zonal gastritis is associated; some, but not all, patients with a duodenal ulcer have acid hypersecretion. Peptic ulcers also complicate conditions characterized by raised gastrin levels. These include Zollinger–Ellison syndrome (a gastrin-producing tumour), hyperparathyroidism (high serum calcium provokes gastrin release) and chronic renal failure (poor gastrin metabolism). Factors that may impair the mucus barrier or otherwise promote peptic ulceration include genetic influences, stress, smoking, diet, environmental factors and drugs, particularly aspirin and other anti-inflammatory analgesics, and corticosteroids.

A characteristic feature of peptic ulcer is epigastric pain which has a variable relationship to meals but is often relieved by antacids. The severity of the pain bears no relationship to the size or severity of the ulceration and many patients with peptic ulcers suffer little more than dyspepsia. Some have no symptoms and the first sign of an ulcer may be one of the complications, such as haemorrhage, perforation, or pyloric obstruction with vomiting.

• General management of peptic ulcer

Endoscopy is the most reliable way of confirming the diagnosis but is usually preceded by barium meal radiography. The presence of *H. pylori* can be determined serologically, by breath test, or by lesional culture or biopsy. Gastric acid studies or the estimation of serum gastrin levels may also be carried out.

Non-drug treatments, particularly bed rest, dietary changes and stopping smoking, and limiting alcohol intake, accelerate the healing of gastric but not duodenal ulcers. Milk, antacids and frequent small meals with no fried foods often relieve symptoms.

Drug treatment is now frequently used. *H. pylori* appears to play a role in many cases, and its elimination with antimicrobials (typically metronidazole plus tetracycline or amoxycillin) and bismuth salts often hastens healing. Drugs that block H_2 receptors also block gastric acid production. H_2-receptor antagonists (H_2RAs) such as cimetidine, ranitidine, famotidine and nizatidine are among the most effective drugs and accelerate the healing, particularly of duodenal ulcers. Also effective are pirenzepine, a selective antimuscarinic, and sucralfate; these may be used in combination with H_2 blockers in intractable cases. Omeprazole, which blocks acid production by inhibiting the parietal cell proton pump mechanism, is frequently effective when H₂RAs fail. Other proton pump inhibitors (PPIs) such as lansoprazole appear most effective against duodenal ulcers. Pirenzepine is an antimuscarinic agent that inhibits gastric acid and pepsin production and aids ulcer healing. Sucralfate and carbenoxolone may also aid ulcer healing. Any of these drug treatments may have to be maintained, as relapses may follow.

Partial gastrectomy is usually reserved for those with complications but is effective and also has the advantage that it eliminates the need for long-term drug treatment. Gastric ulcers are managed by antrectomy with gastroduodenal anastomosis; duodenal ulcers are usually managed with vagotomy and pyloroplasty or antrectomy.

• **Dental aspects of peptic ulcer**

Drugs that cause gastric ulceration, or increase bleeding from such ulcers, should not be given to patients with peptic ulcers. Such drugs include aspirin and other non-steroidal anti-inflammatory analgesics particularly if given with corticosteroids. Cimetidine may delay benzodiazepine clearance but the effect is not clinically significant. Anaemia may also complicate treatment, particularly general anaesthesia.

There are no oral manifestations of peptic ulcer unless there is acid regurgitation, or anaemia from gastrointestinal bleeding, or surgical procedures. Persistent regurgitation of gastric acid as a result of pyloric stenosis can cause severe dental erosion, typically of the palatal aspects of the upper anterior teeth and premolars. Complications of surgery, relevant to dentistry, mainly follow total resections. They include deficiencies of vitamin B₁₂, folate or iron, and attacks of hypoglycaemia, but should not be seen now. Pirenzepine and sucralfate may cause dry mouth, ranitidine erythema multiforme, and omeprazole loss of taste or erythema multiforme.

Though *H. pylori* may be transmitted in saliva, the evidence suggests that dental staff are not at particular risk from *H. pylori* infection.

CANCER OF THE STOMACH

The stomach is one of the most frequent sites of cancer, which typically causes no symptoms until late. The prognosis is poor, with about a 7 per cent 5-year survival rate (Chapter 6). Men are affected nearly twice as often as women. The aetiology of gastric cancer is unclear but may include genetic influences, atrophic gastritis, achlorhydria and, possibly, ingestion of carcinogens. Patients with pernicious anaemia have a raised incidence of gastric cancer.

The symptoms of gastric cancer may closely mimic peptic ulcer, a common complaint being indigestion or vague upper abdominal pain. Later, anorexia, loss of weight, nausea, vomiting or melaena (stools black and tarry with blood) and anaemia may develop. The tumour spreads locally to cause pain, and may obstruct the intestine to cause vomiting, or bile duct to cause jaundice. Jaundice may also be caused by liver metastases and deposits may form in the peritoneum (causing ascites), lungs, bones or brain.

The diagnosis of gastric cancer is usually suggested by radiography but confirmed by gastroscopy and biopsy. Most patients are treated by surgery, but unfortunately, it is frequently only palliative.

• **Dental aspects of stomach cancer**

Anaemia or obstructive jaundice may complicate dental treatment. Pernicious anaemia (*see* Chapter 5) may precede development of gastric cancer.

Oral signs of anaemia can be an initial feature and it is worth emphasizing that iron deficiency in a male should always be regarded with suspicion, since it usually results from chronic haemorrhage, often from the gastrointestinal tract and then not infrequently due to an ulcer or neoplasm. Metastases to the jaw from gastric carcinomas are uncommon. They are usually in the body of the mandible and may cause swelling, pain, paraesthesia, loosening of teeth or sockets that fail to heal, or be found as ragged radiolucent areas, sometimes with resorption of roots. Other rare manifestations are discussed in Chapter 6. Occasionally metastases from a gastric carcinoma may be first detected in a lower cervical lymph node, usually on the left side (Troisier's sign).

THE SMALL INTESTINE

Normal function

The small intestine is the main area of digestion and absorption of food. Digestion depends on intestinal and pancreatic enzymes acting on food previously exposed to salivary amylase and gastric acid and pepsin. Bile salts facilitate the absorption of fats and the fat-soluble vitamins (A, D, E and K); gastric intrinsic factor is needed for the absorption of vitamin B_{12} in the terminal part of the ileum. Iron and folate are absorbed in the duodenum, most other substances in the jejunum.

- ### General aspects of small intestine disease

Malabsorption is the main feature of most of these disorders. Lassitude, weakness, loss of weight or failure to thrive, vitamin deficiencies and anaemia are common. Diarrhoea or steatorrhoea, and sometimes abdominal discomfort, are the main complaints, but in the later stages there are manifestations of chronic deficiencies.

Diseases of the small intestine of most significance include coeliac disease and Crohn's disease, but other causes of malabsorption include surgery, infestations and drugs.

COELIAC DISEASE (GLUTEN-SENSITIVE ENTEROPATHY)

Coeliac disease affects about 1 in 1800 of the population. There is a hypersensitivity or toxic reaction of the small intestine mucosa to the gliadin component of gluten (prolamine) – a group of proteins present in wheat, rye, barley and possibly oats typically on a genetic background of HLA-DQw2. Destruction of villi (villous atrophy) and inflammation follow ingestion of gluten and can result in malabsorption, abdominal pain and steatorrhoea or more subtle symptoms – coeliac disease is one of the great mimics in medicine. Furthermore, many affected individuals are asymptomatic.

Stunting of growth is sometimes conspicuous but, at the opposite extreme, symptoms can be minimal or absent and the diagnosis is made only after some complication develops; indeed, the diagnosis is not uncommonly missed. Recurrent aphthae, anaemia, lymphoma, cancer, osteoporosis or infertility are examples of non-specific effects that may ultimately lead to the diagnosis at almost any age.

- ### General management of coeliac disease

It is important to make a firm diagnosis and institute a gluten-free diet, even in those with minimal symptoms, in order to prevent complications such as lymphoma. The diagnosis of coeliac disease depends on the clinical features, particularly those of malabsorption and its complications. The latter include low blood folate and carotene levels (the screening method of choice) and findings of antibodies to gliadin and to endomysium. These antibodies are not invariably useful; patients may also be IgA deficient and lack antibodies; anti-gliadin antibodies lose specificity with age; and anti-endomysial antibodies are only seen in those with severe mucosal damage and thus fail to detect persons with minimal lesions. Jejunal biopsy should show villous atrophy. The biopsy, if positive, is repeated after a gluten-free diet has been maintained for about 3 months. In children the same procedure is used, except that an additional biopsy is carried out after a test challenge of gluten, as it is essential to establish the diagnosis with certainty from the outset and to eliminate such conditions as self-limiting but prolonged post-infectious gastroenteritis, which can cause a histologically similar lesion. Similar jejunal changes are seen in dermatitis herpetiformis.

Nutritional deficiencies should be rectified and a gluten-free diet adhered to. Patients require continued supervision, as there is often difficulty in keeping to the diet.

- ### Dental aspects of coeliac disease

A surprisingly wide range of foods and beverages contain gluten and care must be taken not to interfere with the gluten-free diet.

Anaemia may complicate dental treatment or predispose to oral lesions. Coeliac disease may be found in up to 5 per cent of patients with recurrent aphthae and should be suspected if there are any other symptoms suggestive of small intestine disease. Other mucosal complaints include glossitis, burning mouth or angular stomatitis. Short stature associated with diarrhoea and enamel defects is particularly suggestive of early onset coeliac disease.

DERMATITIS HERPETIFORMIS

Dermatitis herpetiformis is an uncommon chronic skin disease related to coeliac disease. It usually affects males past middle age, and causes an itchy papulovesicular eruption, usually on the extensor surfaces of the upper limbs and trunk. It leaves pigmented areas on healing. The coeliac disease is not as severe as in isolated coeliac disease. There may be associations with thyroid disease, gastric achlorhydria and pernicious anaemia, and lymphoma.

Diagnosis is established by demonstrating deposits of IgA at the papillae at the epithelial basement membrane zone (BMZ), with papillary tip microabscesses and a sub-epithelial split. Anti-endomysial antibodies may be detectable.

Serum immune complexes are often found, but decline if the patient is put on a gluten-free diet which, if strictly adhered to, may be of considerable benefit.

- ## Dental aspects of dermatitis herpetiformis

Oral lesions in dermatitis herpetiformis are usually innocuous but may be erythematous, vesicular, purpuric or sometimes erosive, and are most likely to be confused with pemphigoid. Coeliac-type enamel defects may rarely be seen. Indomethacin should be avoided, since it may exacerbate the condition.

Patients are usually managed with dapsone, which rarely causes a lichenoid eruption, or sulphapyridine or sulphamethoxypyridazine, which may cause erythema multiforme. Rarely, dermatitis herpetiformis is a complication of internal cancer (*see* Chapter 6).

LINEAR IgA DISEASE

Linear IgA disease (LAD) is a rare variant of dermatitis herpetiformis, in which the IgA deposits are linear at the BMZ, but coeliac disease is rare. There may be association with lymphoma.

Similar oral manifestations to dermatitis herpetiformis may be seen, and LAD is most likely to be confused with pemphigoid. A variant seen in childhood is termed *chronic bullous dermatosis of childhood*.

The diagnosis and treatment are as for dermatitis herpetiformis, though the IgA deposits at the epithelial basement membrane zone are linear deposits of IgA, and a gluten-free diet is not required.

CROHN'S DISEASE (REGIONAL ENTERITIS OR ILEITIS)

Crohn's disease is an inflammatory disease of unknown cause which, with ulcerative colitis, is one of a spectrum of diseases that have many features in common and are termed chronic inflammatory bowel disease. Crohn's disease appears to be a heterogeneous group of disorders probably caused by commensal bacteria in persons with a genetically determined dysregulation of mucosal T-lymphocytes, the inflammatory response being mediated by various factors such as tumour necrosis factor alpha. Susceptibility appears to be related to a locus on chromosome 16. The micro-organisms involved are unknown and many have been implicated. *Mycobacterium paratuberculosis* is one of the latest bacteria to be incriminated, but it appears unlikely that this is of major importance.

Microscopically, a submucosal chronic inflammatory infiltrate with non-caseating granulomas is found. Crohn's disease can affect any part of the gastrointestinal tract but especially the ileocaecal region, typically with ulceration, fissuring and fibrosis of the wall. The manifestations of Crohn's disease depend on its severity and the site affected. Small intestinal involvement may cause abdominal pain that often mimics appendicitis, with malabsorption or abnormal bowel habits such as alternating diarrhoea and constipation. Colonic Crohn's disease may mimic ulcerative

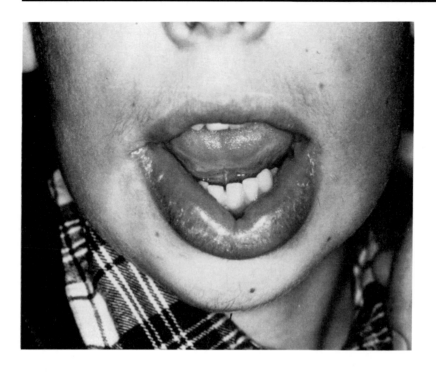

Fig. 9.1 Facial and labial swelling in Crohn's disease

colitis and is frequently associated with chronic perianal disease. Oral involvement is discussed below.

Complications include gastrointestinal obstruction, internal or external fistulas, perianal fissures, abscesses, troublesome arthralgia and sometimes renal damage (renal stones or infections). There is also a slightly greater predisposition to small bowel carcinoma.

• General management of Crohn's disease

Haematological examination may show deficiencies of iron, folate or vitamin B_{12}. The ESR and levels of acute phase proteins such as C-reactive protein and seromucoid are usually raised but the serum potassium, zinc and albumin are depressed. Different subpopulations have serum perinuclear antineutrophil cytoplasmic antibodies, or antierythrocyte autoantibodies. These investigations however, are non-specific and the diagnosis of Crohn's disease is confirmed by sigmoidoscopy, rectal mucosal biopsy and radiography. Rectal biopsies often show typical granulomas when Crohn's disease affects either the large or small intestine.

Barium enemas of large and small bowel, or barium meal and follow-through, are required. The major differential diagnoses include ulcerative colitis, tuberculosis, ischaemic colitis, infections, infestations such as giardiasis, and lymphoma.

Management includes correction of nutritional deficiencies, but there is no specific treatment. Sulphasalazine or corticosteroids may be useful in acute disease; olsalazine and mesalazine are newer alternatives which lack sulphonamide side-effects. Any of these may be supplemented with metronidazole, and azathioprine may be used in unresponsive patients. Surgery (usually resection) becomes necessary at some stage in most patients with intestinal Crohn's disease, but nearly 50 per cent relapse within 10 years of operation and, overall, treatment is unsatisfactory. Recent studies using monoclonal antibodies directed against tumour necrosis factor alpha, suggest that such therapies may be beneficial.

• Dental aspects of Crohn's disease

Dental management may be complicated by any of the problems associated with malabsorption or by corticosteroid or other immunosuppressive treatment. Oral lesions may be caused by Crohn's disease itself, by associated nutritional defects, or may be coincidental. Orofacial granulomatosus, sarcoidosis and tuberculosis are the main differential diagnoses.

Oral lesions of Crohn's disease include ulcers, facial or labial swelling (*Fig. 9.1*), mucosal tags or 'cobblestone' proliferation of the mucosa. Oral effects of malabsorption such as angular stomatitis may also be seen. Some of these patients may have asymptomatic intestinal disease, or develop intestinal disease later. Melkersson–Rosenthal syndrome (facial swelling, facial palsy and fissured tongue) and cheilitis granulomatosa may possibly also be incomplete manifestations of Crohn's disease. Patients with atypical ulcers, especially when they are large, linear and ragged, or those with recurrent facial swellings, should have biopsy of the mucosa in addition to other investigations, particularly chest radiography, serum angiotensin-converting enzyme levels, serum ferritin and vitamin B_{12}, red cell folate and intestinal radiography. Biopsies in oral Crohn's disease typically show granulomas and lymph-oedema and in their absence diagnosis is somewhat speculative. Microscopically similar granulomatous lesions may also be seen in the absence of systemic disease and may possibly result from reactions to some foods or medicaments. This condition has been termed 'orofacial granulomatosis' but this should not be confused with midfacial (midline) granuloma syndrome (Chapter 21). Reactions to foods should be excluded by dietary modification but where there is gut Crohn's disease, systemic medication is required. Intralesional injection of corticosteroids may help the facial swelling resolve.

An increased prevalence of caries in Crohn's disease has also been reported.

PEUTZ–JEGHERS SYNDROME (*see Table 9.13*)

SHORT BOWEL SYNDROME

Short bowel syndrome, where the small intestine is short, may be congenital, or caused by surgery. Numerous metabolic defects may be seen, particularly vitamin and mineral deficiencies leading to osteomalacia and fractures. Premature tooth loss has been described.

THE PANCREAS

ACUTE PANCREATITIS

Acute pancreatitis may be precipitated by gallstone disease, alcoholism, hypercalcaemia, hyperlipidaemia, viral infections such as mumps, drugs such as corticosteroids or phenothiazines, or various other factors.

Acute pancreatitis causes acinar damage and activation of enzymes leading to local fat necrosis and systemic effects such as severe abdominal pain, nausea, vomiting and shock. Mild pancreatitis usually resolves in a few days, but in fulminating pancreatitis the patient is severely ill with retroperitoneal haemorrhage, pleural effusion and paralytic ileus. Metabolic complications include hypocalcaemia, hyperbilirubinaemia, hyperglycaemia and raised serum levels of alkaline phosphatase, the transaminases, amylase and lipase. Radiology and ultrasonography aid the diagnosis.

The mortality in acute pancreatitis is 15–25 per cent. Treatment of shock and metabolic complications and relief of pain are essential.

CHRONIC PANCREATITIS

Chronic pancreatitis is of similar aetiology to acute pancreatitis; gallstone disease and alcoholism are frequently contributory factors but malnutrition, hyperparathyroidism, haemochromatosis, hyperlipidaemia, carcinoma, cystic fibrosis and other factors may be implicated.

Chronic pancreatitis results in acinar atrophy and deterioration in both endocrine and exocrine function. Abdominal pain is severe. Chronic dull pain is punctuated by episodes of acute pancreatitis. Many patients have abnormal glucose tolerance or frank diabetes mellitus, and weight loss is common.

Exocrine dysfunction is confirmed by a decline in the volume, bicarbonate content and enzyme content of pancreatic secretions. Serum levels of amylase and lipase are often raised; faecal levels of chymotrypsin are depressed. Pancreatic steatorrhoea is suggested by high faecal fat and undigested faecal meat fibres.

Radiography demonstrates pancreatic calcification, especially in alcoholic pancreatitis, and the diagnosis may be supported by barium meal, duodenography, cholangiographic findings and endoscopy.

Management includes analgesics, treatment of diabetes and the oral administration of pancreatic enzymes to aid digestion.

• Dental aspects of pancreatitis

Factors predisposing to or resulting from pancreatitis that might influence dental management include:

1. Bleeding due to vitamin K malabsorption (Chapter 4).
2. Alcoholism (Chapter 24).
3. Hyperparathyroidism (Chapter 14).
4. Diabetes mellitus (Chapter 14).
5. Cystic fibrosis (Chapter 8).
6. Narcotic abuse because of severe pain.

PANCREATIC TUMOURS

Pancreatic carcinoma appears to be increasing in incidence and is now about one-tenth as common as bronchogenic carcinoma. Carcinomas frequently involve the head of the pancreas and invade locally to cause biliary obstruction, pancreatitis and diabetes mellitus. Extra-pancreatic complications such as peripheral vein thrombosis (thrombophlebitis migrans) are also common. Radiography or percutaneous transhepatic cholangiography may be of diagnostic help.

Pancreatic carcinoma has the worst prognosis of any cancer (*see* Chapter 6). It is usually treated surgically, often with a bypass to relieve obstructive jaundice for as long as possible.

• Dental aspects of pancreatic carcinoma

In many cases the poor prognosis of pancreatic cancer may significantly influence the dental treatment plan (Chapter 6). Biliary obstruction may lead to bleeding tendencies, especially if there are hepatic metastases, and diabetes mellitus may be an added complication.

PANCREATIC TRANSPLANTATION

Pancreatic transplantation is in its infancy but is associated with all the problems that accompany immunosuppression (Chapter 20).

THE LARGE INTESTINE

ULCERATIVE COLITIS

Ulcerative colitis is an inflammatory disease of part or the whole of the large intestine and frequently of the rectum. The aetiology is unknown but psychosomatic symptoms are often associated. Women are slightly more frequently affected, particularly young adults.

Typical features are painless bloody diarrhoea with stools containing intermixed mucus. In severe cases there is abdominal pain, fever, anorexia and weight loss. Extra-abdominal signs of ulcerative colitis may be minimal unless there are complications such as iron deficiency anaemia caused by blood loss. However, arthralgia, uveitis, finger clubbing, erythema nodosum and other skin lesions such as pyoderma gangrenosum may be troublesome. An increase in platelets and some clotting factors may lead to thromboembolism. Various types of liver disease may complicate ulcerative colitis. The most serious complication is, however, carcinoma of the colon, which is up to 30 times more frequent than in the general population.

• General management of ulcerative colitis

Apart from routine examinations, all patients must have sigmoidoscopy and rectal biopsy to establish the diagnosis. Colonoscopy is also necessary if any polyps are seen radiographically. Patients with early onset colitis or with disease persisting for more than 10 years are most likely to develop colonic carcinoma and regular colonoscopy is needed.

Treatment includes drugs containing 5-aminosalicylic acid, that is sulphasalazine or 5-aminosalicylic acid itself (mesalazine or olsalazine) and local corticosteroids, often by enema. Patients on 5-aminosalicylic acid may develop headaches and blood dyscrasia and therefore should have regular blood counts. A high fibre diet is indicated and any anaemia needs treatment.

Systemic steroids or azathioprine may be required in acute exacerbations. If symptoms are really severe, the response to medical treatment is poor, or complications such as pyoderma gangrenosum or haemorrhage develop, colectomy may be indicated. This also eliminates the risk of malignant change and is curative.

- **Dental aspects of ulcerative colitis**

Management complications may include anaemia and those associated with corticosteroid therapy.

Oral manifestations in ulcerative colitis are rare but include pyostomatitis gangrenosum (chronic ulceration), pyostomatitis vegetans (multiple intra-epithelial microabscesses), discrete haemorrhagic ulcers or lesions related to anaemia. Since uveitis, skin lesions and mouth ulcers can be found in ulcerative colitis, it is important to differentiate it from Behçet's syndrome (Chapter 21).

DIVERTICULAR DISEASE

Diverticular disease includes both diverticulosis (diverticula of the large intestine) and diverticulitis (inflammation of the diverticula), but these can rarely be reliably distinguished. The disorder is common, affecting up to 25 per cent of adults over middle age, and involves particularly the descending and pelvic colon. Diverticular disease may result from a low fibre diet.

Diverticular disease may be asymptomatic but is often accompanied by dyspepsia, abdominal pain, constipation and flatulence.

Complications include pericolic abscess, perforation or fistula formation.

Management includes a high fibre diet and reassurance. There are no management problems in dentistry, although codeine should be avoided.

IRRITABLE BOWEL SYNDROME (SPASTIC COLON)

This is a common cause of recurrent abdominal pain in which there is increased tone and activity of the colon, abnormal bowel habits and other symptoms. It may affect up to 30 per cent of the population and is the most common cause of referral to gastroenterologists. There is frequently a positive family history and patients frequently have anxious personalities. Many also have migraine or psychogenic oral symptoms such as pain–dysfunction syndrome, sore tongue or atypical facial pain (Chapter 19).

A high fibre diet is said frequently to be effective in controlling the bowel symptoms but many patients use antispasmodics such as loperamide or an antimuscarinic such as dicyclomine. Dry mouth may then be a problem.

FAMILIAL POLYPOSIS COLI

This is an autosomal dominant condition in which multiple adenomatous polyps affect the rectum and colon. Carcinomatous change usually supervenes. Familial polyposis coli is a feature of Gardner's syndrome (*Table 9.13*) with multiple exostoses and osteomas of the jaws which also appear to be more common in patients with non-familial colorectal cancer than in the general population.

CARCINOMA OF THE COLON

Carcinoma of the colon is common. The peak incidence is in the sixth or seventh decades and the tumour usually arises in the rectum or pelvic (sigmoid) colon. Carcinoma of the colon may cause abdominal pain, change in bowel habit, weight loss or complications such as anaemia, intestinal obstruction or perforation.

Abdominal examination may reveal a mass. Sigmoidoscopy and barium enema are needed and colonoscopy may be required. Surgical resection is the usual treatment, while radiotherapy may be useful for dealing with pain from recurrences. Spread is frequently to the liver. The 5-year survival rate is overall about 30 per cent (*see* Chapter 6).

- **Dental aspects of carcinoma of the colon**

Anaemia resulting from chronic intestinal haemorrhage can cause oral signs or symptoms or complicate dental management. Mandibular osteomas may, as mentioned earlier, be markers of an increased risk of colorectal cancer.

ANTIBIOTIC-ASSOCIATED (PSEUDOMEMBRANOUS) COLITIS

Most of the orally administered antimicrobials can cause diarrhoea, but clinically significant colitis is rare. The most severe type was staphylococcal enterocolitis, usually caused by prolonged heavy doses of tetracyclines, particularly after bowel surgery. Now that the cause is recognized, this type of colitis has become rare.

Lincomycin and clindamycin cause pseudomembranous colitis more frequently than other antibiotics, as a result of proliferation of toxigenic strains of clostridia, particularly *Clostridium difficile*, which are resistant to low concentrations of these antibiotics. However, pseudomembranous colitis is not known to follow clindamycin in a single dose, which is now recommended for the prophylaxis of infective endocarditis as an alternative to penicillin. Other antibiotics usually allow the survival of more competitors to *Clostridium difficile*, which cannot so readily proliferate as a consequence. Even so, other antimicrobials, including the penicillins, can cause colitis occasionally.

Clinically, pseudomembranous colitis is characterized by painful diarrhoea and passage of mucus. In some cases, in elderly debilitated patients especially, there is passage of blood and pseudomembranous material (necrotic mucosa), occasionally resulting in death.

Pseudomembranous colitis usually responds to oral vancomycin or metronidazole.

BIBLIOGRAPHY

Aine L., Maki M. and Reunala T. (1992) Coeliac-type dental enamel defects in patients with dermatitis herpetiformis. *Acta Dermatol. Venereol. (Stockh.)* **72**, 25–7.

Arens R. and Reichman B. (1992) Grooved palate associated with prolonged use of orogastric feeding tubes in premature infants. *J. Oral Maxillofac. Surg.* **50**, 64–5.

Bartlett J.G. (1996) Antibiotic selection in sinusitis. *Arch. Otolaryngol. Head Neck Surg.* **122**, 422–3.

Baudetpommel M., Albuisson E., Kemeny J.L., Falvard F., Ristori J.M. et al. (1994) Early dental loss in Sjögren's syndrome – histologic correlates. *Oral Surg. Oral Med. Oral Pathol.* **78**, 181–6.

Beutner E.H., Kumar V. and Chorzelski T.P. (1989) Screening for celiac disease. *N. Engl. J. Med.* **320**, 1087–8.

Black M.J.M. and Gunn A. (1990) The management of Frey's syndrome with aluminium chloride hexahydrate antiperspirant. *Ann. R. Coll. Surg. Engl.* **72**, 49–52.

Bombardieri S., Bencivelli W., Vitali C. and Scully C. European Community Study Group of Diagnostic Criteria for Sjögren's Syndrome (1994) Diagnostic criteria for Sjögren's syndrome. In Homma M., Sugai S., Tojo T., Miyasaka N. and Akizuki M. (eds), *Proceedings of the Fourth International Symposium. Sjögren's syndrome – state of the art.* New York, Kugler Publications, pp. 73–6.

Burton J. and Scully C. (1998) The lips. In Champion R.H., Burton J. and Ebling F.J.G. (eds), *Textbook of Dermatology*, 6th edn. Oxford, Blackwell (in press).

Cataldo E., Covino M.C. and Tesone P.E. (1981) Pyostomatitis vegetans. *Oral Surg. Oral Med. Oral Pathol.* **52**, 172.

Cawson R.A., Spector R.G. and Skelly A.M. (1995) *Basic Pharmacology and Clinical Drug Use in Dentistry*, 6th edn. Edinburgh, Churchill Livingstone.

Challacombe S.I., Scully C., Keevil B. et al. (1983) Serum ferritin in recurrent oral ulceration. *J. Oral. Pathol.* **12**, 290–9.

Chan S., Scully C., Prime S.S. et al. (1991) Pyostomatitis vegetans: oral manifestations of ulcerative colitis. *Oral Surg. Oral Med. Oral Pathol.* **72**, 689–92.

Cooke W.T. and Holmes G.K.T. (1984) *Coeliac Disease.* Edinburgh, Churchill Livingstone.

DiAlberti L., Porter S.R., Speight P.M., Scully C. et al. (1997) Presence of human herpesvirus-8 variants in the oral ulcer tissues of HIV-infected individuals. *J. Infect. Dis.* **175**, 703–7.

Epstein J.B. and Scully C. (1992) The role of saliva in oral health and the causes and effects of xerostomia. *J. Can. Dent. Assoc.* **58**, 217–21.

Epstein J.B., Stevenson-Moore P. and Scully C. (1992) Management of xerostomia. *J. Can. Dent. Assoc.* **58**, 140–3.

Gaukroger M.C. (1992) Cervicofacial necrotising fasciitis. *Br. J. Oral Maxillofac. Surg.* **30**, 111–14.

Getchell T.V. (Ed) (1991) *Smell and Taste*. Raven Press, New York.

Gill Y. and Scully C. (1990) Orofacial odontogenic infections: review of microbiology and current treatment. *Oral Surg. Oral Med. Oral Pathol.* **70**, 155–8.

Grattan C.E.H. and Scully C. (1986) Oral ulceration: a diagnostic problem. *Br. Med. J.* **292**, 1093–4.

Gray R.L.M. (1978) Pigmented lesions of the oral cavity. *J. Oral Surg.* **36**, 950–5.

Hugot J-P., Laurent P., Gower Rousseau C. *et al.* (1996) Mapping of a susceptibility locus for Crohn's disease on chromosome 16. *Nature* **379**, 821–3.

Hunter I.P., Ferguson M.M., Scully C., Galloway A.R., Main A.N.H. and Russell R.I. (1993) Effects of dietary gluten elimination in patients with recurrent minor aphthous stomatitis and no detectable gluten enteropathy. *Oral Surg. Oral Med. Oral Pathol.* **75**, 595–8.

Iwu C.O. (1990) Ludwig's angina: report of seven cases and review of current concepts in management. *Br. J. Oral Maxillofac. Surg.* **28**, 189–93.

Jarvinen V., Meurman J.H., Hyvarinen H. *et al.* (1988) Dental erosion and upper gastrointestinal disorders. *Oral Surg. Oral Med. Oral Pathol.* **65**, 298–303.

Jarvinen V., Rytomaa I. and Heinonen O.P. (1991) Risk factors in dental erosion. *J. Dent. Res.* **70**, 942–7.

Jones I.H. and Mason D.K. (1990) *Oral Manifestations of Systemic Disease*, 2nd edn. London, Ballière Tindall.

Kinsner J.B. and Shorter R.G. (1982) Recent developments in 'non-specific' inflammatory bowel disease. *N. Engl. J. Med.* **306**, 775–837.

Lamey P.I., Carmichael F. and Scully C. (1985) Oral pigmentation, Addison's disease and results of screening. *Br. Dent. J.* **158**, 297–305.

Leading Article (1984) An irritable mind or an irritable bowel? *Lancet* **ii**, 1249–50.

Leading Article (1989) A lump in the throat. *Lancet* **i**, 534.

Leading Article (1989) Xerostomia and its management. *Lancet* **i**, 884.

Leading Article (1991) Oral granulomatosis. *Lancet* **38**, 20–1.

Li T.J., Chen X.M., Wang S.Z. *et al* (1996) Kimura's disease; a clinicopathologic study of 54 Chinese patients. *Oral Surg. Oral Med. Oral Pathol.* **82**, 549–55.

Lu D.P. (1982) Halitosis: an etiologic classification, a treatment approach, and prevention. *Oral Surg. Oral Med. Oral Pathol.* **54**, 521–6.

Marsh M.N. (1995) The natural history of gluten sensitivity: defining, refining and re-defining. *Q.J. Med.* **85**, 9–11.

Mathieu D., Neviere R., Teillon C. *et al.* (1995) Cervical necrotizing fasciitis; clinical manifestations and management. *Clin Infect Dis.* **21**, 51–6.

Matsuda O., Makiguchi K., Ishibashi K. *et al.* (1992) Long-term effects of steroid treatment on nephrotic syndrome associated with Kimura's disease and a review of the literature. *Clin. Nephrol.* **37**, 119–23.

Meurman J.K., Toskala J., Nuutinen P. *et al.* (1994) Oral and dental manifestations in gastroesophageal reflux disease. *Oral Surg. Oral Med. Oral Pathol.* **78**, 583–9.

Michels V.V., Mokri B., Piergras D.G. and Perry H.O. (1995) Brief report; a familial syndrome of arterial dissections with lentiginosis. *N. Engl. J. Med.* **332**, 576–9.

Mutlu S., Porter S., Richards A., Porter K., Maddison P. and Scully C. (1991) Periodontal health in Sjögren's syndrome. In Gold S.I., Midda M. and Mutlu S (eds), *Recent Advances in Periodontology*, Vol II: *Proceedings of the 4th Meeting of the International Academy of Periodontology*. Amsterdam, Elsevier, pp. 205–8.

Norris A.H., Krasinskas A.M., Salhany K.E. and Gluckman S.J. (1996) Kikuchi–Fujimoto disease: a benign cause of fever and lymphadenopathy. *Am. J. Med.* **171**, 401–5.

Pavli P., Cavanaugh J. and Grimm M. (1996) Inflammatory bowel disease: germs or genes? *Lancet* **347**, 1198.

Porter S.R. and Scully C. (1991) Aphthous stomatitis: overview of aetiopathogenesis and management. *Clin. Exp. Dermatol.* **16**, 235–43.

Porter S.R. and Scully C. (1994) Periodontal aspects of systemic disease – some therapeutic aspects. In Lang N.P. and Karring T. (eds), *Proceedings of the 1st European Workshop on Periodontology*. Berlin, Quintessence, pp. 415–38.

Porter S.R. and Scully C. (1994) Periodontal aspects of systemic disease – classifications. In Lang N.P. and Karring T. (eds), *Proceedings of the 1st European Workshop on Periodontology*. Berlin, Quintessence, pp. 375–414.

Porter S.R. and Scully C. (1996) *Innovations and Developments in Non-Invasive Oral Health Care*. Northwood, Science Reviews.

Porter S.R., Scully C. and Flint S.R. (1988) Haematological status in recurrent aphthous stomatitis compared with other oral disease. *Oral Surg. Oral Med. Oral Pathol.* **66**, 41–4.

Rasmussen P. and Espelid I. (1980) Coeliac disease and dental malformation. *J. Dent. Child.* **47**, 424.

Rooney T.P. (1984) Dental caries prevalence in patients with Crohn's disease. *Oral Surg. Oral Med. Oral Pathol.* **57**, 623–4.

Rustgi A.K. (1994) Hereditary gastrointestinal polyposis and non-polyposis syndromes. *N. Engl. J. Med.* **331**, 1694–702.

Sanderson J.D., Moss M.T., Tizard M.L. *et al.* (1992) *Mycobacterium paratuberculosis* DNA in Crohn's disease tissue. *Gut* **33**, 890–6.

Scully C. (1982) The mouth in general practice. *Dermatol. Practice* **1**, 19–29.

Scully C. (1982) Serum β microglobulin in recurrent aphthous stomatitis and Behçet's syndrome. *Clin. Exp. Dermatol.* **7**, 61–4.

Scully C. (1983) An update on mouth ulcers. *Dental Update* **10**, 141–52.

Scully C. (1986) Sjögren's syndrome: review of immunopathogenesis: clinical and laboratory features and management in relation to dentistry. *Oral Surg. Oral Med. Oral Pathol.* **62**, 510–23.

Scully C. (1988) *The Dental Patient.* Oxford, Heinemann.

Scully C. (1989) *The Mouth and Perioral Tissues.* Oxford, Heinemann.

Scully C. (1989) Oral parameters in the diagnosis of Sjögren's syndrome. *Clin. Exp. Rheumatol.* **7**, 113–18.

Scully C. (1989) *Patient Care: a Dental Surgeon's Guide.* London, British Dental Association

Scully C. (1990) Oral medicine: mouth ulcers. In Bell C.J. (ed), *Heinemann Dental Handbook.* Oxford, Heinemann, pp. 297–407.

Scully C. (1991) Oral component of Sjögren's syndrome. In Betail G. and Sauvezie B. (eds), *Le Syndrome de Gougerot Sjögren.* Paris, Merck Sharp Dohme Chibret, pp. 41–58.

Scully C. (1992) Non-neoplastic diseases of the major and minor salivary glands: a summary update. *Br. J. Oral Maxillofac. Surg.* **30**, 244–7.

Scully C. (1995) Prevention of oral mucosal disease. In Murray J.J. (ed), *Prevention of Oral and Dental Disease,* 3rd edn. Oxford, Oxford University Press, pp. 160–72.

Scully C. (1998) The oral cavity. In Champion R.H., Burton J. and Ebling F.J.G. (eds), *Textbook of Dermatology,* 6th edn. Oxford, Blackwell (in press).

Scully C. and Cawson R.A. (1986) Common dental disorders. *Med. Int.* **2**, 1129–33.

Scully C. and Cawson R.A. (1986) White, red and pigmented patches. *Med. Int.* **2**, 113–142.

Scully C. and Matthews R.W. (1983) Mouth ulcers. *Dental Update* **26**, 693–700.

Scully C. and Porter S.R. (1989) Recurrent aphthous stomatitis: current concepts of aetiological pathogenesis and management. *J. Oral Pathol. Med.* **18**, 21–7.

Scully C. and Porter S.R. (eds) (1990) Oral medicine. In: *Medicine International* **76**, 3145–9.

Scully C. and Porter S.R. (1992) Oral medicine: 2. Disorders affecting the oral mucosa (part 1). *Postgrad. Dentist* **2**, 109–13.

Scully C. and Porter S.R. (1993) Oral medicine: 2. Disorders affecting the oral mucosa (part 2). *Postgrad. Dent.* **3**, 142–7.

Scully C. and Porter S.R. (1993) Oral medicine: 3. Salivary disorders. *Postgrad. Dentist* **3**, 150–3.

Scully C. and Porter S.R. (1993) Oral medicine: 4. Orofacial pain. *Postgrad. Dentist* **3**, 186–8.

Scully C. and Porter S.R. (1994) The mouth 2: Signs and symptoms of oral disease. *Dermatol. Pract.* **2**, 14–17.

Scully C. and Porter S.R. (1997) The clinical spectrum of desquamative gingivitis. *Sem. Cut. Med. Surg.* **16**, 308–13.

Scully C. and Shepherd J. (1986) *Slide Interpretation in Oral Diseases and Oral Manifestations of Systemic Diseases.* Oxford, Oxford University Press.

Scully C., Cawson R.A. and Griffiths M.J. (1990) *Occupational Hazards to Dental Staff.* London, British Dental Journal.

Scully C., Porter S.R. and Greenman J. (1994) What to do about halitosis (Editorial). *Br. Med. J.* **308**, 217–18.

Scully C., Russell R.I., Cochran K.M. *et al.* (1982) Crohn's disease of the mouth; an early indicator of intestinal involvement. *Gut* **23**, 198–201.

Shanahan F. and Weinstein W.M. (1988) Extending the scope of celiac disease. *N. Engl. J. Med.* **319**, 782–3.

Soll A.H. (1996) Medical treatment of peptic ulcer disease. *J. Am. Med. Assoc.* **275**, 622–9.

Sreebny L.M. and Schwartz S.S. (1986) A reference guide to drugs and dry mouth. *Gerodontology* **5**, 75–99.

Stratakis C.A., Carney J.A., Lin J-P. *et al.* (1996) Carney complex, a familial multiple neoplasia and lentiginosis syndrome. *J. Clin. Invest.* **97**, 699–705.

Strober W. and James S.P. (1986) The immunologic basis of inflammatory bowel disease. *J. Clin. Immunol.* **6**, 415–33.

Targan S.R. and Murphy L.K. (1995) Clarifying the causes of Crohn's. *Nature Med.* **1**, 1241–3.

Thompson W.G. (1984) The irritable bowel. *Gut* **25**, 305–20.

Trau H. (1982) Peutz–Jeghers syndrome and bilateral breast carcinoma. *Cancer* **50**, 788–92.

Vitali C., Bencivelli W., Chiellini S., De Vita S., Sciuto M. *et al.* (1994) Sensitivity and specificity of tests for ocular and oral involvements in Sjögren's syndrome. *Ann. Rheum. Dis.* **53**, 637–47.

Vitali C., Bombardieri S., Moutsopoulos H., Scully C. and European Study Group on Diagnostic Criteria for Sjögren's Syndrome (1996) Assessment of the European classification criteria for Sjögren's syndrome in a series of clinically defined cases: results of a prospective multicentre study. *Ann. Rheum. Dis.* **55**, 116–121.

Vitali C., Moutsopoulos H.M., Bombardieri S., Scully C. and European Community Study Group of Diagnostic Criteria for Sjögren's Syndrome (1994) In Homma M., Sugai S., Tojo T., Kiyasaka N. and Akizuki M. (eds), *Proceedings of the Fourth International Symposium. Sjögren's syndrome – state of the art.* New York, Kugler, pp. 351–5.

Walmsley R.S., Ibbotson J.P., Chahal H. *et al.* (1996) Antibodies against *Mycobacterium paratuberculosis* in Crohn's disease. *Q. J. Med.* **89**, 217–21.

Wiesenfeld D., Ferguson M.M., Mitchell D.N. *et al.* (1985) Orofacial granulomatosis: clinical and pathological analysis. *Q. J. Med.* **213**, 101–13.

Worsae N., Christensen K.C. and Schiodt M. (1982) Melkersson–Rosenthal syndrome and cheilitis granulomatosa. *Oral Surg. Oral Med. Oral Pathol.* **54**, 404–13.

Wray D. and Scully C. (1986) The sore mouth. *Med. Int.* **2**, 1134–7.

Wright K.B., Holan G., Casamassimo P.S. et al. (1991) Alveolar bone loss in two children with short bowel syndrome receiving total parenteral nutrition. *J. Periodontol.* **62**, 272–5.

10

Liver disease

Key points

- Liver disease is important because of:
    bleeding tendencies,
    drug intolerance,
    possible viral causes.
- Liver disease may manifest with jaundice, pale faeces, dark urine, spider naevi, leuconychia, palmar erythema, gynaecomastia, clubbing, sialosis, Dupuytren's contracture, or tremor.
- Drug intolerance is a problem mainly in relation to general anaesthesia, but even a small dose of diazepam may be hazardous in liver disease.
- In patients with liver disease, other drugs to be avoided include aspirin, carbamazepine, diazepam and other sedatives, erythromycin estolate, MAOI, NSAIDs and tetracyclines.
- Viral hepatitis is important since it is due to blood-borne viruses which pose an infection risk, and there is liver dysfunction.
- Viral hepatitis relevant to dentistry may be caused by hepatitis B virus (HBV), C (HCV), D (HDV) or G (HGV).
- Viral hepatitis B carries a small but significant early mortality rate (1%) and a significant morbidity, mainly from cirrhosis, chronic hepatitis and liver cancer.
- Some forms of non-A, non-B hepatitis, such as hepatitis C, may also have similar morbidity and mortality, with an even greater risk of chronic hepatitis.
- Hepatitis D may be associated with hepatitis B, and cause a fulminant hepatitis.
- Groups at high risk of hepatitis virus carriage include:
    Patients with acute or chronic hepatitis.
    Persons who spent their childhood in countries outside Europe, North America, Australia and New Zealand, and particularly those from Vietnam.
    Injecting drug users, especially if suffering from hepatitis.
    Male homosexuals or bisexuals.
    Hospital staff who have had acute hepatitis.
    Inmates of custodial or mental institutions who have had acute hepatitis.
    Persons who have had acute hepatitis more than 6 weeks after blood transfusion.
    Persons who have had acute hepatitis after being in countries outside Europe, North America, Australia or New Zealand between 6 weeks and 6 months previously.
    Persons with chronic active hepatitis.
    Sexually promiscuous persons.
- Before infection control procedures and immunization were implemented, dental clinical staff, particularly those involved in surgical procedures, were at risk especially from HBV.
- Hepatitis B immunization is recommended for all dental clinical staff.
- Hepatitis B vaccine is a recombinant vaccine of HBsAg, which gives protective antibody levels after three doses in 85–95% of healthy adults for at least 3 years.

- Persons positive for hepatitis B surface antigen (HB$_s$Ag) are infective if also HB$_e$Ag positive.
- Those who have HB$_s$Ag should later be screened again at 3 months, and if still positive at 9 months are 'chronic carriers'.
- Drugs may also damage the liver. Among those used in dentistry and implicated are halothane, paracetamol, erythromycin estolate, tetracyclines, and ketoconazole.
- Halothane should never be given within 3 months of a previous halothane anaesthetic, nor repeatedly, nor to patients with unexplained jaundice or pyrexia after exposure to halothane.
- Jaundice has many causes other than infections and drugs, including particularly gall bladder disease, liver metastases, and biliary obstruction by pancreatic carcinoma.
- Postoperative jaundice may be caused by drugs, viral hepatitis, haemolysis, or unrelated liver disease. In Gilbert's disease – a benign enzyme defect – jaundice may follow starvation for general anaesthesia.

The main functions of the liver are in the metabolism, breakdown and excretion of drugs and endogenous materials, the formation of some plasma proteins, including some components of the clotting mechanism, and of complement, and the storage of substances such as vitamin B$_{12}$.

Effects of liver disease

Problems in the dental management of patients with liver disease are related to:

1. impaired drug detoxification;
2. bleeding tendencies;
3. transmission of viral hepatitis.

Liver diseases fall into three broad groups but there is some overlap (*Table 10.1*). The main groups of patients with liver disease are those who abuse alcohol or drugs, those from the developing world, those who have been exposed to unscreened blood or blood products and the sexually promiscuous.

Liver diseases can have many effects (*Table 10.2*). Impaired degradative and excretory activity in parenchymal liver disease often results in the accumulation of drugs and metabolites in the body. Impaired drug metabolism means that CNS depressants such as sedatives, analgesics and general anaesthetics may be potentiated and can even

Table 10.1 Causes of liver disease

- Congenital hyperbilirubinaemia
  Rhesus incompatibility
  Prematurity
  Biliary atresia
  Gilbert's syndrome
  Crigler–Najjar syndrome
  Others (*Table 10.3*)
- Parenchymal liver disease (hepatocellular disease)
  Viral hepatitis
  Chronic hepatitis
  Cirrhosis (often alcohol)
  Primary biliary cirrhosis
  Drug-induced hepatitis
  Others
- Extrahepatic biliary obstruction
  Gallstones
  Carcinoma of pancreas
  Others

cause coma. Even the maximum safe dose of local anaesthetics is lower than in healthy persons. Bilirubin, the breakdown product of haemoglobin, is normally conjugated in the liver to produce a water-soluble form for excretion. This bilirubin ester is excreted in bile and colours the faeces. If bilirubin is not conjugated (enzyme defect or parenchymal liver disease) or excreted (biliary obstruction), it accumulates in the body and colours the skin and mucous membranes (jaundice or icterus). Failure of the bilirubin to reach the

Table 10.2   Manifestations of liver diseases

Disorder	Main diseases	Consequences	Clinical features
Impaired bilirubin metabolism	Congenital hyperbilirubinaemia Hepatocellular disease	Hyperbilirubinaemia	Jaundice
Impaired bilirubin excretion	Extrahepatic obstruction Hepatocellular disease Pale stools	Hyperbilirubinaemia Bilirubinuria	Jaundice Dark urine
Impaired excretion of bile salts	Extrahepatic obstruction Hepatocellular disease	Rise in serum alkaline phosphatase and 5' nucleotidase Fat malabsorption and malabsorption of fat-soluble vitamins (especially vitamin K) Prolonged prothrombin time	Pruritus Fatty stools Bleeding tendencies
Impaired liver cell metabolism	Hepatocellular disease	Impaired clotting factor synthesis and prolonged prothrombin time Impaired albumin synthesis Impaired drug metabolism Rise in serum transaminases Portal venous hypertension Disorganized liver structure Cirrhosis Bleeding from oesophageal varices	Bleeding tendencies Oedema Coma or neurological disorders Splenomegaly

intestine (obstructive diseases) results in pale faeces but dammed-back bilirubin spills over into, and darkens, the urine.

Bile salts, which are needed for the absorption of fats, are also held back and the faeces therefore become fatty. Malabsorption of fats also causes impaired absorption of fat-soluble vitamins such as vitamin K and this, with depressed synthesis of plasma proteins including most clotting factors, causes the consequent bleeding tendency. Other factors, such as excess fibrinolysins, aggravate the bleeding tendency and both the prothrombin and activated partial thromboplastin times are prolonged (Chapter 4).

Accumulation of bile salts is thought to be responsible for the itching, nausea, anorexia and vomiting seen in some forms of liver disease. Glucose metabolism is also disturbed and there may be disorders of calcium and sex steroid metabolism.

Chronic liver disease is also associated with obstruction to the portal circulation leading to portal hypertension, oesophageal varices and the risk of fatal gastrointestinal haemorrhage. Portal obstruction can lead to hepatic encephalopathy and tremor (liver flap), and chronic bleeding may cause anaemia. Cutaneous features may include purpura, telangiectasia (spider naevi) and palmar erythema, and sometimes finger clubbing and leuconychia (opaque white nails). Gynaecomastia and testicular atrophy may be present. Dupuytren's contracture of the 4th and 5th fingers, and sialosis, may be seen in chronic alcoholism, though there are also other reasons for these conditions.

Liver function tests

Liver damage is reflected by changes in liver function tests (LFTs), particularly by a rise in various enzymes released into serum (*Table 10.3*). Serum levels of aspartate transaminase (AST, sometimes called serum glutamine-oxaloacetate transaminase or SGOT), alanine transaminase (ALT, sometimes called serum glutamic pyruvate transaminase or SGPT) and gamma-glutamyl transpeptidase (GGT) are often raised in parenchymal liver disease: GGT is particularly raised in alcoholic liver disease. Rises in the levels of these enzymes may, however, also be seen if there is tissue damage elsewhere. Biliary canalicular enzymes such as 5'-nucleotidase and alkaline phosphatase may be increased in the serum in obstructive jaundice, but again the enzymes are not totally specific.

Table 10.3 Liver function tests

Test	Basis	Abnormalities
Urine bilirubin	Water-soluble conjugates enter urine	Positive in most patients with jaundice except unconjugated hyperbilirubinaemia
Serum		
Bilirubin	Bilirubin is product of haem breakdown	Bilirubin rises because of overproduction, or obstruction
Aspartate aminotransferase	Leaks from damaged liver, heart or muscle	Rises in liver, heart or muscle damage
Alanine aminotransferase	Found mainly in liver	Rises in liver disease
Alkaline phosphatase	Found in biliary canaliculi, osteoblasts, intestinal mucosa, placenta	Rises in pregnancy, liver disease, bone disease
5′ Nucleotidase	Found in liver, thyroid and bone	Rises in biliary obstruction
Gamma glutamyl transpeptidase	Found in liver, kidneys, pancreas, prostate	Rises in alcoholism, most liver diseases, pancreatitis, diabetes, myocardial infarct
Albumin	Produced by liver	Falls in liver disease, nephrotic syndrome, gastrointestinal disease
Caeruloplasmin		Rises in Wilson's hepatolenticular degeneration

CONGENITAL DISORDERS ASSOCIATED WITH JAUNDICE (HYPERBILIRUBINAEMIA)

Transient jaundice is common in neonates but usually of little consequence. More severe neonatal jaundice can be caused by prematurity or rhesus incompatibility and can lead to kernicterus (damage to the basal ganglia of the brain). This can be fatal or cause epilepsy or choreoathetosis (with or without mental defect) and deafness in survivors. Somewhat less severe congenital jaundice can result from biliary atresia or be intrahepatic. It rarely causes kernicterus but may lead to portal hypertension, hepatic coma or respiratory infection.

Rare familial hepatic disorders characterized by jaundice are summarized in *Table 10.4*. The most common of this group is Gilbert's syndrome in which the serum level of total (but not conjugated) bilirubin is raised; bilirubin does not enter the urine and other liver functions are quite normal. Gilbert's syndrome is benign. However if patients starve, take alcohol or have a general anaesthetic, they may become jaundiced. After an anaesthetic the jaundice may be confused with the many other, more serious causes of postoperative jaundice (*see Table 10.15*). Other benign congenital disorders are rare, but include the Dubin–Johnson and Rotor syndromes. The familial disorders cause little difficulty except for the need to differentiate them from more serious liver disease. The Crigler–Najjar syndrome is more serious and can cause kernicterus as the

Table 10.4 Features of congenital hyperbilirubinaemias

	Gilbert's syndrome	Crigler–Najjar syndrome	Dubin–Johnson syndrome	Rotor syndrome
Prognosis	Usually benign	Usually lethal	Benign	Benign
Bilirubinaemia	Unconjugated	Unconjugated	Conjugated	Conjugated
Pigment in urine	—	—	+	+
Associated problems	—	Kernicterus	—	—

bilirubin levels rise, and the condition is usually fatal in early childhood.

- **Dental aspects of congenital jaundice**

The more serious disorders may lead to a bleeding tendency and impaired drug metabolism (*see below*). Disorders associated with an early rise in serum levels of conjugated bilirubin (mainly rhesus disease and biliary atresia) can cause dental hypoplasia and a greenish discoloration of the teeth.

ACQUIRED (PARENCHYMAL) LIVER DISEASE

The most common acquired causes of liver disease are summarized in *Table 10.1*. Many of the disorders may significantly affect dental management, but only general aspects are considered here. Further details are given under the specific disorders.

- **Dental aspects of parenchymal liver disease**

Impaired drug detoxification and excretion
The effects of drugs in parenchymal liver disease are not entirely predictable. Factors determining the response include the type and severity of the liver disease, as well as induction of hepatic drug-metabolizing enzymes by previous medication. Drugs, particularly the barbiturates, liable to cause respiratory depression are especially dangerous.

Brain metabolism is abnormal and the brain becomes more sensitive to a variety of drugs. Encephalopathy or coma can thus be precipitated by sedatives, hypnotics, tranquillizers or opioids. The effects may also be enhanced by reduced protein-binding of the drug resulting from hypoalbuminaemia.

Tetracyclines, erythromycin estolate, chlorpromazine, monoamine oxidase inhibitors and phenylbutazone which, in varying degrees, are hepatotoxic should be avoided. Clindamycin, desflurane, metronidazole and paracetamol should be used in lower than normal doses. Alternative drugs are shown in *Table 10.5*.

Local anaesthesia is safe given in normal doses, prilocaine more so than lignocaine, and relative analgesia is preferable to intravenous sedation with a benzodiazepine. General anaesthesia, if unavoidable, must be given by a specialist anaesthetist. Premedication with opioids must be avoided; pethidine and phenoperidine appear to be fairly well tolerated but benzodiazepines are preferred. Benzodiazepines are preferable to thiopentone for induction; isoflurane or sevoflurane are preferable to halothane (*see below*: Halothane hepatitis).

Suxamethonium (Scoline) is best avoided since the impaired cholinesterase activity in liver disease causes increased sensitivity to this neuromuscular blocker. Nitrous oxide with pethidine or phenoperidine appears to

Table 10.5	**Drugs contraindicated and alternatives in patients with liver disease**	
	Contraindicated	*Use instead*
Analgesics	Aspirin	Paracetamol*
	Codeine	
	Mefenamic acid	
	Opioids	
	Indomethacin	
Antimicrobials	Tetracyclines	Penicillin
	Erythromycin estolate	Erythromycin stearate
	Talampicillin	Amoxycillin
Anaesthetics	Methohexitone	Isoflurane
	Thiopentone	Desflurane
	Halothane	Sevoflurane
		Prilocaine
Muscle relaxants	Suxamethonium	Tubocurarine
Antidepressants	Monoamine oxidase inhibitors	Tricyclics*
Central nervous system depressants	Barbiturates	Pethidine*
	Opioids	Temazepam*
	Phenothiazines	
Corticosteroids	Prednisone	Prednisolone
Others	Diuretics	
	Oral contraceptives	
	Methyldopa	
	Biguanides	
	Lomotil	
	Liquid paraffin	
	Anticoagulants	
	Anticonvulsants	

*Acetoaminophen: give smaller dose.

be suitable for anaesthesia but it is essential to avoid hypoxia.

Bleeding tendencies
Impaired haemostasis leads to haemorrhage. Patients with parenchymal liver disease can therefore present serious problems if surgery is needed, and a clotting screen is therefore indicated. If the prothrombin time is prolonged, vitamin K_1 10 mg parenterally (phytomenadione) should be given daily for several days preoperatively in an attempt to improve haemostatic function. If there is an inadequate response as shown by the prothrombin time, a transfusion of fresh blood or plasma may be required. Repeated gastrointestinal bleeding may cause anaemia (Chapter 5) or be fatal.

Anticoagulants can cause uncontrollable haemorrhage since clotting factor synthesis is depressed and broad-spectrum antibiotics (at least in theory) may further reduce vitamin K availability by destroying the gut flora. Aspirin and most other non-steroidal anti-inflammatory analgesics such as indomethacin should be avoided because they aggravate the haemorrhagic tendency and because of the risk of gastric haemorrhage in those with portal hypertension or those with peptic ulcers, which are not uncommon in liver disease (*Table 10.5*).

Other complications
There may be alcoholism (Chapter 24), autoimmune disease, hepatitis B, C or D antigen carriage or diabetes (Chapter 14). Acute renal failure may complicate hepatic failure (hepatorenal syndrome) but the precise mechanism is obscure. If a jaundiced patient must undergo major surgery, aggressive therapy is indicated using intravenous fluids and diuresis with mannitol, in order to avoid this complication.

VIRAL HEPATITIS

The term 'viral hepatitis' usually refers to liver infection by hepatitis A, hepatitis B with or without delta agent, or non-A non-B hepatitis (particularly hepatitis C) viruses. However, hepatitis viruses A, B, C, D, E and G have now been recognized. Most, except hepatitis A and E, constitute a cross-infection

Table 10.6   Causes of viral hepatitis
• Hepatitis A virus
• Hepatitis B virus
• Non-A non-B viruses (hepatitis C, G and E particularly)
• Delta agent (hepatitis D)
• Epstein–Barr virus (infectious mononucleosis)
• Herpes simplex
• Cytomegalovirus
• Coxsackie B virus
• Yellow fever

risk in dentistry as they are transmitted parenterally. Other viruses are occasionally responsible (*Table 10.6*). Some hepatitis viruses may be associated with liver cancer or can be responsible for aplastic anaemia.

Hepatitis B is discussed first because of its importance in dentistry, but in the absence of a vaccine as yet, hepatitis C may become a more serious problem.

Hepatitis B (serum hepatitis, homologous serum jaundice)

This infection is endemic throughout the world, especially in institutions, in cities and in poor socioeconomic conditions. It is especially common in the developing world. Worldwide some 300 million persons are chronically infected. The prevalence of carriers varies considerably, being low (about 0.2 per cent) in Western Europe and North America, rising to 20 per cent in southern and eastern Europe, up to 40 per cent in some parts of West Africa and even higher in Indo-China. Africa, South-East Asia and South America are the areas of highest endemicity. Over 75 per cent of some populations such as Australian aborigines (hence the term 'Australia antigen') are carriers. The incidence of hepatitis B has been increasing worldwide, but now seems to be declining in some developed countries.

Spread of hepatitis B is mainly parenteral (via unscreened blood or blood products, particularly by intravenous drug abuse, and by tattooing/ear-piercing), sexually (especially among male homosexuals) and perinatally. Hepatitis B virus has been transmitted to patients and staff in health care facilities. Apart from health care workers, those in the

Table 10.7 Viral hepatitis: clinical features and biochemical changes

Stage	Clinical features	Serum bilirubin	Aspartate transaminase	Alanine transaminase	Alkaline phosphatase
Prodrome	Anorexia Lassitude Nausea Abdominal pain	N or ↑	↑	↑↑	N or ↑
Clinical hepatitis	As above plus Jaundice Pale stools Dark urine Pruritus Fever Hepatomegaly	↑	↑	↑↑↑	N or ↑

Arrows indicate a value above normal (N).

armed forces, missionaries and aid workers, and persons travelling to the developing world are at risk from infection.

The disease has an incubation period of 2–6 months, and has an acute mortality of less than 2 per cent. In a very few outbreaks where there is also infection with hepatitis D virus the death rate has been as high as 30 per cent.

Clinical aspects of hepatitis B
The effects of hepatitis B virus (HBV) infection range from subclinical infections without jaundice (anicteric hepatitis) in the vast majority of cases, to fulminating hepatitis, acute hepatic failure and death. Most patients recover completely and suffer no untoward effect, apart perhaps from some persistent malaise.

The prodromal period of 1–2 weeks is characterized by anorexia, malaise and nausea. Muscle pains, arthralgia and rashes are more common in hepatitis B than hepatitis A and there is often fever. As jaundice becomes clinically evident the stools become pale and the urine dark due to bilirubinuria. The liver is enlarged and tender, and pruritus may be troublesome (*Table 10.7*). Serum enzyme estimations are useful in diagnosis: aspartate transaminase (AST) and alanine transaminase (ALT) are raised in proportion to the severity of the illness. Alkaline phosphatase, alpha-fetoprotein and serum bilirubin levels are also raised.

In the absence of complications, infection with hepatitis B confers immunity. A high proportion of staff working in developing countries or in institutions for the mentally handicapped developed antibody to hepatitis B surface antigen in spite of a low incidence of overt hepatitis. This suggests that active immunity can be acquired naturally.

Complications of hepatitis B
Carrier state: In most patients who contract hepatitis B, viraemia precedes the clinical illness by weeks or months and lasts for some weeks thereafter before clearing completely. Hepatitis B progresses to a carrier state, in which virus persists within the body for more than 6 months, in 5–10 per cent, more frequently in anicteric infections or those contracted early in life. Carriers may remain positive for up to 20 years, although some 5–10 per cent of carriers lose the hepatitis antigen each year. The carrier state may not be suspected clinically. However, certain groups of patients, especially those who have received blood products and those who have immune defects, are predisposed to the carrier state. These 'high risk' groups are shown in *Table 10.8*. They are also liable to contract other blood-borne infections such as HIV. Most carriers are healthy but others, especially those with persistently abnormal liver function tests, develop chronic liver disease.

Chronic hepatitis: Chronic liver disease can affect up to 20 per cent and appears especially to complicate insidious hepatitis B with mild or absent jaundice but continued malaise. The very young and old are particularly at risk, as

---

Table 10.8   Viral hepatitis – high risk groups for hepatitis B

- Patients receiving blood products or multiple plasma or blood transfusions (e.g. haemophilia, thalassaemia) (especially in the Far East or Africa)
- Immunosuppressed or immunodeficient patients (e.g. HIV-infected, post-transplantation or due to malignant disease)
- Residents and staff of long-stay institutions (especially for the mentally handicapped)
- Health care and laboratory personnel (especially surgeons)
- Intravenous drug abusers
- Sexually active individuals (especially male homosexuals)
- Patients from the developing world (especially Africa and Asia)
- Tattooing and acupuncture (especially in the Far East)
- Certain other disorders (e.g. Down's syndrome, polyarteritis nodosa)
- Consorts of patients with hepatitis or any of the above groups
- Some chronic liver diseases

---

are those who have persistent serum markers (HBsAg, HBeAg, and anti-HBc and DNA polymerase, *see Table 10.9* for details).

Cirrhosis (see below).

Hepatocellular carcinoma: Epidemiological evidence has implicated hepatitis B virus (HBV) in the aetiology of hepatoma as a consequence of the cirrhosis. HBV nucleic acid has also been detected in this tumour.

Polyarteritis nodosa (see Chapter 21).

Serological markers of hepatitis B
Electron microscopy shows three types of particle in serum from patients with hepatitis B. The Dane particle probably represents intact hepatitis virus, and consists of an inner core containing DNA and core antigens (HBcAg), and an outer envelope of surface antigen (HBsAg). The smaller spherical forms and the tubular forms represent excess HBsAg. The other antigen from hepatitis B is the e antigen (HBeAg). Serological markers are useful in diagnosis and are of prognostic value (*Table 10.9*).

Hepatitis B surface antigen and antibody: HBsAg (Australia antigen, hepatitis associated antigen, hepatitis B antigen) is a non-infectious protein found transiently in those with acute hepatitis B, and persists in carriers and in some who are non-infectious.

In a typical case of hepatitis B, HBsAg develops 20–100 days after exposure, is detectable in the serum for 1–120 days and then disappears. The serum becomes negative for HBsAg about 6 weeks after the onset of clinical jaundice and in most instances antibody (anti-HBs) develops and is detectable in the serum for many years thereafter. Persistence of HBsAg beyond 13 weeks of the clinical illness often implies a carrier state is developing. The presence of anti-HBs in the absence of HBsAg implies recovery and immunity. Vaccination with hepatitis B vaccine, which consists of HBsAg, elicits an anti-HBs response.

Hepatitis B e antigen and antibody: The e antigen (HBeAg) is a soluble protein found only in serum that is also HBsAg-positive. However, only about 25 per cent of those who are HBsAg-positive are also HBeAg-positive and infectious. HBeAg is indicative of active disease and high infectivity. If HBeAg persists beyond about 4 weeks of the onset of symptoms the patient will probably remain infectious and develop chronic liver disease.

Table 10.9   Serum markers of hepatitis B infection in relation to progress of disease

	HBsAg	Anti-HBs	HBeAg*	Anti-HBe	HBcAg	Anti-HBc	DNA polymerase*
Late incubation	+	–	+	–	Liver only	–	++
Acute hepatitis	++	–	±	–	Liver only	++	+
Recovery (immunity)	–	++	–	+	–	+	–
Asymptomatic carrier state	++	–	–	±	–	++	±
Chronic active hepatitis	++	–	+	–	–	+	±

+ = Serum level raised.
*Presence implies high infectivity.

Development of antibody to HBeAg (anti-HBe) and loss of HBeAg usually indicates complete recovery and loss of infectivity. Asymptomatic HBsAg carriers often possess anti-HBe, and are usually a lower infective risk than those with HBeAg and DNA polymerase (super-carriers). Absence of HBeAg has usually indicated low infectivity but *pre-core mutants* of HBV have now been identified which are infective but show no HBeAg.

Hepatitis B core antibody: The core antigen of the Dane particle is found in liver biopsies in acute hepatitis B but not in serum. Serum antibody to HBcAg (anti-HBc) is a sensitive marker of viral replication indicating current or recent infection. Anti-HBc associated with anti-HBs appears to indicate recovery and immunity to hepatitis. However, if anti-HBs is absent, anti-HBc suggests the carrier state or chronic hepatitis.

DNA polymerase: The core of the Dane particle contains the enzyme DNA polymerase which appears transiently in the serum early in the course of viral B hepatitis. If demonstrable in HBsAg carriers it, like HBeAg, appears to imply high infectivity.

• General management of hepatitis B

Patients with hepatitis may benefit from bed rest and a high carbohydrate diet and should avoid hepatotoxins such as alcohol. Normal human immunoglobulin may confer some protection against hepatitis B but the evidence is weak. Any such protection presumably depends on the titre of antibody to hepatitis B (anti-HBs), which varies between batches of sera.

Passive immunity may be temporarily conferred by high titre hepatitis B immunoglobulins (HBIG) but is only indicated for non-immune groups at risk or after accidental exposure, when it should be given with active immunization (hepatitis B vaccine). The degree and duration of protection are, however, uncertain and it is not known whether immunoglobulin affects the sequelae of hepatitis B infection.

Active immunity as conferred by the hepatitis B vaccine (*see below*) is the most effective prophylaxis but may not protect against newly reported (pre-core) variants. For the treatment of *chronic* hepatitis B inter-

feron alpha is used, and adenine arabinoside and aciclovir are under trial.

Sources of infection by hepatitis B in the dental environment

Although pure parotid saliva does not contain HBsAg, saliva collected from the oral cavity may contain hepatitis B antigens and nucleic acid (presumably derived from serum) and may be a source for non-parenteral transmission. However, the risk of transmission by this route appears to be low except where there is very close contact, as in families or children's nurseries or sexual contact, or possibly needle-stick injuries. Hepatitis B can also be transmitted by human bites.

Blood, plasma or serum can be infectious: indeed, as little as 0.0000001 ml of HBsAg-positive serum can transmit hepatitis B. The main danger is from needlestick injuries and some 25 per cent of these may transmit HBV infection if the instrument has been used on HBV-infected patients.

Risk of infection by hepatitis B virus in dental personnel

About 1 in 1000 of the UK population are HBsAg carriers. Even among *high risk* patients attending dental hospitals (*Table 10.8*) less than 10 per cent are HBsAg carriers and 75 per cent of these are probably non-infectious (HBeAg-negative). There is clear evidence of unvaccinated dentists and other dental personnel contracting hepatitis, but several reports indicate that the risk is fairly low, now that precautions are taken. Recent surveys in Scandinavia and Israel have failed to show a risk to general dental practitioners significantly greater than that to the population at large, but there is still a greater risk for oral surgeons and periodontologists, and for those working with high-risk patients probably because of needlestick injuries.

Vaccination against hepatitis B has substantially reduced this risk and there are now few cases of hepatitis B among British dental staff. Good cross-infection control also reduces the risk.

Risk of transmission of HBV infection to patients

Dental procedures have transmitted hepatitis B to patients, although recent studies suggest that if adequate precautions are taken the dental surgery is no longer a significant source of transmission.

In earlier studies, HBsAg carriage was found in about 1 per cent of dental practitioners and up to 20 per cent of oral surgeons, who have occasionally transmitted the infection to their patients.

Practitioners ill with hepatitis should stop dental practice until fully recovered. Testing for HBeAg may prove useful in identifying those individuals likely to spread hepatitis B, and HBeAg-positive dental surgeons may well be advised to discontinue practice (see Chapter 11). Other HBsAg-positive personnel should follow the precautions outlined in Chapter 11, and must wear protective clothing, gloves and mask.

Hepatitis B vaccination
The current vaccine against HBV infection is a recombinant vaccine of HBsAg. After vaccination, anti-HBs develops and confers protection against HBV infection. Vaccination also protects indirectly, against hepatitis D. Immediate side-effects from the vaccine are minimal and no long-term reactions have been reported. Vaccination is recommended for all clinical dental staff, especially those working with high-risk groups, and for those travelling to high prevalence areas. Protection probably persists for at least 3–5 years, but thereafter, booster immunization may be needed. Occasional HBV variants are *not* protected against by the vaccine.

- **Dental management of the patient with jaundice, hepatitis, or a history of either**

Jaundice is not a disease *per se* but the manifestation of several diseases. Although jaundice usually signifies liver disease, the possibility that jaundice is a result of haemolytic anaemia should be considered.

In the presence of clinical jaundice or where, in the absence of jaundice, there are abnormal liver function tests, operative intervention should be avoided unless imperative. The responsible physician should be consulted for the diagnosis and for advice on management of dental treatment. The main problems in management (bleeding tendencies and drug sensitivity) have been outlined above.

A more frequent problem for the dental surgeon is the patient with a past history of jaundice who requires dental treatment. It is wise in this event to try to establish the probable diagnosis. Jaundice just after birth is common, usually physiological and rarely of consequence. Jaundice during childhood is often caused by hepatitis A – also of little consequence. Jaundice in the teenager or young adult may be due to viral hepatitis (A, B, C, D or non-A non-B). Jaundice in middle age or later is more likely to be obstructive.

It is not practical to screen all patients with a history of jaundice for viral carriage, and even if it were possible, most carrier states follow anicteric hepatitis and would therefore not be suspected. Further, failure to detect HBsAg does not confirm absence of infectivity for hepatitis B, unless there is other evidence suggesting past infection and immunity (the presence of anti-HBs, and anti-HBe or anti-HBc). Testing will not usually exclude hepatitis C carriage or other infections such as HIV.

The groups *most* likely to be carrying HBV are those with a recent history of hepatitis (often male homosexuals or intravenous drug abusers or both), or patients from Africa or South East Asia. Such patients may also be carrying other infections such as HIV. Venepuncture, where necessary, should be carried out in conformity with the current code of practice for cross-infection control. The bottle should be clearly labelled and the necessary laboratory request forms completed before venepuncture. Equipment necessary for venepuncture should be laid out on a plastic or metal tray, so that there is no contamination of working surfaces, and sodium isocyanurate should be readily available for disinfection in the event of spillage of blood.

The operator should be experienced in venepuncture and should wear a gown and disposable rubber gloves. Ten millilitres of blood are withdrawn into a plastic 20 ml syringe or into a vacuum syringe. The needle must not be resheathed but removed with a needle removal device and immediately discarded into a suitable impermeable disposal container. The blood is gently introduced into the glass bottle with care not to contaminate its outer surface. The bottle is closed and sealed securely in a plastic bag (coloured red or yellow) labelled as *infected* or

Table 10.10 Comparative features of more common forms of viral hepatitis relevant to dentistry

	Hepatitis A (infectious hepatitis)	Hepatitis B (serum hepatitis)	Hepatitis C (Non-A non-B-hepatitis)*	Hepatitis D (delta agent)
Incubation	2–6 weeks	2–6 months	2–22 weeks	?
Main route of transmission	Faecal–oral	Parenteral	Parenteral	Parenteral
Severity	Mild	May be severe	Moderate	Severe
Complications	Rare	Relatively few Chronic liver disease Hepatoma Polyarteritis nodosa Chronic glomerulonephritis	Many Chronic liver disease Hepatoma Other complications	Can cause fulminant hepatitis
Carrier state possible	No	Yes	Yes	Yes
Acute mortality	0.1 per cent	1–2 per cent	?	?

*Several forms of NANB exist (E, F, G)

biohazard. The syringe, mask and gloves are discarded into a plastic bag and similarly labelled.

• Management of patients infected with HBV

It is important to avoid penalizing virus-positive patients by refusing them treatment since such actions may lead patients to conceal the fact that they may be positive or at risk. Furthermore, since most positive patients are unidentified, refusal to treat known carriers would not significantly reduce the risk to the operator.

Asymptomatic carriers of HBsAg: Although asymptomatic carriers of HBsAg may be infective, those whose serum is anti-HBe-positive/DNA-polymerase-negative are a *very* low risk.

Asymptomatic carriers whose serum is HBeAg-positive/DNA-polymerase-positive are the highest risk and may have other problems that influence their management (for example, HIV infection or drug abuse) and thus then may need to be managed in hospital dental departments that have appropriate facilities.

Patients with acute hepatitis B: If patients are known to be incubating hepatitis B or are in the acute or convalescent stages of hepatitis, dental treatment should be deferred where possible until after recovery is complete. Virus is usually cleared by about 3 months after symptomatic recovery and then serological examination should be carried out to detect HBsAg and HBeAg carriage.

Essential emergency dental care during incubation or acute hepatitis should be carried out in a hospital department. Due regard must be taken for the fact that the liver damage may influence dental treatment.

Symptomatic carriage of HBsAg: Patients with HBsAg carriage who also have liver or other disease should be treated in a hospital department as indicated above.

Hepatitis D

Hepatitis D virus (HDV) or delta agent (δ agent) is an incomplete RNA virus carried within the hepatitis B particle and will only replicate in the presence of HBsAg. HDV is found worldwide and is endemic especially in the Mediterranean littoral and among intravenous drug abusers. It is not endemic in Northern Europe or the USA, but some haemophiliacs and others have acquired the infection and the prevalence is rising. The incubation period is unknown. HDV spreads parenterally, mainly by shared hypodermic needles. Risk groups are as for HBV (*Tables 10.8 and 10.10*). HDV has been transmitted to patients and staff in health care facilities.

HDV infection may coincide with hepatitis B or superinfects patients with chronic hepatitis B. Infection may produce a biphasic pattern with double rises in liver enzymes, and bilirubin. HDV infection does not necessarily differ clinically from hepatitis B but it can cause fulminant disease with a high mortality rate. HDV antigen and antibody can now be assayed: δ antigen indicates recent infection; δ antibody indicates chronic hepatitis or recovery. Vaccination against HBV protects indirectly against HDV.

Hepatitis C

Hepatitis C accounts for at least 90 per cent of cases of post-transfusion non-A non-B hepatitis (NANBH) and is responsible for much sporadic viral hepatitis, particularly in intravenous drug abusers, among whom its prevalence is rising. By contrast, transfusion-associated hepatitis C is declining and will presumably decline rapidly now that blood is routinely tested for it. Hepatitis C has a similar incubation period to hepatitis B (usually less than 60 but up to 150 days). The illness is usually less severe and shorter than hepatitis B, but many more (25–80 per cent) have abnormal liver function tests after one year and many go on to chronic liver disease and liver cancer. Hepatitis C is responsible for a substantial proportion of patients with chronic liver disease and may account for a significant number of those who were thought to have autoimmune hepatitis. Patients infected with HCV are, in about 15 per cent of cases, also infected with hepatitis G virus (HGV). HCV may be associated with oral lichen planus in some populations.

Serological tests (ELISA) are available to detect the hepatitis C virus, but anti-HCV IgG is usually not detectable until 1–3 months after the acute infection and may take up to a year to appear. A more sensitive method using the polymerase chain reaction (PCR) to detect viral sequences has also been developed but is not suitable for mass screening. The timing of its application is also critical as viraemia in HCV fluctuates. Radioimmunoassay underestimates the prevalence of HCV and testing for hepatitis C antigen by PCR suggests that most of those who are seropositive by immune assay are viraemic and (despite the presence of antibody) are infective.

Carriers of hepatitis C and any other form of non-A non-B hepatitis should be managed with the precautions recommended for HBV or HIV carriers (*see below*). The hepatitis C virus has been found in saliva and infection has followed a human bite. HCV has been transmitted to patients and staff in health care facilities. HCV is transmitted in about 10% of needlestick injuries involving HCV-contaminated instruments. There has been a raised prevalence of HCV infection in some dental populations studied. There is as yet no vaccine against hepatitis C but interferon alpha may help.

Hepatitis G

HGV accounts for nearly 20 per cent of non-A non-B hepatitis in the USA, and most of these patients are also infected with HCV. About 1.5 per cent of healthy blood donors in the USA are infected with HGV, and it is of high prevalence in intravenous drug users.This is clearly a transmissible virus but the resultant infection if it produces clinical hepatitis tends to be less severe than hepatitis C. HGV appears to respond to interferon alpha.

Chronic hepatitis

Chronic hepatitis is a term applied to two inflammatory diseases with quite different prognoses, *chronic persistent hepatitis* and *chronic active hepatitis*.

Chronic persistent hepatitis

Chronic persistent hepatitis is benign, often of unknown aetiology but sometimes complicating viral hepatitis or other diseases (*Table 10.11*).

The main features are persistent lassitude and fatigue, intolerance of fats and alcohol, and an enlarged tender liver. Laboratory investigations show raised serum transaminases but normal levels of bilirubin, alkaline phosphatase, albumin and immunoglobulins. The diagnosis is confirmed by liver biopsy.

The prognosis is good and no specific treatment is required. However, complete recovery may take some years. Hepatotoxic agents should be avoided.

Table 10.11 Causes of chronic hepatitis		
Causes	*Chronic active hepatitis*	*Chronic persistent hepatitis**
Hepatitis B, or C	+	+
Autoimmune	+	–
Alcoholism	+	+
Inflammatory bowel disease	–	+
Wilson's disease	+	–
Alpha₁-antitrypsin deficiency	+	–
Aspirin	+	+
Cytotoxic agents	–	+
Halothane	+	–
Isoniazid	+	+
Methyldopa	+	+
Paracetamol	+	+

*Chronic persistent hepatitis may follow chronic active hepatitis.

Chronic active hepatitis

Chronic active hepatitis, by contrast, is a serious condition that frequently leads to cirrhosis. Chronic active hepatitis may be immunologically mediated (so-called lupoid hepatitis) or caused by various other factors (*Table 10.11*).

Lupoid hepatitis mainly affects women and is asymptomatic or causes mild fatigue. It may, however, be associated with arthralgia, diabetes, thyroiditis, haemolytic anaemia, ulcerative colitis, renal tubular acidosis, pulmonary infiltration or amenorrhoea. There is often a Cushingoid appearance, hepato-splenomegaly and recurrent episodes of acute hepatitis with jaundice. Lupoid hepatitis is characterized by negative HBsAg, hyperim-munoglobulinaemia G, smooth muscle autoantibodies, antinuclear antibodies, lupus erythematosus (LE) cells and HLA B8/DR3.

Chronic active hepatitis caused by hepatitis B virus mainly affects males, especially those who have been frequently exposed to this virus (e.g. some homosexuals), some immigrants and the immunologically compromised. The condition may be asymptomatic or have features of chronic liver disease but only moderate rises in serum bilirubin, transaminases and immunoglobulins. In contrast to lupoid hepatitis, smooth muscle autoantibodies are not a prominent feature. Serological findings include positive HBsAg, HBeAg and anti-HBc. This type of hepatitis may progress to cirrhosis or hepatoma.

- **General management of chronic active hepatitis**

Prednisolone is effective mainly for lupoid hepatitis. Corticosteroids may be used alone or with azathioprine in chronic active hepatitis and hepatotoxic agents should be avoided. Interferon alpha is indicated for HBeAg-positive patients.

- **Dental aspects of chronic active hepatitis**

Hepatotoxic agents, aspirin and paracetamol should be avoided. Other management problems include:

1. Chronic liver disease.
2. HBV or HCV carriage.
3. Corticosteroids.
4. Complicating disorders such as other autoimmune diseases, diabetes, Wilson's disease or alpha₁-antitrypsin deficiency.

There are no common oral problems in chronic active hepatitis but Sjögren's syndrome is relatively common in the lupoid hepatitis variant and oral lichen planus may develop.

Hepatitis A (infectious hepatitis)

Hepatitis A is endemic throughout the world, particularly being found in children in the developing world and where socioeconomic and living conditions are poor. Worldwide there are an estimated 1.4 million cases each year. Infection is less common in the developed world, where up to 70 per cent have no immunity by adulthood; such persons are at risk of infection if they travel to areas where the infection is common. In these groups, infection is seen mainly in adults. Spread is largely by the faecal–oral route, by the consumption of contaminated water or food, particularly raw shellfish. For example, nearly 300 000 persons were infected in one outbreak in Shanghai, originating from contaminated clams. The infection can also be transmitted sexually and by close person to person contact, and in body fluids including saliva. Persons in the armed forces, food handlers, healthcare workers, sewage workers and travellers to areas of high endemicity are at greatest risk.

The incubation period is 2–6 weeks but the disease is frequently subclinical or anicteric and has a mortality of less than 0.1 per cent. Infectious hepatitis usually affects children and gives long-lasting immunity and, since many adults have had the infection, there is little risk of a further attack if subsequently exposed to the virus.

The clinical features of hepatitis A are similar to those of hepatitis B but muscle pains, rashes and arthralgia are rare (*Table 10.10*). Recovery is usually uneventful, the blood and faeces become non-infective during or shortly after the acute illness and there is no evidence either of a carrier state or of the progression of hepatitis A to chronic liver disease.

The diagnosis can be confirmed by demonstrating serum antibodies to the virus (HAAb). No treatment is usually needed.

Normal human immunoglobulin may prevent or attenuate the clinical illness, but does not necessarily prevent infection. It is used mainly in sporadic outbreaks. A vaccine is available for prophylaxis in travellers to Asia, South America and Africa, where there is a high endemic rate. A combined vaccine against HAV and HBV is now available.

• Hepatitis A and dentistry

Hepatitis A is excreted for only about 2–3 weeks – or the latter half of the incubation period until a few days after the onset of jaundice. There appears to be no evidence of transmission of hepatitis A in dentistry.

Hepatitis E

The hepatitis E virus, which is an unenveloped single-stranded RNA virus transmitted enterically and causing a disease similar to hepatitis A, is epidemic in India, South East Asia, parts of the CIS and Africa. It has a high mortality (up to 40 per cent) in pregnant women.

Hepatitis E is not known to be transmitted during dentistry.

CIRRHOSIS

Cirrhosis is a late result of parenchymal liver damage, leading to fibrosis, nodular regener-

---

Table 10.12   Causes of cirrhosis

- Adults
  Idiopathic (cryptogenic)
  Alcoholism
  Hepatitis B
  Hepatitis C
  Chronic active hepatitis
  Primary biliary cirrhosis
  Wilson's disease
  Alpha$_1$-antitrypsin deficiency
  Haemochromatosis
  Congestive cardiac failure
- Children
  Cystic fibrosis
  Chronic active hepatitis
  Wilson's disease
  Alpha$_1$-antitrypsin deficiency
  Galactosaemia

---

ation and vascular derangement. Cirrhosis is a non-specific reaction to a wide variety of factors (*Table 10.12*). The aetiology is, however, known in only relatively few cases: most are idiopathic (cryptogenic cirrhosis) or, increasingly frequently, alcoholic, but cirrhosis can also be a sequel to hepatitis B and C.

Cirrhosis chiefly affects the middle-aged or elderly. The main features result from hepatocellular damage or portal venous hypertension (*Table 10.13*) but cirrhosis is frequently asymptomatic in the earlier stages. Anorexia, malaise

---

Table 10.13   Cirrhosis – clinical features

- Jaundice
- Oedema
    Ascites
    Swollen ankles
- Gastrointestinal haemorrhage
- Mental confusion
- Hepatomegaly
- Splenomegaly
- Finger clubbing
- Skin manifestations
    Spider naevi
    Palmar erythema
    Opaque nails
    Sparse hair
- Other occasional manifestations
    Parotid swelling
    Gynaecomastia
    Bleeding (liver failure)
    Portal hypertension and varices

and weight loss are common. Jaundice, hepatosplenomegaly, ascites, gastrointestinal haemorrhage, palmar erythema, spider naevi, finger clubbing, opaque nails, pigmentation, fluid retention, bruising, gynaecomastia, testicular atrophy and other features may be present. Alcoholic cirrhosis may have associated parotid swelling (sialosis), Dupuytren's contracture, gastric ulceration or pancreatitis.

Laboratory tests are non-specific with no consistent pattern of abnormalities. Serum bilirubin levels, immunoglobulins, transaminases and alkaline phosphatase may be raised. Serum albumin is often low. Haematological abnormalities include a prolonged prothrombin time, anaemia, macrocytosis, thrombocytopenia and sometimes leucocytosis.

Cirrhosis is a serious disorder with complications which include:

1. Portal-systemic encephalopathy, which can be precipitated by drugs, gastrointestinal haemorrhage or a high protein diet and lead to coma.
2. Haemorrhage from oesophageal varices causing anaemia or death. Blood may be vomited (haematemesis.)
3. Ascites.
4. Diabetes mellitus.
5. Hepatoma.
6. Peptic ulceration.

*   **General management of cirrhosis**

Any identifiable cause should be treated if possible. In those with chronic active hepatitis, interferon, corticosteroids or immunosuppressives may be indicated. Adequate nutrition is maintained and the management is mainly directed towards the prevention and treatment of complications.

*   **Dental aspects of cirrhosis**

Routine dental treatment can usually be carried out without any particular problem. The physician should be contacted if surgery or general anaesthesia is needed. Surgery is hazardous, particularly in view of bleeding tendencies, but also because of diabetes, anaemia, drug therapy, possible HBV or HCV carriage or infection, and poor wound healing. In advanced cirrhosis, surgery, and

particularly general anaesthesia, are so hazardous that the patient should be referred to hospital for treatment.

Alcoholism may be a problem and some patients have sialosis, or tooth erosion from gastric regurgitation. There is an association between liver cirrhosis and oral carcinoma.

PRIMARY BILIARY CIRRHOSIS

Primary biliary cirrhosis (PBC) is a rare, progressive, inflammatory disorder of intrahepatic bile ducts. It begins with non-suppurative destructive cholangitis and jaundice, and culminates in cirrhosis. The vast majority of patients with PBC are middle-aged women. Patients may be asymptomatic for many years but eventually complain of weakness, lethargy, weight loss, pale stools and dark urine, jaundice and pruritus. The biochemical features also resemble those of obstructive jaundice. Complications include skin pigmentation and xanthomas, osteomalacia, or the complications of any chronic liver disease. PBC may be complicated by other connective tissue diseases, particularly systemic sclerosis (scleroderma) or Sjögren's syndrome. Most patients have serum autoantibodies to mitochondria and hyperimmunoglobulinaemia.

*   **General management of PBC**

Cholestyramine is often needed to relieve pruritus. Vitamins A, D and K are required (intramuscularly) and oral medium-chain triglycerides improve nutrition. Penicillamine may be of benefit by lessening fibrosis.

*   **Dental aspects of PBC**

Patients with PBC may present similar management problems to those with other parenchymal liver diseases but, in addition, penicillamine may cause thrombocytopenia. Sjögren's syndrome complicates 70 per cent or more cases of PBC (Chapter 9); telangiectasias may be seen, and oral lichen planus is an occasional complication. Penicillamine occasionally causes polymyositis (Chapter 16), pemphigus or myasthenia, and may also cause lichenoid lesions, oral ulceration and loss of taste; zinc supplements may then help.

Table 10.14	Drug and chemically related liver damage	

Dose-related liver damage	Non-dose-related liver damage
Alcohol	Halothane
Tetracyclines	Sulphonamides
Ketoconazole	Erythromycin estolate
Paracetamol	Anti-thyroid drugs
Methyldopa	Phenytoin
Isoniazid	Nitrofurantoin
Methyltestosterone and	Phenylbutazone
anabolic steroids	Phenothiazines
Vinyl chloride and carbon	
tetrachloride	

DRUG-INDUCED LIVER DISEASE

Many drugs, especially alcohol, may induce liver damage. In some cases this is a predictable dose-related effect, while in others the damage is unpredictable and may be related to an immunological reaction.

Dose-related damage may be induced especially by alcohol, tetracyclines, carbon tetrachloride or paracetamol, but many other drugs may be responsible (*Table 10.14*).

Damage that is unpredictable and may be immunologically mediated is induced by many other drugs (*Table 10.14*), especially halothane, the phenothiazines and sulphonamides.

- **Dental aspects of drug-induced liver disease**

The major problems in dentistry are those created by the tetracyclines, erythromycin estolate, halothane and, possibly, aspirin.

Tetracyclines: The extent of liver damage is related to the blood levels and the danger of hepatotoxicity is therefore increased if there is impaired urinary excretion. However, there is a risk of liver damage only if massive doses of tetracyclines are administered.

Erythromycin estolate: Erythromycin estolate is potentially hepatotoxic but the effect is reversible when the drug is stopped. Erythromycin stearate is not hepatotoxic.

Halothane hepatitis
Abnormal liver function tests and occasionally jaundice or liver failure may follow any

general anaesthetic and may result from such factors as contaminated infusions or the stress of surgery (*see Table 10.15*), so that it is difficult to establish the relationship of hepatic reactions to the anaesthetic agent itself. The frequency of reactions to halothane is at a level low enough to have very little impact on postoperative mortality and morbidity.

However, halothane can undoubtedly cause hepatitis which may follow a single exposure in 1 in 35 000 cases. Transient impairment of liver function appears after halothane as after other anaesthetics, but liver damage is more common

- especially when anaesthetics are given repeatedly at intervals of less than 3 months;
- in middle-aged females;
- in the obese.

There also appears to be a genetic susceptibility. The reaction may be some form of hypersensitivity but the precise mechanism is uncertain and pre-existing liver disease does *not* appear to be a contributory factor.

Clinically, halothane hepatitis causes pyrexia developing after a week postoperatively. Malaise, anorexia and jaundice may then appear, and if jaundice is severe, the prognosis is very poor.

Unfortunately there are no dependable criteria or laboratory tests to indicate when halothane is truly contraindicated. Serum antibodies reacting with halothane-altered liver membrane determinants have been reported in about 75 per cent of patients, but as with antibodies to penicillin, few patients have a reaction on a further exposure.

Halothane should therefore never be given repeatedly, or within a period of 3 months, and never to any patient who has had malaise, pyrexia or jaundice after exposure to it.

Newer halogenated anaesthetic agents: Enflurane and particularly, isoflurane, desflurane and sevoflurane, do not induce hepatitis in those who have had an episode of halothane hepatitis. In many hospitals these have, despite cost, replaced halothane, particularly to carry out several operations on the same patient at short intervals

Aspirin and Reye's sydrome
There is some evidence that the use of aspirin in children who have an upper respiratory tract infection, chickenpox, influenza or other

viral infections, may rarely precipitate liver damage with encephalopathy (Reye's syndrome). Aspirin is therefore contraindicated for children under 12, except for certain specific diseases. Paracetamol in moderate dosage only is now the preferred analgesic and antipyretic in most circumstances.

Since this precaution seems to have been widely implemented the mortality from Reye's syndrome has declined significantly and the disease has become rare. In the period 1989/1990 there were only 7 confirmed cases in the UK and Ireland.

LIVER CANCER

Many tumours in the liver are metastases and often cause jaundice and wasting. Most tumours arise from the stomach, lung, breast, colon or uterus. Hepatocellular carcinoma is common in Africa, South East Asia, Japan and some Mediterranean countries – mainly areas of high endemicity for hepatitis B and C. Ultrasound, isotope scans and biopsy are often needed to establish the diagnosis. Treatment is unsatisfactory and usually consists of surgical resection; the prognosis is invariably poor.

EXTRAHEPATIC BILIARY OBSTRUCTION

The main causes of obstructive jaundice are gallstones and carcinoma of the pancreas (*see Table 10.1*). Obstructive jaundice is characterized by pruritus, dark urine and pale stools. There is a rise in serum bilirubin esters, alkaline phosphatase, 5'-nucleotidase, gamma-glutamyl transpeptidase and transaminases.

• Dental aspects of obstructive jaundice

The main danger in surgery on the patient with obstructive jaundice is excessive bleeding resulting from vitamin K malabsorption. Surgical intervention should be deferred wherever possible in the presence of jaundice until haemostatic function returns to normal. If surgery is essential, vitamin K_1 should be given parenterally at a dose of 10 mg daily for several days in an attempt to correct the bleeding tendency (Chapter 4).

General anaesthesia in a severely jaundiced patient can lead to renal failure (hepatorenal syndrome). If general anaesthesia is unavoidable it must be given by a specialist anaesthetist; hypotension must be avoided and the anaesthetist will usually give an intravenous infusion of mannitol to cause osmotic diuresis and help prevent renal complications.

Obstructive jaundice in the neonate may result in green teeth.

GALLSTONES

Gallstones are a frequent problem, especially with advancing age. Cholesterol-containing stones are the most common. The aetiology is usually unclear but some patients on clofibrate, oral contraceptives or oestrogens appear to be susceptible. Pigment gallstones may complicate chronic haemolytic anaemias (hereditary spherocytosis, thalassaemia or sickle cell anaemia).

Gallstones are often asymptomatic. Passage of the stones into the bile ducts, however, may precipitate acute cholecystitis, biliary colic, obstructive jaundice or acute pancreatitis.

• General management of obstructive jaundice due to gallstone disease

Cholecystectomy is usually indicated in obstructive jaundice due to gallstones, but lithotripsy and medical treatment with chenodeoxycholic acid have a place in the treatment of asymptomatic stones.

• Dental aspects of obstructive jaundice due to gallstone disease

Oral surgical intervention should be deferred wherever possible in the jaundiced patient in view of the risk of haemorrhage. Other potential problems, such as the hepatorenal syndrome, have been discussed above.

POSTOPERATIVE JAUNDICE

Postoperative jaundice was mentioned in Chapter 2. It is a problem of some importance

Table 10.15   Causes of postoperative jaundice

- Increased bilirubin load
    Haemolysis due to haemolytic anaemia or
    incompatible transfusions
    Resorption of blood from large haematoma
- Hepatocellular disease
    Halothane and other drug-induced hepatitis
    Gilbert's syndrome
    Viral hepatitis
    Shock
    Sepsis
- Obstructive jaundice
    Bile duct damage
    Gallstone disease
    Pancreatitis

and may be caused by several factors (*Table 10.15*).

LIVER TRANSPLANTATION

Liver transplantation is now increasingly used as treatment for patients with end-stage liver disease such as liver failure, biliary atresia, metabolic disease or malignancy.

Patients with a liver transplant can have multiple medical and other problems, particularly those related to immunosuppression (infections, adverse drug effects) and liver failure (bleeding tendencies, impaired drug metabolism).

- **Dental aspects of liver transplantation**

Before transplantation there should be a full oral and dental evaluation and careful attention to oral and dental disease, bearing in mind that after transplantation the patient will be chronically immunosuppressed and at risk from infection. General anaesthesia should be avoided, but if unavoidable, must only be given in hospital with appropriate expertise and facilities. Any invasive dental treatment should only be carried out after consultation with the responsible physician and with due consideration to the bleeding tendency (Chapter 4), any infectious risk and impaired drug metabolism. It is best to prevent the patient swallowing blood, as this may lead to encephalopathy. Drugs such as sedatives, aspirin and paracetamol are also

best avoided. A full preventive oral health care programme should be instituted.

Following transplantation, elective dental care is best deferred until after 3 months. Oral hygiene and preventive care must be maintained at a high standard. General anaesthesia should be avoided and, if necessary, should only be given in hospital with appropriate expertise and facilities. If any invasive procedures are likely to be necessary the responsible physician should be consulted with particular respect to the need for antibiotic cover, corticosteroid cover and any bleeding tendency. Any infectious risk should also be considered.

Children needing liver transplants may have retarded tooth eruption and discoloured and hypoplastic teeth. Gingival hyperplasia may be seen in patients on cyclosporin or some other drugs.

BIBLIOGRAPHY

Bagg J. (1995) Viral hepatitis. In Porter S.R. and Scully C. (eds), *Oral Health Care for Those with HIV Infection and Other Special Needs*. Northwood, Science Reviews, pp. 75–80.
Blogg C.E. (1986) Halothane and the liver: the problem revisited and made obsolete. *Br. Med. J.* **292**, 1691–2.
Bouchier A.D. (1981) Diagnosis of jaundice. *Br. Med. J.* **283**, 1282.
Brown B.R. (1985) Halothane hepatitis revisited. *N. Engl. J. Med.* **313**, 1347–8.
Cawson R.A., Spector R.G. and Skelly A.M. (1995) *Basic Pharmacology and Clinical Drug Use in Dentistry*, 6th edn. Edinburgh, Churchill Livingstone.
Centers for Disease Control (1982) Hepatitis B vaccine safety: report of an inter-agency group. *Morbidity Mortality Wkly Rep.* **31**, 465–7.
Di Bisceglie A.M. (1996) Hepatitis G virus infection: a work in progress. *Ann. Intern. Med.* **125**, 772–3.
Editorial (1986) Halothane-associated liver damage. *Lancet* **i**, 1251–2.
Epstein J.B., Porter S.R. and Scully C. (1992) Non-A, non-B hepatitis and dentistry. *Am. J. Dentistry* **5**, 49–56.
Esteban J.I., Gomez J., Martell M. *et al.* (1996) Transmission of hepatitis C by a cardiac surgeon. *N. Engl. J. Med.* **334**, 555–60.
Farrell G., Prendergast D. and Murray M. (1985) Halothane hepatitis. *N. Engl. J. Med.* **313**, 1310–14.
Gelman S. (1986) Halothane hepatotoxicity again? *Anesth. Analg.* **65**, 831–4.
Gerberding J.L. (1996) The infected health care provider. *N. Engl. J. Med.* **334**, 594–5.
Harpaz R., Von Seidlein L., Averhoff F.M. *et al.* (1996) Transmission of hepatitis B virus to multiple patients

from a surgeon without evidence of inadequate infection control. *N. Engl. J. Med.* **334**, 549–54.

Hibbs J., Rosenfeld S., Feinstone S.M. *et al.* (1992) Hepatitis/aplasia syndrome; non-A, non-B, non-C? *J. Am. Med. Assoc.* **267**, 2051–4.

Hosey M.T., Gordon G., Kelly D.A. *et al.* (1995) Oral findings in children with liver transplants. *Int. J. Paediatr. Dent.* **5**, 29–34.

Klein R.S., Freeman K., Taylor P.E. *et al.* (1991) Occupational risk for hepatitis C among New York City dentists. *Lancet* **338**,1539–42.

Kuo MY-P., Hahn L-J., Hong C-Y. *et al.* (1993) Low prevalence of hepatitis C virus infection among dentists in Taiwan. *J. Med. Virol.* **40**, 10–13.

Little J.W. and Rhodus N.L. (1992) Dental treatment of the liver transplant patient. *Oral Surg.* **73**, 419–26.

Majewski R.F., Hess J., Kabani S. *et al.* Dental findings in a patient with biliary atresia. *J. Clin. Pediatr. Dent.* **18**, 33–7.

Matthews R.W., Dowell T.B. and Scully C. (1987) Acceptance of hepatitis vaccination by auxiliary dental personnel. *Hlth Trends* **19**, 22–7.

Matthews R.W., Hislop S. and Scully C. (1986) The prevalence of hepatitis B markers in high risk dental patients. *Br. Dent. J.* **161**, 294–6.

Matthews R.W., Scully C. and Dowell T.B. (1986) Acceptance of hepatitis B vaccine by general dental practitioners in the United Kingdom. *Br. Dent. J.* **161**, 371–3.

Morisaki I., Abe K., Tong L.S.M. *et al.* (1990) Dental findings of children with biliary atresia: report of seven cases. *J. Dent. Child.* May, pp. 220–3.

Nunn J. Hepatic disease. In Porter S.R. and Scully C. (eds), *Oral Health Care for Those with HIV Infection and Other Special Needs.* Northwood, Science Reviews, pp. 153–5.

Porter S.R. and Scully C. (1990) Non-A, Non-B hepatitis and dentistry. *Br. Dent. J.* **168**, 257–61.

Porter S.R. and Scully C. (1996) *Innovations and Developments in Non-Invasive Oral Health Care.* Northwood, Science Reviews.

Porter S.R., Scully C. and Samaranayake L.P. (1994) Viral hepatitis: an update in relation to dental practice. *Oral Surg. Oral Med. Oral Pathol.* **78**, 682–95

Richards A., Rooney J., Prime S. and Scully C. (1994) Primary biliary cirrhosis: sole presentation with rampant dental caries. *Oral Surg. Oral Med. Oral Pathol.* **77**, 16–18.

Samaranayake L.P., Scully C., Dowell T. B. *et al.* (1988) New data on the acceptance of the hepatitis B vaccine by dental personnel in the United Kingdom. *Br. Dent. J.* **164**, 74–7.

Schiff E.R., de Medina M.D., Kline S.N. *et al.* (1986) Veterans Administration cooperative study on hepatitis and dentistry. *J. Am. Dent. Assoc.* **113**, 390–6.

Scully C. (1985) Hepatitis B: an update in relation to dentistry. *Br. Dent. J.* **159**, 321–8.

Scully C. (1988) *The Dental Patient.* Oxford, Heinemann.

Scully C. (1989) *The Mouth and Perioral Tissues.* Oxford, Heinemann.

Scully C. (1989) *Patient Care: a Dental Surgeon's Guide.* London, British Dental Journal.

Scully C. (1997) The dental profession. In Collins C.H. and Kennedy D.A. (eds), *Occupational Blood Borne Infections.* CAB International, pp 133–58.

Scully C. and Porter S.R. (1994) Infection control in dentistry. *Curr. Opin. Infect. Dis.* **7**, 488–92.

Scully C. and Samaranayake L.P. (1992) *Clinical Virology in Dentistry and Oral Medicine.* Cambridge, Cambridge University Press.

Scully C., Cawson R.A. and Griffiths M.J. (1990) *Occupational Hazards to Dental Staff.* London, British Dental Journal.

Scully C., Matthews R., Dowell T. and Griffiths M. (1986) Use of the airotor in hepatitis B surface antigen carriers. *Br. Dent. J.* **161**, 355–6.

Scully C., Pantlin L., Samaranayake L.P. *et al.* (1990) Increasing acceptance of hepatitis B vaccine by dental personnel but reluctance to accept hepatitis B carrier patients. *Oral Surg. Oral Med. Oral Pathol.* **69**, 45–7.

Scully C., Potts A.J.C., Hamburger J. *et al.* (1985) Lichen planus and liver diseases: how strong is the association? *J. Oral Pathol.* **14**, 224–6.

Sims W. (1980) The problem of cross-infection in dental surgery with particular reference to serum hepatitis. *J. Dent.* **8**, 20–6.

Svirsky J.A. (1989). Dental management of patients after liver transplantation. *Oral Surg. Oral Med. Oral Pathol.* **67**, 541–6.

Taylor T.W.S. (1986) Halothane and the liver. *Br. Med. J.* **293**, 335.

Zaia A.A., Graner E., Almeida O.P.D. *et al.* (1993) Oral changes associated with biliary atresia and liver transplantation. *J. Clin. Paediatr. Dent.* **18**, 39–42.

Zuckerman A.J. (1982) Priorities for immunization against hepatitis B. *Br. Med. J.* **284**, 686–8.

11

Infections and infection control

Key points

- Most oral infections are odontogenic, a sequel to caries. Mucosal infections are predominantly viral and in children, particularly where general hygiene is poor.
- Oral fluids can contain a range of micro-organisms, and saliva can be the vehicle for transmission of a range of agents, especially herpes viruses, enteroviruses and hepatitis viruses.
- The most serious relevant transmissible infections are blood-borne viruses such as HIV and hepatitis viruses, and respiratory pathogens, notably tuberculosis.
- Serious transmissible infections are most likely in:
  Injecting drug users
  Patients who have attended clinics for sexually transmitted diseases
  Male homosexuals and bisexuals
  Immunocompromised persons
  Vagrants
  Persons from parts of the developing world
- Infections are transmissible in dentistry unless infection control measures are continually practised.
- Blood-borne viruses are most readily transmitted by sharps (needlestick) injuries, or use of infected blood, blood products, or tissues. Bites are occasionally a route.
- All members of the dental team have a duty to ensure that all necessary steps are taken to prevent cross-infection, in order to protect their patients, colleagues and themselves and their families.
- The routine practice adopted for *all* dental patients must be sufficient to prevent cross-infection (universal precautions) with blood borne agents
- Gloves should be worn routinely by all dentists, students, hygienists and close support dental staff.
- Wash hands before gloving, and after gloves are removed. Cuts and abrasions should be protected with waterproof dressings and/or double gloving as appropriate.
- Gloves must be changed if punctured, and after treatment.
- When aerosols or tooth fragments are generated masks and eye protection should be worn, high volume aspiration used and waste should go into a central drain or sanitary suction unit.
- *Clean* white coats, or clean surgical gowns must be worn, changed if contaminated and not taken into any food/drink area.
- All 3-in-1 syringe tips, handpieces and ultrasonic scaler tips should be changed after use, and cleaned and autoclaved before re-use.

- Ultrasound scaler handpiece ends, which cannot be sterilized, must be thoroughly cleaned and disinfected before re-use.
- Cling-film should be placed over control buttons, operating light handles, ultrasonic scaler handpieces and 3-in-1 syringe bodies, and changed or decontaminated after every patient.
- Work surfaces should be protected with cling-film or other disposable material and changed after every patient.
- All 'sharps' must be disposed of in rigid containers.
- Inoculation injuries are the most likely source of cross-infection. Resheathing of needles should be avoided wherever possible.
- When cleaning an operation area or instruments, heavy-duty gloves should be worn.
- In the event of accidental injury to the operator:
  1. Ensure that the accident is not repeated.
  2. Wash the wound.
  3. Test the patient's serum for hepatitis B antigens and enquire about possible HIV positivity.
  4. If the patient's serum is negative, there is probably no problem.
  5. If the patient's serum is positive, consult a microbiologist immediately for advice.

Many infections, particularly viral, affect the mouth, pharynx or perioral area. Most cause lesions of limited duration, and where hygiene is poor, are seen mainly in children. Many have little influence on dental treatment though they may pose a small occupational risk to dental staff. In the developed countries adults not infrequently are non-immune, and thus these infections are now being seen more in adults.

Other infections, especially viral hepatitis, HIV infection and other sexually transmitted diseases, are much more common in the developing than the developed world. In developed countries they are mainly diseases of adults, particularly those who are promiscuous, and of urbanization and travel. These infections are an occupational hazard unless infection control is good, and can significantly influence dental management.

Table 11.1 Infectious diseases: incubation times and period of infectivity

Incubation period	Disease	Incubation period	Period of infectivity
<1 wk	Diphtheria	2–5 d	Until treated
	Gonorrhoea	2–5 d	Until treated
	Scarlet fever	1–3 d	3 weeks after onset of rash
1–2 wk	Measles	7–14 d	4 days after onset of rash
	Pertussis	7–10 d	21 days after onset of symptoms
2–3 wk	Chickenpox	14–21 d	Until all lesions scab
	Mumps	12–21 d	7 days after onset of sialadenitis
	Rubella	14–21 d	7 days after onset of rash
3 wk	Hepatitis A	2–6 wk	Usually non-infective at diagnosis
	Hepatitis B	2–6 mth	About 3 mth after jaundice resolves*
	Hepatitis non-A, non-B†	?	?*
	HIV	Up to 5 yr	?*
	Infectious mononucleosis	30–50 d	?*
	Syphilis	10–90d	Until treated*

*Carrier states exist.
†Several viruses responsible, including hepatitis C, D, E, F and G viruses (*see* Chapter 10).

Table 11.2 Synopsis of infectious diseases*

Disease	Cause	Major manifestations	Main oral manifestations	Laboratory diagnosis	Specific treatment used†	Specific management problems
AIDS	HIV	Opportunistic infections Tumours Encephalopathy	Cervical lymphadenopathy Candidosis Hairy leukoplakia Kaposi's sarcoma	Lymphopenia HIV serology	Protease and reverse transcriptase inhibitors may help	Cross-infection Bleeding tendency Immune defect
Cat scratch disease	*Bartonella henselae*	Tender papule, regional lymph nodes enlarge, mild fever	Cervical lymphadenopathy	Leucocytosis, ESR raised, skin test	Antibiotics (erythromycin)	—
Chickenpox (varicella)	Varicella zoster virus	Rash evolves through macule, papule, vesicle and pustule: rash crops and is most dense on trunk	Oral ulcers	Complement fixation antibody titres (not usually needed)	Zoster immune globulin in high-risk patients	Problems of dissemination in immunologically compromised patient
Diphtheria	*Corynebacterium diphtheriae*	Tonsillar or pharyngeal exudate; cervical lymph nodes enlarged	Tonsillar exudate, palatal palsy	Culture	Antitoxin: penicillin	Respiratory obstruction, myocarditis, palatal paralysis
Erysipelas	*Streptococcus pyogenes*	Rash (confluent erythema and oedema)	—	Culture	Penicillin	Cross-infection
Hand-foot-and-mouth disease	Usually Coxsackie virus A strains	Rash, stomatitis, minor malaise	Oral ulceration (usually mild)	Serology	None	Highly infective; myocarditis rarely
Hepatitis	Hepatitis A, B and non-A non-B viruses	Jaundice, malaise, pale stools, dark urine	—	Serology	Immune globulin	Cross-infection liver damage (*see* Chapter 10)
Herpangina	Usually Coxsackie virus A strains	Fever, sore throat, enlarged cervical lymph nodes	Vesicles and ulcers on soft palate	Serology	None	Differential diagnosis from herpes simplex: myocarditis rarely
Herpes simplex	Herpes simplex virus type 1 or 2	Fever, oral ulceration, cervical lymph node enlargement	Gingivostomatitis, herpes labialis, erythema multiforme	Serology	Aciclovir may help**	Dissemination in immunologically compromised patient
Herpes zoster (shingles)	Varicella zoster virus	Rash like chickenpox but limited to dermatome	Oral ulceration in zoster of maxillary or mandibular division of trigeminal nerve. Ulcers in palate and pinna of ear in Ramsay–Hunt syndrome	Not needed	Aciclovir plus zoster immune globulin in high-risk patients**	Severe pain during and after attack Eye involvement in ophthalmic zoster: may be underlying neoplasm
Impetigo	Streptococci and/or staphylococci	Rash (bullous) spreading to other areas rapidly	Lesions on lips may resemble recurrent herpes labialis	Culture	Topical chlortetracycline or flucloxacillin	Cross-infection or dissemination: acute nephritis

Disease	Organism	Clinical features	Oral/other signs	Laboratory diagnosis	Treatment	Complications/Notes
Infectious mononucleosis	Epstein–Barr virus	Fever, lymph node enlargement, pharyngitis	Tonsillar exudate, palatal petechiae, oral ulceration	Blood film, Monospot test, Paul–Bunnell test	—	Airway obstruction
Lyme disease	Borrelia burgdorferi	Arthritis, neurological and rash	Facial palsy	Serology	Tetracycline	Heart block in some
Measles	Measles virus	Rash (maculopapular), fever, acute respiratory symptoms	Koplik's spots, pharyngitis	Not usually needed	Immune globulin in high-risk patients	Pneumonia, especially in immunologically compromised patient
Mucocutaneous lymph node syndrome	Not known	Rash – hands and feet, desquamation, lymph node enlargement	Strawberry tongue, labial oedema, pharyngitis	—	—	Myocarditis or infarction
Mumps	Mumps virus	Fever, malaise, parotitis	Sialadenitis, trismus, papillitis at salivary duct orifices	Complement fixing antibody titres to S and V antigens rise: not usually needed	—	Differential diagnosis of salivary swelling; rarely myocarditis
Mycoplasmal pneumonia (atypical pneumonia)	Mycoplasma pneumoniae (Eaton agent: PPLO)	Sore throat, fever, pneumonia	Erythema multiforme occasionally later	Culture, complement fixing antibodies, cold agglutinins	Erythromycin or tetracycline	Respiratory complications
Whooping cough (pertussis)	Bordetella pertussis	Cough, fever	Occasionally ulceration of lingual fraenum	Culture	Amoxycillin for secondary infection	Respiratory complications
Poliomyelitis	Polio virus	Paralyses	—	Serology	—	Respiratory involvement
Rubella	Rubella virus	Rash (mainly macular), fever, enlarged posterior cervical lymph nodes	Pharyngitis ± palatal petechiae	Serology	—	Pregnant staff; Congenital rubella
Scarlet fever	Streptococcus pyogenes	Sore throat, fever, rash (macular), enlarged cervical nodes	Tonsillar exudate, Strawberry tongue	Culture, Antistreptolysino titre	Penicillin	Rheumatic fever, Acute glomerulonephritis, cross-infection
Toxoplasmosis	Toxoplasma gondii	Glandular fever type of syndrome	Sore throat	Sabin–Feldman dye test	Sulphonamide plus pyrimethamine	Differential diagnosis of cervical lymphadenopathy

*Infections discussed elsewhere include tuberculosis (Chapter 8), AIDS (Chapter 20), gonorrhoea and syphilis (Chapter 11).
†Also supportive care.
**or famciclovir.

Table 11.1 summarizes the incubation periods and *Table 11.2* the features of many of the more common infections. The few which are characterized mainly by oral symptoms or which significantly influence dental care are discussed here. Others are discussed in Chapters 8, 10, 20 and 26.

VIRAL INFECTIONS

HERPESVIRUSES

The herpes viruses are DNA viruses that are transmitted mainly in saliva and other body fluids, cause a short-lived primary clinical or more often subclinical infection, and remain latent thereafter. Reactivation is often because of immunosuppression, and recrudescence can lead to fairly protracted illness. Some of the viruses can be oncogenic.

Herpes simplex (human herpesviruses type 1 and 2)

Primary oral infection with herpes simplex virus (HSV) typically causes acute gingivostomatitis, fever, cervical lymph node enlargement and irritability. This is a common infection of young children but may be misdiagnosed as 'teething', or may be subclinical. The virus is usually type I *herpes simplex* virus which apparently thereafter remains latent, often in the trigeminal ganglia. A growing number of oral or oropharyngeal infections appear to be caused by type 2 herpes simplex virus, which traditionally causes genital infections.

The virus can be spread by saliva and occasionally causes painful whitlows in dental staff not previously exposed to it (*Fig. 11.1*).

Primary herpetic gingivostomatitis is limited to the mouth and resolves within about 10 days but, in immunosuppressed patients or in those with eczema, disseminated infection may result. Aciclovir is effective against HSV but many patients present with disease too far advanced to benefit. Aciclovir is, however, essential to control infection in immunocompromised patients. In other patients, treatment is usually limited to supportive care such as adequate fluid intake, antipyretics and analgesics (paracetamol/acetoaminophen usually) and good oral hygiene by mouth cleansing and the use of

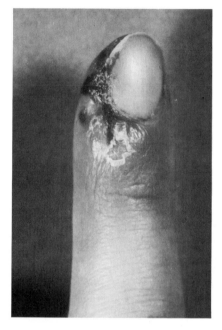

Fig. 11.1 Herpetic whitlow (herpes simplex infection) in a dental surgeon who worked without gloves

aqueous chlorhexidine (0.2 per cent) mouthwashes.

Many patients suffer no consequence once the primary infection resolves. Recurrent infections appear later in up to 30 per cent of patients and typically affect the mucocutaneous junction of the lip (herpes labialis; cold sores). Recurrences, which are often precipitated by factors such as exposure to systemic infections, sunlight, trauma, stress or menstruation respond well to 5 per cent aciclovir cream applied early or penciclovir. Intraoral recurrences appear as ulcers, and seem to be more likely after trauma, such as in the palate, or in immunocompromised patients (such as in leukaemia or HIV infection). Aciclovir may be indicated but HSV is now showing resistance in some cases, and famciclovir or even forscarnet may be required.

Herpetic infection is by no means exclusively a disease of childhood and adults are often affected since immunity may not have been acquired in early life. Those who develop herpetic infection in adult life may have particularly severe and prolonged systemic illness.

Varicella and zoster (human herpesvirus 3)

Chickenpox

Primary infection with the varicella zoster virus causes chickenpox – usually a trivial illness in childhood but often with oral ulceration. It is most common below the age of 10 years, by which time most children have become immune by natural infection. The infection spreads readily by droplets and via the airborne route. The characteristic rash, which is centripetal, and passes through stages that are macular, papular, vesicular and pustular before scabbing, differentiates chickenpox from other causes of oral ulceration. Patients are infectious from 1 to 2 days before the rash, until the rash scabs and dries. Complications are seen mainly in immunocompromised persons who may develop disseminated or haemorrhagic varicella. Adults, especially those who are pregnant or who smoke, are at risk from fulminating varicella pneumonia.

There is also a risk to the fetus and neonate if the mother contracts chickenpox. In the first 20 weeks of pregnancy, a congenital varicella syndrome, with microcephaly, cataracts, growth retardation and limb hypoplasia may result, and the mortality rate is high. Later in pregnancy, chickenpox may result in zoster in an otherwise healthy infant. Chickenpox around the time of delivery may cause severe and even fatal infection of the neonate.

Varicella zoster immunoglobulin, or aciclovir, may thus be indicated for non-immune persons who are pregnant or immunocompromised. A vaccine is becoming available.

Zoster

The virus remains latent within dorsal root ganglia and usually causes no further problems. However, reactivation may occur, especially in the elderly or immunocompromised, and can lead to shingles (zoster), which involves the dermatome supplied by

the sensory nerve affected (*Plate 9*). In some 8–10 per cent of cases zoster reflects an underlying immunodeficiency state, sometimes as result of HIV disease or a neoplasm, particularly a lymphoma.

Severe pain and a rash similar to chickenpox, but localized to the dermatome, characterize zoster; the pain may persist after the rash heals (post-herpetic neuralgia, Chapter 19). Zoster of the maxillary or mandibular divisions of the trigeminal nerve may cause facial pain (sometimes simulating toothache) and oral ulceration – unilateral and in the distribution of the nerve involved.

Those with ophthalmic zoster should have an urgent ophthalmological opinion. In immunocompromised patients who are not immune but are exposed to the virus, it is important to consider giving protection with zoster immunoglobulin or vaccine. Treatment of zoster is with aciclovir by mouth, but intravenous administration is needed in immunodeficient patients, particularly in those with HIV infection for whom it can be a life-threatening disease.

Epstein–Barr virus (human herpesvirus 4)

Glandular fever is a syndrome in which fever, malaise and lymph node enlargement are the main features. Several infectious agents (HIV, cytomegalovirus, human herpesvirus 6, *Toxoplasma gondii*) can cause this (*Table 11.3*) but the most frequent is the Epstein–Barr virus (EBV) (infectious mononucleosis; IM). This virus also has epidemiological associations with Burkitt's and some other lymphomas and nasopharyngeal carcinoma.

EBV is found in saliva during infectious mononucleosis and for several months thereafter, and is often in saliva of immunocompromised persons. Infection appears to be

Table 11.3 Causes of glandular fever syndrome

- Infectious mononucleosis
- HIV infection
- Cytomegalovirus infection
- Toxoplasmosis
- Infectious lymphocytosis
- Human herpesvirus 6 infection
- Rarely: acute leukaemia; brucellosis

spread by close oral contact, such as kissing, but infectivity is low. The disease is common among young adults and often subclinical or unrecognized, especially in children.

Infectious mononucleosis (IM) is protean in its manifestations. Children suffer mainly from lymphadenopathy, sore throat and fever. Adolescents often have a vague illness with malaise and a low fever but little lymphadenopathy. A high fever with rubelliform rashes and occasionally jaundice characterizes the febrile type of IM. In the anginose type, the throat is sore with soft palate petechiae and a whitish exudate on the tonsils, and pharyngeal oedema may threaten the airway. The glandular type of IM is characterized by general, especially cervical, lymph node enlargement and splenomegaly.

Complications of infectious mononucleosis include persistent fatigue, mild liver dysfunction, ECG changes, depression, neurological syndromes, oral ulceration and, rarely, nephritis, pancreatitis or lung infiltration. Ampicillin and amoxycillin very frequently cause a maculopapular rash which is not a manifestation of penicillin allergy, affecting the extensor surfaces of the limbs (*Fig. 11.2*).

Characteristic of IM are an excess of atypical lymphocytes (mononucleosis) in the blood: these may cause confusion with leukaemia but for the absence of its features such as anaemia. These cells may also be seen in, for example, viral hepatitis or chickenpox. Occasionally in IM there is mild neutropenia or thrombocytopenia.

A wide variety of serological changes are typical of IM, including transient heterophil antibodies, persistent EBV antibodies and a false-positive Wassermann reaction. *Heterophil antibodies* are IgM antibodies that agglutinate sheep and horse red blood cells: the Paul–Bunnell test for IM employs sheep erythrocytes but rapid methods are available to detect heterophil antibodies to horse red blood cells by detecting agglutination on a glass slide (Monospot test). Heterophil antibodies usually develop during the first or second week of the illness (60 per cent of patients), and by 4 weeks up to 90 per cent of patients have a titre before absorption of 224 (or 28 after absorption). The titre then declines and disappears over 3–6 months.

EBV antibodies include those to viral capsid antigen. This antibody is produced early, the

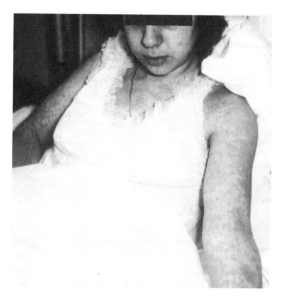

Fig. 11.2 Rash following the administration of ampicillin to a patient with infectious mononucleosis

titre peaks at about 4 weeks and the antibody persists for many years.

- **General management of infectious mononucleosis**

No specific treatment is available, but as there frequently is malaise and fatigue the patient may benefit from bed rest. Systemic corticosteroids are required if there is severe pharyngeal oedema which hazards the airway. Some also advise the use of penicillin since nearly 20 per cent of patients have concurrent beta-haemolytic streptococcal pharyngeal infection. Tinidazole may improve the sore throat.

- **Dental aspects of infectious mononucleosis**

Infectious mononucleosis is an important cause of enlarged cervical lymph nodes which must be distinguished particularly from those caused by local infections, HIV, leukaemia or lymphomas. Rarely, infectious mononucleosis is clinically atypical and enlarged lymph nodes have been removed for biopsy. Unfortunately, the lymph node histopathological changes in infectious mononucleosis closely resemble those in lymphomas and an expert opinion is needed. A useful precaution in such cases is to have a haematological examination and a test for heterophil antibodies.

Within the mouth, the most typical manifestation of infectious mononucleosis is a confluent creamy exudate in the fauces (to be distinguished from diphtheria) and fine petechiae at the junction of the hard and soft palate. The latter are occasionally seen in other viral infections such as rubella and HIV. Occasionally there is mucosal or gingival ulceration. EBV may also cause sialadenitis (*see below*) and in immunocompromised persons EBV may be shed in high titres in saliva and associated with hairy leukoplakia (Chapter 20) or lymphomas.

Chronic Epstein–Barr Virus (EBV) disease
It is now recognized that EBV infection is not invariably an acute self-limiting infection. Some patients have persistent symptoms for months or years, which may be related to chronic EBV infection because of inadequate antibody production against nuclear antigen, and impaired ability to generate EBV-specific cytotoxic T-lymphocytes, with weak lympho-proliferative responses. This infection mostly affects women aged 25–40, symptoms are vague – such as malaise, fatigue and fever – and most have a negative Paul–Bunnell test. There may be an association with HLA-D7 and with atopic disease. Treatment is not satisfactory, but intravenous gammaglobulin, and aciclovir, are under trial.

Caution must be exercised before assigning this diagnosis since several patients have eventually been shown to have other diagnoses such as SLE, ankylosing spondylitis or lymphoma. The syndrome resembles multiple sclerosis and 'myalgic encephalitis' (chronic fatigue syndrome; epidemic neuromyasthenia) in many respects.

Duncan's disease
A rare group of patients, with specifically demonstrable defects in antibodies to EBV nuclear antigens, have Duncan's disease (sex-linked lymphoproliferative syndrome), characterized by severe mononucleosis, immunoblastic sarcoma or lymphoma.

Burkitt's lymphoma
Burkitt's lymphoma is found predominantly in Africa, in children before the age of 12 years. It appears to be related to EBV in association with malaria. Massive swellings affect particularly the mandible, with pain, paraesthesia and bone destruction causing tooth mobility, jaw radiolucencies and destruction of the lamina dura. Burkitt's lymphoma may also be seen outside of Africa and can be a complication of HIV disease. Chemotherapy is remarkably effective.

Cytomegalovirus (human herpesvirus 5)

Cytomegalovirus (CMV) is a ubiquitous herpesvirus. Most primary infections with CMV are asymptomatic but some produce a glandular fever illness. Thereafter CMV remains latent in oropharyngeal and other epithelial cells and may be reactivated by immunosuppression and other factors. Under these circumstances disseminated infection may result, causing CMV retinitis in particular – often leading to blindness. CMV infection is a particular problem in HIV disease (Chapter 20).

The main other problem identified in relation to CMV is the potential to cause fetal damage similar to that caused by rubella (TORCH syndrome). CMV is thereafter excreted by the neonate in urine and saliva for many months.

Antiviral therapy for CMV includes ganciclovir or foscarnet.

TORCH syndrome
*T*oxoplasmosis, *r*ubella, *c*ytomegalovirus and *h*erpes simplex virus infection of the pregnant mother, especially in the first trimester, can cause fetal damage, sometimes lethal. This TORCH syndrome may at its lesser extent cause mild hearing loss, but it can also result in learning disability, pneumonitis, cardiac malformations, micro-ophthalmia, microcephaly, jaundice and low birth weight. Similar defects can be produced by infection with HIV, parvovirus, enteroviruses, varicella zoster virus, influenza, EBV, syphilis, malaria, listeriosis and possibly HIV.

Human herpesvirus 6

Human herpesvirus 6 (HHV-6) is a T-cell lymphotropic herpes virus which is almost invariably contracted within the first two years of life via oropharyngeal secretions, and thereafter remains latent. HHV-6 causes a febrile illness, sometimes with a macular or papular rash on the face and/or trunk (exanthema subitum; roseola infantum), mild diarrhoea, cough, oedematous eyelids and occasionally meningitis or meningo-encephalitis or blood dyscrasias (particularly granulocytopenia) or hepatitis. Infection in later life may produce a glandular fever syndrome, persistent lymph-adenopathy, chronic fatigue syndrome, or hepatitis. Immunocompromised patients may develop pneumonitis, retinitis, encephalitis or bone marrow failure and HHV-6 may have a cofactorial role in HIV infection. There are suggested but certainly unproven associations with multiple sclerosis and various neoplasms.

Foscarnet is active against HHV-6, but aciclovir and ganciclovir are not.

There are no specific oral lesions reported, though erythematous papules may be seen on the soft palate and uvula (Nagayama's spots) and in the pharynx. There are no known implications apart from those associated with the infective risk and complications. Cervical lymphadenopathy is detectable in about one-third of patients.

HHV-7 and HHV-8

These are recently discovered viruses. HHV-7 is T-lymphotropic and may cause rashes, and HHV-8 is B-lymphotropic and may be an agent responsible for Kaposi's sarcoma and sarcoidosis.

MEASLES

Measles is an acute viral illness transmitted by droplet infection, with an incubation period of about 10–14 days. Whitish spots in the buccal mucosa (Koplik's spots) herald the onset of an illness consisting of fever, coryza, conjunctivitis and a maculopapular rash.

Complications include bronchitis, pneumonia, otitis media, convulsions and encephalitis. The latter leaves a neurological deficit in up to 40% and has a mortality of 15%. Subacute sclerosing panencephalitis (SSPE) is a late complication. Mortality is highest in infants, complications in chronically ill or malnourished children.

Immunization is indicated in early childhood (Appendix 3 to this chapter).

RUBELLA (GERMAN MEASLES)

Rubella is a highly infectious, usually mild viral disease spread by droplet infection, with an incubation period of about 14–21 days. In children, rubella causes a fairly trivial illness characterized by a macular rash starting on the face and behind the ears, mild fever, sore throat and enlarged lymph nodes (including the posterior auricular and sub-occipital posterior cervical nodes). In adults it may cause arthritis or arthralgia. However, it can seriously damage or kill the fetus, and thus females should be immunized as children (Appendix 3). As a consequence of this, most rubella is now seen in young males.

Congenital rubella

Infection during the first trimester of pregnancy causes damage to the fetus ranging from deafness to death. If the fetus survives, mental handicap, retinopathy and cataracts, cardiac malformations and deafness may result (major rubella syndrome). The affected infant may also have liver damage, bone defects and thrombocytopenic purpura and is also infective. The virus is excreted, particularly in the urine, for months after birth (*see* TORCH syndrome).

Prevention of congenital rubella
Immunization of non-immune prepubertal females against rubella is the most effective prophylaxis. Antibody titres should be measured. The haemagglutination inhibition (HAI) test for rubella antibodies is rapid, reliable, rises within 48 hours of illness or immunization and persists for years. The HAI test is useful to differentiate past infection from acute illness. Serum should be obtained within 2 days of the onset of the illness or within 2 weeks of exposure to the virus. If this acute serum is not available, complement fixation tests or assay of rubella-specific IgM antibody is required (*Table 11.4*).

Rubella immunization should be given to those who are seronegative, not pregnant and unlikely to become pregnant within the following 2 months. Health care staff should be immunized in order to avoid the risk of transmitting rubella to pregnant patients. Immunity is long-lasting.

Table 11.4 Management of pregnant patient after contact with rubella

Suspected rubella infection of patient	*Suspected contact with rubella*

1. Test acute serum for HAI antibody to rubella
2. If HAI positive in acute serum, reassure
  If HAI continues negative, reassure
3. If HAI negative but then rises, offer termination or rubella immunoglobulin
	1. Test acute serum for HAI antibody to rubella
	2. Test serum of the contact for rubella. If HAI negative, reassure
	3. If pregnant woman has rubella antibodies already, reassure
	4. If pregnant woman has no immunity and contact is rubella or suspected, re-test patient's sera for HAI
	  If HAI continues negative, reassure
	  If HAI becomes positive, offer termination or rubella immunoglobulin

HAI, haemagglutination inhibition.

Because of the danger to the fetus, pregnant patients exposed to, or developing, rubella or a similar rash should have serological investigation.

Acquired rubella

Rubella has little oral significance. Enlarged cervical lymph nodes, particularly the posterior cervical ones, facial rash and occasionally oral petechiae are the orofacial manifestations. There is a risk to non-immune pregnant female dental staff and, in such cases, expert medical advice should be sought (*Table 11.4*). No antiviral treatment is available. Unfortunately, rashes resembling rubella (rubelliform rashes) are not uncommon, particularly with enterovirus infections, and a clinical diagnosis of rubella may not always be accurate unless confirmed serologically. Females who imagine they have had rubella (and thus think they are immune) may in fact be non-immune and at risk.

MUMPS

Mumps is a common viral infection involving particularly the major salivary glands – usually the parotids. It is usually caused by the mumps virus, occasionally by adenoviruses or echoviruses, and is spread by droplet infection. The incubation period is 14–21 days and mumps is transmissible from 2 or 3 days before parotitis appears until several days after.

One or both parotids become enlarged and tender, with trismus, and oedema and erythema of the orifice of the parotid duct (papillitis). The other major salivary glands may also be affected, but rarely, in the absence of parotitis. Mumps should always be considered in the differential diagnosis of acute swellings of salivary glands, particularly in the young (Chapter 9).

Complications of mumps are uncommon but include particularly pancreatitis, meningo-encephalitis (and sometimes deafness), orchitis and oophoritis. The latter conditions rarely cause sterility, even if bilateral. Nevertheless, mumps immunization is carried out in childhood.

Other forms of infectious sialadenitis

Parotitis is now a recognized manifestation of HIV disease, especially in children (Chapter 20). Recurrent parotitis in other children and adolescents may be caused by cytomegalovirus, or may be associated with EBV or other agents. Bacterial sialadenitis is usually an ascending infection secondary to a dry mouth (Chapter 9).

PAPILLOMAVIRUSES

Human papillomaviruses (HPV) are ubiquitous viruses that cause warts and other epithelial lesions, affecting skin and mucosae. These are usually chronic benign lesions and include genital warts (*see below*), common warts and others. The viruses are transmissible mainly by close contact.

Over 75 HPV types are now recognized. Some are closely associated with specific lesions, and some appear to be associated with malignant disease. For example HPV-16, 18 and 33 appear to be associated with cervical carcinoma.

Some HPV cause oral lesions such as warts (verruca vulgaris) and papillomas. Heck's disease (focal epithelial hyperplasia) is an unusual condition, caused by specific HPV (types 13 and 32) in certain ethnic groups such as Inuits and American Indians. HPV can also cause lesions in HIV disease. Local surgery, or podophyllum resin have been the usual treatments, though interferon alpha is now being used.

Genital warts (condylomata acuminata)

Some 65 per cent of sexual contacts of patients with genital warts (condylomata acuminata) develop warts after an incubation period that may exceed 2 years. Genital warts are caused by HPV and may be found on the penis, vulva or vagina or perianally, or may be unseen in the meatus of the urethra. Oral and perioral lesions may develop and are infectious. Oral condylomata acuminata can be a manifestation of HIV disease.

MOLLUSCUM CONTAGIOSUM

This viral infection spreads easily among children, and in adults may be sexually transmitted. Characteristic umbilicated papules may be seen on the face and, rarely, intra-orally. Oral molluscum contagiosum can be a manifestation of HIV disease. Local treatment with trichloracetic acid is effective.

BACTERIAL INFECTIONS

DIPHTHERIA

Diphtheria immunization is carried out in early childhood as this is a potentially lethal infection (Appendix 3). In developed countries, because of the absence of diphtheria in much of the community, natural immunity is lacking, and thus immunization is essential for protection. Although preventable by immunization, diphtheria continues to be seen from time to time, mainly where immunization has been neglected, and it has recently re-emerged in Eastern Europe. Many adults in developed countries lack immunity; one recent study showed 38 per cent of UK adults to be susceptible.

Corynebacterium diphtheriae multiplies mainly on the pharyngeal mucous membranes to produce an inflammatory reaction, surface necrosis and exudate (pseudomembrane). Diphtheritic pseudomembrane may spread to the palate or rarely on to the oral mucosa. The membrane is creamy-yellow or grey, firmly attached and associated with faucial oedema. There is a mild sore throat but disproportionate cervical lymph node enlargement which in severe cases produces a bull-neck appearance. Nasal, laryngeal or tracheal diphtheria are variants.

C. diphtheriae produces exotoxin which, when absorbed, causes myocardial, adrenal and neurological damage. Palatal paralysis is one of the earliest neuropathies and develops during the third week of the illness. Any suggestion of diphtheria must be taken seriously and medical advice immediately obtained. Swabs should be taken for bacterial culture, the immunity to diphtheria established and antibiotics (usually penicillin) given. Diphtheria antitoxin is needed if the patient has not been actively immunized. Patients are infectious for up to 4 weeks but carriers may shed bacilli longer. Spread is by droplet infection and through fomites.

TUBERCULOSIS (*see* Chapter 8)

NON-TUBERCULOUS MYCOBACTERIAL (NTM) INFECTIONS (*see also* p.158)

Mycobacteria other than *M. tuberculosis* have been recognized as causing four main types of disease: skin infections and abscesses, pulmonary disease, disseminated infection and cervical lymphadenopathy. NTM are responsible for some cases of cervicofacial lymphadenopathy, mainly in immunocompetent individuals, but now increasingly in immunocompromised patients. Occasional cases of NTM causing salivary masses have been reported.

M. avium, M. kansasii, M. fortuitum, M. malmoense, M. scrofulaceum and *M. intracellulare* are the most common NTM and by far the most frequent are infections with the *M. avium* complex (*M. avium/M. intracellulare*) (MAC). Water, soil and dust appear to be the source of infection in most cases but the organisms are widespread in wild and domestic animals. NTM are not thought to be transmissible between humans.

Clinical lymphadenitis is seen most commonly in pre-school females who have unilateral cervical lymphadenopathy, typically in the submandibular or high jugular nodes, and has the appearance of a 'cold abscess'. NTM is the usual cause in children under 12 years, but TB is more common in older patients. Tuberculins from several different mycobacteria are now available to assist diagnosis. Absence of fever or tuberculosis, a positive tuberculin test, and failed response to conventional antimicrobials are highly suggestive but definitive diagnosis is by culture or polymerase chain reaction of biopsy material obtained by fine needle aspiration or open biopsy. Most NTM are resistant to standard anti-tubercular medication (Chapter 8) and, though it is possible that clarithromycin or clofazimine may have some effect, excision of affected nodes is recommended.

BUCCAL CELLULITIS

Buccal cellulitis is an uncommon but distinctive infection characterized by swelling, tenderness, induration and warmth of the cheek soft tissues in the absence of an adjacent oral or skin lesion. Almost invariably seen in children under the age of 5 years, most infections are caused by *Haemophilus influenzae* type B which may spread by bacteraemia, by lymphatics from, for example, otitis media, or more probably from direct invasion through the oral mucosa. A minority develop meningitis. Blood and cerebrospinal fluid cultures should be taken and treatment with intravenous cefuroxime started.

CAT SCRATCH DISEASE

Infection with the Gram-negative bacillus *Bartonella* (*Rochalimaea*) *henselae*, which is carried long term by cats, may cause lymphadenitis. Most common in children, in the cervical region, the typical case presents with a tender papule about 3–10 days after contact with the animal, and this is followed by cervical lymphadenopathy after up to 6 weeks (*Plate 10*). Systemic features vary from none to a mild flu-like illness and only very rarely are there more serious sequelae such as encephalitis. The condition is usually self-limiting.

The diagnosis is made from the history and examination, supplemented with a skin test and lymph node aspiration or incision biopsy. Treatment is rarely needed but erythromycin can be effective.

EPITHELIOID ANGIOMATOSIS

Epithelioid (bacillary) angiomatosis is a manifestation of infection with *Bartonella* (*Rochalimaea*) *henselae*, seen mainly in immunosuppressed patients. In HIV infected persons, a similar lesion may also be caused by *B. quintana*. Lesions resemble Kaposi's sarcoma both clinically and histologically, though staining with Warthin–Starry silver stain shows the causal organisms in epithelioid angiomatosis, and the condition responds to a 3-week course of erythromycin. Tetracycline is an alternative.

OTHER BACTERIAL INFECTIONS (*see* Chapter 26)

KAWASAKI'S DISEASE (*see* Chapter 3)

SEXUALLY TRANSMITTED BACTERIAL DISEASES

There is a rising incidence of many sexually transmitted (venereal) diseases, with oral lesions in some cases. Some groups are at especially high risk (*Table 11.5*), especially sexually promiscuous young adults. More than one of these diseases, such as viral hepatitis or infection with herpes simplex or HIV, may be associated in the same patient.

Table 11.5   High-risk groups for sexually transmitted diseases

---

- Homosexuals, bisexuals and promiscuous heterosexuals
- Prostitutes
- Drug addicts and alcoholics
- Armed forces
- Merchant seamen
- Aircrew
- Frequent business travellers
- Learning disability
- Sexual partners of the above groups

It is important to note that these diseases are not highly contagious but require the intimate contact with the mucosa or body fluids of an infected person, or breaches of epithelium across which infected fluids (including blood) or tissues are transmitted. They are not normally transmitted by the airborne route or by social contact.

SYPHILIS

Syphilis, caused by *Treponema pallidum*, is a serious sexually transmitted disease that may damage the cardiovascular or nervous systems, and fetus, and can be fatal. The incidence of syphilis is currently rising, and in HIV infection it can present as a particularly atypical severe form of the disease (lues maligna).

Primary syphilis

The incubation period of syphilis is about 3 weeks (range 10–90 days). Over 80 per cent of cases are in homosexual men. Primary infec-tion with *T. pallidum* causes a chancre (primary or Hunterian chancre) which begins as a small, firm, pink typically single macule (usually on the glans penis or vulva), changes to a papule and then ulcerates to form a painless round ulcer with a raised margin and indurated base. Untreated chancres heal in 3–8 weeks but are highly infectious and are associated with enlarged painless regional lymph nodes. Primary chancres occasionally involve the lips or tongue.

• **Management of primary syphilis**

Diagnosis of syphilis is by dark-ground microscopy of the lesional exudate, and serol-ogy. Exudate from the chancre should be examined for treponemes by dark-ground microscopy. In oral lesions, the diagnosis can be confused by oral commensal treponemes. To minimize confusion therefore, specific fluoresceinated antibodies should be used or oral lesions should be thoroughly swabbed with sterile gauze or cotton wool to remove as many contaminating oral bacteria as possi-ble, then gently but thoroughly scraped with an instrument such as a sterile plastic spatula. The scraping is then transferred to a slide, covered with a coverslip and examined as quickly as possible by dark-ground microscopy. If the lesion is a chancre, many large but slender, regular, helical forms with a leisurely rotational movement across the field should be seen. A negative test does not rule out syphilis, though this investigation is important as serology is often negative at this stage (*Table 11.6*). Biopsy may be uninforma-tive and is unlikely to be diagnostic unless specific antibodies are used.

Procaine penicillin 600 000 units intramus-cularly daily for 14 days (or tetracycline 500 mg orally four times a day, or doxycy-cline 100 mg orally twice a day for 14 days or erythromycin) should be given. Patients must be followed up clinically and serologically for 2 years and contacts traced.

Secondary syphilis

Secondary syphilis follows the primary stage after 6–8 weeks but a chancre may still be

Table 11.6   Serological tests for syphilis*

	Stage of disease					
	Primary		Secondary		Tertiary	
Test	*U*	*T*	*U*	*T*	*U*	*T*
Non-specific tests						
VDRL	Become +ve late	–ve	+ ve	–ve	Usually + ve	± ve
Specific tests						
FTA-Abs, TPHA, TPI	Become + ve early	+ ve	+ ve	+ ve	+ ve	± ve

U, Untreated; T, treated.
*For explanation of abbreviations see text

present. It is in this stage that classically oral lesions appear but these are seen in only about one-third of patients. As in the primary stage, the mucosal lesions are highly infectious.

Signs and symptoms of secondary syphilis are often non-specific with fever, headache, malaise, a rash (characteristically, symmetrically distributed coppery maculopapules on the palms) and generalized painless lymph node enlargement with unusual enlargement of the epitrochlear nodes. Painless oral ulcers (mucous patches and snailtrack ulcers) are the typical oral lesions at this stage.

- **Management of secondary syphilis**

Mucosal lesions should be examined for *T. pallidum* as described above. Blood should be taken for serological examination and is often positive (*see below* and *Table 11.6*). Treatment is as for primary syphilis (*see below*; Herxheimer reaction).

Tertiary syphilis

If untreated, syphilis progresses to a tertiary stage 3–10 or more years after infection in about 30 per cent of patients. The remainder are, however, serologically reactive and are said to have latent syphilis. The characteristic lesion is the gumma, a localized granuloma varying in size from a pin head to several centimetres. Gummas break down to form deep punched-out ulcers affecting skin or mucosa. Skin gummas heal with depressed shiny scars (tissue-paper scars). Mucosal gummas may destroy bone, particularly the palate, or involve the tongue. Bone gummas

may affect the long bones (especially the tibia – 'sabre tibia') or skull, producing lytic lesions and periostitis with new bone formation. Gummas are non-infectious.

The main oral manifestation of late stage syphilis is, however, leukoplakia, particularly of the dorsum of the tongue, which has a high potential for malignant change.

Cardiovascular syphilis, which affects only about 10 per cent of patients, is a late complication and causes aortitis, coronary arterial stenosis or aortic aneurysms (Chapter 3). A similar number of patients develop neurosyphilis (Chapter 17) sometimes with sensorineural deafness.

- **Management of tertiary syphilis**

The diagnosis of tertiary syphilis is confirmed by serology. Treatment is with procaine penicillin, 600 000 units daily for 3 weeks, and lifelong follow-up. Systemic corticosteroids are given at the start of antibiotic therapy in order to reduce the possibility of a Jarisch–Herxheimer reaction (febrile reaction often with exacerbation of the local syphilitic lesions).

Congenital syphilis

Syphilis in the pregnant patient (after the fifth month) may result in infection of the fetus. Congenital syphilis is now almost unknown in Great Britain but is a rare cause of mental handicap, deafness and blindness. It typically results in a saddle nose (*Plate 11*), and Hutchinson's teeth – screw-driver shaped incisors. Affected children are highly infectious until about 2 years of age. Penicillin is the usual treatment.

Serological tests for syphilis

Non-specific (reaginic) tests: These tests are useful for screening but false-positive results may be seen when the immune system is up-disturbed, such as in autoimmune disease, HIV infection or malaria. The VDRL (Venereal Disease Research Laboratory) test – a flocculation test which is positive in all treponematoses (e.g. yaws, bejel, pinta) is usually used but the rapid plasma reagin (RPR) card test, automated reagin test (ART) and toluidine red treated serum test (TRUST) are also used. A positive VDRL appears towards the end of primary syphilis and remains positive in untreated secondary or tertiary syphilis. The VDRL usually becomes negative in treated syphilis, 1–2 years after treatment (*see Table 11.6*).

False-positive VDRL results can be caused by technical faults or several diseases (*Table 11.7*), but the VDRL is useful as a simple screening test.

Specific tests: Specific tests overcome the problem of the false-positive results found in the VDRL caused by non-related diseases, but still cannot differentiate syphilis from other treponemal diseases such as yaws or bejel in those from tropical and semi-tropical countries.

Specific tests include the fluorescent treponemal antibody (absorbed) (FTA-Abs) test, the treponemal haemagglutination (TPHA) test and the treponemal immobilization (TPI) test.

Specific tests become positive during primary and remain positive through untreated secondary or tertiary syphilis, as does the VDRL. However, in contrast to the VDRL, most of the specific tests remain positive even in treated syphilis.

Both specific and non-specific tests are therefore used in each case to distinguish those with active syphilis from those who have had syphilis which has been effectively treated (*see Table 11.6*).

GONORRHOEA

Gonorrhoea is about 15 times more common than syphilis but less common than other sexually transmitted diseases such as non-specific urethritis (NSU). Gonorrhoea is caused by *Neisseria gonorrhoeae* and usually causes urethritis or proctitis in males, and urethritis or endocervicitis in females. Dysuria and urethral or vaginal discharge are the common symptoms, and an important complication is urethral stenosis. However, gonorrhoea in all sites is frequently asymptomatic, a fact that increases the chances of transmission.

- **General management of gonorrhoea**

Diagnosis depends on laboratory tests including Gram-stained smears (to show the Gram-negative diplococci within leucocytes), bacterial culture and sensitivity tests. Repeated smears or culture may be required, particularly in female contacts. Serological tests are uninformative.

Penicillin is usually still the drug of choice in the UK and is often given as 2 g ampicillin plus 1 g probenecid as a single oral dose. Patients hypersensitive to penicillin can be treated with co-trimoxazole, 4 tablets 12-hourly for 2 days.

Penicillin-resistant strains of *N. gonorrhoeae* may be resistant also to many other antibiotics: spectinomycin 2–4 g i.m. should then be used.

- **Dental aspects of gonorrhoea**

In contrast to the high incidence of urethral gonorrhoea, oral lesions appear to be rare. Fellatio is probably the main cause of such infections, but it has been shown that saliva normally strongly inhibits the growth of *N. gonorrhoeae*. There is no direct evidence for pharyngeal-to-pharyngeal or for pharyngeal-to-genital transmission.

The oropharynx seems to be the most frequently affected oral site, especially perhaps in male homosexuals. The tonsils

---

Table 11.7   Causes of false-positive VDRL tests

- Technical faults
- Infections such as viral pneumonia, tuberculosis, malaria, leptospirosis
  (VDRL +ve for 6 months)
- After immunizations
  (VDRL +ve for 6 months)
- Connective tissue disease
  (VDRL +ve for more than 6 months)

become red and swollen with a greyish slough and there is regional lymphadenitis. Lesions in other parts of the oral mucosa are described as showing fiery erythema and oedema, sometimes with painful superficial ulceration. The inflamed mucosa may also be covered with a yellowish or greyish exudate, which when detached may leave a bleeding surface. The severity of the symptoms may vary widely and in extreme cases there may be painful oral or pharyngeal ulceration, cervical lymphadenitis, fever and malaise. However, the infection may be asymptomatic, and the throat appear normal.

Though a rarity, gonococcal stomatitis may be suspected when there is acute stomatitis and/or pharyngitis (a) without features ascribable to other oral diseases; (b) with severe but ill-defined inflammation or painful ulceration; (c) in a young adult; and especially (d) with a history of recent oro-genital or oro-anal contact.

A throat swab should be taken in suspected cases and Gram-staining should show polymorphs containing Gram-negative diplococci. Confirmation is by culture and identification of *N. gonorrhoeae*, as saprophytic neisseriae are common in the mouth. Penicillin is effective in 97 per cent of oropharyngeal infections. There is no evidence that oral gonococcal infections can be transmitted by coughing and droplet infection, or by saliva to the dentist (especially if normal cross-infection control is practised), except if the dentist works with ungloved hands or has a needle-stick injury. Furthermore, dental procedures on an infected patient will not produce haematogenous spread or deep infection.

PARASITIC INFECTIONS

TOXOPLASMOSIS (*see also* p.539)

Toxoplasmosis is a parasitic infection caused by *Toxoplasma gondii*. The parasite infects cats and appears in faeces, from which it can be transmitted to man directly or via uncooked meat.

The most common orofacial lesion is cervical lymphadenopathy. The condition is usually self-limiting but there may be some fever and malaise. Congenital toxoplasmosis is one cause of the TORCH syndrome (*Plate 12*).

Diagnosis is helped by serology using the Sabin–Feldman dye test or an ELISA. Fine needle aspiration cytology of an affected lymph node may be helpful. Treatment when required is with pyrimethamine and sulphadimidine.

OTHER INFECTIONS

FUNGAL INFECTIONS (*see* Chapter 20)

HIV AND AIDS (*see* Chapter 20)

NON-SPECIFIC URETHRITIS

Non-specific urethritis (NSU) is relevant to dentistry in that it may be a feature of Reiter's disease (Chapter 16).

VIRAL HEPATITIS (*see* Chapter 10)

INFECTION CONTROL

There is no doubt that infections have been transmitted in the dental surgery from patient to dental staff, and from dental staff to patient. Mostly these have been airborne transmissions of respiratory viruses, but blood-borne viral and other infections have

Table 11.8 Infections known to have been transmitted to dental patients

- Hepatitis B virus
- HIV
- Herpes simplex virus
- *Pseudomonas aeruginosa*
- *Mycobacterium tuberculosis*

been transmitted in the past (Chapters 8, 10, 20) (*Table 11.8*). Organizations such as the national dental associations have produced guidelines for cross-infection control.

Universal precautions

Everyone should be protected from blood-borne infections – the infections of most concern. Such measures must protect staff members from patients and patients from staff members. The essentials are summarized in *Table 11.9* and in Appendix 1 to this chapter. In many countries dental staff now also have a legal responsibility to cease practice where they are involved in exposure-prone procedures, and seek advice if they believe they may be infected with blood-borne viruses (*see* Appendix 2 to this chapter).

Equipment
All working surfaces should be covered with disposable material. Disposable instruments should be used wherever possible and local anaesthetic cartridges and needles must *never* be re-used for any other patient. Used equipment should be clearly identified as infected and always handled with gloves before discarding into an impervious container, or washing and autoclaving.

Sterilization
Instruments, needles etc. must be placed in an impervious container before sterilization or incineration, and must be labelled as infec-

Table 11.9 Precautions to prevent transmission of blood-borne viral infections in the dental surgery

1. All patients should be regarded as potentially infectious.
2. All dental staff should wear gloves, protective eye-wear, mask and gown. Staff with any exposed skin wounds must ensure those are covered.
3. All working surfaces should be covered with plastic sheeting or cling film.
4. Wherever possible, disposable instruments should be used.
5. To avoid any possible aerosol spread of HBV, HIV, other viruses and opportunistic organisms, ultrasonic scalers should not be used. Air-rotors should be used with a rubber dam.
6. Avoid needle-stick injuries: needles should not be bent, broken or removed from disposable syringes without protection.
7. Intraoral radiographs can be taken, provided each film pack is wrapped in a sealable plastic envelope before use. The cone of the X-ray machine should be wrapped in plastic sheeting or cling film.
8. A portable suction system should be used and a metal container used as a spitoon.
9. Dental impressions can be taken using a silicone-based material. The dental laboratory should have notice of a patient's high-risk status. Before pouring up, the impressions should be soaked in 2% glutaraldehyde for 1 h, rinsed and then immersed in 2% glutaraldehyde for a further 3 h. The dimensional stability of impressions is not affected by this process.
10. All disposable instruments and waste should be placed in puncture-resistant sharps containers (e.g. burn-bins) and double wrapped in plastic bags. The outer bag should be labelled as a biohazard containing contaminated waste. These should then be incinerated.
11. All non-disposable instruments that can be sterilized should first be physically cleaned in detergent and warm water and then sterilized. This can either be by saturated steam or by hot air. Boiling water is not sufficient. All non-disposable instruments that cannot be autoclaved should be soaked in 2% glutaraldehyde for 1 h, washed in detergent and warm water to remove all debris, and then left to soak in 2% glutaraldehyde; this should be left for 3 h at least.
12. All external surfaces of equipment and contaminated working surfaces should be cleaned with freshly prepared sodium hypochlorite at a concentration of 10 parts/10^6 available chlorine (1 in 10 dilution of household bleach). This should be left on the surfaces for 30 min before rinsing off. Metallic surfaces can be sterilized with 2% glutaraldehyde solution; this should be left on for 3 h. Non-exposed surfaces can be simply washed down with hypochlorite or glutaraldehyde.
13. All non-disposable garments can be washed in a conventional automatic washing machine, provided the washing cycle includes a 10 min period of 90°C water temperature.

Table 11.10   Disinfectants active against hepatitis viruses and HIV

Disinfectant	Concentration	Trade names	Shelf life	Comments
Hypochlorite	10% of stock solution	Chloros, Domestos, Milton	Prepare fresh	Corrosive to metals
Glutaraldehyde	2%	Cidex	14 days	Care: may burn skin or mucosa

tive. Disposable instruments, dressings etc. should be incinerated. Heavy domestic rubber gloves should be worn during instrument cleaning. Non-disposable instruments should be rinsed in an effective disinfectant (*Table 11.10*) and sterilized immediately by autoclaving (134 °C for 3 min) or hot air (160 °C for 1 h). In hospital practice, ethylene oxide gas (10 per cent concentration in carbon dioxide) at 55–69 °C for 8–10 h can be used. It should be emphasized that solutions of ethyl or isopropyl alcohol, quaternary ammonium compounds or chlorhexidine are unreliable for inactivating viruses. *Boiling instruments in a dental boiling water bath for 30 minutes is also unreliable.*

Non-disposable instruments and dental impressions that cannot be sterilized by heat should be disinfected by immersion for at least 1 h (preferably overnight) in a suitable disinfectant such as 10 per cent hypochlorite (*Table 11.9*).

Working areas are disinfected with hypochlorite (1 per cent available chlorine). Since some viruses remain stable in blood stains for up to 6 months at room temperature, spillage of blood should be disinfected by dropping a napkin on the area and flooding it with hypochlorite.

Protection of dental staff
All staff must be educated about the possible dangers of hepatitis, HIV and other infections, their modes of transmission and the precautions necessary to prevent cross-infection, particularly vaccination against HBV. **Every member of dental staff has a legal and moral duty to ensure that all necessary steps are taken to prevent cross-infection to protect the patient, colleagues and themselves**. It is recommended that all members of the dental team should be fully immunized appropriately for the job they do and all should be confirmed as satisfactorily

immunized against HBV. Immunocompromised staff should probably be absolved from the responsibility of treating infected patients. A formal follow-up procedure should be introduced for the re-calling of all staff members.

Should the skin be punctured by an instrument that has been used on a patient, the area of skin should be liberally rinsed in water and the advice of the nearest Public Health Laboratory or hospital microbiologist sought. Where appropriate, blood from the patient on whom the instrument was used, and from the wounded person, should be tested for HBeAg, HCV, HDV and HIV antibodies to determine the possible risks.

Routine safe working practice
Safe working practices will ensure that staff and patients are protected from transmission of infections from blood and body fluids. The most effective measure in avoiding infection is extreme precaution against accidental cuts and pricks from instruments or needles. Protective clothing, namely surgical gown, gloves, mask and eye protection should be worn at *all* times during the treatment of all patients and also during the disinfection and cleaning of instruments and dental surgery. Surgical gloves alone do not provide adequate protection against viruses. They are readily perforated, often microscopically, and should be changed between patients. Gloves, masks and other protective clothing must not be worn or taken elsewhere, unless in an impervious container clearly labelled as infective. Clothing should be autoclaved before laundering. These precautions are summarized below.

1. Always cover cuts and grazes with waterproof dressings.
2. Wear gloves if there is any chance of contact with blood or body fluids. Gloves

must always be worn for clinical treatment by all personnel when touching blood, saliva, teeth or mucous membranes or items that have been in contact with them. Between each patient the gloves are removed, hands washed and a new pair of gloves put on before proceeding. When wearing gloves contact with inanimate objects should be avoided as far as possible. When gloves are torn, cut or punctured, they must be removed immediately, hands thoroughly washed and regloving accomplished before completion of the dental procedure.

3. If there is a risk of splashes of blood or body fluid also wear masks and protective spectacles or goggles. Masks should be worn whenever dental aerosol or tooth fragments are generated. Eye protection should be worn by staff treating patients whenever dental aerosol or tooth fragments are generated. Patients should always be given eye protection during treatment. Eye washing facilities should be available in all clinical and laboratory areas in the event of an accident.

4. Dispose of needles, syringes and injection tray immediately into sharps containers – only resheath local anaesthetic syringe needles using an appropriate sheath-holding device:
   • do not resheath phlebotomy needles but place these in a sharpsafe box for disposal;
   • dispose carefully of all surgical sharps, glass items, burs, wire etc., ensuring the sharpsafe box is no more than three-quarters full, and available in all areas where sharps are being used.

5. Take extreme care with sharp instruments.

6. Consider all working practices – are there any ways of amending procedures to avoid or reduce the handling of needles and sharp instruments?
   • Make sure working clothing is clean. Contaminated clothing (e.g. blood-stained) must be changed *immediately*.
   • Hands should be washed thoroughly when entering or leaving clinical areas and before eating or drinking. Soap dispensers and taps should be operated by the elbows or wrists not gloves or hands.

• All specimens for laboratory tests should be placed in appropriate containers and sealed into plastic bags separate from the request form. The bagged container and request form should then be sealed in a second bag for transportation to the laboratory.
• Do not eat, drink, comb hair, brush teeth or apply cosmetics in clinical areas, including clinical laboratories (cloakrooms should be used).

Specific precautions

Before a session
Run water through each of the dental unit water systems (3-in-1 syringe, air-rotor coolants etc.), according to manufacturers' recommendations.
   Clean and disinfect with detergent

• working surfaces
• dental equipment

Reduce to a minimum the number of items of equipment and instruments laid out ready for use.
Only keep out supplies of frequently used materials and where possible cover with lids.
   Instruments: Wherever possible, instruments should be sterilizable or disposable. *All instruments*, including handpieces, must have been sterilized before use and should be laid on a sterile or clean tray using the appropriate sterile or clean working technique.
Cling-film should be placed across the dental chair control buttons, operating light handles, ultrasonic scaler handpiece and 3-in-1 syringe bodies. The film must be changed or decontaminated with sanitizer solution after every patient.

During a clinical session
In the surgery high and low contamination zones must be defined and the surgery arranged accordingly.
A small area around the patient, designated Zone A, includes the dental unit and extends to include the waste disposal bag. Only essential equipment, instrument, materials and personnel should remain in or enter this area of potential high contamination. Attach an open yellow bag for waste to hang from a worktop or wall close to the operator and ensure a sharpsafe box is accessible. The

contents of the remainder of the treatment area (Zone B) should be kept to a minimum.

Open cuts and fresh abrasions to the skin should be covered with a waterproof dressing.

Touching anything other than essential items with contaminated gloves/hands should be avoided.

A good working posture should be maintained to reduce facial contamination from the patient's mouth.

High volume suction should be used to reduce dental aerosols.

Blood or body fluid spillage must be dealt with as soon as it happens. Hypochlorite granules can be sprinkled over the spillage. Alternatively, disposable tissues can be placed over the spillage and then strong hypochlorite poured on to paper towels which are placed over the spill and left for 30 minutes.

Clearing up and cleaning after each patient
It is during the clean up and disposal stage that the greatest risk of injury or infection occurs. It is advisable to wear heavy-duty rubber gloves and to wash them during clean-up procedures to reduce the spread of infection.

Remove sharps first and place in a sharp-safe box. For instruments, follow the procedure outlined for sterilization and disinfection below.

Sterilize detachable handpieces, ultrasonic scalers, aspiration tips and 3-in-1 tip.

Disinfect the chair, bracket table, including body of the 3-in-1 syringe, slow speed motor and the holder, operating light and spittoon.

Wipe all surfaces with detergent or hypochlorate. Remove any residual cement or impression material from handles etc., and wipe area with detergent chloros. Anything likely to be contaminated with blood, wipe thoroughly with strong hypochlorite.

Infection control management of patients undergoing general anaesthesia

The procedures for patients undergoing anaesthesia should, in general, be no different than for any other patient in the clinical environment. The only additional precautions which must be taken are as follows.

1. Whenever possible, suspected or confirmed high-risk patients should be treated at the end of the operating session.
2. Floors and surfaces must be cleaned after each session.
3. All theatre linen should be treated as 'high risk'.
4. Theatre clothes, including footwear, *must not* be worn outside the department. Clothes *must* be changed if there is any spillage of blood or any other body fluids.
5. Theatre personnel must wear masks during procedures and while recovering patients. Masks and caps must be worn at all times by main theatre personnel.
6. Theatre nurses wearing uniforms must wear protective disposable aprons over them when treating patients and making beds.
7. Uniforms must not be worn outside.
8. Cardigans must not be worn whilst working in the unit.
9. Use small sharps boxes and discard either daily or weekly.
10. The scrub nurse and nurse(s) recovering patients must wear eye protection. Clinicians carrying out surgical procedures should also wear eye protection. Suitable eye protection must be given to patients undergoing surgery under general anaesthesia or sedation.

General notes on the use of disinfectants and sterilization

Sterilization of all items is the aim. Sterilization with disinfectants is difficult to achieve. Some items may have to be disinfected because they cannot withstand routine processes or sterilization such as autoclaving, e.g. anaesthetic masks.

- Chemical agent – be careful to choose the correct agent, e.g. chlorhexidine is ineffective against HBV: hypochlorite solution should be used.
- Concentration – disinfectants *must* be used at the correct concentration. Effectiveness decreases with
  (a) age – check expiry dates;
  (b) use – make up fresh solutions according to manufacturers' instructions.
- Cleaning – reduces the numbers of micro-organisms before disinfection. Retained

blood, saliva, dental materials and oils will reduce the effectiveness of disinfectants.

- Contact – ensure that instruments are in full contact with disinfectant.
- Correct time – for effective disinfection follow manufacturers' instructions for immersion times.
- Container – clean all containers before use.
- Care – many disinfectants are strong chemicals which may corrode metal instruments and damage fabrics. Care should be taken to avoid skin contact. Inhalation of fumes can be harmful; disinfectants should be kept in covered containers.

Autoclaving
Autoclaving is the method of choice for most instruments. There are two main types:

1. Small, non-porous load:
   suitable for unwrapped instruments;
   unperforated metal boxes need to be upturned to allow steam penetration and must be closed on removal from the autoclave;
   only distilled water should be used when re-filling;
   do not allow to boil dry;
   approximate cycle time 15 minutes – this includes 134 °C at 32 lb/sq in for a minimum of 3 minutes. Indicators must be used with each load.
2. Post-vacuum, porous load:
   suitable for dressings and wrapped instruments.

In order to ensure autoclave functioning correctly, sterilization indicators must be incorporated into every load.

Disinfectants in use

1. Environmental disinfectants:
Sodium hypochlorite 10 000 ppm of available chlorine.
   Uses: For disinfection of areas contaminated with blood. Contact time: 20 minutes at least.

Detergent Chloros – 0.1% v/v of detergent (e.g. Lapols liquid detergent) and sodium hypochlorite equivalent to 1000 ppm of available chlorine (hypochlorite).

Uses: Disinfection of work surfaces. Use undiluted for swabbing down. Allow to dry.

Durr 212 disinfectant with cleaning agent: 20 ml is mixed with 1 litre of water to make a 2% solution. Undiluted solution has a shelf life of 2 years. Diluted solution should be changed daily.
   Uses: Disinfection of articles which cannot be autoclaved. Immerse for at least 20 minutes. In case of known inoculation risk patients, immersion should be for at least 3 hours.

Phenolic type solution, e.g. Orotol: 50 ml added to 1 litre of water.
   Uses: Disinfecting and cleaning of suction apparatus.

Following immersion in disinfectants all items must be *thoroughly* rinsed, especially hollow items, before being used in the mouth.

2. Skin surface antiseptics
Povidone-iodine 7.5% surgical scrub (Betadine surgical scrub).
   Uses: Hand- and glove-washing before and after clinical procedures. Rinse hands and dry thoroughly with disposable hand towel.

Chlorhexidine 4% surgical scrub (Hibiscrub).
NB: For staff who are allergic to iodine.
   Uses: As above, but note that gloves become sticky after washing with Hibiscrub.

Chlorhexidine gluconate 0.2% mouthwash (Corsodyl)
   Uses: Mouthwash before surgical procedures in the mouth; inhibits formation of plaque.

70% alcohol-impregnated swabs (Medi-swabs)
   Uses: Skin preparation before injection. Allow to dry before commencing procedure.

BIBLIOGRAPHY

American Thoracic Society (1990) Diagnosis and treatment of disease caused by nontuberculous mycobacteria. *Am. Rev. Respir. Dis.* **142**, 940–53.

Asano Y., Yoshikawa T., Suga S. *et al.* (1994) Clinical features of infants with primary human herpesvirus 6 infection (exanthem subitum, roseola infantum). *Pediatrics* **93**, 104–8.

BDA Advisory Sheet A12 (1996) *Infection Control in Dentistry.* London, British Dental Association.

Birnbaum W., Dinsdale R., Dowell T., Howard C., Scully C. and Shovelton D. (1991) *The Control of Cross-infection in Dentistry*. BDA Advice Sheet A12. London, British Dental Association.

Borysiewicz L.K., Haworth S.J., Cohen J. *et al.* (1986) Epstein–Barr virus specific immune defects in patients with persistent symptoms. *Q. J. Med.* **58**, 111–21.

Chang Y., Cesarman E., Pessin M.S. *et al.* (1994) Identification of herpesvirus-like DNA sequences in AIDS-associated Kaposi's sarcoma. *Science* **266**, 1865–9.

Chartrand S.A. and Harrison C.J. (1986) Buccal cellulitis revisited. *Am. J. Dent.* **140**, 891.

Cox H.J., Brightwell A.P. and Riordan T. (1995) Non-tuberculous mycobacterial infections presenting as salivary gland masses in children: investigation and conservative management. *J. Laryngol. Otol.* **109**, 525–30.

Di Alberti L., Ngui S.L., Porter S.R. *et al.* (1997) Presence of human herpesvirus-8 variants in oral tissues of HIV-infected persons. *J. Infect. Dis.* **175**, 703–7.

Di Alberti L., Piattelli A., Artese L. *et al.* (1997) Human herpesvirus 8 variants in sarcoid tissue. *Lancet* **350**, 1655–61.

Dinsdale R.C.W. (1985) *Viral Hepatitis, AIDS and Dental Treatment*. London, British Dental Journal.

Editorial (1980) Tests for infectious mononucleosis. *Br. Med. J.* **1**, 1153–4.

Epstein J.B. and Scully C. (1991) Herpes simplex virus in immunocompromised patients: growing evidence of drug resistance. *Oral Surg. Oral Med. Oral Pathol.* **72**, 47–50.

Epstein J.B. and Scully C. (1993) Cytomegalovirus: a virus of increasing relevance to oral medicine and pathology. *J. Oral Pathol. Med.* **22**, 348–76.

Finegold S.M. (1988) Legionnaire's disease – still with us. *N. Engl. J. Med.* **318**, 571–3.

Fotos P.G., Westfall H.N., Snyder I.S. *et al.* (1985) Prevalence of Legionella-specific IgG and IgM antibody in a dental clinic. *J. Dent. Res.* **64**, 1382–5.

Giunta J.L. and Fiumara N.J. (1986) Facts about gonorrhea and dentistry. *Oral Surg. Oral Med. Oral Pathol.* **62**, 529.

Grattan C.E.H., Small D., Kennedy C.T.C. et al. (1986) Oral herpes simplex infection in bullous pemphigoid. *Oral Surg. Oral Med. Oral Pathol.* **61**, 40–3.

Guess H.A., Broughton D.D., Metton L.J. *et al.* (1985) Epidemiology of herpes zoster in children and adolescents. *Pediatrics* **76**, 512–17.

Kalman C.M. and Laskin O.L. (1986) Herpes zoster and zosteriform herpes simplex virus infections in immunocomptent adults. *Am. J. Med.* **81**, 775.

La Placa M., Re M.G., La Placa and Cevenini R. (1991) Sexually transmitted diseases. *Microbiologica* **14**, 267–78.

Laskaris G. (1996) Oral manifestations of infectious diseases. *Dent. Clin. N. Amer.* **40**, 395–423.

Lusso P. (1996) Human herpesvirus 6 (HHV-6). *Antiviral. Res.* **31**, 1–21.

Macey-Dare L.V., Kocjan G. and Goodman J.R. (1996) Acquired toxoplasmosis of a submandibular lymph node in a 9-year-old boy diagnosed by fine-needle aspiration cytology. *Int J. Paediatr. Dent.* **6**, 265–9.

Matthews R.W., Scully C. and Dowell T.B. (1989) Attitudes and practices regarding control of cross-infection in general dental practice. *Health Trends* **21**, 10–12.

Maurin M., Birtles R. and Raoult D. (1997) Current knowledge of *Bartonella* species. *Eur. J. Clin. Microbiol. Dis.* **16**, 487–506.

Ogden G.R. and Kerr M. (1989) Mucocutaneous lymph node syndrome (Kawasaki disease). *Oral Surg. Oral Med. Oral Pathol.* **67**, 569–72.

Porter S.R. and Scully C. (1996) *Innovations and Developments in Non-Invasive Oral Health Care*. Northwood, Science Reviews.

Porter S.R., El-Maaytah M., Afonso W., Scully C. and Leung T. (1995) Cross-infection compliance of UK dental staff and students. *Oral Dis.* **1**, 198–200.

Salisbury D.M. and Begg N.T. (1996) *Immunisation against Infectious Disease*. London, HMSO.

Samaranayake L.P. and Scully C. (1988) Oral disease and sexual medicine. *Br. J. Sexual Med.* **15**, 138–43, 174–80.

Scully C. (1985) Ulcerative stomatitis, gingivitis and rash: a diagnostic dilemma. *Oral Surg. Oral Med. Oral Pathol.* **59**, 261–3.

Scully C. (1988) Viruses and salivary gland disease. *Oral Surg. Oral Med. Oral Pathol.* **66**, 179–82.

Scully C. (1988) *The Dental Patient*. Oxford, Heinemann.

Scully C. (1989) Infectious diseases in oral medicine. In Millard H.D. and Mason D.K. (eds), *Perspectives on 1988 World Workshop on Oral Medicine*. Chicago, Year Book, pp. 131–212.

Scully C. (1989) *The Mouth and Perioral Tissues*. Oxford, Heinemann.

Scully C. (1989) Orofacial herpes simplex virus infections. *Oral Surg. Oral Med. Oral Pathol.* **68**, 701–10.

Scully C. (1989) *Patient Care: a Dental Surgeon's Guide*. London, British Dental Association.

Scully C. (1991) Infection and infectious diseases. *Curr. Opin. Dent.* **1**, 375–6.

Scully C. (1995) Infections. In Millard H.D. and Mason D.K. (eds) *1993 World Workshop on Oral Medicine*. Ann Arbor, University of Michigan Press, pp. 27–89.

Scully C. (1996) New aspects of oral viral diseases. *Current Topics in Pathology*, 90. Berlin, Springer Verlag, pp. 30–96.

Scully C. (1997) The dental profession. In Collins C.H. and Kennedy D.A. (eds) *Occupational Blood Borne Infections*. CAB International, pp. 133–58.

Scully C. and Bagg J. (1992) Viral infections in dentistry. *Curr. Opin. Dent.* **9**, 8–11.

Scully C. and Porter S.R. (1994) Infection control in dentistry. *Curr. Opin. Infect. Dis.* **7**, 488–92.

Scully C. and Samaranayake L.P. (1992) *Clinical Virology in Dentistry and Oral Medicine*. Cambridge, Cambridge University Press.

Scully C., Blake C., Griffiths M.J. and Levers B.G.H. (1994) Protective wear and instrument sterilisation disinfection in UK general dental practice. *Health Trends* **26**, 21–2.

Scully C., Cawson R.A. and Griffiths M.J. (1990) *Occu-*

pational Hazards to Dental Staff. London, British Dental Journal.

Scully C., Cox M., Prime S.S. *et al.* (1988) Papilloma viruses: the current status in relation to oral disease. *Oral Surg. Oral Med. Oral Pathol.* **65**, 526–32.

Scully C., Eckersall D., Emond R.T.D. *et al.* (1981) Serum amylase isoenzymes in mumps: estimation of salivary and pancreatic isozymes by isoelectric focussing. *Clin. Chim. Acta* **113**, 281.

Scully C., Porter S.R. and Epstein J. (1992) Compliance with infection control procedures in a dental hospital clinic. *Br. Dent. J.* **173**, 20–3.

Scully C., Prime S. and Maitland N. (1985) Papilloma-viruses: their possible role in oral disease. *Oral Surg. Oral Med. Oral Pathol.* **60**, 166–74.

Smith O.P., Prentice H.G., Madden G.M. *et al.* (1990) Lingual cellulitis causing upper airways obstruction in neutropenic patients. *Br. Med. J.* **300**, 24.

Stewart M.G., Starke J.R. and Coker N.J. (1994) Nontuberculous mycobacterial infections of the head and neck. *Arch. Otolaryngol Head Neck Surg.* **120**, 873–6.

Sumi Y., Kaneda T. and Nagasaka T. (1987) Toxo-plasmosis of the preauricular and cervical lymph nodes. *J. Oral Maxillofac. Surg.* **45**, 978–9.

Tabi M. and Strauss E. (1985) Chronic Epstein–Barr virus disease: a workshop held by the National Inst. of Allergy and Infectious Diseases. *Ann. Intern. Med.* **103**, 951–4.

Tramont E.C. (1995) Syphilis in adults: from Christopher Columbus to Sir Alexander Fleming to AIDS. *Clin. Infect. Dis.* **21**, 1361–71.

Welliver R.C. (1986) Allergy and the syndrome of chronic Epstein–Barr virus infection. *J. Allerg. Clin. Immunol.* **78**, 278.

Wood P.R. (1992) *Cross-Infection Control in Dentistry. A Practical Illustrated Guide.* London, Mosby–Wolfe.

Wray D., Scully C., Rennie J. S. *et al.* (1980) Major and minor salivary gland involvement in *Mycoplasma pneumoniae* infection. *Br. Med. J.* **1**, 1421.

Wright J.E. (1989) Cervical lymphadenitis in childhood: which antibiotic agent? *Med. J. Aust.* **150**, 150–1.

APPENDIX 1 TO CHAPTER 11

A TO Z OF RECOMMENDED PROCEDURES FOR INFECTION CONTROL

Alginate bowls
Clinical bowls only to be used. After use, clean, rinse and dry.

Amalgam carriers (plastic or metal)
Ensure free of amalgam, clean, dismantle, autoclave, store dry.

Anaesthetic equipment (GA) (e.g. laryngoscope, props, masks)
Follow manufacturers' instructions – autoclave where possible, otherwise immerse in Durr 212 2% solution for 60 minutes, rinse in water, store dry.

Aspirators – mobile type
See Suction apparatus

Autoclave
Damp dust outer casing and door seal daily. Wipe handle and controls with suitable detergent. Check distilled water level before use. Run regular tests.

Beakers
Disposable recommended

Bibs
Use disposable where possible. Plastic bibs – clean with water and detergent chloros then allow to dry.

Broaches
Plain or barbed – dispose into sharpsafe box.

Bur brush
Autoclave at end of each session.

Burs – clinical polishing and abrasive items, dentine pin drill
Clean thoroughly, using an ultrasonic bath or bur brush if appropriate. Autoclave and dry thoroughly. Surgical cases use pre-packed sterile burs.

Butterfly sponge pack
Wash under running water then autoclave, store dry but moisten before use. Not disposable.

Cheatle forceps
Clean, autoclave, store in a clean and dry place.

Composition bath
Empty, discard any material remaining. Wipe with detergent chloros after each patient.

Containers – glass, plastic
Clean with detergent, rinse and dry.

continued

Crown and bridge remover
 Autoclave.
Crown forms
 Tried in but unused – disinfect in Durr 212 2% solution.
Curing light
 Wipe tip and outer casing with surface disinfectant.
Dappens pot – glass or plastic
 See Containers. For inoculation risk, use plastic disposable type.
Denture brushes
 Autoclave.
Drawers and cupboards
 Clean weekly using detergent Chloros and allow to dry.
Endodontic RCT instruments
 Use pre-sterilized, otherwise collect a set of root canal instruments and autoclave them immediately before use. After use, clean in ultrasonic bath, arrange items in endobox and sterilize.
Face bows
 Remove wax and debris. Wipe with a suitable disinfectant.
Floors
 If blood spillage, clean as for work surfaces.
Forceps
 As for instruments, but use pre-sterilized packs where possible.
Gauze, e.g. swabs, throat packs
 Use pre-sterilized packs and dispose of carefully in clinical waste bag.
Glass
 Slab – wipe clean immediately after use then wash with water and detergent, rinse and dry.
 Tumbler – clean then autoclave. Disposable mouthwash cup preferred.
Glasses (protective)
 After use clean with water and detergent and store dry.
Gloves
 Non-sterile gloves are available for use when working with patients or handling dirty instruments.
 Sterile gloves should be reserved for use with surgical cases.
 Domestic gloves should be used for cleaning purposes.
Gowns
 Disposable – paper. Cotton to laundry.
Gutta percha points
 Disposable.
Handpieces
 Faults: Sterilize before returning to the workshop.
 Laboratory: Wipe with surface disinfectant after use on patient's dentures or appliances.
 Bracket for handpieces: Wipe all surfaces with disinfectant between patients.
Hand washing
 Use wrist or elbow to operate water tap. Use liquid soap, antiseptic scrub, e.g. Betadine, Hibiscrub in warm water, rinse thoroughly and dry on paper towel. Surgical procedures special washing technique. Cover all cuts and grazes.
Impression composition
 Wrap in gauze (sufficient for one patient). Discard after use.
Impression trays
 Metal: Trays not used after trying in the mouth should be sterilized.
 Disposable: Impression material together with disposable trays must be discarded into yellow plastic bags.
Instrument trays
 After clearing, wipe with detergent Chloros. Re-lay with cling-film.
Lead apron
 Wipe with detergent chloros and allow to dry.
Local anaesthetic kit
 Syringe (metal): Wash, place in ultrasonic bath – autoclave (store dry).

continued

Cartridges: Store in manufacturers' packages until loading. Do not touch 'needle end'. Check expiry date. After use dispose in sharpsafe container.

Needle: Do not break seal until needed. Resheathing – *see* Needles below. Dispose in sharpsafe container.

Metal instruments (non-surgical) and matrix retainers
Autoclave – store in clean and dry container.

Mirror (handheld face mirror)
Wipe with water and detergent Chloros.

Mixers
Use on tray, wipe with detergent at end of each session.

Nail brushes
Use prepacked sterilized.

Needles
Disposable needles must *never* be re-used on another patient. Resheathing of any needles should be avoided wherever possible.

Needlestick injury
Rinse wound under running water, encourage bleeding and then protect. Immediately report injury to member of staff in charge and follow Sharps Policy

Occlusal plane guide
Clean, disinfect with detergent Chloros.

Operating light
Switch off light. Wipe with detergent Chloros. Do not over-wet. Do not wet back of light when warm.
Light switch – protect with cling-film.

Orthodontic items
Autoclave whenever possible – if not, then immerse in Durr 212 2% solution for 20 minutes, rinse thoroughly. Pliers with box joints should be blown dry after rinsing. Store dry.

Paper points
Autoclave. Use pre-sterilized packs or use a suitable autoclave cycle.

Photographic items – cheek and lip retractors, intra-oral mirrors
Clean then disinfect.

Plastic items, i.e. instruments, spatulas, etc.
Check if item is meant to be disposed of or not. If not, clean and immerse in Durr 212.

Pliers
Oil joint if necessary, then as for orthodontic items.

Pulp tester
Switch off. Clean and disinfect probe tip. Wipe casing with surface disinfectant.

Reamers
See Endodontic RCT instruments.

Repairs, relines, rebases
Appliances or dentures from inoculation risk patients which need to be repaired or relined should be immersed in a 2% solution of Durr 212 for 30 minutes and rinsed before proceeding.

Resuscitation kit
As for anaesthetic equipment and mask.

Ribbon gauze
Pre-sterilized packs from CSSD.

Rubber dam equipment
Clamp, clamp forceps: Clean and autoclave.
Frame, metal or plastic, punch: Wipe with detergent Chloros.

Scalpel blades
Use pre-packed sterile. Remove blade using artery forceps, and place immediately into sharpsafe box.

Scissors
Clean, check for sharpness, oil if necessary, autoclave.

Shade guide
Check manufacturers' guidance. Unless otherwise indicated, wipe or dip in a suitable detergent, store dry.

continued

Sharp items
After use they *must* be placed in sharpsafe containers provided, together with other discarded 'sharp' items such as scalpel blades, hypodermic and endodontic syringes, burs, root canal instruments.

Silver points
Autoclave.

Skin preparation for venepuncture
Wipe area with 70% alcohol swab.

Spatulae
Physically clean, autoclave or disinfect.

Specimens
Containers should be identified with patient's name and hospital number before use. For high-risk patients both the specimen and request card should carry a recognizable hazard label, 'Danger of Infection'. Gloves must be worn at all times by all staff involved in the collection of specimens from any patient. The specimen bottle and request card should be placed in separate compartments of the double-sleeved plastic specimen bag. All patients' specimens should be double bagged for transport to the laboratory.

Spittoon
After each patient: Flush through with water, wipe outside of bowl with damp tissue, check no debris or blood spots.
After each session: As for 'After each patient' plus put half cupful of Orotol solution in bowl and leave.

Stainless steel instruments
See Metal instruments. These should not come into contact with hypochlorite.

Suction apparatus
(a) Before each patient:
Routine cases: Check that the system works by drawing through clean water and set up new or sterile tips.
Surgical cases: Set up new or sterile tubing and sterile tips.
Mobile aspirator: Quarter fill bottle with strong hypochlorite solution (or Orotol) but *not* detergent Chloros which may froth.
(b) After each patient:
Routine cases: Remove tips for disposal or autoclaving. Wipe down tubing with detergent Chloros.
Surgical cases: As for routine cases then remove tubing for cleaning and sterilization or disposal.
Mobile aspirator: Carefully empty contents of bottle into main drainage system, flush away with running water.
(c) End of day:
Suction tips: Draw water through on unit then remove. Check metal or hard plastic for cleanliness inside and outside. Autoclave.
Central suction: Flush with 1 litre of water. Wearing rubber gloves – remove waste trap filter, clean and replace then run Orotol through tubing.
Clean and disinfect suction equipment before sending for repair.

Sutures
Use pre-sterilized packs. Dispose of needle into sharpsafe box.

Syringes
(a) Cartridge – dismantle and autoclave. Chip-clean metal tube outside and inside (by removal of any debris with wire and then irrigation with Durr 212 solution). Autoclave bulb and tube.
(b) Hypodermic – pre-sterilized and disposable.
(c) Impression
(i) disposable;
(ii) metal with disposable tips – autoclave;
(iii) automixing syringes – suitable disinfectant.
(d) Three-in-one – autoclave tip. Handle and bracket holder – wipe with detergent Chloros.

continued

Thermometers

After use immerse in Durr 212 2% solution for 20 minutes – rinse and store dry in safe place.

Toothbrushes

Preferably use patient's own brush – demonstration brushes used in a patient's mouth should be given to the patient to take home. Denture brushes should be cleaned and autoclaved.

Trolleys

Before use – wipe with detergent Chloros.

Ultrasonic bath

Used to clean instruments before sterilization.

Ultrasonic scalers

As for metal instruments tips.

Venepuncture

First wipe the site with an alcohol swab. Take care not to spill any blood. If minor spillage does take place, mop up immediately then wipe affected area with sodium hypochlorite 10 000 ppm. Dispose of needle with syringe directly into sharpsafe box and other items into clinical waste bag. Provide dressings to cover injection site immediately following withdrawal of the needle.

Wax knife

Clean off wax, wipe with detergent Chloros and autoclave if possible.

Work surfaces

Before clinical session: Wipe with detergent Chloros on fresh cloth or paper towel.

After each patient: Wipe with detergent Chloros. For blood-contaminated surfaces apply liberal amount of strong hypochlorite and then dry.

Willis bite gauge

As for metal instruments – autoclave.

X-ray equipment

X-ray machine: Switch off machine – wipe with detergent Chloros.

Cassettes: Wipe with detergent Chloros after use.

File holders: Wash to remove saliva then autoclave. Alternative is immerse in Durr 212 2% solution for 20 minutes.

X-ray films

Following removal from the mouth, dry the film. The empty film packet should be discarded as clinical waste. Wash hands.

Inoculation risk patients: Seal each intra-oral film in a plastic bag ready for use.

After exposure: Film can be removed from plastic bag (without it touching the contaminated outside) and then processed as normal.

APPENDIX 2 TO CHAPTER 11

GENERAL DENTAL COUNCIL: PROFESSIONAL CONDUCT AND FITNESS TO PRACTISE

MAY 1996: PARAGRAPH 30

It is the ethical responsibility of dentists who believe that they themselves may have been infected with HIV, hepatitis viruses or other blood-borne viruses to obtain medical advice, including any necessary testing and, if found to be infected, to submit to regular medical supervision. Their medical supervision will include counselling, in particular, in respect of any changes in their practice which might be considered appropriate in the best interests of protecting their patients. It is the duty of such dentists to act upon medical advice they have been given, which may include the necessity to cease the practice of dentistry altogether, to exclude exposure prone procedures* or to modify their practice in some other way. By failing to obtain appropriate medical advice or to act upon the advice that has been given to them, dentists who know they are, or believe that they may be infected with HIV, hepatitis viruses or other blood-borne viruses and might jeopardize the wellbeing of their patients are behaving unethically and contrary to their obligations to patients. Behaviour of this kind may raise a question of serious professional misconduct.

---

*Exposure prone procedures are defined as 'those where there is a risk that injury to the worker may result in the exposure of the patient's open tissues to the blood of the worker. These procedures include those where the worker's gloved hands may be in contact with sharp instruments, needle tips or sharp tissues (spicules of bone or teeth) inside a patient's open body cavity, wound or confined anatomical space where the hands or finger-tips may not be completely visible at all times'.

APPENDIX 3 TO CHAPTER 11

IMMUNIZATION SCHEDULE

Vaccine	Age	Comments
Diphtheria/tetanus/ pertussis (D/T/P), *Haemophilus meningitidis* b and poliomyelitis (polio)	1st dose at 2 mth 2nd dose at 3 mth 3rd dose at 4 mth	Primary course
Measles/mumps/rubella (MMR)	At 12–15 mth	Or any age over 12 mth
Booster DT and polio; second dose MMR	At 3–5 yr	3 years after completion of primary course
Bacille Calmette–Guerin (BCG)	At 10–14 yr	At infancy if high risk
Booster DT and polio	At 13–18 yr	—
High-risk groups	As required	HBV, HAV, influenza, pneumococcal vaccine

12

Skin diseases

Key points

- Several skin diseases can present with oral and other mucosal lesions.
- Ectodermal dysplasia can cause hypodontia and salivary gland hypoplasia.
- Epidermolysis bullosa can cause mouth blistering, ulceration and scarring.
- Multiple basal cell naevi syndrome (Gorlin's syndrome) can present with odontogenic keratocysts, skeletal anomalies and basal cell naevi.
- Gardner's syndrome can present with colonic polyps which undergo malignant change, other malignant tumours and osteomas involving the jaws.
- Neurofibromatosis, tuberous sclerosis and Sturge–Weber syndrome are phakomatoses that present with ocular, mucocutaneous and neurological disorders, sometimes including epilepsy.
- Pemphigus is a potentially lethal autoimmune disease that often heralds in the mouth with ulcers, but then involves the skin.
- Pemphigoid is an autoimmune disorder affecting mucosae and/or skin. Oral lesions are common; ocular lesions should be ruled out, as they may scar.
- Erythema multiforme is a reaction usually to herpes virus, mycoplasma or drugs. Oral, ocular, genital and/or skin lesions may be seen.
- Lichen planus is a common mucocutaneous disorder which is usually idiopathic but may arise after drug use, especially after NSAIDs, and is sometimes related to dental restorations.
- Lichen planus or similar lesions may be seen in graft-versus-host disease, in HIV disease and in some chronic liver diseases.
- Topical immunosuppressive therapy often controls skin diseases but systemic treatment may be required.
- Corticosteroid treatment of skin or oral lesions may suppress adrenocortical activity.

Several skin diseases can involve the mouth or may influence dental treatment. Oral lesions sometimes herald some skin diseases or may be the main manifestation. The most serious diseases are pemphigus, erythema multiforme and mucous membrane pemphigoid. These, and other conditions with oral manifestations, or those relevant to dental management, are included here. Many of the skin diseases are treated with topical corticosteroids some of which may, if used for prolonged periods, cause adrenocortical suppression (Chapter 14).

GENETIC DISORDERS

ECTODERMAL DYSPLASIA

Ectodermal dysplasia is a relatively common sex-linked dermatosis characterized by hypoplasia or agenesis of a wide variety of dermal appendages, including the teeth. Sweat glands may fail to form and heat control is then defective (hypohidrotic ectodermal dysplasia). The nails may also be defective and the skin somewhat fragile. Either, or in extreme cases both, the deciduous and permanent dentition may fail to form (anodontia) and as a consequence there is hypoplasia of the jaws. Teeth are more often few in number (hypodontia) and those present may be of simple conical form. Minor salivary glands may fail to form.

There are many variants described. In typical cases, the hair is fine, blond and scanty (hypotrichosis), especially in the tonsure region, and the eyelashes and eyebrows may be absent. Frontal bossing, a depressed nasal bridge and, if the teeth are absent, a prematurely senile (nutcracker) profile with protuberant lips may be seen. Ectodermal dysplasia rarely causes management problems apart from those related to the oral manifestations of the disease.

EPIDERMOLYSIS BULLOSA

Epidermolysis bullosa is an uncommon bullous disease affecting skin and mucosae. There are several forms of epidermolysis bullosa which show different patterns of inheritance and vary greatly in severity. The severe form appears soon after birth; milder forms do not become apparent until adolescence or later (*Table 12.1*). An acquired form, with antibodies against collagen VII, is also recognized. Rare cases are associated with poikiloderma congenitale (Weary–Kindler syndrome) and may present with early-onset periodontitis or desquamative gingivitis.

Vesicles and bullae form in response to mild or insignificant trauma and may lead to disabling scarring. One characteristic effect of the latter severe type is to transform the hands into fingerless stumps.

• **Management**

Potent corticosteroids may help to prevent blister formation and some success has been reported with vitamin E and with phenytoin.

Table 12.1   The main types of epidermolysis bullosa

	Onset	Main sites of lesions[a]	Oral mucosal lesions	Dental defects	Nail defects	Scarring	Inheritance
I. Non-scarring types							
Simplex[b]	Neonatal onwards	Hands and feet and elbows	Rarely	No	No	No	AD
Letalis[c]	Birth	Widespread	Yes[d]	Yes	Severe	No	AR
II. Scarring types							
Dermolytic dominant (Dystrophic)[e]	Childhood	Extremities; may be haemorrhagic	Uncommon	No	Yes	Yes Soft scars	AD
Dermolytic recessive (Polydysplastic)[g]	Birth or infancy	Widespread	Severe, mutilating	No	Destruction	Mutilating[f]	AR

AD, Autosomal dominant; AR, autosomal recessive.
[a]Usually also any site of trauma.
[b]May improve by puberty: commonest type.
[c]Usually fatal in neonatal period or childhood. Also known as Herhliz disease.
[d]Vermilion border of lips spared: lesions are perioral and perinasal. May be corneal lesions.
[e]A cemental defect has been reported but destruction and loss of teeth from caries and periodontal care is a typical result of inability to brush the teeth.
[f]Typically leads to destruction of hands and feet. Oesophageal stricture may lead to aspiration into airway.
[g]Rare and lethal.

- ### Dental aspects of epidermolysis bullosa

Management problems include:

1. Oral scarring and severe microstomia.
2. Blistering after dental treatment.
3. Bullae on the face or in the airway if intubation is attempted.

Early preventive dental care is extremely important. Blistering, erosions and aggravation of scarring following dental treatment (however carefully carried out) may possibly be reduced by giving a short preoperative course of corticosteroids such as 30 mg of prednisolone orally an hour before treatment, again on the following day, and then tapering the dose off over the next 3 days. If the duration of administration is short the steroid should cause no complications. Some also suggest the use of antimicrobials to cover surgery in these patients.

Hypertension secondary to renal disease is not uncommon and therefore general anaesthesia should be avoided where possible. If it must be used, the face should be protected with petroleum jelly gauze and intubation should be oral rather than nasal. Iron deficiency anaemia is common and may need correction before general anaesthesia is given (Chapter 5).

Intravenous ketamine has proved a useful anaesthetic in these patients. Atropinics are often needed to control excessive salivation. Intramuscular injections can cause sloughing and adhesive tapes easily traumatize the epidermis; these should therefore be avoided.

Within the mouth the buccal sulcus may become obliterated by scar tissue with the tongue bound down to the floor of the mouth. Scarring can also obliterate the normal papillated surfaces of the tongue. Since even 'normal' tooth-brushing can cause ulceration, adequate oral hygiene is almost impossible to achieve and dental diseases such as caries and periodontal disease may become rampant. Enamel hypoplasia may be seen.

Rarely, squamous cell carcinoma can complicate the oral lesions.

MULTIPLE BASAL CELL NAEVI SYNDROME

The multiple basal cell naevi syndrome (Gorlin–Goltz syndrome) consists of multiple

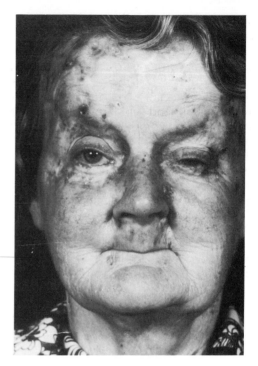

Fig. 12.1 Gorlin's syndrome: multiple basal cell naevi and typical facies

basal cell naevoid carcinomas of early onset, odontogenic keratocysts, anomalies of the vertebrae and ribs and a variety of other abnormalities.

The syndrome is inherited as an autosomal dominant trait with poor penetrance. Multiple naevoid basal cell naevi over the nose, eyelids, cheeks and elsewhere are often an early sign and there may also be pitting of the palms or soles. Skin lesions appear in childhood or adolescence. Multiple odontogenic keratocysts develop. The facial appearance is characterized by frontal and temporoparietal bossing, a broad nasal root, prominent supra-orbital ridges and a degree of mandibular prognathism (*Fig. 12.1*). Bifid ribs, vertebral defects with kyphoscoliosis and short fourth metacarpals may be noted. Other associated abnormalities may include calcification of the falx cerebri, mental handicap or cerebral tumours.

Pseudohypoparathyroidism has been described in some patients and there is also a slightly greater incidence of diabetes mellitus. Cardiac lesions may be present.

GARDNER'S SYNDROME (FAMILIAL ADENOMATOUS POLYPOSIS COLI)

Gardner's syndrome is an autosomal dominant trait of poor penetrance characterized by the association of multiple osteomas, skin fibromas and epidermoid cysts, and pigmented ocular fundus lesions with colonic polyposis.

The skin lesions, which affect any part, include fibromas, desmoid tumours, epidermoid cysts or lipomas. Multiple osteomas appear in adolescence and characteristically involve the jaws, facial skeleton or frontal bone but can affect any bone. Compound odontomes and dental anomalies may be associated.

Multiple polyps of the colon and rectum almost invariably undergo malignant change. Colonic resection is usually required; desmoid tumours often arise in the abdominal wall scar. Thyroid, adrenal and biliary carcinomas may also develop.

COWDEN'S SYNDROME

This is an autosomal dominant condition of multiple hamartomas, with a predisposition to carcinoma of the breast, thyroid or colon. Skin and mucosal papules precede the onset of malignant disease. Other lesions include keratoses on the palms and soles, and sometimes learning disability. When associated with cerebellar hypertrophy the syndrome is known as Cowden–Lhermitte syndrome.

THE PHAKOMATOSES

The phakomatoses (neurodermatoses) are hereditary hamartomatous autosomal dominant disorders affecting the skin and nervous system. Sporadic cases are not uncommon. The fourth member of this group, cerebroretinal angiomatosis, is not discussed here.

Neurofibromatosis, type I (von Recklinghausen's disease)

Neurofibromatosis type I is a simple autosomal dominant condition in which there are tumours of the nerve sheath (neurilemmomas or neurofibromas), sometimes in vast numbers, and often patches of skin hyperpigmentation (café-au-lait spots). The nerve sheath tumours may be disfiguring but are often asymptomatic unless pressure effects develop. When the tumours involve the spinal nerve roots and compress the spinal cord, pressure effects can be serious. In addition, there is a greater frequency of cerebral gliomas.

Neurofibromatosis type II is characterized by bilateral acoustic neuromas, which can cause deafness and any of the symptoms of cerebellopontine angle lesions (*see* Chapter 17) but the skin lesions of type I are lacking.

Oral mucosal neurofibromatosis is uncommon and more typically associated with endocrine disorders (MEA type III, *see* Chapter 14). Complications may include mental handicap and epilepsy in a minority. Sarcomatous change may develop in about 10 per cent of severely affected patients.

Tuberous sclerosis (Bourneville's disease; epiloia)

Tuberous sclerosis is a simple autosomal dominant trait linked to chromosomes 9 or 16, characterized by epilepsy, mental defects, and skin adenoma sebaceum and leaf-shaped depigmented naevi. The skin lesions are not adenomas but fibromas which are typically distributed in a butterfly pattern across the cheeks, bridge of the nose, forehead and chin (*Plate 13*). Oral lesions include hyperplastic gingivitis and pit-shaped defects in the teeth of both dentitions. Dental management may be complicated by cardiac or renal involvement, or by endocrinopathies – particularly diabetes mellitus – in addition to epilepsy and sometimes learning disability.

Sturge–Weber syndrome

Sturge–Weber syndrome (encephalotrigeminal angiomatosis) is characterized by an angiomatous defect (hamartoma) which is usually in the upper part of the face and also within the skull. The occipital lobe of the brain is then usually involved but the parietal and frontal lobes of the brain may be affected if the lower face is involved by the angioma.

Clinically, there are convulsions, hemiplegia and often learning disability. When the vascular naevus involves the face it usually extends to the underlying oral mucosa and gingivae which are red and sometimes hyper-plastic, and also to the alveolar bone. Dental surgery in the area affected by the haemangioma may be complicated by profuse haemorrhage and should therefore only be attempted in hospital.

ACQUIRED SKIN DISORDERS

PEMPHIGUS

Pemphigus is characterized by widespread formation of vesicles and bullae followed by ulceration (*Fig. 12.2*). The majority of patients are middle-aged women. Pemphigus vulgaris is the most frequent variant. It is an uncommon disease which affects the skin and mucous membranes and, in the absence of treatment, is usually fatal.

Pemphigus has the most clearly defined autoimmune pathogenesis of any disease affecting the mouth. The initiating cause is unclear though, in a small minority, drugs such as penicillamine, captopril or rifampicin have been implicated. The main immunological finding is circulating antibodies to the desmoglein-3 of intercellular attachments (desmosomes) of epithelial cells. These IgG antibodies, and complement components, can also be localized by immunostaining around the epithelial cells. The loss of adherence of these cells to one another (acantholysis), with resulting destruction of the epithelium, is the essential feature of the disease. *Pemphigus vulgaris* is the term used to describe pemphigus that is associated with acantholysis in the supra-basal epithelium. Where there is acantholysis more superficially, the condition is termed *pemphigus foliaceus* but does not affect the mouth.

Clinically, pemphigus vulgaris is characterized by thin-roofed vesicles or bullae which frequently first affect the oral mucosa. Stroking the skin with a finger may induce vesicle formation in an apparently unaffected area or cause a bulla to extend (Nikolsky's sign), but this is rarely positive in the mouth. The course of the disease varies from fulminating to relatively chronic but when initially affecting the oral mucosa can be expected to involve the skin within a few weeks or months at most. If untreated, pemphigus is fatal as a result of extensive skin damage leading to fluid and electrolyte loss, and often infection.

- ### Management of pemphigus vulgaris

Acute cases need immediate immunosuppressive treatment. Rapid diagnosis is therefore essential and the following means are available.

Direct smears: Smears, preferably (but not easily) obtained from vesicle fluid or from a recently ruptured vesicle, should show acantholytic (Tzanck) cells which are detached epithelial cells, round in shape as a result of contraction of the cytoplasm. Tzanck cells are not specific and their absence does not exclude the diagnosis of pemphigus. Confirmation of the diagnosis can be made by immunofluorescence to demonstrate a coating of antibody (immunoglobulin) and/or complement around the acantholytic cells.

However, biopsy is essential to confirm the diagnosis and for this purpose the specimen should be halved to enable both immuno-

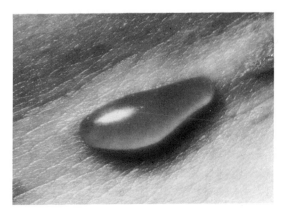

Fig. 12.2 Pemphigus: these bullae are large and flaccid and arose where the skin was rubbed (Nikolsky's sign) beneath the edge of the brassière

Table 12.2 Immunostaining in skin and oral mucosal diseases

Disease	Direct immuno-fluorescence	Epithelial location	Indirect immuno-fluorescence	Type of antibody[a]	Main epithelial antigen
Pemphigus vulgaris	Yes	Intercellular	Yes	IgG	Desmoglein
Paraneoplastic pemphigus	Yes	Intercellular[b]	Yes	IgG	Desmoplakin
IgA pemphigus	Yes	Intercellular	Yes	IgA	?Desmocollin
Bullous pemphigoid	Yes	Basement membrane area	Yes	IgG	BP1
Mucous membrane pemphigoid	Yes	Basement membrane area	Rarely	IgG	BP2
Angina bullosa haemorrhagica	No	—	No	—	—
Dermatitis herpetiformis	Yes	Basement membrane area	No	IgA	?
Linear IgA disease	Yes	Basement membrane area	No	IgA	?
Systemic lupus erythematosus	Yes	Basement membrane area	Yes	ANA	NR
Chronic discoid lupus erythematosus	Yes	Basement membrane area	No	ANA	NR
Lichen planus	Frequently	Basement membrane area	No	(usually fibrin)	?
Chronic ulcerative stomatitis	Yes	Basal cell layer	No	IgG / ANA	?

[a]Usually with complement deposits; ANA, antinuclear antibody.
[b]Transitional epithelium.
NR, not relevant.
BP, bullous pemphigoid.

fluorescent and light microscopy to be carried out. Immunofluorescent examination can be carried out by the direct method using fluorescein conjugated anti-human IgG and anti-complement (C3) sera on the frozen specimen or on exfoliated cells. In the indirect method, the patient's serum is incubated with normal mucosa, which is then labelled with fluorescein-conjugated, anti-human globulin. This method detects circulating antibodies but is more cumbersome and less sensitive than the direct method, and involves unnecessary killing of an animal (*Table 12.2*).

Light microscopy on a paraffin section is usually distinctive and shows supra-basal cleft formation and intra-epithelial vesicles containing free-floating acantholytic cells.

The usual treatment of pemphigus is with corticosteroids plus azathioprine to reduce the amount of corticosteroids needed in some cases. Even with 100–150 mg daily of azathioprine, 40–80 mg daily of prednisolone may be required. Gold may be used. Cyclophosphamide or methotrexate may be used instead of azathioprine.

With current methods of treatment the mortality may be about 8 per cent, usually secondary to immunosuppression. Long-term remission of pemphigus has been reported in some patients following high-dose immuno-suppressive treatment but many require prolonged therapy.

Variants which are considerably less common and largely of less serious prognosis include pemphigus vegetans (a variant of pemphigus vulgaris), and erythematosus (a variant of pemphigus foliaceus). As with other autoimmune diseases, related disorders may be present and pemphigus may be associated, for example, with lupus erythematosus, inflammatory bowel disease, or with thymoma and myasthenia gravis, but this is uncommon. Rarely pemphigus is induced by a drug such as rifampicin (Chapter 25). Pemphigus associated with cancer, especially lymphoproliferative disorders, in another part of the body (paraneoplastic pemphigus) is associated with IgG antibodies against desmoplakin in transitional epithelium. Oral lesions are almost invariable in this condition. One other variant of pemphigus is associated with IgA antibodies to intercellular substance (possibly to desmocollin) of stratified squamous epithelium (IgA pemphigus).

Mucous membrane pemphigoid (cicatricial or ocular pemphigoid)

Mucous membrane pemphigoid, often called 'benign', is a bullous disease. It results from loss of attachment of the epithelium to the connective tissue. The underlying mechanism appears to be the production of autoantibodies to some component of the epithelial basement membrane, and it is becoming evident that the term pemphigoid includes a number of diseases with autoantibodies directed to different basement membrane proteins. The common variant has antibodies against bullous pemphigoid antigen 2 (BPZ) but the oral type has antibodies against epiligrin.

Unlike pemphigus vulgaris, circulating autoantibodies are demonstrable in the serum in relatively few patients. Localization of immunoglobulins along the line of the epithelial basement membrane can be shown in fewer than 50 per cent but complement components may be demonstrable in about 80 per cent.

Clinically, mucous membrane pemphigoid usually affects older patients than those with pemphigus vulgaris and women between 50 and 70 are predominantly affected.

Intact vesicles or bullae are more likely to be seen in mucous membrane pemphigoid than in pemphigus vulgaris. The distribution of these lesions is often characteristic in that the gingivae are particularly affected. Mucous membrane pemphigoid is therefore an important cause of so-called 'desquamative gingivitis'. Sometimes the blisters fill with blood and then must be distinguished from generalized or localized oral purpura (Chapter 4). Scarring after healing of the bullae is rare in the mouth but in other sites, particularly the eyes or larynx, is a serious complication.

The progress of the disease is typically indolent and lesions may remain restricted to one site, such as the mouth, for several years or possibly never develop elsewhere, depending on the type. However, ocular involvement is the most dangerous manifestation since it can impair or destroy sight. Laryngeal or oesophageal stenosis secondary to scarring can also develop.

• **Management of pemphigoid**

The diagnosis must be confirmed by biopsy. The section should be halved and a frozen section should be tested for localization of immunoglobulins or complement components along the basement membrane (*see Table 12.2*)

since it can be difficult otherwise to differentiate from conditions such as pemphigus, dermatitis herpetiformis, linear IgA disease, and acquired epidermolysis bullosa. The paraffin sections show separation of the epithelium from the underlying connective tissue which is often infiltrated by inflammatory cells, often with many eosinophils.

The danger of ocular involvement is regarded by some as an indication for giving systemic corticosteroids to all patients having mucous membrane pemphigoid. However, it is by no means certain that any individual patient will develop ocular lesions, or if they do, it may be some years after the appearance of oral lesions. Regular observation is, however, essential and if there is any suspicion of ocular involvement, referral to an ophthalmologist is essential. Oral lesions can often be adequately controlled by potent topical corticosteroids such as a beclomethasone spray and this avoids the complications of systemic treatment. Dapsone or systemic corticosteroids may be needed for more severe cases.

Oral pemphigoid-like lesions have occasionally been reported in association with internal cancers (Chapter 6) or the use of certain drugs, such as penicillamine (Chapter 25).

Bullous pemphigoid is essentially a skin disease. It rarely affects the mouth but immunologically (apart from more readily detectable serum antibodies) and histologically does not appear to differ from mucous membrane pemphigoid. There are occasional associations with diabetes or psoriasis.

DERMATITIS HERPETIFORMIS AND LINEAR IgA DISEASE (*see* Chapter 9)

ERYTHEMA MULTIFORME

Erythema multiforme primarily affects young males and is characterized by recurrent mucosal and/or cutaneous lesions. Ocular, genital or oral mucous membranes may be involved together or in isolation. The typical skin lesion is the target or iris lesion (*Fig. 12.3*) in which there are concentric erythematous rings affecting particularly the hands and feet. However, virtually any type of rash can

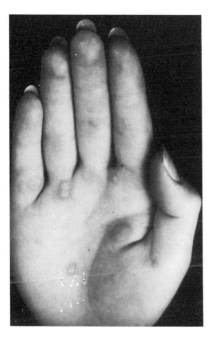

Fig. 12.3 Erythema multiforme: classic target or iris lesions

---

Table 12.3 Erythema multiforme: possible causes

- Micro-organisms
  Herpes simplex virus[a]
  Mycoplasma
- Drugs[b]
  Barbiturates
  Carbamazepine
  Chlorpropamide
  Codeine
  Hydantoins
  Penicillins
  Phenylbutazone
  Salicylates
  Sulphonamides
  Tetracyclines
  Thiazides
- Others
  Pregnancy
  Irradiation
  Internal malignancy

Most important causes are shown in italics.
[a]Most common cause of recurrent EM.
[b]Most drugs have at some time been implicated in EM.

---

develop (hence erythema *multiforme*) and bullae may cause confusion, especially with pemphigoid. Severe cases with multiple mucosal involvement and fever are termed *toxic epidermal necrolysis* (TEN), or *Stevens–Johnson syndrome*. TEN is the term often used when there is very extensive skin detachment and the condition is drug-induced. TEN has a poor prognosis – with a mortality of up to 40 per cent. Stevens–Johnson syndrome is a less severe form. The distinction between TEN and Stevens–Johnson syndrome is *very* unclear.

The aetiology of erythema multiforme is uncertain but it has been suggested that it may be an immune complex disorder in which the antigens can be as diverse as various micro-organisms, particularly herpes simplex virus, mycoplasma, or drugs (*Table 12.3*). Herpes simplex appears to be responsible for most erythema multiforme that is limited to the mouth.

TEN and Stevens–Johnson syndrome are often drug-related. Although drugs have for long been known to be an important precipitating cause, mere coincidence is difficult to exclude and it is not easy in reported cases to be certain whether the drug was given before the onset of the disease or in an attempt at treatment. However, TEN and Stevens–Johnson syndrome are well-authenticated as reactions particularly to sulphonamides, but also to anticonvulsant agents (including carbamazepine), oxicam, NSAIDs, allopurinol, chlormezanone (a minor tranquillizer), and corticosteroids, although they are rare complications of these drugs.

• Management of erythema multiforme

Diagnosis can be difficult when the disease is limited to the mouth. Typical features are grossly swollen, crusted and blood-stained lips, and widespread superficial oral ulceration with ill-defined margins. Vesicles or bullae, though rarely seen in the mouth, may be obvious on the skin. When these oral lesions are associated with ocular and dermal lesions the diagnosis can be made largely on clinical grounds.

Other suggestive features are recent use of drugs (particularly sulphonamides), or recent infections, particularly by herpes simplex or *Mycoplasma pneumoniae*. The latter may result in formation of cold agglutinins which have been reported in erythema multiforme.

Biopsy can be useful, particularly to exclude other more serious diseases such as early-onset pemphigus, but otherwise the histological features, though said to be diagnostic, are variable.

Treatment is unsatisfactory. An ophthalmological opinion should be obtained if the conjunctivae are involved. Oral lesions can be symptomatically managed with topical corticosteroids, chlorhexidine (0.2 per cent) or lignocaine gel to ease the pain. Healing usually takes 10–14 days. Severe erythema multiforme may necessitate hospital admission as feeding may be difficult. Systemic corticosteroids are frequently given but may not give anything more than symptomatic relief. Aciclovir is indicated if herpes simplex is involved.

LICHEN PLANUS

Lichen planus is a common skin disease which frequently involves the oral mucosa. It affects up to 2 per cent of the population, mainly those over 40 years of age. The aetiology of lichen planus is unknown. There is evidence for an immunopathogenesis in lichen planus with a dense T-lymphocyte infiltrate causing the lesion, though the provoking antigen is unidentified. Lesions similar or identical to lichen planus (lichenoid lesions) can be related to dental restorations, particularly amalgam, and to drug reactions, particularly to non-steroidal anti-inflammatory agents, gold, antimalarials, and methyldopa. Other drugs responsible for lichenoid lesions are shown in the Appendix to Chapter 25. Lichenoid lesions frequently complicate graft-versus-host disease (Chapter 6) (*Table 12.4*).

There are rare associations of lichen planus with various autoimmune disorders and neoplasms, and in persons of Mediterranean extraction lichen planus may sometimes be associated with chronic liver disease and hepatitis C virus infection. Reported associations of oral lichen planus with diabetes mellitus and hypertension have not been confirmed however, and there is doubt whether the so-called Grinspan syndrome of lichen planus, diabetes mellitus and hypertension is an entity or is simply aleatoric, or related to drug treatment.

Oral lichen planus has a small malignant

Table 12.4 Occasional associations of lichenoid lesions

- Drugs
- Graft-versus-host disease
- Chronic liver disease
- HIV

potential. Approximately 1 per cent of cases may develop malignant change after 10 years.

Up to 70 per cent of patients with cutaneous lichen planus have demonstrable oral lesions but only about 10 per cent of patients presenting with oral lichen planus have skin involvement. Skin lesions are usually small polygonal purplish or violaceous itchy papules particularly affecting the flexor surfaces of the wrist, and also elsewhere such as on the shins (*Plate 14*) or periumbilically but rarely, if ever, on the face. Examination with a lens may show a fine lacy white network of striae (Wickham's striae) on these papules. Lesions may be seen on the genitals or involving the nails.

• **Dental aspects of lichen planus**

Oral lesions can persist for years although the skin lesions frequently resolve within a few months. Oral lesions in lichen planus include macroscopic striae (the most common feature), papules, white plaques, atrophic areas or erosions. The latter are sore. Oral lesions characteristically are bilateral and sometimes strikingly symmetrical. They affect particularly the posterior part of the buccal mucosa, but may also involve the tongue, gingivae or other sites. Gingival lesions may be atrophic ('desquamative gingivitis') and need to be differentiated from somewhat similar lesions seen in other conditions such as mucous membrane pemphigoid.

A drug history should be taken in order to exclude possible reactions. Clinical examination may show typical oral and/or other lesions but if there is any doubt about the diagnosis a biopsy is needed, particularly to differentiate lichen planus from lupus erythematosus, chronic ulcerative stomatitis or keratosis. Lichenoid lesions may be seen in some chronic liver disease, and in graft-versus-host disease.

Oral lesions need no treatment if they are asymptomatic but topical corticosteroids such as hydrocortisone hemisuccinate, betamethasone, beclomethasone, clobetasol or fluocinonide can be useful in symptomatic lichen planus, especially for severe erosive lesions, often with an antifungal. Exceptionally severe lichen planus sometimes responds only to intralesional or systemic corticosteroids. Other drugs such as vitamin A analogues (e.g. etretinate), dapsone or cyclosporin are used only rarely.

Mercury amalgam-associated oral lesions
Some studies have shown an association between oral lichenoid lesions and dental amalgams and suggest that replacement of this material with non-metallic alternatives may sometimes cause the lesions to resolve. Dental amalgam can become embedded in the mucosa to produce a pigmented patch (amalgam tattoo). These may provoke a localized foreign body reaction, but in 40 per cent of cases there is no reaction. Though it is usual to regard these pigmented patches as amalgam tattoos on the basis of their clinical and microscopic appearances, X-ray energy spectroscopy shows that a variety of other materials from endodontic preparations, toothpastes and even impression media may be responsible.

Possible systemic toxic effects of mercury are discussed in Chapter 17 and possible risks to a fetus in Chapter 14. Trace amounts of mercury are absorbed from amalgam and can be detected in the oral mucosa, but do not cause any local reaction and are too small in amount to have any systemic effect (Chapter 17).

CHRONIC ULCERATIVE STOMATITIS

This presents clinically with an appearance similar to erosive lichen planus. Antinuclear antibodies against epithelial basal cells appear to distinguish it from lichen planus. It may respond to hydroxychloroquine.

PSORIASIS

Psoriasis is a common chronic inflammatory skin disorder causing pruritic erythematous papules and plaques predominantly on the scalp, elbows and knees, and pitting lesions of the nails. There is a strong genetic background with HLA-Cw6 and HLA-DR7, and associations with stress and alcoholism. Management may include ultraviolet light therapy, topical applications of tars, steroids or retinoids, and in severe cases systemic medication with methotrexate, cyclosporin or retinoids.

There may be a higher prevalence of erythema migrans and fissured tongue, particularly in pustular psoriasis and, in rare cases, erythematous, or white oral patches may be seen. The temporomandibular joint is involved in up to 60 per cent of patients with psoriatic arthritis. Oral complications of the therapy of psoriasis, such as gingival hyperplasia from cyclosporin, may be seen.

DESQUAMATIVE GINGIVITIS

This term is the clinical description of chronically desquamated, and occasionally sore, gingivae. Initially thought to be due to the menopause, this is now recognized to be caused mainly by pemphigoid or lichen planus, though a number of other mucocutaneous disorders and other causes may be responsible (*Table 12.5*).

Table 12.5   Causes of desquamative gingivitis
• Lichen planus • Pemphigoid • Chronic ulcerative stomatitis • Dermatitis herpetiformis • Linear IgA disease • Pemphigus • Erythema multiforme • Pyostomatitis vegetans

OTHER SKIN DISORDERS

These are discussed elsewhere in the text (Chapter 21).

BIBLIOGRAPHY

Anhalt G.J., Kim S.C., Stanley J.R. *et al.* (1990) Paraneoplastic pemphigus. An autoimmune mucocutaneous disorder associated with neoplasia. *N. Engl. J. Med.* **323**, 1729–35.

Barrett A.W., Scully C. and Eveson J.W. (1993) Erythema multiforme involving gingiva. *J. Periodontol* **64**, 910–13.

Block M.S. and Gross B.D. (1982) Epidermolysis bullosa dystrophica recessive. *J. Oral Maxillofac. Surg.* **40**, 753–8.

Cawson R.A., Spector R.G. and Skelly A.M. (1995) *Basic Pharmacology and Clinical Drug Use in Dentistry*, 6th edn. Edinburgh, Churchill Livingstone.

El-Kabir M.A., Scully C., Porter S., MacNamara E. and Porter K. (1993) Liver disease and oral lichen planus in English patients. *Clin. Exp Dermatol.* **18**, 12–16.

Harris S.A. and Large D.M. (1984) Gorlin's syndrome with a cardiac lesion and jaw cysts with some unusual histological features. *Int. J. Oral Surg.* **13**, 59–64.

Kwiatkowski D.J. and Short M.P. (1994) Tuberous sclerosis. *Arch Dermatol.* **130**, 348–54.

Pindborg J.J. (1980) Diseases of the skin. In Jones J.H. and Mason D.K. (eds), *Oral Manifestations of Systemic Disease*. London, Saunders.

Pindborg J.J., Murti P.R., Bhonsle R.B. *et al.* (1984) Oral submucous fibrosis as a precancerous condition. *Scand. J. Dent. Res.* **92**, 224–9.

Porter S.R. and Scully C. (1996) *Innovations and Developments in Non-Invasive Oral Health Care*. Northwood, Science Reviews.

Porter S.R., Cawson R.A., Scully C. and Eveson J.W. (1996) Multiple hamartoma syndromes presenting with oral lesions. *Oral Surg. Oral Med. Oral Pathol.*

Porter S.R., Malamos D. and Scully C. (1986) Mouth–skin interface. *Dent. Update* **32**, 94–6.

Robinson C.M., DiBiase A.T., Leigh I.M. *et al.* (1996) Oral psoriasis. *Br. J. Dermatol.* **134**, 347–9.

Roujeau J.C., Kelly J.P., Naldi L. *et al.* (1995) Medication use and the risk of Stevens–Johnson syndrome or toxic epidermal necrolysis. *N. Engl. J. Med.* **333**, 1600–7.

Scully C. (1980) Oral mucosal lesions in association with epilepsy and cutaneous lesions: Pringle–Bourneville syndrome. *Int. J. Oral Surg.* **10**, 68.

Scully C. (1980) The orofacial manifestations of the neurodermatoses. *J. Dent. Child.* **47**, 255.

Scully C. (1982) Serum IgG, IgA, IgM, IgD and IgE in lichen planus: no evidence for a humoral immunodeficiency. *Clin. Exp. Dermatol.* **7**, 163–7.

Scully C. (1988) *The Dental Patient*. Oxford, Heinemann.

Scully C. (1989) *The Mouth and Perioral Tissues*. Oxford, Heinemann.

Scully C. (1989) *Patient Care: a Dental Surgeon's Guide*. London, British Dental Association.

Scully C. and Elkom M. (1985) Lichen planus: review and update on pathogenesis. *J. Oral Pathol.* **14**, 431–58.

Scully C. and Porter S.R. (1988) The mouth and the skin. In Verbov J.L. (ed.), *New Clinical Applications in Dermatology*, vol. 8: *Relationships in Dermatology*. Lancaster, MTP Press, pp. 1–34.

Scully C. and Porter S.R. (1997) The clinical spectrum of desquamative gingivitis. In Eisen D. (ed.), *Seminars in Cutaneous Medicine and Surgery* **16**, 308–13.

Scully C., Almeida O.D.P. and Welbury R. (1994) Oral lichen planus in childhood. *Br. J. Dermatol.* **131**, 131–3.

Scully C., Beyli M., Feirrero M. *et al.* (1998) Update on oral lichen planus: a European consensus on aetiopathogenesis and management. *Crit. Rev. Oral Biol. Med* **9**, 1–37.

Scully C., Cawson R.A. and Griffiths M.J. (1990) *Occupational Hazards to Dental Staff*. London, British Dental Journal.

Sondergaard J.O., Bulow S., Jarvinen H. *et al.* (1987) Dental anomalies in familial adenomatous polyposis coli. *Acta Odontol. Scand.* **45**, 61–3.

Traboulisi E.I., Krush A.J., Gardner E.F. *et al.* (1987) Prevalence and importance of pigmented ocular fundus lesions in Gardner's syndrome. *N. Engl. J. Med.* **316**, 661–7.

Weits-Binnerts J.J., Hoff M. and van Grunsven M.F. (1982) Dental pits in deciduous teeth; an early sign in tuberous sclerosis. *Lancet* **ii**, 1344–5.

Wiebe C.B., Silver J.G. and Larjava H.S. (1996) Early onset periodontitis associated with Weary–Kindler syndrome: a case report. *J. Periodontol.* **67**, 1004–10.

Zhu J.F., Kaminski M.J., Pulitzer D.R. *et al.* (1996) Psoriasis; pathophysiology and oral manifestations. *Oral Diseases* **2**, 135–44.

13

Genitourinary and renal disease

Key points

- Renal disease may manifest with nocturia and hypertension.
- Renal patients may have a bleeding tendency, usually due to platelet dysfunction.
- Renal patients may have impaired drug excretion, a problem mainly when general anaesthesia is contemplated.
- Avoid NSAIDs (including aspirin), opioids, aminoglycosides and tetracyclines in renal patients, and consider reducing the dose of other drugs.
- Patients on haemodialysis may be heparinized and should receive oral health care the day after dialysis, when the anticoagulant activity has abated.
- Avoid the use of the vascular access arm when performing venepuncture.
- The other main problems are in relation to the immunosuppression given for a kidney transplant. Dental treatment should be completed well *before* the transplant operation if possible.
- Patients with transplants are, particularly during the immediate postoperative period, liable to present a number of complications to dental treatment; in particular:
    need for a corticosteroid cover;
    liability to infection;
    bleeding tendency (if on anticoagulants);
    gingival hyperplasia if on cyclosporin.
- Oral health is important as transplant patients are particularly liable to the same fungal and viral infections and other complications seen in patients on chemotherapy for malignant disease.
- Erythromycin is contraindicated in transplant patients since it impairs cyclosporin metabolism and increases its toxicity.

The common diseases of the genitourinary tract are infections, usually of the bladder or urethra.

GENITOURINARY INFECTIONS

These are particularly seen in females and usually have little relevance for dental care, although the symptoms may cause the patient to defer treatment for a few days. However, such infections often suggest that the patient is sexually active and if infections are frequent or persistent *may* suggest the person is at risk from sexually transmitted diseases (Chapter 11).

CANCER

Cervical cancer is the most common neoplasm of the genitourinary tract, and has a relatively poor prognosis. It is most common in sexually active persons, especially those who smoke cigarettes and particularly in the lower socioeconomic classes. It is now recognized to be associated with certain human papillomaviruses, often transmitted sexually (Chapter 11).

Bladder cancer is mostly seen in smokers and presents with haematuria and/or urinary obstruction. The latter is also a common manifestation of prostatic hyperplasia and carcinoma. Metastases occasionally involve the jaws.

RENAL DISEASE

This chapter concentrates mainly on renal disease. Renal function is required to maintain normal body fluid volumes and composition and for the excretion of many metabolites and drugs. Several of the renal disorders pose special problems of dental management. Some previously fatal chronic renal diseases can also now be managed successfully, so that the number of patients with chronic renal disease and those treated with renal transplants who may require dental care, is growing.

Loss of renal function may be caused by pre-renal conditions such as renal hypoperfusion in severe shock or haemorrhage, by renal disease, or by post-renal disorders such as obstruction of renal outflow by calculi, prostatic hypertrophy or tumour. The main diseases affecting the kidneys include chronic glomerulonephritis, chronic pyelonephritis, congenital renal anomalies, hypertension and diabetes.

CHRONIC RENAL FAILURE AND RENAL TRANSPLANTATION

Loss of renal function may lead to renal failure. Chronic renal failure (CRF) results from progressive and irreversible renal damage as shown by a low glomerular filtration rate (GFR) persisting for more than 3 months.

CRF is asymptomatic at first, but later there is significant impairment of all renal functions with effects on virtually all body systems. The symptoms and signs depend on the degree of

Table 13.1 Chronic renal failure: clinical features

- Metabolic
  Nocturia and polyuria
  Thirst
  Glycosuria
  Increased serum urea, creatinine, lipids and uric acid
  Electrolyte disturbances
  Secondary hyperparathyroidism
- Cardiovascular
  Hypertension
  Congestive cardiac failure
  Pericarditis
  Cardiomyopathy
  Atheroma
- Gastrointestinal
  Anorexia
  Nausea and vomiting
  Hiccoughs
  Peptic ulcer and gastrointestinal bleeding
- Neuromuscular
  Weakness and lassitude
  Drowsiness leading to coma
  Headaches
  Disturbances of vision
  Sensory disturbances
  Tremor
- Dermatological
  Pruritus
  Bruising
  Hyperpigmentaton
- Haematological
  Bleeding
  Anaemia
  Lymphopenia
- Immunological
  Liability to infections

renal malfunction. Early features are nocturia and anorexia, and raised serum levels of nitrogenous compounds such as urea and creatinine (azotaemia), from normal metabolic processes. Advanced CRF is complicated by many problems (*Table 13.1*), the term 'uraemia' being applied to the clinical and biochemical syndrome (end-stage renal disease, ESRD). Hypertension is common. A wide range of protein metabolites and electrolytes such as sodium and potassium, hydrogen ions and hormones such as parathyroid hormone accumulate. Hormone production by the kidneys falls, lack of active vitamin D (1,25-dihydroxycholecalciferol) causes renal osteodystrophy, and lack of erythropoietin causes anaemia.

Renal osteodystrophy: Bone disease in CRF is predominantly caused by secondary hyperparathyroidism and deficiency of 1,25 dihydroxycholecalciferol (vitamin D_3). Phosphate retention in CRF leads to depression of plasma calcium levels and subsequently increased parathyroid activity (secondary hyperparathyroidism). Parathyroid hyperplasia may eventually become adenomatous and irreversible (tertiary hyperparathyroidism). Phosphate retention may also interfere with vitamin D metabolism, and calcium absorption is thereby reduced, further contributing to the osteodystrophy. Vitamin D metabolism is also impaired by the renal disease. Renal osteodystrophy appears to cause increasing symptoms after the start of regular dialysis.

Patients may therefore be treated with a low phosphate diet, calcium carbonate, vitamin D_3 or its synthetic analogue or intravenous clodronate to inhibit bone resorption. Parathyroidectomy may be necessary (Chapter 14).

Anaemia is caused by lack of erythropoietin, blood loss in the gut, haemolysis, toxic suppression of the bone marrow and hypersplenism. Recombinant erythropoietin, particularly if supplemented with androgens, is the preferred treatment for anaemia. Blood transfusions are best avoided in view of the risk of transmitting hepatitis and other viruses.

- **General management**

Renal function may remain relatively adequate for long periods if the progress of the renal lesion is slow, but any stress, infection or urinary tract obstruction may precipitate symptoms. Initial management aims to lower the level of blood urea, electrolytes etc. by dietary control, but dialysis or transplantation becomes essential if function deteriorates to ESRD. Despite the tendency to inexorable deterioration, complications such as uncontrolled hypertension, congestive cardiac failure, infections, urinary tract obstruction and biochemical disturbances should be promptly treated where possible.

General management therefore includes:

1. Low protein diet.
2. Potassium restriction.
3. Salt or water control.

4. Dialysis, peritoneal or renal, followed when appropriate and possible by renal transplantation.
5. Treatment of symptoms and complications such as hiccough, vomiting, fits and calcium loss.
6. Prevention of further renal damage (antibiotics or antihypertensives).

Dialysis aims to reduce the manifestations of ESRD and can totally rehabilitate up to 20 per cent of patients but it cannot prevent all complications and is itself associated with some adverse effects Intermittent peritoneal dialysis (IPD) has been superseded by continuous ambulatory peritoneal dialysis (CAPD) or continuous cyclic peritoneal dialysis (CCPD) but haemodialysis is often eventually required. Haemodialysis is carried out, often at home or as an outpatient, for two to three 6-hourly sessions per week. An arteriovenous fistula is created surgically at the wrist to facilitate the introduction of infusion lines. The patient is heparinized during dialysis in order to keep both the infusion lines and the dialysis machine tubing patent. Control of infection is of paramount importance during haemodialysis as infection with hepatitis viruses or HIV or other blood-borne agents is possible. Over 70 per cent of patients on haemodialysis survive at least 5 years. Renal transplantation may then become necessary.

- **Dental aspects of chronic renal failure**

The main management problems are with patients in CRF and with the immunosuppressed post-transplant patient who has had severe CRF and has been dialysed. Treatment may be complicated by:

1. Bleeding tendencies and anticoagulant therapy (Chapter 4).
2. Impaired drug excretion.
3. Corticosteroid or other immunosuppressive therapy (Chapter 14).
4. Hypertension (Chapter 3).
5. Infections or clotting at arteriovenous shunts.
6. Infections with hepatitis B, or other viruses (Chapters 10 and 11).
7. Anaemia (Chapter 5).
8. Renal osteodystrophy.

Table 13.2 Drugs apart from general anaesthesia that may be contraindicated and alternatives for use in patients with chronic renal failure[a]

Safe (No dosage change usually required)	Fairly safe (Dosage change only in severe renal failure)	Less safe (Dosage reduction indicated[b] even in mild renal failure)	Avoid (Best avoided in any patient with renal failure)
Antimicrobials			
Cloxacillin	Ampicillin[c]	Aciclovir[c]	Cephaloridine
Doxycycline	Amoxycillin	Aminoglycosides	Cephalothin
Erythromycin	Benzylpenicillin	Cephalosporins[d]	Sulphonamides
Flucloxacillin	Clindamycin	Fluconazole	Tetracyclines[e]
Fucidin	Co-trimoxazole	Vancomycin	
Ketoconazole	Lincomycin		
Minocycline	Metronidazole		
Phenoxymethyl Penicillin			
Rifampicin			
Local anaesthetics			
Lignocaine			
Analgesics	Codeine	Paracetamol/acetaminophen	NSAIDs and aspirin
		Pethidine and opioids	
CNS-active drugs			
Chloral hydrate	Barbiturates		
Diazepam	Phenothiazines	Antihistamines	

[a]Many other drugs unlikely to be used in dentistry may be contraindicated: check the literature.
[b]Severe renal failure – GFR <10 ml/min; moderately severe renal failure – GFR <25 ml/min; mild renal failure – GFR <50 ml/min.
[c]Systemic aciclovir.
[d]Except cephaloridine and cephalothin, which are contraindicated.
[e]Except doxycycline and minocycline.

9. Dysrhythmias predisposed to by hyperkalaemia.
10. The underlying disease.

Bleeding tendencies
Haemostasis is poor in CRF as a result mainly of impaired platelet adhesiveness and function, and defective von Willebrand's factor. There may be lowered platelet Factor III (thromboxane) and raised prostacyclin (prostaglandin I), leading to poor platelet aggregation and vasodilatation. The bleeding time is often prolonged though there is no defined clotting defect. Patients on haemodialysis are also heparinized during dialysis but the effect is brief.

Careful haemostasis should therefore be ensured if oral surgical procedures are necessary (Chapter 4). Dialysis improves platelet function. Therefore dental treatment is best carried out on the day after dialysis, when there has been maximal benefit from the dialysis and the effect of the heparin has worn off, but the haematologist should first be consulted. Should bleeding be prolonged, desmopressin (DDAVP) may achieve haemostasis for up to 4 hours. If this fails, cryoprecipitate may be effective, has a peak effect at 4–12 hours and lasts up to 36 hours. Conjugated oestrogens may aid haemostasis: the effect takes 2–5 days to develop but persists for 30 days.

Impaired drug excretion
Many drugs are excreted mainly by the kidney and may therefore have undesirably enhanced or prolonged activity if doses are not reduced in renal failure. Some drugs such as tetracycline, cephaloridine, phenacetin, phenylbutazone and aminoglycosides are directly nephrotoxic. Tetracyclines can also cause nitrogen retention and worsen renal function.

Few of the drugs likely to cause complications in CRF are used in dentistry. Lignocaine, diazepam and opioids are mainly metabolized by the liver. However, antimicrobials, analgesics, hypnotics and general anaesthetics may need to be given in lower doses (*Table 13.2*) and, except in emergency, should be prescribed only after consultation with the renal physician.

Fluorides: Fluorides can usually safely be given topically for caries prophylaxis but it is probably best to avoid systemic fluorides because of doubt about fluoride excretion by damaged kidneys.

Antimicrobials: Erythromycin, cloxacillin, fucidin and can be given in standard dosage. The doses of penicillins other than phenoxymethyl penicillin and flucloxacillin, metronidazole and cephaloridine, should be reduced, since very high serum levels may be toxic to the central nervous system. Benzylpenicillin has a significant potassium content and may also be neurotoxic and may therefore be contraindicated. The anti-anabolic effect of most tetracyclines can cause increasing nitrogen retention and acidosis in CRF and thus they should be avoided, but doxycycline and minocycline can be safely given.

Analgesics: Excretion of aspirin and other non-steroidal anti-inflammatory analgesics is delayed and in any event, gastrointestinal irritation and bleeding may be associated with CRF. Aspirin should therefore be avoided. Analgesics that can be safely used in renal disease include codeine and dihydrocodeine.

Hypnotics and sedatives: Diazepam or chloral hydrate can be used. Long-acting barbiturates (phenobarbitone) are contraindicated since their excretion is delayed. Chlordiazepoxide may cause depression and lethargy in patients with CRF and is best avoided. Antihistamines or drugs with antimuscarinic side-effects may cause dry mouth or urinary retention.

Anaesthetics: Local anaesthesia is safe unless there is a severe bleeding tendency. General anaesthesia should only be carried out in hospital by a specialist anaesthetist. Some of the difficulties with general anaesthesia are that patients with CRF are highly sensitive to the myocardial depressant effects of halothane or cyclopropane, and may develop hypotension at moderate levels of anaesthesia. Myocardial depression and cardiac dysrhythmias are especially likely in those with poorly controlled metabolic acidosis and hyperkalaemia. Enflurane is metabolized to potentially nephrotoxic organic fluoride ions and therefore should only be used with caution if other nephrotoxic agents are used concurrently. Isoflurane and sevoflurane are probably safer. Induction with methohexitone followed by very light general anaesthesia with nitrous oxide is generally the technique of choice. In dental practice local anaesthesia should be used, with relative analgesia if necessary.

Other drugs: Antacids containing magnesium salts should not be given as there may be magnesium retention. Antacids containing calcium or aluminium bases may impair absorption of penicillin V and sulphonamides. Cholestyramine, sometimes used in CRF, may also interfere with the absorption of penicillins. Many renal patients are on antihypertensive therapy, digoxin and diuretics (Chapter 3), which may also complicate management. Some have peptic ulceration which is a further contraindication to aspirin.

Hypertension

Hypertension is common in CRF and may affect dental treatment, and these patients are also liable to atherosclerosis. Angiotensin-converting enzymes are indicated to treat the hypertension.

Infections

Infections are poorly controlled by the patient with CRF, especially if immunosuppressed, and may spread locally as well as giving rise to septicaemia or distant contiguous spread. They also accelerate tissue catabolism causing clinical deterioration. Infections can be difficult to recognize as signs of inflammation are masked. Haemodialysis predisposes to blood-borne viral infections such as hepatitis virus infection. Tuberculosis is also more frequent in patients on dialysis, but is usually extra-pulmonary and therefore does not constitute a risk to dental staff.

Odontogenic infections should be treated vigorously (*Table 13.2*). Dental surgery may need to be covered by antibiotic prophylaxis in view of the susceptibility of patients with CRF to infections, especially at the arteriovenous fistula. These patients may therefore need to be managed with precautions similar to others at risk from infective endocarditis (Chapter 3). An alternative is to give 400 mg teicoplanin i.v. during dialysis, which gives cover for at least a day.

The veins of the forearms and the saphenous veins are lifelines for patients on regular haemodialysis. If, therefore, the dentist has to give (for example) intravenous diazepam or midazolam, or take blood, other veins such as those at or above the elbow should be used in case there is consequent fistula infection or thrombophlebitis. Patients with indwelling peritoneal catheters are not considered at risk from infection during dental treatment.

Anaemia

CRF is invariably complicated by anaemia which is a contraindication to general anaesthesia if the haemoglobin is below 10 g/dl.

Postoperative complications

Major surgical procedures may be complicated by hyperkalaemia as a result of tissue damage, acidaemia and blood transfusion. Hyperkalaemia predisposes to dysrhythmias and may cause cardiac arrest. Dialysis is deferred postoperatively if possible since heparinization is required.

Underlying diseases and complications

Consideration must be given to the effect on dental management of underlying diseases, such as diabetes (Chapter 14), systemic lupus erythematosus, polyarteritis nodosa (Chapter 21), myelomatosis and amyloidosis (Chapter 6), or complications such as peptic ulceration (Chapter 9).

Common complaints are of a dry mouth, halitosis and a metallic taste. Insidious oral bleeding and purpura can also be a manifestation. The salivary glands may swell, salivary flow is reduced, there are protein and electrolyte changes and there is calculus accumulation.

In children with CRF, growth is usually retarded and tooth eruption may be delayed. There may be malocclusion and enamel hypoplasia with brownish discoloration but tetracycline staining of the teeth should no longer be seen. A *lower* caries rate and less periodontal disease have been reported in children with CRF.

Osseous lesions include loss of the lamina dura, osteoporosis and osteolytic areas (renal osteodystrophy). Secondary hyperparathyroidism may lead to giant cell lesions. There may be abnormal bone repair after extractions, with socket sclerosis. A variety of mucosal lesions may be seen. The oral mucosa may be pale because of anaemia, and there may be oral ulceration.

RENAL TRANSPLANTATION

Renal transplantation is now commonplace and graft survival can be as high as 90 per cent at one year with an overall mortality of less than 5 per cent. Patients need to be immunosuppressed, usually with a corticosteroid plus a steroid-sparing drug such as azathioprine or now more commonly cyclosporin, to prevent graft rejection.

Patients with renal transplants may still have some of the problems of those with CRF; the above management considerations may therefore apply. More important, patients with a transplant are immunocompromised and liable to infection (Chapter 20) and may need steroid supplementation or antimicrobial cover during dental treatment (Chapter 14). This applies probably for at least two years post-transplantation. Carriage of hepatitis viruses is common, and patients should be kept away from sources of infection (Chapter 11).

Rarely dental infections may spread, with serious complications such as cavernous sinus thrombosis or metastatic infections, and oral bacteria are an important source of bacteraemias. Oral candidosis may be persistent, especially in the immunosuppressed patient, or mixed bacterial plaques may

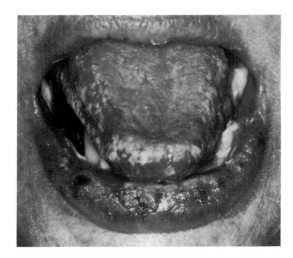

Fig. 13.1 Thrush 'pseudomembranous candidosis' frequently implies an underlying disease, in this instance immunosuppression with corticosteroids and azathioprine in a patient who has a renal transplant for chronic renal failure caused by diabetes mellitus

develop on the oral mucosa. Oral candidosis can usually be managed with topical nystatin, amphotericin or miconazole (*Fig. 13.1*). Mixed bacterial oral mucosal plaques may respond to the appropriate antibiotic, trypsinization and possibly to an aqueous chlorhexidine (0.2 per cent) mouthwash. Some patients carry enterococci in plaque. Other oral infections such as herpes simplex or zoster, cytomegalovirus, Epstein–Barr virus, mycoses and toxoplasmosis, to which the immuno-suppressed patient is prone, are discussed in Chapter 20. Oral herpes simplex and zoster infections can be prevented, deferred or ameliorated by prophylactic low dose oral aciclovir.

Patients on immunosuppressive treatment after renal transplantation have a greatly increased incidence of malignant disease, particularly lymphomas and, to a lesser extent, skin, cervical and lip cancer. In other patients hairy leukoplakia, leukoplakia or Kaposi's sarcoma have been reported. Cyclosporin may cause gingival hyperplasia as may nifedipine or other calcium-channel blockers which are frequently used to control hypertension. Dental pulp narrowing has been noted, apparently a corticosteroid effect.

THE NEPHROTIC SYNDROME

The nephrotic syndrome is characterized by massive proteinuria with hypoalbuminaemia, oedema and hyperlipidaemia. The main causes of nephrotic syndrome are minimal change disease, diabetic nephropathy and systemic lupus erythematosus.

Oedema, especially of the face, genitals and lower limbs, and transudates in serous cavities (especially the peritoneal cavity) may result. Loss of immunoglobulins (especially IgG) in the urine predisposes to infections, often pneumococcal. Initially there is neither hypertension nor raised blood urea, but the serum cholesterol is high. Loss of cholecalcif-erol-binding protein may lead to vitamin D deficiency, secondary hyperparathyroidism and bone disease. Loss of antithrombin III and increased Factor VIII may cause increased blood coagulability and result in thromboses.

Treatment is aimed at reducing proteinuria, controlling infections, preventing throm-boembolic complications and removing or treating the basic cause of the nephrotic syndrome. Treatment may include corticos-teroids together with a low salt but high protein diet. Prophylactic antimicrobials may also be given.

• **Dental aspects of nephrotic syndrome**

Many of the considerations in the manage-ment of the patient in chronic renal failure are also applicable to the nephrotic patient. The nephrotic syndrome occasionally is seen in Kimura's disease (Chapter 9).

Drugs: Long-term corticosteroid therapy is the main problem (Chapter 14).

Infections: Treatment with corticosteroids and other factors such as electrolyte imbal-ance, hypoproteinaemia and hypoimmuno-globulinaemia predispose to infections.

Cardiovascular and haematological disorders: Patients with the nephrotic syndrome are susceptible to cardiovascular disease (atheroma) because of hypercholesterolaemia. The blood concentrations of Factor VIII, fibrinogen and other clotting factors are also raised, leading to a hypercoagulable state. This may lead to spontaneous thromboses, especially in patients treated with corticos-teroids. Immobilized patients are often, there-fore, treated with heparin.

RENAL STONES

Renal stones are not uncommon. They may be seen on radiography or cause symptoms of renal colic or secondary renal damage. Although no underlying systemic disease is usually identified, stones may complicate gout, hyperparathyroidism, hyperoxaluria, cystinosis or renal tubular acidosis. There is no known predisposition to salivary calculi or dental calculus formation in these patients.

BIBLIOGRAPHY

Brenner B.M. and Rector F.C. (1991) *The Kidney*, 4th edn. Philadelphia, Saunders.
Buckley D.J., Barrett A.P., Koutts J. and Stewart J.H. (1986) Control of bleeding in severely uraemic patients undergoing oral surgery. *Oral Surg.* **61**, 546–9.
Cawson R.A. Spector R.G. and Skelly A.M. (1995) *Basic Pharmacology and Clinical Drug Use in Dentistry*, 6th edn. Edinburgh, Churchill Livingstone.

Ciechanover M. (1980) Malrecognition of taste in uraemia. *Nephron* **26**, 20–2.

DiRossi S.S. and Glick M. (1996) Dental considerations for the patient with renal disease receiving hemodialysis. *J. Am. Dent. Assoc.* **127**, 211–19.

Eigner T.L., Jastak J.T. and Bennett W.M. (1986) Achieving oral health in patients with renal failure and renal transplants. *J. Am. Dent. Assoc.* **113**, 612–6.

Epstein S.R., Mandel I. and Scopp I.W. (1980) Salivary composition and calculus formation in patients undergoing hemodialysis. *J. Periodontol.* **51**, 336–9.

Fillastre J.P. and Godin M. (1980) Prescribing for patients with renal failure. *Medicine (UK)* **25**, 1299–303.

Fraser C.G. (1985) Urine analysis: current performance and strategies for improvement. *Br. Med. J.* **291**, 321–5.

Hruska K.A. and Teitelbaum S.L. (1995) Renal osteodystrophy. *N. Engl. J. Med.* **333**, 166–74.

Jaffe E.C., Roberts G.J., Chantler C. *et al.* (1990) Dental maturity in children with chronic renal failure assessed from dental panoramic radiographs. *J. Int. Assoc. Dent. Child.* **20**, 54–8.

Janson R.A. (1980) Treatment of the bleeding tendency in uraemia with cryoprecipitate. *N. Engl. J. Med.* **303**, 318–22.

Kellett M. (1983) Oral white plaques in uraemic patients. *Br. Dent. J.* **154**, 366–8.

King G.N., Fullinfaw R., Higgins T.J. *et al.* (1993) Gingival hyperplasia in renal allograft recipients receiving cyclosporin-A and calcium antagonists. *J. Clin. Periodontol.* **20**, 286–93.

King G.N., Healy C.M., Glover M.T. *et al.* (1994) Prevalence and risk factors associated with leukoplakia, hairy leukoplakia, erythematous candidiasis, and gingival hyperplasia in renal transplant recipients. *Oral Surg. Oral Med. Oral Pathol.* **78**, 718–26.

King G.N., Healy C.M., Glover M.T. *et al.* (1995). Increased prevalence of dysplastic and malignant lip lesions in renal transplant recipients. *N. Engl. J. Med.* **332**, 1052–7.

Krekeler G., Whilms H. and Akuamoa-Boateng E. (1980) Inflammatory pathology in the dental system in renal transplantation. *Int. J. Oral Surg.* **9**, 383–6.

Leading Article (1988) Is routine urinalysis worthwhile? *Lancet* **i**, 747.

London N.J., Farmery S.M., Will E.J. *et al.* (1995) Risk of neoplasia in renal transplant patients. *Lancet* **346**, 403–6.

Milam S.B. and Cooper R.L. (1983) Extensive bleeding following extractions in a patient undergoing chronic hemodialysis. *Oral Surg. Oral Med. Oral Pathol.* **55**, 14–16.

Mitwalli A. (1991) Tuberculosis in patients on maintenance dialysis. *Am. J. Kidney Dis.* **18**, 579–82.

Nasstrom K., Forsberg B., Petersson A. *et al.* (1985). Narrowing of the dental pulp chamber in patients with renal disease. *Oral Surg. Oral Med. Oral Pathol.* **59**, 242–6.

Nunn J. (1995) Renal disease. In Porter S.R. and Scully C. (eds), *Oral Health Care for Those with HIV Infection and Other Special Needs.* Northwood, Science Reviews, pp. 143–52.

Porter S.R. and Scully C. (1996) *Innovations and Developments in Non-Invasive Oral Health Care.* Northwood, Science Reviews.

Scully C. (1988) *The Dental Patient.* Oxford, Heinemann.

Scully C. (1989) *The Mouth and Perioral Tissues.* Oxford, Heinemann.

Scully C. (1989) *Patient Care: a Dental Surgeon's Guide.* London, British Dental Association.

Scully C., Cawson R.A. and Griffiths M.J. (1990) *Occupational Hazards to Dental Staff.* London, British Dental Journal.

Seale L., Jones C.J. and Kathpalia S. (1985) Prevention of herpes virus infections in renal allograft recipients by low dose oral acyclovir. *J. Am. Med. Assoc.* **254**, 3435–8.

Shasha S.M. (1983) Salivary content in hemodialysed patients. *J. Oral Med.* **38**, 67–70.

Smyth C.J., Halpenry M.K. and Ballagh S.J. (1987) Carriage rates of enterococci in the dental plaque of haemodialysis patients in Dublin. *Br. J. Oral Maxillofac. Surg.* **25**, 21–33.

Sowell S.B. (1982) Dental care for patients with renal failure and renal transplants. *J. Am. Dent. Assoc.* **104**, 171–7.

Stoufi E.D., Sonis S.T. and Shklar G. (1986) Significance of the head and neck in late infection in renal transplant recipients. *Oral Surg. Oral Med. Oral Pathol.* **62**, 524–8.

Tolefson T. and Johansen J.R. (1985) Periodontal status in patients before and after renal allotransplantation. *J. Periodont. Res.* **20**, 227–36.

Ziccardi V.B., Saini J., Demas P.N. *et al.* (1992) Management of the oral and maxillofacial surgery patient with end-stage renal disease. *J Oral Maxillofac. Surg.* **50**, 1207–12.

14

Endocrine conditions

Key points

These appear in advance of the discussion of each endocrine gland.

The endocrine system is a widespread system consisting of glands that exert their effects, usually at some distance, by means of chemicals (hormones) secreted into the circulation. Endocrine and nervous control mechanisms thus normally maintain homeostasis. The endocrine system is not absolutely distinct from the nervous system however; rather there is a coordinated neuroendocrine system, most apparent in the hypothalamus, that acts as the highest integrative centre for the system.

The function of an endocrine gland can be assessed by measuring the hormone in the plasma, the hormone or a metabolite in the urine, dynamic tests of hormone secretion or regulation, levels of hormone receptors, or effects on the target tissues. The main control of the endocrine system is via the hypothalamus and pituitary gland, but some glands react to local concentrations of hormones or other substances. Some endocrine functions are also mediated by tissues and organs that were not originally recognized as endocrine in nature; for example, the chemical 1,25-dihydroxycholecalciferol, secreted by the kidney and active in calcium homeostasis, has a hormonal function.

THE HYPOTHALAMUS AND PITUITARY

Key points

- Antidiuretic hormone production can be disturbed after a head injury or for several other reasons.
- Gigantism and acromegaly can result from anterior pituitary hyperfunction, with headaches and visual loss, and often diabetes and hypertension. The mandible becomes prognathic.

The hypothalamus is the part of the brain that controls pituitary function. It is itself under the control of higher centres, and is inhibited by the hormone somatostatin (octreotide). This hormone has been used clinically to treat salivary fistulae, since it reduces salivary secretion without affecting amylase. The hypothalamus controls the pituitary by means of various hypophysiotropic hormones.

Table 14.1   Pituitary hormones

Hormone	Effects
Anterior pituitary	
Growth hormone (GH)	Growth (diabetogenic)
Thyroid-stimulating hormone (TSH)	Stimulates thyroid hormone synthesis and release
Adrenocorticotrophin (ACTH)	Stimulates glucocorticoid synthesis and release
Prolactin	Lactation
Luteinizing hormone (LH)	Gonadotrophin
Follicle-stimulating hormone (FSH)	Gonadotrophin
Melanocyte-stimulating hormone (MSH)	Pigmentation
Posterior pituitary	
Antidiuretic hormone (ADH)	Water reabsorption in renal distal tubules and collecting ducts
Oxytocin	Lactation Uterine contraction

The posterior pituitary (neurohypophysis) is a downgrowth from the base of the brain and is connected by neurones with the hypothalamus. The posterior pituitary stores two hormones produced by the hypothalamus – vasopressin (antidiuretic hormone, ADH) and oxytocin – and neurophysin. The anterior pituitary (adenohypophysis) originates as an outgrowth from the stomatodeum (Rathke's pouch). It produces several hormones (*Table 14.1*) and controls many metabolic activities.

Although anatomically distinct from the hypothalamus, the anterior pituitary falls under its influence by factors passing through a portal venous system. Feedback control influences both the amount of hypothalamic hormone secreted and the response of the pituitary to a particular hypothalamic hormone.

POSTERIOR PITUITARY HYPOFUNCTION

Diabetes insipidus

Diabetes insipidus is a rare disease caused either by lack of antidiuretic hormone (ADH)

secretion (cranial diabetes insipidus) or renal insensitivity to ADH action (nephrogenic diabetes insipidus). This results in the production of an excessive volume of dilute urine, and thirst.

Cranial diabetes insipidus is more common and can be caused by trauma, a tumour or vascular disease in the region of the hypothalamus or pituitary, or it may be idiopathic. The disorder may be temporary – especially after head injuries. Polyuria and persistent thirst are the main features, but a lesion in the hypothalamic area may also cause pressure on the optic chiasma leading to visual defects, or raised intracranial pressure and headaches.

The diagnosis of diabetes insipidus is established by assessing the relation of plasma to urine osmolality and by demonstrating inability to concentrate the urine during a water-deprivation test. Skull radiographs, MRI, visual field charting and also tests of anterior pituitary function are used to assess the local extent of disease.

Diabetes insipidus is treated with the ADH-like peptide desmopressin or other drugs having an antidiuretic action such as chlorpropamide or carbamazepine.

• Dental aspects of diabetes insipidus

Dentistry is usually uncomplicated by this disorder except for dryness of the mouth. Transient diabetes insipidus can be a complication of head injury. Carbamazepine used in the treatment of trigeminal neuralgia may have an additive effect with other drugs used to treat diabetes insipidus.

Syndrome of inappropriate antidiuretic hormone secretion (SIADH)

Excessive ADH levels may be caused by head injury or other intracranial lesions, some tumours (especially some lung cancers), or drugs (carbamazepine, chlorpropamide, vinca alkaloids, tricyclics). They occasionally follow maxillofacial or head injuries, general anaesthesia, or even elective maxillofacial surgery, possibly because of trigeminal stimulation. The SIADH is characterized by water retention, overhydration causing confusion, behavioural disturbances, ataxia and dysphagia. Diagnosis is by finding hyponatraemia with a concentrated urine and high

Table 14.2   Hypopituitarism – clinical effects

Sequence of development of hormone defects	*Effects*
1. LH FSH	Impotence Amenorrhoea Infertility Loss of pubic hair
2. GH	Impaired growth in child
3. Prolactin	Failure of lactation if post-partum (Sheehan's syndrome)
4. ACTH	Hypoadrenocorticism
5. TSH	Hypothyroidism

For abbreviations *see Table 14.1.*

plasma and urinary ADH and an abnormal water excretion test. Patients with SIADH are treated with fluid restriction, corticosteroids or demeclocycline.

ANTERIOR PITUITARY HYPOFUNCTION

The usual causes of hypopituitarism are local hypothalamic or pituitary lesions. There may be individual or more frequently multiple hormone deficiencies. The results of hypopituitarism (*Table 14.2*) are essentially hypofunction of the target glands, the gonads, thyroid or adrenal cortex.

Surgery may be needed if there are tumours, cranial nerve defects or hydrocephalus. Substitution therapy is needed for deficiency states.

- **Dental aspects of hypopituitarism**

General anaesthesia is usually contraindicated since there may be no TSH (leading to hypothyroidism) or ACTH (leading to hypoadrenocorticism). Patients are at risk from adrenal crisis and hypopituitary coma.

Hypopituitary coma may be precipitated by stress (trauma, surgery, general anaesthesia or infection), much in the way that an adrenal crisis may be caused. Hypopituitary coma may also be precipitated by sedatives or hypnotics.

Hypopituitary coma should be treated with an immediate intravenous injection of 200 mg hydrocortisone sodium succinate. Blood

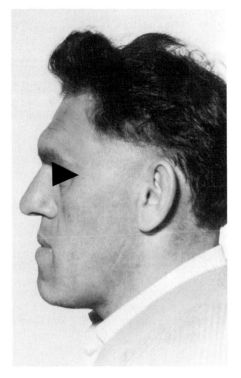

Fig. 14.1 Acromegaly

should be taken for assay of glucose, thyroid hormones and cortisol, and 25–50 g dextrose should be given intravenously if there is hypoglycaemia. Oxygen should be given by face mask, medical assistance summoned and emergency admission to hospital arranged.

ANTERIOR PITUITARY HYPERFUNCTION

Growth hormone excess: gigantism and acromegaly

Overproduction of growth hormone by an anterior pituitary adenoma causes gigantism before the epiphyses have fused, and acromegaly thereafter. In gigantism all the organs, soft tissues and skeleton enlarge. In acromegaly, only those bones with growth potential such as the mandible can enlarge, but again there is thickening of the soft tissues with prominence of the supraorbital ridge, coarse oily skin, thick spade-like fingers, and deepening of the voice. Acromegaly is one of the few endocrine diseases that can be instantly recognized – even in a passer-by in the street – by the appearance of the face and hands (*Fig. 14.1*). However, many cases go unrecognized for long periods. These disorders may be complicated by diabetes mellitus, hypertension, cardiomyopathy, hypercalcaemia and osteoarthrosis. Life expectancy is shortened by cardiovascular, cerebrovascular or other disease such as colonic carcinoma. Local pressure effects from the pituitary tumour may cause hypopituitarism, compression of the optic chiasma (leading to visual field defects) and raised intracranial pressure with severe headache.

• **Diagnosis and management of growth hormone excess**

Facial photographs may clearly demonstrate the increasingly coarse features. Skull radiography (to demonstrate pituitary – sella turcica – enlargement), CT and MRI scans, visual field assessment (to detect optic chiasma involvement), glucose tolerance tests (to exclude diabetes and to assess the plasma growth hormone response), levels of growth hormone and insulin-like growth factor 1 (IGF-1/SM-C) and assessment of remaining pituitary function are required. The sella may also be enlarged by hypothalamic masses or cysts, aneurysms, primary hypothyroidism or hypogonadism, raised intracranial pressure, or the empty sella syndrome. The latter is caused by herniation of a sac of leptomeninges into the sella and is typically seen in obese multiparous women who are hypertensive and may occasionally suffer from spontaneous CSF rhinorrhoea. Though the rhinorrhoea may warrant surgical correction, no other treatment is indicated for the empty sella syndrome.

The pituitary adenoma in growth hormone excess may be resected trans-sphenoidally or the whole gland may have to be irradiated. Hypopituitarism or diabetes insipidus follow such treatment. Bromocriptine or octreotide (an analogue of the hypothalamic release-inhibiting hormone somatostatin) may be used but are rarely effective alone.

• **Dental aspects of growth hormone excess**

Mandibular enlargement leads to class III malocclusion with spacing of the teeth and thickening of all soft tissues, but most conspicuously of the face (*Fig 14.1*). Orthognathic surgery may therefore be needed and fatalities have followed such surgery in the past, because of airways obstruction. The paranasal air sinuses are enlarged and the skull thickened. Sialosis may be seen. Otherwise, dental management may be complicated by:

1. Blindness.
2. Diabetes mellitus.
3. Hypertension.
4. Cardiomyopathy and dysrhythmias.
5. Hypopituitarism.
6. Kyphosis and other deformities affecting respiration may make general anaesthesia hazardous. The glottic opening may be narrowed and the cords' mobility reduced. A goitre may further embarrass the airway.
7. Thromboembolic phenomena.

Rarely, acromegalics have Cushing's syndrome or hyperparathyroidism due to associated multiple endocrine adenoma syndrome.

ACTH excess (*see* Cushing's syndrome)

ADRENAL CORTEX

Key points

- Adrenocortical hypofunction may be caused by adrenal disease, is often autoimmune and sometimes associated with other endocrinopathies, or iatrogenic suppression by corticosteroids.
- Corticosteroids absorbed systemically suppress adrenocortical function.

- The suppression may persist for up to 2 years after the steroid treatment.
- Such patients cannot respond adequately to the stress of trauma, operation or infection.
- Stress may cause collapse in adrenal crisis.
- Injected and oral corticosteroids are most potent at causing adrenocortical suppression.
- Systemic steroids may interfere with adrenocortical responses, within one week.
- History, blood pressure, chest radiograph, blood glucose, faecal occult blood and weight should be checked before starting a patient on systemic steroids, and a warning card given.
- Steroids are best given on alternate mornings to minimize the adrenocortical suppression.
- Steroids must not be abruptly withdrawn.
- Patients on, or recently on, steroids therefore need steroid supplementation before operations.
- Patients on, or recently on, steroids need supplementation if there is intercurrent infection or illness.
- Contraindications to steroids include hypertension, diabetes, peptic ulceration and tuberculosis.
- Adrenocortical hyperfunction leads to obesity with fat redistribution (moon face) and hypertension, and sometimes psychoses, skin striae and osteoporosis.

The adrenal cortex produces a series of corticosteroids, mainly the glucocorticoids cortisol (hydrocortisone) and corticosterone, and the mineralocorticoid, aldosterone. Glucocorticoid production is stimulated by adrenocorticotropic hormone (corticotropin) from the anterior pituitary gland and cortisol exerts a negative feedback on the pituitary. Adrenocorticotropic hormone arises from a precursor, pro-opiomelanocortin (POMC), and is released in response to hypothalamic activity, with a diurnal rhythm (peak early morning, nadir on retiring), stress, fever, hypoglycaemia and eating.

ADRENOCORTICAL HYPOFUNCTION

Adrenocortical hypofunction may lead to hypotension, shock and death if the individual is stressed as, for example, by operation. Rarely it may be due to a congenital defect in the biosynthesis of corticosteroids (congenital adrenal hyperplasia), occasionally by acquired adrenal disease (primary hypoadrenocorticism) or more commonly by adrenocorticotrophic hormone (ACTH; corticotrophin) deficiency (secondary hypoadrenocorticism) by the iatrogenic suppression of adrenocortical function associated with the use of systemic corticosteroids.

Primary hypoadrenocorticism (Addison's disease)

Hypoadrenocorticism is a rare disease characterized by atrophy of the adrenal cortices and failure of secretion of cortisol and aldosterone. In most cases there are circulating autoantibodies to the adrenal cortex. Patients with autoimmune Addison's disease also have a higher incidence of other endocrine deficiencies (*see below*) and, occasionally, chronic mucocutaneous candidosis is associated. Other causes such as adrenal tuberculosis, histoplasmosis (occasionally secondary to HIV infection), malignancy, haemorrhage, sarcoidosis, amyloidosis or adrenalectomy for metastatic breast cancer are even more rare.

Lack of cortisol predisposes to hypotension and hypoglycaemia. The hypothalamopituitary axis is stimulated by the low serum cortisol and there is therefore increased release of pro-opiomelanocortin which has ACTH and melanocyte stimulating hormone (MSH) activity. Lack of aldosterone leads to

Table 14.3	Hyper- and hypoadrenocorticism – clinical features

Hyperadrenocorticism	*Hypoadrenocorticism*
Weakness	Weakness
Weight gain	Weight loss
Truncal obesity	Skin and mucosal pigmentation
Hypertension	Hypotension
Hirsutism	Anorexia, nausea and vomiting
Amenorrhoea	
Cutaneous striae	
Personality changes	

sodium depletion, reduced extracellular fluid volume and hypotension. Patients with hypoadrenocorticism therefore suffer from fatigue and weakness, lethargy, anorexia, nausea, vomiting, diarrhoea, hyperpigmentation, weight loss, dizziness and postural hypotension (*Table 14.3*).

More important, the lack of adrenocortical reserve makes patients vulnerable to any stress such as infection, injury, surgery or anaesthesia, though they may be asymptomatic otherwise. The main complication of hypoadrenocorticism is an acute adrenal crisis (Addisonian crisis or shock). Acute adrenal crisis is characterized by collapse, bradycardia, hypotension, profound weakness, hypoglycaemia, vomiting and dehydration. This may be the first manifestation of the disease and results from failure of the adrenocortical response to stress.

Secondary adrenocortical insufficiency

Secondary adrenocortical insufficiency is caused by corticosteroid therapy or ACTH deficiency as a result of hypothalamic or pituitary disease. Secondary adrenocortical insufficiency may therefore be associated with other endocrine defects, but there is no hyperpigmentation (ACTH levels are low) and blood pressure is virtually normal (aldosterone secretion is normal).

Congenital adrenal hyperplasia

Congenital adrenal hyperplasia is the term given to a group of rare autosomal recessive inborn errors of corticosteroid metabolism characterized by lack of cortisol (adrenal insufficiency) and androgen excess. Aldo-

sterone secretion is also lacking in some of these disorders.

Nelson's syndrome

This rare syndrome may affect up to 40 per cent of persons who have had bilateral adrenalectomy, usually to control breast cancer metastases or Cushing's syndrome. This results in increasing pituitary activity and sometimes adenoma formation. Large amounts of ACTH are released and there is cutaneous pigmentation. Some 10 per cent develop oral pigmentation.

• Diagnosis and management of hypoadrenocorticism

The blood pressure should be measured, as hypotension is frequent. Blood should be taken for plasma cortisol estimation (10 ml in lithium heparin orange tube, or plain tube) at 8.00 or 9.00 a.m. In hypoadrenocorticism the basal cortisol level is usually lower than 100 nmol/l, but in early disease the cortisol levels may still be in the low normal range and therefore a short tetracosactrin (Synacthen) test (ACTH stimulation) is indicated, as described below. Plasma electrolytes are normal in many cases, unless a crisis is imminent, but the plasma sodium level may be low and the potassium raised. There is often also hypoglycaemia.

Estimation of serum ACTH levels differentiates primary (ACTH raised, usually above 200 ng/l) from secondary (ACTH low or normal) hypoadrenocorticism.

Other investigations include radiography or CT scans of the skull (for pituitary abnormalities), chest (for tuberculosis) or abdomen (for adrenal calcification suggestive of tuberculosis or a mycosis). Serum should be tested for autoantibodies to various tissues – especially endocrine glands. Most patients are treated with oral hydrocortisone and fludrocortisone.

The Synacthen test: Plasma is collected before and 30 minutes after 250 μg of tetracosactrin (synthetic ACTH: Synacthen) is injected intramuscularly or intravenously. In health the plasma cortisol level normally doubles from at least 200 nmol/l to more than 500 nmol/l after tetracosactrin. In hypoadrenocorticism the basal cortisol level is low and does not rise by more than 200 nmol/l after tetracosactrin is given.

- ### Dental aspects of hypoadrenocorticism

The danger of dental treatment in the patient with hypoadrenocorticism is of precipitating hypotensive collapse, and therefore corticosteroids must be given preoperatively. This is discussed more fully below under the section on systemic corticosteroid therapy, the most frequent cause of hypoadrenocorticism.

Pigmentation of the mucosae of a brown or black colour is seen in over 75 per cent of patients with Addison's disease, but is not a feature of corticosteroid-induced hypoadrenocorticism or of hypoadrenocorticism secondary to hypothalamopituitary disease. Hyperpigmentation is related to high levels of MSH and affects particularly areas normally pigmented or exposed to trauma (for example in the buccal mucosa at the occlusal line, or the tongue, but also the gingivae). Other causes of oral pigmentation (Chapter 9) (especially racial pigmentation) need to be differentiated but, though it is a rare cause, Addison's disease must be considered particularly if there is hypotension, weakness, weight loss, anorexia, nausea, vomiting or abdominal pain.

The diagnosis is established by (a) assay of plasma fluorogenic corticosteroids (cortisol) which in hypoadrenocorticism are lower than 6 μg/100 ml (170 nmol/l) at 8.00 to 9.00 a.m. and (b) failure of synthesis of cortisol in response to ACTH stimulation (Synacthen test).

SYSTEMIC CORTICOSTEROID THERAPY

Corticosteroids are used either to replace missing hormones (in Addison's disease or after adrenalectomy) or for immunosuppression (*Table 14.4*). Corticosteroids can therefore mask the presence of many serious diseases that may influence dental care as well as causing suppression of the adrenocortical response to stress.

Complications of systemic corticosteroid therapy
Long-term systemic use of corticosteroids can

Table 14.4	Some uses of systemic corticosteroids
Allergic disorders	Asthma
Connective tissue disorders	Rheumatoid arthritis (rarely)
	Systemic lupus erythematosus
Renal disorders	Nephrotic syndrome
	Renal transplants
Gastrointestinal disorders	Ulcerative colitis
	Crohn's disease
Blood dyscrasias	Idiopathic thrombocytopenia
	Lymphocytic leukaemia
	Lymphoma
Adrenal insufficiency	Addison's disease
	Adrenalectomy
	Hypopituitarism
Mucocutaneous diseases	Pemphigus

cause many side-effects (*Fig. 14.2*), often beginning soon after the start of treatment (*Table 14.5*). The most significant effect is suppression of ACTH secretion, leading to adrenal atrophy and failure to respond to stress. Corticosteroids in high doses also cause a significant morbidity or mortality,

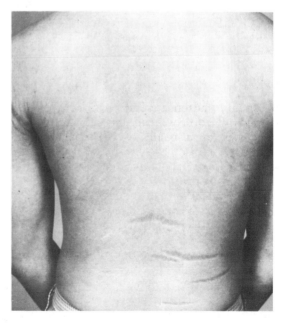

Fig. 14.2 Systemic corticosteroid therapy causes several complications, including cutaneous striae, as here

Table 14.5   Complications of systemic corticosteroid therapy

Metabolic	Hypothalamic–pituitary–adrenal suppression
	Impaired glucose tolerance, or diabetes mellitus
	Growth retardation
	Loss of sodium and potassium
	Osteoporosis
	Fat redistribution (moon face and buffalo hump)
Immunosuppressive	Increased susceptibility to infections
Cardiovascular	Hypertension
	Myocardial infarction
	Cerebrovascular accidents
Gastrointestinal	Peptic ulcer
Neurological	Mood changes
	Psychosis
	Cataracts
Dermatological	Acne
	Striae
	Bruising
	Neoplasms

particularly from infection, perforated or bleeding peptic ulcers, diabetes and hypertension and their complications. However, the more immediately obvious effects are of cushingoid weight gain around the face (moon face) and hirsutism. In children there may be growth retardation.

These complications may be reduced but not abolished if steroids are given on alternate days. Thus, once the desired therapeutic effect of the steroid is achieved by daily administration, there should be a transition to giving the entire 48 hour dose as a single early morning dose on alternate days.

Corticosteroids and suppression of adrenal function

Corticosteroids are an essential part of the body's response to stresses such as trauma, infection, general anaesthesia or operation. At times of stress there is normally increased corticosteroid production and the size of the response is related to the degree of stress. In the absence of such a response there is rapidly developing hypotension, collapse and death.

The hypothalamus is in overall control of adrenocortical function by producing releasing factors that stimulate the pituitary to release adrenocorticotrophic hormone (ACTH

or corticotrophin). ACTH stimulates the production of adrenal corticosteroids. Circulating steroids control hypothalamic activity by a negative feedback mechanism.

The function of the hypothalamic–pituitary–adrenocortical axis (HPA) is disrupted if the pituitary or adrenal cortex ceases to function as a result of trauma, surgery or disease, or if exogenous corticosteroids are given. Administration of corticosteroids results in negative feedback to the hypothalamus, reduced ACTH secretion and consequent adrenocortical atrophy. The adrenal cortex is then unable to produce the necessary steroid response to stress, and acute adrenal insufficiency (adrenal crisis) is precipitated.

Suppression of the HPA axis becomes deeper as the dose of steroids exceeds physiological levels (more than about 7.5 mg/day of prednisolone), but especially if treatment is prolonged. However, adrenal function may even be suppressed for up to a week after cessation of steroid treatment lasting only 5 days. If steroid treatment is for longer periods, adrenal function may be suppressed for at least 30 days and perhaps for 2–24 months after the cessation of treatment. Adrenal suppression is less when the exogenous steroid is given on alternate days or as a single morning dose (rather than as divided doses through the day). Corticotrophin (ACTH) was formerly used in the hope of reducing adrenal suppression, but the response is variable and unpredictable, and wanes with time.

Patients who are to be put on steroids should have baseline evaluations of their:

1. weight;
2. blood pressure;
3. chest radiograph;
4. blood glucose, and possibly
5. occult blood (faecal blood).

Steroids should then be prescribed under the following conditions:

1. There should be no contraindications such as hypertension (*see* Chapter 25).
2. The smallest effective dose should be given.
3. The steroid is best given in the morning on alternate days.
4. The patient must be given a warning card and told of the dangers of withdrawal, and side-effects.

I am a patient on—

STEROID TREATMENT

which must not be stopped abruptly

and in the case of intercurrent illness

may have to be increased

full details are available

from the hospital or general——▶

practitioners shown overleaf

STC1

INSTRUCTIONS

1 **DO NOT STOP** taking the steroid drug except on medical advice. Always have a supply in reserve.

2 In case of feverish illness, accident, operation (emergency or otherwise), diarrhoea or vomiting the steroid treatment **MUST** be continued. Your doctor may wish you to have a **LARGER DOSE** or an **INJECTION** at such times.

3 If the tablets cause indigestion consult your doctor AT ONCE.

4 Always carry this card while receiving steroid treatment and show it to any doctor, dentist, nurse or midwife whom you may consult.

5 After your treatment has finished you must still tell any new doctor, dentist, nurse or midwife that you have had steroid treatment.

Fig. 14.3 Steroid Warning Card: this is a blue card that should be carried at all times by patients on systemic corticosteroids in view of the danger of an adrenocortical crisis and collapse if the patient is subjected to trauma, stress or anaesthesia. (By permission of the Controller of Her Majesty's Stationery Office)

---

5. There should never be abrupt withdrawal of the steroid.
6. The dose should be increased if there is illness, infection, trauma, or operation.

Corticosteroids vary tremendously in their potency as anti-inflammatory agents. As a rough guide, 3 mg of dexamethasone, 3 mg betamethasone, 20 mg prednisone and 80 mg hydrocortisone are about equipotent.

Patients on, or who have been on, corticosteroid therapy within the past 30 days are at risk from adrenal crisis, and those who have been on them during the previous 24 months may be at risk, if they are not given supplementary corticosteroids before and during periods of stress. Patients should be warned of this danger and should carry a steroid card indicating the dosage and the responsible physician (*Fig. 14.3*). Metal bracelets or necklaces with the diagnosis engraved on them are available, for example, from Medic-Alert Foundation, 9 Hanover Street, London W1R 9HF (*see Figs 1.2, 1.3*).

- ## Dental aspects of patients on systemic corticosteroids

Systemic corticosteroids cause the greatest risk of adrenocortical suppression. It is obvious, therefore, that topical steroids should always be used in preference to systemic steroids provided that the desired therapeutic effect is achievable. However, there can also be adrenocortical suppression from extensive application of steroid skin preparations, particularly if occlusive dressings are used.

Adrenocortical function is likely to be suppressed if:

1. The patient is currently on systemic corticosteroids.
2. Corticosteroids have been taken regularly during the previous 30 days.
3. Corticosteroids have been taken for more than 1 month during the past year.

During intercurrent illness or infection, after trauma, or before operation or anaesthesia, these patients require a considerable increase in steroid dosage. Minor operations under local anaesthesia may be covered by giving oral steroids 2–4 hours pre- and postoperatively (100 mg hydrocortisone or 20 mg prednisolone or 4 mg dexamethasone) or, better, by giving intravenous hydrocortisone immediately before operation (*see below*). Intravenous hydrocortisone must be immediately available for use if the patient collapses or the blood pressure falls. General anesthesia must be given only in hospital by a specialist anaesthetist. Cover should be provided, by

Table 14.6 Suggested management of patients with a history of systemic corticosteroid therapy

	No steroids for previous 12 mth	*Steroids taken during previous 12 mth*	*Steroids currently taken*
Conservative dentistry or minor surgery (e.g. single extraction) under LA	No cover required	Give hydrocortisone 200 mg orally,[a] or i.v. preop.[b]	Give hydrocortisone 200 mg orally,[a] or i.v. preop[b] Continue normal steroid medication postop.
Intermediate surgery (e.g. multiple extractions, or surgery under GA)	Consider cover if large doses of steroid were given. Test adrenocortical function (ACTH stimulation test)	Give hydrocortisone[b] 200 mg i.v. preop. and i.m. 6-hourly for 24 h	Give hydrocortisone[b] 200 mg i.v. preop. and i.m. 6-hourly for 24 h. Then continue normal medication
Major surgery or trauma (e.g. maxillofacial surgery)	Consider cover if large doses of steroid were given. Test adrenocortical function (ACTH stimulation test)	Give hydrocortisone[b] 200 mg i.v. preop. and i.m. 6-hourly for 72 h	Give hydrocortisone[b] 200 mg i.v. preop. and i.m. 6-hourly for 72 h. Then continue normal medication

[a]Hydrocortisone orally 2 h preoperatively.
[b]Hydrocortisone sodium succinate (e.g. Ef-Cortelan soluble) or phosphate immediately preoperatively and monitor blood pressure.

giving at least 100–200 mg hydrocortisone sodium succinate intramuscularly or intravenously (with the premedication) and then 6-hourly for a further 24–72 hours (*Table 14.6*). The blood pressure must also be carefully watched during surgery and especially during recovery, and steroid supplementation given immediately if the blood pressure starts to fall. Corticosteroids given by intramuscular injection are more slowly absorbed and reach lower plasma levels than when given intravenously or orally.

Drugs, especially sedatives and general anaesthetics, are a hazard and it is extremely important to avoid hypoxia, hypotension or haemorrhage. Patients may also require special management as a result of diabetes, hypertension, poor wound healing, or infections.

Aspirin and other non-steroidal anti-inflammatory agents should be avoided as they may increase the risk of peptic ulceration in those on corticosteroids. Osteoporosis introduces the danger of fractures when handling the patient.

Topical corticosteroids for use in the mouth are unlikely to have any systemic effect but predispose to oral candidosis.

Susceptibility to infection is increased by systemic steroid use (*see below*) and there is a predisposition to herpes virus infections (particularly herpes simplex). Chickenpox is an especial hazard to those patients who are

not immune and fulminant disease has resulted. Therefore, passive immunization with varicella zoster immunoglobulin is indicated for non-immune patients on systemic corticosteroids (or who have been on them within the previous 3 months) who are exposed to chickenpox or zoster. The immunization should be given within 3 days of the exposure.

Candidosis and bacterial infections also tend to be more frequent and severe. Wound healing is impaired in systemic corticosteroid therapy and wound infections are more frequent. In addition to careful aseptic surgery, prophylactic antimicrobials may, therefore, be indicated.

Long-term and profound immunosuppression may lead to the appearance of hairy leukoplakia, Kaposi's sarcoma, lymphomas, lip cancer or other oral complications (Chapter 20).

ACUTE ADRENAL INSUFFICIENCY

Acute adrenal insufficiency has several causes (*Table 14.7*) and is managed as follows:

1. Lay the patient flat with the legs raised.
2. Give 200 mg hydrocortisone intravenously.
3. Summon medical assistance.
4. Take blood for glucose and electrolyte estimation.

Table 14.7 Causes of hypotensive adrenal crisis

- *In a patient on systemic corticosteroids*
  Trauma
  Operation
  Anaesthesia
  Infection
- *Adrenal disorders* (causes of stress as above)
  Addison's disease
  Post-adrenalectomy
  Waterhouse–Friderichsen syndrome (adrenal
  haemorrhage caused by septicaemia,
  anticoagulants or epilepsy)
  Congenital adrenal hyperplasia
- *Hypopituitarism*

---

5. Give glucose if there is hypoglycaemia (25 g orally or intravenously).
6. Put up an intravenous infusion of normal saline or glucose-saline. Give 1 litre over 2 hours together with 200 mg hydrocortisone sodium succinate, repeating this at 4–6-hourly intervals as required and monitor the blood pressure.
7. Determine and deal with the underlying cause (*Table 14.7*) when the blood pressure has been stabilized. Control of pain and infection are particularly important and steroid supplementation must be continued for at least 3 days after the blood pressure has returned to normal.

Subacute adrenal insufficiency (corticosteroid withdrawal syndrome)

Subacute adrenal insufficiency develops if corticosteroid dosage is reduced too quickly after replacement therapy in postsurgical patients with Cushing's syndrome. Features include lethargy, abdominal pain, hypotension and psychological disturbances. Scaly desquamation of the facial skin, particularly of the forehead, is a characteristic sign. Hydrocortisone replacement needs to be increased if there are signs of adrenal insufficiency.

ADRENOCORTICAL HYPERFUNCTION

Adrenocortical hyperfunction may lead to release of excessive glucocorticoids (Cushing's disease), mineralocorticoids (Conn's syndrome or hyperaldosteronism) or androgens (congenital adrenal hyperplasia).

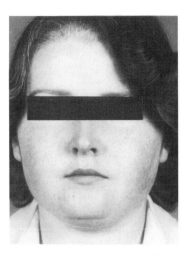

Fig. 14.4 Moon face in a patient with Cushing's syndrome

Cushing's syndrome and disease

Cushing's disease is caused by excess glucocorticoid production by adrenal hyperplasia secondary to excess ACTH production by pituitary adenomas, or occasionally by adrenal or other tumours such as small-cell lung carcinomas which produce ectopic ACTH. A similar clinical picture results where there is ectopic production by a tumour (usually a bronchial carcinoid tumour) of corticotrophin-releasing hormone (CRH). Cushing's syndrome is clinically similar but caused by primary adrenal disease (adenoma or rarely carcinoma or micronodular bilateral hyperplasia). The two terms are often used interchangeably. A similar syndrome is produced by systemic corticosteroid therapy (*Table 14.5*) and, rarely, by the multiple endocrine adenoma syndromes (*see Table 14.19*). The most obvious features are obesity, affecting particularly the face (moon face) (*Fig. 14.4*), interscapular region (buffalo hump) and trunk, but with relative sparing of the limbs. Hypertension has more serious effects and the breakdown of proteins with conversion to glucose leads to hyperglycaemia and diabetes mellitus, osteoporosis, muscle weakness, thinning of the skin, purpura and purplish skin striae. Acne is common and many patients become hirsute. Hyperpigmentation is uncommon and usually suggests that excess ACTH production is the cause.

- ### Diagnosis and management of hyperadrenocorticism

The main differential diagnoses are from severe depression, and alcoholism. Facial photographs may show the development of a moon face. Pituitary MRI or abdominal CT scans may be indicated. The plasma cortisol levels may be informative but are not always raised in Cushing's syndrome and it is better to look for absence of diurnal variation in cortisol levels, which are normally highest early in the morning and lowest at midnight. A corticotrophin-releasing hormone stimulation test should be used and a 24-hour urine collection should be assayed for free cortisol and 17-hydroxycorticosteroid levels which are increased. Another useful screening test is to measure plasma cortisol at 8.00–9.00 a.m. after giving 1 mg dexamethasone orally at midnight to suppress the adrenals temporarily (low dose overnight dexamethasone suppression test). This normally lowers cortisol levels, but in Cushing's syndrome there is no such fall. Other special dexamethasone tests or sampling from the inferior petrosal sinus are needed to distinguish pituitary from adrenal causes of Cushing's syndrome.

Corticotrophin-releasing hormone (CRH) stimulation test: This test depends on the fact that the pituitary is responsive to CRH, whereas adrenal tumours and other tumours producing ectopic ACTH, are not.

Baseline ACTH and cortisol levels are first obtained, CRH is then given. An exaggerated increase in plasma ACTH and cortisol levels is given by patients with pituitary Cushing's disease but not by patients with other types of Cushing's syndrome.

The pituitary tumour in Cushing's disease is treated by trans-sphenoidal microadenectomy and, for those not cured, then by pituitary irradiation. Cyproheptadine or sodium valproate are sometimes used where surgery is inappropriate. The adrenal glands responsible for Cushing's syndrome are usually irradiated or excised though medical treatment with ketoconazole, mitotane, aminoglutethimide or metyrapone has also been effective. About 10 per cent of patients subjected to bilateral adrenalectomy develop pituitary ACTH-producing adenomas with hyperpigmentation and symptoms related to the pituitary tumour (Nelson's syndrome).

Cushing's syndrome secondary to carcinoma of the bronchus is not controllable by surgery. Metapyrone, an inhibitor of hydroxylation in the cortex, can relieve symptoms.

- ### Dental aspects of Cushing's syndrome

There are no specific oral manifestations of Cushing's syndrome or disease, but, though it may be hard to believe, patients have been referred for a suspected dental cause of the swollen face.

Patients once treated are maintained on corticosteroid replacement therapy and then are at risk from an adrenal crisis if subjected to operation, anaesthesia or trauma.

Management complications may therefore include:

1. Need for corticosteroid cover.
2. Hypertension.
3. Cardiovascular disease.
4. Diabetes mellitus.
5. Psychosis.
6. Vertebral collapse or myopathy causing limited mobility.
7. Multiple endocrine adenomatosis (MEA I, *see Table 14.19*).

Hyperaldosteronism

A rare tumour or hyperplasia of the adrenal cortex results in primary hyperaldosteronism (Conn's syndrome). Secondary hyperaldosteronism may complicate cirrhosis, nephrotic syndrome, severe cardiac failure or renal artery stenosis as a result of activation of the renin–angiotensin system.

High aldosterone secretion leads to potassium loss and sodium retention. Loss of potassium often results in muscle weakness, polyuria and polydipsia, and, since it is associated with a metabolic alkalosis, may lead to tetany. Sodium retention leads to hypertension but rarely to oedema.

The aldosterone antagonist spironolactone is given until the affected glands can be excised.

- ### Dental aspects of hyperaldosteronism

In the untreated patient, hypertension and muscle weakness are the main complications.

Competitive muscle relaxants should be used with restraint if a general anaesthetic is needed, as they can cause profound paralysis.

If bilateral adrenalectomy has been carried out, the patient is at risk from collapse during dental treatment and therefore requires corticosteroid cover.

THE ADRENAL MEDULLA

The adrenal medulla secretes noradrenaline and adrenaline, which are normally released in response to hypotension, hypoglycaemia and other stress, their release being regulated by the central nervous system.

PHAEOCHROMOCYTOMA

Phaeochromocytomas are rare, usually benign tumours, producing excessive catecholamines. The tumours most commonly form in the adrenal medulla but may arise in other neuroectodermal tissues such as paraganglia or the sympathetic chain. Phaeochromocytomas may occasionally be associated with neurofibromatosis, or with endocrine tumours, particularly medullary carcinoma of the thyroid and hyperparathyroidism (multiple endocrine adenomatosis: MEA II or III, *see Table 14.19*). There is often then a familial incidence. Up to 25 per cent of persons with von Hippel–Lindau disease (cerebelloretinal haemangioblastomatosis) have phaeochromocytoma.

Typical features of phaeochromocytoma are episodes of anxiety, palpitations, sweating, pyrexia, flushing, fluctuating hypertension, headache and epigastric discomfort. Attacks may be accompanied by tachycardia, dysrhythmias, hypertension and glycosuria.

- **Diagnosis and management of phaeochromocytoma**

Diagnosis of a phaeochromocytoma is supported by finding excessive urinary catecholamines and metabolites such as vanillylmandelic acid (VMA) or metanephrines. Plasma catecholamines (collected at rest in the supine position) may also be increased but are less reliable than urinary assays. The site of the tumour is localized by such techniques as CT, MRI, venous catheterization, arteriography and radionuclide scanning.

The tumour is excised after the blood pressure has been controlled with an alpha-blocking agent, such as phenoxybenzamine, and a beta-blocker.

- **Dental aspects of phaeochromocytoma**

Acute hypertension and dysrhythmias are likely to complicate dental treatment. Elective treatment should therefore be deferred until after surgical treatment of the phaeochromocytoma. If emergency care is required, the blood pressure should first be controlled with alpha- (such as phenoxybenzamine or prazosin) *and then* beta-adrenergic (such as propanolol) blockers. A general anaesthetic must not be given to the uncontrolled patient and it is best to use neuroleptanalgesia using a combination such as droperidol, fentanyl and midazolam. It is best to avoid local analgesics containing adrenaline.

Patients who have had adrenal surgery for phaeochromocytoma may suffer from hypoadrenocorticism, since the adrenal cortex is inevitably damaged at operation. These patients therefore require steroid cover at operation. Phaeochromocytoma is occasionally associated with oral mucosal neuromas (MEA III syndrome, *see Table 14.19*).

THE THYROID

> **Key points**
>
> - Thyroid disease may present with goitre which can endanger the airway.
> - Lingual thyroid may present as a lump in the dorsum containing part or all of the functional thyroid tissue. This is best not excised unless adequate thyroid is present in the neck.
> - General anaesthesia is contraindicated in hypothyroidism and hyperthyroidism.

Key points

The normal thyroid produces two main hormones, thyroxine (T4) and triiodothyronine (T3). These hormones are stored as iodide-rich 'thyroid colloid' and released under the influence of thyroid stimulating hormone (TSH) from the pituitary.

The diagnosis of thyroid disease is mainly made on clinical grounds (*Table 14.8*), from the history and examination, and laboratory tests. There are many such tests but they may give conflicting results and no one alone is sufficiently reliable or comprehensive (*Table 14.9*).

T4 and T3 are bound to plasma proteins and only a small amount is free in plasma. It is, however, the free hormones that are biologically important. The free thyroxine index is useful since measurement of free T4 is difficult. The index is the ratio of T4 to binding protein (binding protein is equivalent to T3 uptake). Thyroid antibody tests, ultrasound and scans using ^{131}I are other common thyroid function tests.

GOITRE

A goitre is an enlarged thyroid gland. A goitre is usually a consequence of thyroid hyperplasia secondary to excessive TSH levels caused by decreased circulating thyroid hormone. Some goitres are congenital and seen in cretinism but most are acquired and seen in Graves' disease, or thyroiditis.

Table 14.8 Hypo- and hyperthyroidism – typical clinical features

Hypothyroidism	Hyperthyroidism
Cold intolerance	Heat intolerance
Decreased sweating	Excess sweating
Dry cold skin	Warm moist skin
Loss of hair	No hair loss
Decreased appetite	Increased appetite
Weight gain	Weight loss
Bradycardia	Tachycardia (atrial fibrillation)
Angina	Heart failure
Hoarseness	No voice change
Slow reactions	Tremor
Constipation	Diarrhoea
Slow cerebration, poor memory	Irritability
Psychosis	Psychosis

Table 14.9 Tests of thyroid function

Test	Hyper-thyroidism	Hypo-thyroidism
Hypothalmic–pituitary–thyroid axis		
Serum TSH	↓	↑[a]
TRH test (release of TSH by TRH)	ND	↓[a]
Thyroid function		
Radio-iodine uptake	↑[b]	ND
Concentration of serum thyroid hormones		
T4	↑	↓
T3	↑	↓
Free thyroxine index	↑	↓
T3 resin uptake	↑	↓
Other tests		
Thyroid autoantibodies	LATS	Thyroglobulin autoantibodies

[a]Depressed in pituitary hypofunction.
[b]Not suppressed by administration of T3.
Note: Basal metabolic rate not now used as a test.
LATS, Long acting thyroid stimulator; ND, not done; arrows indicate raised or lowered values.

Table 14.10   Causes of goitre

- Physiological
    Puberty
    Pregnancy
- Low iodine intake or natural goitrogens (endemic goitre)
- Drugs
    Thiouracil
    Carbimazole
    Potassium perchlorate
    Lithium
    Phenylbutazone
- Thyroid disease
    Graves' disease (toxic goitre)
    Dyshormonogenesis
    Carcinoma
    Hashimoto's thyroiditis

Thyroid cancer is another possible cause (*Table 14.10*).

•   Diagnosis and management of goitre

Thyroid function is assessed to determine whether it is normal (euthyroid), hyperactive (hyperthyroid) or hypoactive (hypothyroid), and the cause of the goitre is sought.

Most goitres do not require surgery but it is indicated if there is a danger of airways obstruction, as shown by cough, voice changes, dyspnoea, tracheal deviation or dysphagia. A large goitre may also need to be reduced for cosmetic reasons.

•   Dental aspects of goitre

Dental management in goitre may be influenced by changes in thyroid function, by the underlying cause of the goitre, or by complications such as respiratory obstruction.

A rare cause of goitre is a medullary carcinoma of the thyroid which can be part of a multiple endocrine adenomatosis syndrome (MEA II and MEA III, *see Table 14.19*). In the latter, numerous small plexiform neuromas are found in the oral mucosa, lips, eyelids and skin. The patient may also have a Marfanoid habitus and diarrhoea.

LINGUAL THYROID

The thyroid develops as a downgrowth from the foramen caecum at the junction of the posterior third with the anterior two-thirds of the tongue. Rarely thyroid tissue remains in this area and may be seen as a lump anywhere in the midline between the foramen caecum and epiglottis. Seen mainly in females, such a lingual thyroid is often asymptomatic but may cause dysphagia, airway obstruction or even haemorrhage. Hypothyroidism may be associated in about one-third of cases and, occasionally, the lingual thyroid becomes malignant. There is a raised incidence of thyroid disease in relatives. Ectopic thyroid tissue has also been recorded in the oropharynx, infra-hyoid region, larynx, oesophagus, heart and mediastinum.

A lingual thyroid may not be suspected until the lump in the tongue has been biopsied or excised and examined histologically, but if possible, should not be excised unless normal functioning thyroid tissue is identified in the neck. The diagnosis can be confirmed by iodine-123 or -131, or technetium-99 uptake in the tongue or by biopsy. The lesion can also be demonstrated by CT scanning *without* contrast or by MRI.

Treatment depends on the size of the lingual thyroid but thyroxine may be needed and if the lump does not regress sufficiently, the lingual thyroid can be ablated, best by surgery, or if the patient is unfit, by iodine-131.

HYPOTHYROIDISM

Hypothyroidism may be primary (thyroid disease) or secondary (hypothalamic or pituitary dysfunction). Most cases of hypothyroidism are associated with autoantibodies to thyroglobulin or thyroid microsomes. Surgical removal of too much thyroid tissue, or destruction by irradiation, are important causes in a previously hyperthyroid patient. Congenital thyroid disorders are rare.

Hypothyroidism is often unrecognized and subclinical hypothyroidism, with raised TSH but normal T4 levels, may be found in up to 10 per cent of postmenopausal females. Hypothyroidism may cause weight gain, lassitude, dry skin, loss of hair, cardiac failure or ischaemic heart disease, anaemia, neurological or psychiatric changes, hoarseness, bradycar-

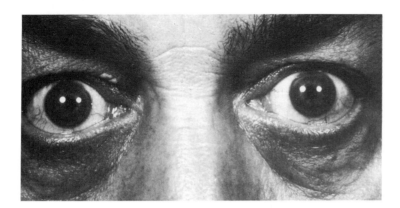

Fig. 14.5 Exophthalmos in hyperthyroidism

dia or hypothermia (*Table 14.8*), and may be complicated by coma. The respiratory centre is hypersensitive to drugs such as opioids or sedatives. Congenital hypothyroidism (cretinism) has similar features, together with an enlarged tongue and mental handicap.

- **Diagnosis and management of hypothyroidism**

The diagnosis is confirmed by demonstrating a reduced free thyroxine index (p. 276). The serum TSH is raised in primary hypothyroidism but depressed in secondary hypothyroidism.

Symptomatic patients are managed with daily oral thyroxine sodium. Treatment is always started slowly, but especially if there is evidence of ischaemic heart disease, as angina, myocardial infarction or sudden death may be precipitated.

- **Dental aspects of hypothyroidism**

The main danger in hypothyroidism is of precipitating myxoedema coma by the use of sedatives (including diazepam), opioid analgesics (including codeine), other tranquillizers and general anaesthetics. These drugs should therefore either be avoided or given in low dose. Hypotension and hypoadrenocorticism may be associated with hypothyroidism and diminished cardiac output and bradycardia are common. Anaemia or ischaemic heart disease (Chapter 3) are often complications. Local anaesthesia is therefore preferable to general anaesthesia.

General anaesthesia, if unavoidable, should be delayed if possible until thyroxine has been started and in any event must be given in hospital by a specialist anaesthetist, since it can precipitate circulatory failure.

Occasional additional problems are associated hypopituitarism and other autoimmune disorders such as Sjögren's syndrome. Povidone-iodine and similar compounds are best avoided.

HYPERTHYROIDISM

Most cases of hyperthyroidism are associated with a diffuse goitre (Graves' disease, primary hyperthyroidism) and thyroid-stimulating autoantibodies. Secondary hyperthyroidism is associated with thyroid nodules or nodular goitre.

Hyperthyroidism causes weight loss, anorexia, vomiting or diarrhoea, anxiety, tremor, sweating, tachycardia and heat intolerance. Eye signs such as lid lag, lid retraction and exophthalmos are also characteristic (*Table 14.8, Fig. 14.5*). Cardiac disturbances such as dysrhythmias (especially atrial fibrillation) or cardiac failure may complicate it, particularly in the older patient.

- **Diagnosis and management of hyperthyroidism**

The diagnosis of hyperthyroidism should be confirmed by determination of the plasma levels of T3 and T4. The free thyroxine index is also raised in hyperthyroidism. The TRH test is negative since raised thyroid hormone levels suppress the response.

Treatment may be medical, with antithyroid drugs or ^{131}I, or surgical. Carbimazole is the usual antithyroid drug. Beta-blockers achieve rapid control of many of the signs and symptoms of hyperthyroidism (since the latter causes sympathetic overactivity) and are useful preoperatively. Care must be taken in stopping beta-blocker treatment, since a thyroid crisis can be precipitated within 4 hours. Antithyroid drugs such as carbimazole can suppress the bone marrow and rarely cause rashes but nearly 50 per cent of patients have a relapse. [131]I is effective, but not infrequently results in hypothyroidism. Surgery is effective, but leads eventually to hypothyroidism in about 30 per cent of cases, but hypoparathyroidism or recurrent laryngeal nerve palsy are now rare complications.

• Dental aspects of hyperthyroidism

Pain, anxiety, trauma or general anaesthesia may precipitate a thyroid crisis in the untreated patient with hyperthyroidism. Thyroid (thyrotoxic) crisis is dangerous and characterized by anxiety, tremor and dyspnoea and can go on to ventricular fibrillation. It may also be precipitated by premature cessation of antithyroid treatment. Medical assistance is essential as treatment of a crisis requires the use of potassium iodide and propylthiouracil, and propranolol or chlorpromazine.

The hyperthyroid patient is especially at risk from general anaesthesia because of the risk of precipitating dangerous dysrhythmias. General anaesthesia must not therefore be given in the dental surgery until the disease is treated. If needed urgently, general anaesthesia should be given by a specialist anaesthetist in hospital. Patients with untreated hyperthyroidism may be also difficult to deal with as a result of heightened anxiety and irritability. The sympathetic overactivity may lead to fainting but the risks of giving adrenaline-containing local anaesthetics in moderate amounts are more theoretical than real. If there is anxiety on this score, prilocaine with felypressin can be given but is not known to be safer. Povidone-iodine and similar compounds are best avoided.

Sedation is desirable since anxiety may precipitate a thyroid crisis. Benzodiazepines may potentiate antithyroid drugs, and nitrous oxide, which is more rapidly controllable, is probably safer for dental sedation.

Medical treatment of hyperthyroidism with carbimazole occasionally leads to agranulocytosis which may cause oral or oropharyngeal ulceration. Otherwise the treated thyrotoxic patient presents no special problems in dental treatment. However, after treatment of hyperthyroidism the patient is at risk from *hypothyroidism* which may pass unrecognized. This point must especially be borne in mind if a general anaesthetic is required.

THE PARATHYROIDS

Key points

- Hypoparathyroidism may present with facial paraesthesiae and twitching in tetany.
- Hyperparathyroidism may cause:
  Giant cell granulomas (central).
  Jaw radiolucencies/rarefaction.
  Loss of lamina dura.
- The essential biochemical feature is a raised serum calcium level. Blood for calcium levels should be collected:
  from the fasting patient;
  early in the morning;
  with tourniquet off (venous stasis and fall in pH alter calcium levels);
  along with serum for albumin assay (albumin levels influence calcium levels).
- Parathyroid hormone (PTH) levels should be assayed, but results may be less helpful than calcium levels.
- Hypertension, dysrhythmias and sensitivity to muscle relaxants mean that hyperparathyroidism is a contraindication to general anaesthesia.

Table 14.11. Parathyroid function tests

	Calcium*	Phosphate*	Alkaline phosphatase	Urea*
Primary hyperparathyroidism				
without bone lesions	↑	↓	N	N
with bone lesions	↑	N or ↓	↑	N or ↑
Secondary hyperparathyroidism				
due to renal failure	N or ↓	N or ↑	N or ↑	↑
due to malabsorption	N or ↓	↓	↑	N
Tertiary hyperparathyroidism				
with bone lesions	↑	N or ↓	↑	N or ↑
without bone lesions	↑	↓	N	N or ↑
Hypoparathyroidism	↓	↑	N	N
Pseudo-hypoparathyroidism	↓	↑	N	N
Pseudo-pseudohypoparathyroidism	N	N	N	N
Vitamin D deficiency	↓	N or ↓	↑	N

*Serum concentrations.
Arrows indicate values above or below normal (N).

The parathyroid glands produce parathyroid hormone (PTH) which regulates a normal plasma calcium level by acting on the kidneys, gastrointestinal tract and bone. PTH secretion is stimulated by a fall in the level of the plasma ionized calcium. PTH increases the renal reabsorption of calcium and decreases phosphate reabsorption. PTH also increases bone resorption: both mineral and matrix are degraded and imino acids such as hydroxyproline thus released are not re-used but excreted in the urine. The excess bone turnover is reflected in a rise in the plasma level of calcium and of the osteoblastic enzyme alkaline phosphatase (*Table 14.11*).

Table 14.12 Clinical features of hypo- and hyperparathyroidism

Hypoparathyroidism	Hyperparathyroidism
Tetany	Renal stones
Epilepsy	Nephrocalcinosis
Candidosis*	Bone resorption
Cataracts*	Peptic ulcer: pain
Psychiatric disorders	Psychiatric disorders
Dental defects*	Polyuria
	Constipation
	Hypertension
	Weakness
	Acute pancreatitis

*Only in some types of congenital hypoparathyroidism.

HYPOPARATHYROIDISM

Thyroidectomy is still the most frequent cause of hypoparathyroidism. The idiopathic form of the disease is rare. Tetany is the classic feature of hypoparathyroidism, with numbness and tingling of arms and legs, facial twitching (Chvostek's sign; contracture of the facial muscles upon tapping over the facial nerve), carpopedal spasms (Trousseau's sign; contracture of the hand and fingers on occluding the arm with a cuff) and even laryngeal stridor. Plasma calcium is low and phosphate often raised (*Tables 14.11, 14.12*). Some cases of idiopathic hypoparathyroidism may be associated with other endocrine defects, particularly hypoadrenalism (poly-endocrinopathy syndrome) and sometimes chronic mucocutaneous candidosis (Chapter 21).

Post-surgical hypoparathyroidism is relatively transient and resolves when the remaining parathyroid tissue undergoes compensatory hyperplasia.

Idiopathic hypoparathyroidism has as its typical features tetany and stridor, cataracts, calcification of the basal ganglia, defects of the teeth and, occasionally, chronic mucocutaneous candidosis and other endocrinopathies – especially hypoadrenocorticism – associated with multiple autoantibodies (Chapter 21).

Pseudohypoparathyroidism is characterized by normal or raised PTH secretion but the tissue receptors do not respond. The clinical features are similar to idiopathic hypoparathyroidism but the patients are short in stature and have small fingers but no defects of the teeth. Similar appearance in patients with normal biochemistry is termed pseudo-pseudohypoparathyroidism.

• **Dental aspects of hypoparathyroidism**

Dental management may be complicated by:

1. Tetany.
2. Epilepsy.
3. Psychiatric problems or mental handicap.
4. Hypoadrenocorticism or other endocrinopathies such as diabetes mellitus.
5. Dysrhythmias.

Oral manifestations of idiopathic (congenital) hypoparathyroidism may include enamel hypoplasia, shortened roots with osteodentine formation, delayed eruption and sometimes chronic mucocutaneous candidosis which can be resistant to antimycotic treatment. There may be facial paraesthesia and facial twitching caused by tetany (Chvostek's sign).

HYPERPARATHYROIDISM

Hyperparathyroidism may be primary, secondary or tertiary.

Primary hyperparathyroidism is usually caused by an adenoma. Rare causes are carcinoma of the parathyroids or the genetic disorder familial hypocalciuric hypercalcaemia, in which there is impaired sensing of plasma calcium by the parathyroids and kidneys.

Hyperparathyroidism is most commonly a disease of postmenopausal women. The main features are hypercalcaemia, renal disease and, less commonly, skeletal disease. Most patients have renal calcifications and often hypertension, dysrhythmias and peptic ulceration (*Table 14.12*). Bone pain, pathological fractures, giant cell tumours, bone rarefaction or pancreatitis are now rare but the expression 'stones, bones and abdominal groans' may still apply to the features of hyperparathyroidism.

Hyperparathyroidism may occasionally be familial and associated with tumours of other endocrine glands (MEA I, II and III).

Measurements of serum calcium require attention to detail since (a) the level must be interpreted in relation to the serum albumin level, and (b) changes may only be intermittent. Ten millilitres of blood should be collected into a plain container, the venepuncture being performed (a) in the fasting patient, and (b) without venous stasis (take the tourniquet off before aspirating). Estimation of serum calcium levels should be repeated several times at intervals of a few days.

In hyperparathyroidism there is hypercalcaemia, the plasma phosphate level is low or normal, the plasma alkaline phosphatase level is normal (unless there is bone involvement, when the level is raised) and urinary calcium excretion is increased (*Table 14.11*).

Parathyroidectomy is usually needed. Medical treatment such as vitamin D (1,25-dihydroxycholecalciferol) is useful in those with severe bone disease.

Secondary hyperparathyroidism is a response to low plasma calcium caused by chronic renal failure or prolonged dialysis, or severe malabsorption, and is increasing in frequency. In contrast to primary hyperparathyroidism, renal stones are uncommon; the main manifestation is bone disease (usually renal osteodystrophy), which often responds to active vitamin D hormone (1,25-DHCC) but not to dietary vitamin D (cholecalciferol). Parathyroidectomy may, however, be needed.

Tertiary hyperparathyroidism follows prolonged secondary hyperparathyroidism which has become autonomous. Parathyroidectomy is then required.

• **Dental aspects of hyperparathyroidism**

Dental treatment in hyperparathyroidism may be complicated by:

1. Hypertension.
2. Cardiac dysrhythmias.
3. Renal disease.
4. Peptic ulcer.
5. Sensitivity to muscle relaxants.
6. Bone fragility.
7. Pluriglandular disease (*see Table 14.19*); MEA I (diabetes or Cushing's syndrome); MEA II or III (phaeochromocytoma).
8. Hepatitis B in secondary or tertiary hyperparathyroidism, resulting from renal dialysis.

Dental changes in hyperparathyroidism, which include loss of the lamina dura, generalized bone rarefaction and giant cell lesions, are late and uncommon. Giant cell lesions of hyperparathyroidism (brown tumours) are rare but histologically indis-

tinguishable from central giant cell granulomas of the jaws. If, therefore, a giant cell lesion is found, particularly in a middle-aged patient or in a patient with renal failure, parathyroid function should be investigated.

THE PANCREAS

> **Key points**
>
> - Diabetes is a condition of impaired carbohydrate utilization (impaired glucose tolerance) caused by insulin resistance or deficiency.
> - A random whole blood glucose above 10 mmol/l or fasting level over about 6.7 mmol/l usually establishes the diagnosis.
> - There are two main types of diabetics: juvenile onset and maturity onset.
> - Diabetic diets should have a constant carbohydrate content.
> - Hypoglycaemic drugs are used for maturity onset diabetics not controllable by diet alone.
> - Insulin is given to juvenile diabetics, subcutaneously, often twice daily.
> - The most certain way of assessing control is by serial measurements of blood glucose, usually by patients testing their own blood with a glucometer.
> - Glycosylated haemoglobin or fructosamine assesses long-term control.
> - Exercise, surgery and infection increase insulin requirements.
> - Hypoglycaemia rapidly arises if a meal is missed.
> - The great danger is hypoglycaemia, because of the risk of brain damage (neuroglycopenia).
> - Under local anaesthesia, always treat early in the morning. Always err on the side of hyperglycaemia.
> - Always consult the physician before considering general anaesthesia.
> - Well-controlled diabetics requiring a simple extraction under general anaesthesia may be managed under a short GA in the early morning, if the patient is going to be able to eat normally soon afterwards

Insulin, produced by the beta-cells of the islets of Langerhans, is the main pancreatic hormone, but several other hormones, such as glucagon, gastrin and vasoactive peptides, are produced.

DIABETES MELLITUS

Diabetes mellitus is the most common endocrine disorder and is the result of an absolute or relative deficiency of insulin from a variety of causes. It is characterized by persistently raised blood glucose levels (hyperglycaemia). Diabetes, if defined as fasting hyperglycaemia, affects at least 2 per

cent of the population but is recognized in only about 50 per cent of those affected and its prevalence appears to be rising. It is especially common in persons of Indian or Pakistani origin, and affects up to one-third of the elderly in those populations.

Diabetes is usually a primary disorder and only a few cases are secondary to diseases such as haemochromatosis or other endocrinopathies (*Table 14.13*). The two main types of primary (idiopathic) diabetes are the less common insulin-dependent juvenile (type I or IDDM) and maturity onset (type II) non-insulin-dependent (NIDDM) forms. Despite the name, about 25 per cent of the latter require insulin.

Table 14.13 Diabetes mellitus – causes

- *Primary*
  Juvenile onset (insulin-dependent, IDDM)
  Genetic type IA
  Autoimmune type IB
  (viral?)
  Maturity onset (non-insulin-dependent, NIDDM)
  Genetic type II non-obese
  Obesity type II obese
- *Secondary to:*
  Pancreatic damage
  Chronic pancreatitis
  Haemochromatosis
  Endocrine abnormalities
  Cushing's syndrome
  Corticosteroid therapy
  Acromegaly
  Phaeochromocytoma
  Glucagonoma
  Somatostatinoma
  Insulin resistance
  Many rare genetic syndromes

Insulin-dependent diabetes generally develops before the age of 25. There may be a viral aetiology; some cases appear to follow an attack of mumps or a Coxsackie virus infection. The disorder is autoimmune in nature and may have a genetic basis. The onset is relatively acute, typically with thirst, polyuria (especially at night), hunger and loss of weight. Lipolysis with increased production of fatty acids leads to over-production of acetoacetate which is converted to the other ketone bodies, hydroxybutyrate and acetone. These cause acidosis and thus hyperventilation. Ketone bodies also appear in the urine (ketonuria). Insulin is required daily for treatment, for life, and diet must be controlled.

Non-insulin-dependent diabetes mainly affects obese, middle-aged patients, often with a family history of diabetes. The causes of type II diabetes are several, and while the genetic basis has been difficult to identify, it is clear that subtypes result from mutations in the glucokinase gene, changes in insulin signalling molecules, defective phosphatidyl-inositol kinases or other mechanisms. The onset of diabetes in type II disease is gradual, but otherwise features are similar to type I diabetes. Most patients with this type of diabetes can be managed on diet and oral hypoglycaemic drugs and though some may need insulin, they are often resistant.

Acute complications of diabetes

The course of diabetes is variable. Many insulin-treated patients are liable to hypoglycaemia, due to an imbalance between food intake and insulin therapy. Some patients, particularly non-insulin-dependent diabetics, are readily controlled, while others are difficult to control (brittle diabetes) and prone to ketosis, severe acidosis and hyperglycaemia (diabetic coma).

Hypoglycaemic coma: Hypoglycaemic coma is usually the result of failure to take food, or overdosage of insulin, hypoglycaemic drugs or alcohol. It is increasing in frequency with the trend towards tighter metabolic control of diabetes. Hypoglycaemic coma is of rapid onset and may resemble fainting. There is adrenaline release, often with anxiety, irritability and disorientation, before consciousness is lost. Occasionally the patient may convulse. The pulse is strong and bounding, and the skin sweaty (*Table 14.14*). Less common causes of hypoglycaemia are shown in *Table 14.15*.

Hyperglycaemic (diabetic ketoacidotic) coma: Hyperglycaemic coma is the result of a relative or absolute deficiency of insulin and, in patients under treatment, may be precipitated by several factors (*Table 14.14*). Diabetic coma usually has a slow onset over many hours, with increasing drowsiness and signs of:

1. Dehydration (dry skin, weak pulse, hypotension).
2. Acidosis (deep breathing).
3. Ketosis (acetone smell on breath, vomiting).

Coma in a diabetic patient is usually due to hypo- or hyperglycaemia but it is important to consider other possible causes of loss of consciousness (Chapter 27). Furthermore, coma in a diabetic may be due to hyperglycaemia in the absence of significant ketosis (hyperosmolar non-ketotic coma) or, rarely, to lactic acidosis.

Management of coma in the diabetic patient
The cause should be established as soon as possible, but hypoglycaemia needs urgent treatment.

If possible, take blood for glucose measurement and if there is any doubt about the

---

Table 14.14 Comparative features of hypo- and hyperglycaemic comas and their treatment

Hypoglycaemic coma	*Hyperglycaemic coma*
Diabetes	
Known usually	May be unrecognized
Insulin	
Too much insulin or too little food or too much exercise or alcohol	Too little insulin, infection, or myocardial infarct
Manifestations	
Adrenaline release causes:	*Acidosis* causes:
Sweaty warm skin	Vomiting
Rapid bounding pulse	Hyperventilation
Dilated (reacting) pupils	Ketonuria
Anxiety, tremor	
Tingling around mouth	
Cerebral hypoglycaemia causes:	*Osmotic diuresis and polyuria* cause:
Confusion, disorientation	Dehydration
Headache	Hypotension
Dysarthria	Tachycardia
Unconsciousness	Dry mouth and skin
Focal neurological signs, e.g. fits	Abdominal pain, acetone breath
Management	
Take blood for sugar estimation	Put up infusion to rehydrate
If conscious give 25 g glucose orally	Take blood for baseline sugar, electrolytes, urea, Hb and
If comatose give 20 mg 20% dextrose	PCV
i.v. and on arousal 25 mg orally	
If unrestrainable for i.v. injection give glucagon 1 mg i.m.	
Call ambulance	Call ambulance

Table 14.15 Causes of hypoglycaemia

- Common (diabetics)
  Excess insulin or oral hypoglycaemic drug
  Missed meal
  Exercise
- Rare (non-diabetics)
  Insulinoma
  Hepatic disease
  Hypoadrenocorticism
  Hypopituitarism
  Functional hypoglycaemia
  Beta-blockers

Table 14.16 Treatment of hypoglycaemia

Patient conscious	*Patient unconscious*
2 teaspoons sugar *or*	20 ml 20% or 50%
3 lumps sugar *or*	dextrose i.v. *or*
3 Dextrosol tablets *or*	1 mg glucagon i.m.
60 ml Lucozade *or*	
15 ml Ribena *or*	
90 ml Cola drink* *or*	
1/3 pt milk	

*Not Diet type.

cause never give insulin but immediately give glucose as a diagnostic test. This will cause little harm in hyperglycaemic coma but will improve hypoglycaemic coma. Insulin, by contrast, can cause severe brain damage or kill a hypoglycaemic patient.

Hypoglycaemia must be quickly corrected or brain damage can result. If the patient is conscious, immediately give 10 g sugar or equivalent glucose solution by mouth (*Table 14.16*). If the patient is comatose, take a blood

sample for glucose estimation (2 ml blood in a yellow cap bottle containing fluoride) and give 10–20 ml of 20–50 per cent sterile dextrose intravenously. If a vein cannot be found, glucagon 1 mg can be given intramuscularly. On arousal, the patient should be given glucose orally.

Hyperglycaemic coma: If it is certain that collapse is due to hyperglycaemic ketoacidotic coma, the first priority is to establish an intravenous infusion line and start rapid

Table 14.17	Chronic complications of diabetes

Circulatory	Atherosclerosis
	  leading to ischaemic heart
	  disease, cerebrovascular disease
	  and peripheral gangrene
	Small vessel disease causing
	  retinopathy and renal damage

Renal	Renal damage and failure
Ocular	Retinopathy Cataracts

Neuropathies	Peripheral polyneuropathy
	Mononeuropathies
	Autonomic neuropathy
	  causing postural hypotension and
	  cardiorespiratory arrest

Infections	Candidosis Staphylococcal infections

rehydration. Blood should be taken for baseline measurements of glucose, electrolytes and pH. Raised plasma ketone body levels can be demonstrated with Ketostix (Ames). Insulin is then started – either 20 units i.m. stat. then 6 units hourly, or 6 U/h as an i.v. infusion. The intravenous infusion is required to correct dehydration, and electrolyte (especially potassium) losses, and to facilitate the administration of insulin. Medical help should be obtained as soon as possible (*Table 14.14*).

Chronic complications of diabetes

Diabetes mellitus may present with dry mouth, impaired vision, polyuria, polydipsia and skin infections or vaginal candidosis. It can also cause serious chronic complications: microangiopathy, macroangiopathy and neuropathy involve the eyes, kidneys, cardiovascular system, peripheral and cerebral vasculature (*Table 14.17*). Ischaemic heart disease, retinopathy, cataracts or renal failure may significantly affect management, and gangrene and amputation of part of the lower extremities are all too common. Autonomic neuropathy is common. Occasionally there are associations with autoimmune disorders, especially Addison's disease.

• Diagnosis of diabetes mellitus

Criteria for the diagnosis of diabetes are a fasting venous plasma glucose of 7.8 mmol/l (140 mg/dl) or random blood glucose higher than 11 mmol/l (200 mg/dl) on more than one occasion, and patients typically have polyuria, polydipsia, polyphagia and glycosuria. Fasting blood glucose levels lower than 6 mmol/l and random blood glucose lower than 8 mmol/l exclude the diagnosis.

Glycosuria is usually indicative of diabetes mellitus but must always be confirmed by blood glucose levels. The absence of glycosuria does not completely exclude diabetes.

A glucose tolerance test is only justified when blood glucose levels are borderline (about 7 mmol/l, fasting) and the clinical picture is not completely convincing. Glucose tolerance testing is now not routinely used since it appears to overdiagnose diabetes; if it is used, then the diagnosis of diabetes should only be made if, after an oral glucose load of 75 g anhydrous glucose, the plasma glucose is at least 11.1 mmol/l (200 mg/dl) on at least two occasions during and at the subsequent 2 hours. Persons with equivocal results are usually termed as having 'impaired glucose tolerance' and some may eventually progress to diabetes.

• Management of diabetes

The objectives of treatment are to maintain the blood glucose at near normal levels and to avoid acute or chronic complications, especially hypoglycaemic attacks. The young generally require insulin as well as dietary control. Elderly, obese diabetics often manage with diet control alone or with diet and oral hypoglycaemic agents – mainly sulphonylureas.

All diabetics should carry a card indicating the diagnosis, treatment schedule and physician in charge. Some diabetics wear a Medic-Alert device (*see Figs 1.2, 1.3*), and all should be advised to do so.

Diet: Diabetics should have meals at regular intervals, with a high fibre and relatively high carbohydrate content but avoiding sugars. The caloric intake should be strictly related to physical activity. The efficacy of the diet is controlled by checking the weight and glucose levels, either by urinalysis, or best by home glucose monitoring.

Insulin: Insulin is given by injection. There is no single standard for patterns of insulin administration. The dose varies widely between patients and also depends on the type of preparation, diet and exercise. Infection or trauma also increase insulin requirements. Nevertheless, there are three broad patterns of insulin use:

1. Conventional insulin therapy: this is one or two injections each day of an intermediate acting insulin (e.g. zinc insulin or isophane insulin), with or without small amounts of soluble (regular) insulin. As the daily output of insulin in a non-diabetic approximates 25 units, the average dose for a diabetic is up to this level. If the diabetes is well controlled, all the insulin is given before breakfast: if not, two-thirds is given then with the remainder at supper.
2. Multiple subcutaneous insulin injections (MSI): this typically involves a single injection of an intermediate, or long-acting insulin (e.g. insulin zinc extended or protamine zinc insulin) at supper, with injections of soluble (regular) insulin before each meal.
3. Continuous subcutaneous insulin infusion (CSII): a subcutaneous pump delivers a continuous basal rate of insulin which must be increased before meals depending on the blood glucose level. Since hypoglycaemia is a real danger, CSII has at present only limited applicability.

Neutral insulins purified to be virtually non-antigenic (monocomponent insulins) and human (recombinant) insulins have been introduced.

Oral hypoglycaemic agents: Sulphonylureas act mainly by stimulating the release of insulin from the pancreas. Chlorpropamide is potent, has a long action (up to 24 hours), is mildly antidiuretic and may predispose to cardiovascular complications by causing fluid retention, and to hypoglycaemia. Chlorpropamide, therefore, is best avoided in the elderly, especially those with cardiovascular disease, as it may worsen congestive cardiac failure. Tolbutamide is short-acting and of lower potency, and since it is less likely to cause unwanted hypoglycaemia in the early morning following a breakfast dose the previous day, it is preferred for the elderly. Gliclazide, glipizide, gliquidone, gliben-

clamide and tolazamide are also available. Sulphonylureas all may enhance, or be enhanced by, aspirin, anticoagulants, monoamine oxidase inhibitors, beta-blockers or clofibrate.

Biguanides (metformin) affect the absorption and metabolism of glucose and reduce appetite but are now used infrequently.

Other drugs include inhibitors of intestinal alpha-glucosidases, such as acarbose, which delay monosaccharide absorption and thus smooth the fluctuations in blood glucose levels. Troglitazone helps overcome insulin resistance.

Surgery: Gastric bypass surgery provides long-term control for obesity and diabetes in adult-onset diabetes, and also alleviates some of the complications.

Self-monitoring of glucose
Insulin-dependent diabetics should measure their own blood glucose levels at least daily, preferably using an instrument to read the blood reagent strips, and measure their urine for ketones daily. Non-insulin-dependent diabetics test their urine for glucose at intervals from daily to once a week and adjust drugs or diet to keep the urine free of glucose.

Long-term assessment of glucose control
This can now be achieved by estimation of the blood level of glycosylated (glycated) haemoglobin (HbA$_1$c). This is normal adult haemoglobin that binds glucose, remains in circulation for the life of the erythrocyte and therefore acts as a cumulative index of diabetic control over the preceding 3 months. Fructosamine is an alternative assay.

• **Dental aspects of diabetes mellitus**

Dental disease and treatment may disrupt the normal pattern of food intake and can interfere with diabetic control. A little forethought will prevent diabetics from collapsing in the waiting room at lunchtime from hypoglycaemia caused by missing a meal. Orofacial infections should be vigorously treated as they may precipitate ketosis. Drugs that can control – aspirin and steroids – must be avoided (Chapter 25).

Routine non-surgical procedures: Routine dental treatment or short minor surgical procedures under local anaesthesia can be

Table 14.18 Management of diabetics requiring general anaesthesia

| | Non-insulin-dependent diabetics[a] | | Insulin-dependent diabetics |
	Minor operations, e.g. few extractions	Major operations, e.g. maxillofacial surgery	Any operation
Before operation	Stop biguanides. If on chlorpropamide, change to tolbutamide 1 week preop.		Stabilize on at least b.d. insulin for 2–3 days preop. One day preop. use only short-acting insulin (Actrapid soluble or neutral)
During operation	Omit oral hypoglycaemic Estimate blood glucose level	Do not give sulphonylurea or subcutaneous insulin on day of operation. Estimate blood glucose level. Set up intravenous infusion of 10 per cent glucose 500 ml containing Actrapid or Leo neutral insulin 10 units plus KCl 1 g at 8.00 a.m. Infuse over 4 h. Estimate blood glucose and potassium levels 2-hourly. Adjust insulin and potassium to keep glucose at 5–10 mmol/l and normokalaemic	
After operation	Estimate blood glucose 4 h postop.	Continue infusion 4-hourly. Estimate blood glucose 4-hourly. Estimate potassium 8-hourly	
When resuming normal diet	Start sulphonylurea or other usual regimen	Stop infusion. Start Actrapid or Leo neutral insulin and over the next 2 days Start sulphonylurea Start normal insulin regimen	

[a]If well controlled, otherwise treat as insulin-dependent.
Adapted from Alberti and Thomas (1979), with permission.

carried out with no special precautions apart from ensuring that treatment does not interfere with eating. The dose of adrenaline used in dental local anaesthetic solution is unlikely to increase blood glucose levels significantly. Treatment is best carried out just after breakfast and routine antidiabetic medication, to allow the diabetic to have lunch.

Surgical procedures: The essential requirement is to avoid hypoglycaemia but to keep hyperglycaemia below levels which may be harmful because of delayed wound healing or phagocyte dysfunction. The desired whole blood glucose levels are therefore 120–180 mg/dl (3–5 mmol/l).

Special management considerations apply to the diabetic who is to undergo anything more than very minor procedures (*Table 14.18*). The main danger to diabetics during operation is that of hypoglycaemia. Therefore, intermediate insulins are usually omitted and treatment is carried out with the patient having an intravenous infusion containing glucose to which, according to the level of plasma glucose, regularly measured, soluble

(regular) insulin can be added as required. The effects of stress and trauma may raise insulin requirements and precipitate ketosis.

Precautions required during oral surgery in diabetics depend mainly on:

1. The type and severity of the diabetes and complications such as autonomic neuropathy that may predispose to hypotension or cardiac arrest.
2. The type of anaesthetic.
3. The extent of surgery.
4. The extent of interference with normal feeding postoperatively.

Many different management regimens have been suggested and each patient requires individual handling: the following therefore provides only general guidelines and the diabetician should always decide the regimen.

Diabetics controlled by diet alone
These diabetics are often obese or elderly with little liability to ketosis and if they are well controlled many can tolerate minor surgical

procedures, such as single extractions under local anaesthetic, without problems. A brief general anaesthetic can be given without special precautions apart from monitoring the urine sugar before the operation and on recovery, at 2-hourly intervals. However, such patients must have the anaesthetic in hospital, so that if ketonuria develops, blood sugar levels can be rapidly estimated.

Not all such patients are necessarily well controlled. In this case, or if more major surgery is planned, the patient should be admitted to hospital preoperatively for assessment and possible stabilization with insulin. The blood sugar should be monitored during and after operation.

Diabetics controlled by diet and oral hypoglycaemics
Patients controlled by oral hypoglycaemic drugs may tolerate minor oral surgical procedures under local anaesthesia, providing that normal meals are not interrupted. Well-controlled patients can safely have short simple procedures carried out under general anaesthesia in hospital without insulin, but the blood glucose should be monitored 2-hourly.

If diabetic control is poor, if the patient is on large doses of drugs or if more major surgery is planned, a suggested regimen is as follows:

1. Chlorpropamide must be stopped at least 3 days, or preferably a week preoperatively because of its prolonged action, and changed to tolbutamide or glibenclamide or, better, to soluble insulin three times daily.
2. Metformin must be stopped at least 2 days preoperatively as it tends to cause lactic acidosis.
3. Admit to hospital 2 days preoperatively for assessment and stabilization.
4. At 8.00 to 9.00 a.m. on the day of operation, blood is taken for glucose estimation and an intravenous infusion line is put up.
5. Infusion of 10 per cent glucose (500 ml) containing 10 mmol potassium chloride and insulin 5 units (if the blood glucose is less than 6 mmol/l) or insulin 10 units (if the blood glucose is higher than 6 mmol/l) appears to be satisfactory. The blood glucose is monitored regularly and

this regimen is continued at 100 ml/h until normal food can be taken orally.
6. The infusion is then stopped and the oral hypoglycaemic restarted.

Diabetics on insulin
Minor surgical procedures under local anaesthesia can be carried out in well-controlled diabetics with no change in the insulin regimen, providing that normal diet has, and can, be taken and that the procedure is carried out within 2 hours of breakfast and the morning insulin injection. In a well-controlled diabetic, minor operations under general anaesthesia, such as simple single extractions, can often be carried out safely by operating early in the morning and withholding both food and insulin until after the procedure.

More protracted procedures such as multiple extractions must only be carried out in hospital, with the following precautions:

1. Patients should be admitted preoperatively for assessment.
2. Before the operation, the patient should be put on soluble insulin and stabilized. Insulin may need to be given twice or three times daily, and control is confirmed by estimation of blood sugar (fasting, midday and before the evening meal).
3. The operation should be carried out early in the morning and booked first in the list, so that any delays in the operation schedule will not impair diabetic control.
4. At 8.00 to 9.00 a.m. blood should be taken for glucose estimation and an intravenous infusion set up giving glucose 10 g, soluble insulin 2 units and potassium 2 mmol/h (GIK infusion), until normal oral feeding is resumed – at which time the patient can be returned to the preoperative insulin regimen.
5. Blood glucose should be monitored at 2–4-hourly intervals until the patient is feeding normally.

General anaesthesia for the diabetic patient
General anaesthesia for the diabetic is a matter for the specialist anaesthetist since it may be complicated especially by:

1. Hypoglycaemia.
2. Chronic renal failure.

3. Ischaemic heart disease.
4. Autonomic neuropathy.

Autonomic neuropathy can lead to postural hypotension and impaired ability to respond to hypoglycaemia. Severe autonomic neuropathy carries a risk of cardiorespiratory arrest if a general anaesthetic is given.

Oral manifestations
There are no specific oral manifestations of diabetes mellitus but even well-controlled diabetics have a slightly more severe periodontal disease than controls. There is some evidence that severe periodontitis may upset glycaemic control. Initially tooth development appears to be accelerated but, after the age of 10 years, is retarded.

A dry mouth may result from dehydration and occasionally there is swelling of the salivary glands (sialosis), possibly due to autonomic neuropathy. The tongue may show glossitis and alterations in filiform papillae or (it is said) there may be burning sensations in the absence of physical changes. Oral mucosal lichenoid reactions may result from the use of chlorpropamide and some other antidiabetic agents (Appendix to Chapter 25). However, the 'Grinspan syndrome' (diabetes, lichen planus and hypertension) may be purely coincidental associations of common disorders probably related to drug use. Chlorpropamide may cause facial flushing.

If control is poor, oral candidosis may develop. Severe diabetes with ketoacidosis predisposes to and is the main cause of mucormycosis originating in the paranasal sinuses and nose (Chapter 20).

HORMONE-SECRETING PANCREATIC TUMOURS

Carcinoma of the head of the pancreas is the most common pancreatic tumour and the carcinoma with the shortest survival time, but hormone-secreting pancreatic tumours are rare.

Glucagonomas are frequently malignant and release large amounts of glucagon, a hormone that causes hyperglycaemia and abnormal glucose tolerance. Estimation of plasma glucagon levels differentiates glucagonomas from diabetes mellitus – the main cause of hyperglycaemia. Glucagon levels may also be raised in patients taking danazol.

A major clinical feature of glucagonoma is a distinctive bullous or pustular skin lesion (necrotic migratory erythema), but there is often also weight loss, anaemia and hypercholesterolaemia. Severe oral lesions have been reported, including bullae, erosions and angular stomatitis

The Zollinger–Ellison syndrome of diarrhoea and duodenal ulceration, due to a gastrin-secreting tumour, may be part of the multiple endocrine adenoma syndrome (MEA I: *Table 14.19*), whilst vasoactive peptides seem to be responsible for the watery diarrhoea, hypokalaemia and achlorhydria (WDHA) syndrome, which often includes hyperglycaemia.

Insulinomas are the most common cause of hypoglycaemia in those not taking insulin.

Table 14.19   Multiple endocrine adenoma syndromes – tissues affected

MEA type	Pituitary	Parathyroid	Thyroid	Adrenals	Pancreas	Others
MEA I (Werner's syndrome)	+++	+++	++	+++ Cushing's	+++ Zollinger–Ellison Insulinoma Others	Carcinoid Lipomas Gastrinoma
MEA II (IIa) (Sipple syndrome)	–	++	+++ Medullary cell Ca in 100%[a]	+++ Phaeochromo-cytoma in 33%	–	Dermal neuroma
MEA III (IIb)	–	–	+++ Medullary cell Ca in up to 80–100%	+ Phaeochromo-cytoma in 70%	–	Oral mucosal neuromas Marfanoid skeletal anomalies Visual disturbances

[a]Causes raised serum calcitonin levels and reduced serum calcium levels.

THE GONADS

Key points

- Oral contraceptives may predispose to thromboembolism, hypertension and liver disease and their action may be impaired by some antibiotics and anticonvulsants.
- Pregnancy is the ideal opportunity to begin preventive dental education.
- Spontaneous abortion is most common in the first trimester, a time when drugs, infections and irradiation also cause most fetal damage.
- Drugs (especially aspirin, tetracyclines, co-trimoxazole, retinoids and CNS depressants) and radiation should be avoided whenever possible during pregnancy, particularly the first trimester.
- Drugs that have been extensively used in pregnant women should be used in preference to newer drugs, and in the smallest effective dose. No drug is safe beyond all doubt.
- In general, most dental treatment is best carried out in the 4th to 6th month of pregnancy (second trimester).
- In the third trimester, avoid general anaesthesia because of the liability of vomiting and do not lay the patient supine, as this may cause hypotension.
- Lactating mothers should avoid aspirin, benzodiazepines and other CNS depressants, co-trimoxazole and tetracyclines.
- The menopause has been wrongly blamed for a number of oral complaints. Hormone replacement therapy, however, appears to reduce alveolar bone loss and gingival bleeding.

ORAL CONTRACEPTIVES

Oral contraceptives are usually mixtures of synthetic oestrogens and progestogens. They may act in several ways, especially by inhibiting ovulation by an action on the hypothalamic–pituitary axis, by altering the composition of uterine cervical mucus and by impeding implantation of the ovum.

The major risk in taking oral contraceptives is the increased incidence of thromboembolic disease (thrombosis of deep veins and coronary or cerebral thrombosis). However, the incidence of cardiovascular or cerebrovascular disease is normally so low in young women that these diseases are still uncommon even with a four- or fivefold increase in incidence in this group.

Hypertension, diabetes, jaundice and liver tumours, usually benign, are amongst the many other disorders increased in incidence in those taking oral contraceptives (*Table 14.20*). Most side-effects are thought to be caused by the oestrogen component, which is now only 50 μg or less.

Table 14.20 Adverse effects of oral contraceptives

- Minor
  - Nausea
  - Depression
  - Loss of libido
  - Breast pain
  - Fluid retention
  - Weight gain
- Moderate
  - Intermenstrual bleeding
- Serious
  - Thromboembolic disease*
  - Hypertension*
  - Myocardial infarction*
  - Gallstones
  - Liver tumours

---

*More frequent in smokers and older women.
Note: Adverse effects are low compared with the risks associated with pregnancy.

• Dental management of patients taking oral contraceptives

Worsening gingivitis and possibly slightly more severe periodontitis may result from

Table 14.21 Some drugs interacting with oral contraceptives to produce risk of pregnancy

- Significantly
  - Anticonvulsants
  - Barbiturates
  - Phenytoin
  - Carbamazepine
  - Primidone
  - Dichloralphenazone
  - Rifampicin
- Slightly (not necessarily significant)
  - Oral antibiotics
  - Ampicillin
  - Amoxycillin
  - Metronidazole
  - Tetracyclines

oral contraceptive use. There may also be a greater risk of dry sockets and, on radiography, there may be jaw radio-opacities or altered trabecular patterns.

The predisposition to myocardial infarction, thromboembolic disease and hypertension theoretically necessitates precautions if operation under general anaesthesia is required. However, if the patient is otherwise well, general anaesthesia in the dental chair is not contraindicated.

In spite of the risk of thromboembolism, the disadvantages of discontinuing oral contraceptives before dental general anaesthesia outweigh the advantages.

Some drugs may interfere with the action of contraceptive pills, usually by increasing the liver metabolism, and as a result may increase the risk of pregnancy. The drugs implicated are shown in *Table 14.21* but are mainly antimicrobials or anticonvulsants. Women prescribed such drugs, for example amoxycillin, other penicillins or tetracyclines, should be advised to use additional contraceptive methods whilst taking the drug and for at least 7 days after (4 weeks in the case of rifampicin).

Oral contraceptives may interact with anticoagulants to disturb anticoagulant control and they can impair the effect of tricyclic antidepressants.

PREGNANCY

Routine dental treatment of pregnant women under local anaesthesia is safe but general anaesthesia, some drugs and possibly radiography may endanger either fetus or mother. Infection control and avoidance of unnecessary drugs are particularly important in this group.

The fetus

Any woman of childbearing age is a potential candidate for pregnancy but may not be aware of pregnancy for 2 or more months, when, unfortunately, the fetus is most vulnerable. Fetal development during the first 3 months (trimester) of pregnancy is a complex process of organogenesis and the fetus is then especially at risk from developmental defects. Ten to twenty per cent of all pregnancies abort at this time, often because of fetal defects. Most developmental defects are of unknown aetiology but, in addition to hereditary influences, infections and drugs, such as alcohol and smoking, can be implicated in some cases. The only safe course of action is therefore to protect the patient as far as possible from infections and to avoid the use of drugs, particularly general anaesthetics, and radiography during the first trimester. In contrast, it is now recognized that folic acid supplements are an important way of minimizing the risk of neural tube defects such as spina bifida, and of facial clefts.

In the second and third trimesters the fetus is growing and maturing but can still be affected by drugs, such as tetracyclines, infections and possibly other factors. Nevertheless, despite the existence of a few disastrous exceptions, notably thalidomide and some retinoids, very few drugs have been *proved* to be teratogenic for humans.

Mercury: Concern has been expressed, particularly in Sweden, about the risk of placental transfer of mercury as a result of exposure to the metal during pregnancy. However, measurements taken at the Department of Odontological Toxicology at the Karolinska Institute on female dental personnel and their newborn babies and non-exposed controls have shown no significant differences in the plasma mercury levels or in the fetal/maternal ratios of mercury levels.

Experimental and clinical data do not suggest that there should be any restriction on use of amalgams or work restriction of dental personnel, provided that work practices are up to accepted standards.

The mother

Pregnancy is a major event in any woman's life and is associated with physiological changes affecting especially the endocrine and cardiovascular systems, and often with changes in attitude, mood or behaviour. Endocrine changes cause nausea and vomiting and deepened pigmentation, particularly of the nipples and sometimes the face (chloasma).

Diabetic control can be difficult, since insulin requirements rise, and pregnant diabetics need specialist attention. Pregnancy is a diabetogenic stress; glycosuria is not uncommon and glucose tolerance is impaired. These disturbances of carbohydrate metabolism usually resolve after pregnancy.

Cardiovascular changes in pregnancy include a rise in both blood volume and cardiac output. Initially there may be a slight fall in blood pressure with the possibility of syncope or postural hypotension. In later pregnancy 10 per cent of patients may become hypotensive if laid supine, when the gravid uterus compresses the inferior vena cava and impedes venous return to the heart (supine hypotension syndrome: *see below*).

The increased cardiac output is associated with tachycardia. Expansion of the blood volume may cause an apparent anaemia but in about 20 per cent of pregnant females true anaemia also develops, mainly because of fetal demands for iron and folate. Most patients are given both of these haematinics. Pregnancy may worsen pre-existing anaemias, especially sickle cell anaemia.

An important complication of pregnancy is hypertension, which leads to increased morbidity and mortality in both fetus and mother. Hypertension may be asymptomatic but, when associated with oedema and proteinuria (pre-eclampsia), may culminate in eclampsia (hypertension, oedema, proteinuria and convulsions) which may be fatal. The fetus is at risk because of possible placental separation or damage leading to prematurity, fetal lung damage or intrauterine death. Hypertensive pregnant patients should therefore rest as much as possible and have antihypertensive treatment.

A further complication of pregnancy is increased blood coagulability which can lead to venous thrombosis, particularly postopera-tively (Chapter 1) or occasionally disseminated intravascular coagulopathy (Chapter 4).

• Dental aspects of pregnancy

Pregnancy is the ideal opportunity to begin a preventive dental education programme and to advise on fluoride administration to the infant. Prenatal fluorides are not indicated as there is little evidence of benefit to the fetus. The teeth do not, of course, lose calcium as a result of fetal demands and there is no reason to expect caries to become more active unless the mother develops a capricious desire for sweets.

Drugs may be teratogenic. Drug treatment should therefore be avoided where possible, especially in the first trimester (*Table 14.22*). Because of the risk of coincidental mishaps it is wise to avoid giving any drugs, possibly even local anaesthetics, and postponing as much treatment as possible until after parturition in those with a history of abortions and those who have at last achieved pregnancy after years of failure. Many women are unaware of being pregnant in the early part of the first trimester and therefore it is preferable to avoid giving any drugs to women of childbearing age, unless absolutely essential.

When drug treatment is unavoidable, penicillin, cephalosporins and erythromycin (stearate or ethyl succinate) are probably safe antimicrobials, while paracetamol and codeine or dihydrocodeine are probably safe analgesics.

General anaesthesia and possibly sedation with diazepam or midazolam are particular hazards and must be avoided in the first trimester and in the last month of pregnancy. In addition, when a general anaesthetic is unavoidable but there is a mishap to the fetus, the mother is likely to blame the anaesthetist, even though this may be quite unjustifiable. Yet another hazard is an increased tendency to vomiting during induction in the third trimester.

Despite such considerations and the results of animal experiments, there is scanty evidence of teratogenic effects in humans from exposure to general anaesthetic agents. It is possible that barbiturates and benzodiazepines are teratogenic but the greater risk is late in pregnancy when they may induce respiratory depression in the fetus. Nitrous

Table 14.22 Drugs contraindicated and alternatives in pregnancy

	To be avoided	*Preferable*
Analgesics	Aspirin	Paracetamol
	Mefenamic acid	
	NSAIDs	
	Dextropropoxyphene	
	Pentazocine	
	Diamorphine	
Antimicrobials	Tetracyclines	Penicillin
	Fluconazole	Erythromycin
	Aminoglycosides	Cephalosporins
	Co-trimoxazole	
	Sulphonamides	Sulphisoxazole
	Rifampicin	
	Metronidazole	
	Ganciclovir	
Premedication	Long-acting benzo-	Temazepam
	diazepines (e.g.	
	diazepam)	
	Opioids	
Anaesthesia	Barbiturates	Nitrous oxide
	Prilocaine	Halothane
Others	Retinoids	
	Antidepressants	
	Carbamazepine	
	Corticosteroids	
	Danazol	
	Povidone-iodine	
	Thalidomide	
	Colchicine	

oxide, though able to interfere with vitamin B_{12} and folate metabolism, does not appear to be teratogenic though it is advisable to limit the duration of exposure.

NSAIDs may cause closure of the ductus arteriosus in utero, and fetal pulmonary hypertension, as well as delaying or prolonging labour. Aspirin, in addition, causes a platelet defect. Co-trimoxazole may cause neonatal haemolysis, and at least in theory, prilocaine can cause methaemoglobinaemia. Corticosteroids can suppress the fetal adrenals, and if given, a steroid cover is needed for labour. It is best to avoid metronidazole, or use a low dose, and to avoid azole antifungals, opioids, ganciclovir and povidone-iodine. Tetracyclines may cause tooth discoloration. Possible teratogens that should be avoided include carbamazepine, phenytoin, co-trimoxazole, and, of course, thalidomide (which is occasionally used to treat aphthae).

Radiography should be avoided, especially in the first trimester, even though dental radiography is unlikely to be a significant risk. Nevertheless, if essential, patients must wear a lead apron and exposure must be minimal.

Dental treatment is best carried out during the second trimester, but the same precautions still apply. Advanced restorative procedures are probably best postponed until the periodontal state improves after parturition and prolonged sessions of treatment are better tolerated. In the third trimester the supine hypotension syndrome may result if the patient is laid flat. The patient should therefore be put on one side to allow venous return to recover. Elective dental care should be avoided in the last month of pregnancy, as it is uncomfortable for the patient. Moreover, premature labour or even abortion may also be ascribed, without justification, to dental treatment.

In some pregnant women gingivitis is aggravated (pregnancy gingivitis) or may even result in a pyogenic granuloma at the gingival margin (pregnancy epulis). These conditions typically arise after the second month, and resolve on parturition. In a few women subject to recurrent aphthae, ulcers may stop (or occasionally become more severe) during pregnancy.

Hazards to pregnant dental staff
Chronic exposure to inhalational anaesthetic agents or mercury vapour, and exposure to infections by some viruses, such as cytomegalovirus or rubella, may pose occupational risks to non-immune pregnant dental staff (Chapter 11).

LACTATION

Since drugs may pass from mother to fetus, care should be taken in their use (*Table 14.23*). Cephalexin is a useful antimicrobial as it is not secreted in the milk. Fluoride passes into breast milk and if the local water supply contains more than 1 mg/l fluoride, supplements are not indicated for the breast-fed infant.

PREMATURITY

Lengthening survival rates of premature infants have revealed several long-term

Table 14.23 Drugs contraindicated and alternatives in lactating mothers

	May be contraindicated	Use instead
Analgesics	Aspirin (high dose)	Aspirin (low dose)
	Dextropropoxyphene	Codeine
	Diflunisal	Diclofenac
		Mefenamic acid
		Paracetamol
Anti-microbials	Tetracyclines	Penicillins
	Co-trimoxazole	Erythromycin
	Metronidazole	Rifampicin
	Sulphonamides	Cephalosporins
	Aminoglycosides	
	Fluconazole	
	Ganciclovir	
Premedication	Atropine	Benzodiazepines (low dose)
	Chloral hydrate	Phenothiazines (low dose)
Others	Beta-blockers	
	Antidepressants	
	Barbiturates	
	Etretinate	
	Carbamazepine	
	Povidone-iodine	
	Corticosteroids (high dose)	Corticosteroids (low dose)

sequelae, including orofacial defects. Some 20–55 per cent of affected children have enamel hypoplasia, compared with 2 per cent of controls. Factors involved range from birth trauma to infections or metabolic and nutritional disorders. Calcium disturbances are also common.

Laryngoscopy can damage the unerupted maxillary anterior teeth and intubation with an oropharyngeal tube can cause grooving of the anterior maxillary ridge. Fortunately, the latter has few serious consequences.

THE MENOPAUSE

The menopause is the termination of a woman's productive life and is marked by cessation of menstrual periods. The menopause can start at any age between 40 and 55 years.

In most women the menopause is not associated with serious physical or emotional complications. Some gain weight, lose some muscle tone and may develop a few hairs on the chin or upper lip. Hot flushes, when the patient feels a wave of heat passing over the body, are, however, common. Flushes may be momentary or last several minutes and their frequency is very variable. Hot flushes appear to be caused by vasomotor instability and may sometimes be controlled by oestrogens (hormone replacement therapy: HRT).

Psychological disorders are not uncommon in the menopause. They are usually mild and include dizziness and insomnia, but depression or paranoia may develop.

• Dental aspects of the menopause

The menopause has been blamed for many problems, although age itself is usually responsible. This period of life is, however, associated with emotional disturbances and stresses, particularly, no doubt, partly as a result of the changing pattern of family life. Depression is relatively common at this time.

Atypical facial pain and oral dysaesthesias are most common but there is little evidence of benefit from steroid sex hormones (Chapter 19). Dryness of the mouth and so-called desquamative gingivitis are not hormonal in origin. Sjögren's syndrome, lichen planus and mucous membrane pemphigoid are all more common in the middle-aged or older, and particularly in females.

HORMONE REPLACEMENT THERAPY

Replacement of reduced oestrogen secretion after menopause or oophorectomy, orally or implanted (hormone replacement therapy; HRT), slows the development of osteoporosis, and reduces the risk of osteoporotic fractures, as well as reducing overall mortality.

HRT also appears to reduce gingival bleeding and tooth loss in older women, as well as alveolar bone resorption, and improves salivary flow and buffering capacity. Overall, however, HRT appears not to improve oral complaints such as discomfort.

MULTIPLE ENDOCRINE ADENOMA (MEA)

MEA syndromes, also known as the multiple endocrine neoplasia (MEN) syndromes, are rare autosomal dominant diseases affecting several endocrine glands (*Table 14.19*). Their main relevance to dentistry is the presence in type III of oral mucosal neurofibromas, particularly along the margins of the tongue. These tumours may lead to the diagnosis of this potentially lethal disease. All, however, can cause difficulties in dental management as a result of the endocrine overactivity.

ENDOCRINE AND METABOLIC MANIFESTATIONS OF CANCER AND OTHER DISEASES

Tumours of various kinds, especially bronchial carcinoma, can be the site of ectopic production of polypeptide hormones or other biologically active substances producing various symptoms or signs (*see* Appendix to this chapter).

Facial flushing is characteristic of carcinoid syndrome due to overproduction of 5-hydroxytryptamine but is sometimes also seen in phaeochromocytoma, where there is release of sympathomimetic enzymes.

Hirsutism is seen in some patients with Cushing's syndrome, hyperthyroidism, acromegaly, adrenal or ovarian tumours. In polycystic ovary syndrome it is usually caused by excess testosterone and there is infertility and oligomenorrhoea.

Impotence is usually caused by psychogenic reasons, but diabetes, drugs, malignant disease and a range of other conditions may be responsible.

Gynaecomastia is typically caused by drugs such as oestrogens, marihuana, cimetidine or digoxin, but may result from chronic liver disease, haemodialysis, thyroid disease, or tumours (lung, adrenal, testicular).

BIBLIOGRAPHY

Alberti K.G.M.M. and Thomas D.J.B. (1979) The management of diabetes during surgery. *Br. J. Anaesth.* **51**, 693–710.

Bainton R. (1986) Interaction between antibiotic therapy and contraceptive medications. *Oral Surg. Oral Med. Oral Pathol.* **61**, 453–5.

Blinkhorn A.S. (1981) Dental preventive advice for pregnant and nursing mothers – sociological implications. *Int. Dent. J.* **31**, 14–22.

Brunt L.M. and Wells S.A. (1985) The multiple endocrine neoplasia syndromes. *Invest. Radiol.* **20**, 916–7.

Catellani J.E., Harvey S., Erickson S.T. *et al.* (1980) Effect of oral contraceptive cycle on dry socket (localized alveolar osteitis). *J. Am. Dent. Assoc.* **101**, 777–80.

Chiodo G.T. and Rosenstein D.I. (1985) Dental treatment during pregnancy: a preventive approach. *J. Am. Dent. Assoc.* **110**, 365–8.

Chow A.W. and Jewesson P.J. (1985) Pharmacokinetics and safety of antimicrobial drugs during pregnancy. *Rev. Infect. Dis.* **7**, 287–313.

Cook D.M. and Kendall J.W. (1980) Cushing syndrome: current concepts of diagnosis and therapy (Medical Progress). *West. J. Med.* **132**, 111–22.

Diaz-Arias A.A., Bickel J.T., Loy T.S. *et al.* (1992). Follicular carcinoma with clear cell change arising in lingual thyroid. *Oral Surg. Oral Med. Oral Pathol.* **74**, 206–11.

Downs A.T., Crisp T. and Ferretti G. (1995) Hunter's syndrome and oral manifestations. *Pediatr. Dent.* **17**, 98–100.

Editorial (1980) Corticosteroids and hypothalamic–pituitary–adrenocortical function. *Br. Med. J.* **280**, 813–14.

Editorial (1985) Measuring serum calcium. *Br. Med. J.* **290**, 728–9.

Findler M., Mazor Z., Galili D. *et al.* (1993) Dental treatment in a patient with malignant pheochromocytoma and severe uncontrolled high blood pressure. *Oral Surg. Oral Med. Oral Pathol.* **75**, 290–1.

Fuks A.B., Kaufman E. and Galiti D. (1980) Comprehensive dental treatment under general anaesthesia for patients with homocystinuria. *J. Dent. Child.* **102**, 340–2.

Gibson J. and McGowan D.A. (1996) Oral contraceptives and antibiotics. *BDJ Launchpad* **3**, 10–13.

Gislen G., Nilsson K.O. and Matsson L. (1980) Gingival inflammation in diabetic children related to degree of metabolic control. *Acta Odontol. Scand.* **38**, 241–6.

Glick M. (1989) Glucocorticosteroid replacement therapy: a literature review and suggested replacement therapy. *Oral Surg. Oral Med. Oral Pathol.* **67**, 614–20.

Grossi S.G., Skrepcinski F.B., De Carlo T. *et al.* (1997) Treatment of periodontal disease in diabetics reduces glycated hemoglobin. *J. Periodontol.* **68**, 713–19.

James V.H.T. (ed) (1992) *The Adrenal Gland*. Raven Press, New York.

Jashi J.V. (1980) A study of interaction of low dose combination oral contraceptive with ampicillin and metronidazole. *Contraception* **22**, 643–52.

Keith O., Flint S. and Scully C. (1989) Lingual abscess in a patient with anorexia nervosa. *Br. Dent. J.* **167**, 71–2.

Kinirons M.J. and Glasgow J.F.T. (1985) The chronology of dentinal defects related to medical findings in hypoparathyroidism. *J. Dent.* **13**, 346–9.

Laine M. and Leimola-Virtanen R. (1996) Effect of hormone replacement therapy on salivary flow rate, buffer effect and pH in perimenopausal and post-menopausal women. *Arch. Oral Biol.* **41**, 91–6.

Lamey P.J., Carmichael F. and Scully C. (1985) Oral pigmentation, Addison's disease and the results of screening for adrenocortical insufficiency. *Br. Dent. J.* **158**, 297–8.

Levin J.A., Muzyka B.C. and Glick M. (1996) Dental management of patients with diabetes mellitus. *Compend. Contin. Dental Educ.* **17**, 82–90.

Luyk N.H., Anderson J. and Ward-Booth R.P. (1985) Corticosteroid therapy and the dental patient. *Br. Dent. J.* **159**, 12–17.

Mazze R.I. (1986) Nitrous oxide during pregnancy. *Anaesthesia* **41**, 897–9.

McAndrew P.G., Nicholl A.D.J. and Beck P.R. (1982) The syndrome of inappropriate antidiuretic hormone secretion. *Br. J. Oral Surg.* **20**, 256–9.

Murrah V.A. (1985) Diabetes mellitus and associated oral manifestations: a review. *J. Oral Pathol.* **14**, 271–81.

Nathan D.M. (1993) Long-term complications of diabetes mellitus. *N. Engl. J. Med.* **328**, 1676–85.

Newrick P.G., Bowman C., Green D., O'Brien I.A.D., Porter S.R., Corrall R.J.M. and Scully C. (1991) Parotid secretion in diabetic autonomic neuropathy. *J. Diabetic Complications* **5**, 35–7.

Norderyd O.M., Grossi S.G., Machtei E.E. *et al.* (1993) Periodontal status of women taking postmenopausal estrogen supplementation. *J Periodontol.* **64**, 957–62.

Orth D.N. (1995) Cushing's syndrome. *N. Engl. J. Med.* **332**, 791–803.

Paganini-Hill A. (1995) The benefits of estrogen replacement therapy on oral health. *Arch. Intern. Med.* **155**, 2325–9.

Pories W.J., Swanson M.S., MacDonald K.G. *et al.* (1995) Who would have thought it? An operation proves to be the most effective therapy for adult-onset diabetes mellitus. *Ann. Surg.* **222**, 339–52.

Porter S.R. and Scully C. (1996) *Innovations and Developments in Non-Invasive Oral Health Care*. Northwood, Science Reviews.

Porter S.R., Eveson J.W. and Scully C. (1995) Enamel hypoplasia secondary to candidiasis endocrinopathy syndrome. *Pediatr Dent.* **17**, 216–9.

Reichlin S. (1984) *The Neurohypophysis. Physiological and Clinical Aspects*. New York, Plenum Press.

Scully C. (1979/80) Orofacial manifestations of disease. 5: Endocrine and metabolic disorders and iatrogenic disease. *Dent. Update* **7**, 175; *Hosp. Update* **6**, 9.

Scully C. (1988) *The Dental Patient*. Oxford, Heinemann.

Scully C. (1989) *The Mouth and Perioral Tissues*. Oxford, Heinemann.

Scully C. (1989) *Patient Care: a Dental Surgeon's Guide*. London, British Dental Association.

Scully C., Cawson R.A. and Griffiths M.J. (1990) *Occupational Hazards to Dental Staff*. London, British Dental Journal.

Seow W.K. (1986) Oral complications of premature birth. *Aust. Dent. J.* **31**, 23–9.

Smith B.K., Haug R.H., Shepard L. *et al.* (1991) Management of the oral and maxillofacial surgery patient on anabolic steroids. *J. Oral Maxillofac. Surg.* **49**, 627–32.

Smith N.J.D. (1982) Dental radiography during pregnancy. *Br. Dent. J.* **152**, 346.

Spinell C., Ricci E., Berti P. and Miccoli P. (1995) Postoperative salivary fistula; therapeutic action of octreotide. *Surgery* **117**, 117–18.

Taylor G.W., Burt B.A., Becker M.P., Genco R.J., Shlossman M., Knowler W.C. and Pettitt D.J. (1996) Severe periodontitis and risk for poor glycemic control in patients with non-insulin-dependent diabetes mellitus. *J. Periodontol.* **67**, 1085–93.

Wang P.H. and Korc M. (1995) Searching for the holy grail: the cause of diabetes. *Lancet* **346** (suppl), 4.

Whelan J., Redpath T. and Buckle R. (1982) The medical and anaesthetic management of acromegalic patients undergoing maxillofacial surgery. *Br. J. Oral Surg.* **20**, 77–83.

Williams J.D., Slupchinsku O., Sclafani A.P. *et al.* (1996). Evaluation and management of the lingual thyroid gland. *Ann. Otol. Rhinol. Laryngol.* **105**, 312–6.

Williamson L.W., Lorson E.L and Osbon D.B. (1980) Hypothalamic–pituitary–adrenal suppression after short-term dexamethasone therapy for oral surgical procedures. *J. Oral Surg.* **38**, 20–8.

Wilson J.D. and Foster D.W. (eds) (1992) *William's Textbook of Endocrinology*. Philadelphia, Saunders.

APPENDIX TO CHAPTER 14

ENDOCRINE AND METABOLIC EFFECTS OF SOME CANCERS

Substance released	*Most common tumours responsible*	*Disease caused*	*Features*
ACTH	Bronchial carcinoma Bronchial carcinoid Phaeochromocytoma Pancreatic carcinoma Parotid carcinoma	Cushing's syndrome	*see* p. 273
Antidiuretic hormone (ADH)	Bronchial carcinoma Hodgkin's disease Pancreatic carcinoma	SIADH	*see* p. 264
Parathormone (PTH) and prostaglandins	Almost any squamous cell carcinoma Renal carcinoma Breast cancer	Hypercalcaemia	Vomiting, constipation, polyuria, polydipsia, psychosis, abdominal pain
Thyroid stimulating hormone (TSH)	Trophoblastic tumours	Hyperthyroidism	*see* p. 278
Human chorionic gonadotrophin (HCG)	Pancreatic carcinoma Hepatoblastoma Breast cancer	Precocious puberty	
Erythropoietin	Fibroids Breast cancer Adrenal tumours Bronchial carcinoma Hepatoma Phaeochromocytoma	Polycythaemia	
Gastrin	Pancreatic carcinoma	Zollinger–Ellison syndrome	Multiple small-intestinal ulcers Diarrhoea
5-hydroxytryptamine and other vasoactive substances	Ileocaecal carcinoma Bronchial carcinoma	Carcinoid syndrome	Symptoms mainly if there are hepatic metastases Flushing, bronchospasm, diarrhoea Right-sided valvular heart lesions (especially pulmonary stenosis)

15

Metabolic conditions and nutrition

Key points

- Inborn errors of metabolism are rare disorders, not commonly relevant to dentistry, but often associated with neurological defects and learning disability.
- *Suxamethonium sensitivity* is a genetic condition in which suxamethonium is contraindicated, as the patient metabolizes this muscle relaxant very slowly.
- Patients with liver, renal or muscle disease, and those who have been burned, may be sensitive to suxamethonium.
- *Malignant hyperthermia* (malignant hyperpyrexia) is a genetic disorder in which general anaesthetics, muscle relaxants and other agents may be contraindicated.
- Oral infections may precipitate an episode of hyperthermia in malignant hyperthermia.
- Preoperative preparation with dantrolene can prevent malignant hyperthermia in susceptible persons.
- *Neuroleptic malignant syndrome* is a disorder in which hyperthermia follows the use of certain antidepressants and CNS-active drugs such as phenothiazines.
- *Hyperlipoproteinaemias* are a group of disorders characterized by high blood lipids which predispose to premature arteriosclerosis and ischaemic heart disease.
- *Porphyrias* are inborn errors of haem metabolism in which lignocaine, prilocaine, barbiturates, benzodiazepines and other agents may be contraindicated.
- *Obesity* predisposes to a range of problems including cardiovascular disease and diabetes. Jaw wiring is now an uncommon treatment for obesity.
- *Malnutrition* can lead to immunodeficiency and oral problems such as ulcers, angular stomatitis and glossitis, occasionally to sialosis or cancrum oris.

INBORN ERRORS OF METABOLISM

A vast number of rare metabolic disorders result from inherited enzyme defects. Most are recessive traits which do not appear unless both parents are heterozygous carriers. The disease appears in one in four (in statistical terms) of the offspring of heterozygous parents, often as a result of marriage of first cousins.

All but a few of the inborn errors of metabolism are rare and unlikely to be encountered in dental practice. Many inborn errors are associated with mental handicap or neurological disease. Some have a particularly high prevalence in certain racial groups. Many are quite innocuous (for example, hereditary pentosuria) but others, especially suxamethonium sensitivity, malignant hyperpyrexia, hyperlipoproteinaemias and porphyria, although rare, can seriously complicate dental management and especially general anaesthesia, and others, such as haemochromatosis, homocystinuria and glycogen storage diseases, can also be relevant. This section includes the inborn errors of metabolism most significant in dentistry. Others are tabulated in the Appendix to this chapter.

It must be repeated that most of these disorders will be encountered rarely in general practice, although in certain situations – especially in paediatric clinics or institutions for the handicapped – they are more common.

SUXAMETHONIUM SENSITIVITY

Suxamethonium (Scoline) is a depolarizing neuromuscular blocker acting similarly to acetylcholine. This agent has a brief action due to its rapid destruction by the plasma cholinesterase, and is therefore widely used for muscle relaxation during the induction of general anaesthesia.

About 1 in 3000 patients are abnormally sensitive to its action because of a defect in plasma cholinesterase. This is an autosomal recessive trait. If given suxamethonium, patients with this defect remain paralysed for several hours and unable to breathe. They therefore die unless artificially ventilated until the drug action abates.

Abnormal sensitivity to suxamethonium may also result from some other diseases (*Table 15.1*, Appendix to Chapter 25) or may be some sort of hypersensivity reaction.

Patients with suspected suxamethonium sensitivity must not be given it with a general anaesthetic in the dental surgery but should be referred to hospital for specialist attention. Local anaesthetic action is sometimes prolonged.

MALIGNANT HYPERTHERMIA (MALIGNANT HYPERPYREXIA)

Malignant hyperthermia is a rare inherited condition affecting about 1 in 12 000 children and 1 in 40 000 adults. It is characterized by a rapid rise in temperature when the patient has a general anaesthetic or another drug that can trigger an attack. The most common trigger is the combination of a halogenated volatile anaesthetic with succinyl choline. The mortality rate, in the absence of treatment, may approach 80 per cent.

Males are predominantly affected and 40 per cent of reported cases have been in children under 14 years of age. Two forms of malignant hyperthermia are recognized – an autosomal dominant type where the individuals are normal between attacks, and a recessive type affecting young boys who have various congenital abnormalities including short stature. Patients with myotonia congenita, myotonic dystrophy, central core disease and Evan syndrome (proximal wasting; short stature; kyphoscoliosis) are particularly susceptible.

The main drugs liable to precipitate malignant hyperthermia are the potent inhalational anaesthetic agents such as halothane, and muscle relaxants including suxamethonium and curare-like (non-depolarizing) agents.

Table 15.1 Conditions in which the action of suxamethonium may be prolonged

- Inherited suxamethonium sensitivity (Scoline sensitivity)
- Myopathies
  Malignant hyperpyrexia
  Dystrophia myotonica and myotonia congenita
  Myasthenia gravis
- Liver disease
- Renal disease
- Burns
- Drugs
  Trasylol
  Cyclophosphamide
  Procaine
  Phenothiazines
  Pancuronium
  Cytotoxic drugs

Table 15.2 Drugs contraindicated and alternatives in malignant hyperpyrexia in susceptible subjects

	Contraindicated	*Safe to use*
Premedication	Atropinics	Diazepam
General anaesthetics	Halothane	Methohexitone
	Ether	Thiopentone
	Cyclopropane	Nitrous oxide
	Ketamine	
	Enflurane	
Muscle relaxants	Suxamethonium	Pancuronium
	Curare	
Antidepressants	Tricyclic antidepressants	
	Monoamine oxidase inhibitors	

Intravenous anaesthetic agents are usually safe (*Table 15.2*).

Malignant hyperpyrexia has been reported after administration of nitrous oxide but this is extremely rare. The brevity of most dental general anaesthetics is possibly a factor that makes hyperpyrexial reactions rare in dentistry.

Local anaesthesia is safe. Amide local anaesthetic agents, including lignocaine and prilocaine, were thought to be weak triggering agents, but this has been dismissed.

Inquiry into the family history is essential before giving a general anaesthetic as there are no absolutely reliable predictive tests. Unfortunately, absence of reaction to a previous anaesthetic does not exclude the possibility of a reaction on the next occasion. The syndrome may develop after a single anaesthetic exposure or after several uneventful exposures.

The importance of the family history is emphasized by the fact that a dental patient reported to the writers had had 14 relatives die under general anaesthesia. Understandably, this patient was less than enthusiastic about the idea of a general anaesthetic for dental purposes.

In a member of an affected family, raised serum creatine kinase and pyrophosphate levels are indicative of susceptibility, but nearly one-third of patients have normal levels of creatine kinase. Excessive in vitro response of muscle to halothane, suxamethonium or caffeine, and raised myophosphorylase A levels, may be detected but muscle biopsy is necessary for these tests.

The onset of malignant hyperthermia may be detected by poor muscular relaxation after induction of anaesthesia or complete failure of the jaw to relax after suxamethonium has been given. However, it is controversial whether masseter spasm is a reliable early sign. Suxamethonium, unlike pancuronium or vecuronium, causes jaw stiffness in many normal children, but intense muscle spasm may be significant.

There is a rise in temperature with tachycardia or dysrhythmias and hypotension. Late complications include pulmonary oedema, acute renal failure and disseminated intravascular coagulation. Malignant hyperthermia is a medical emergency with a high mortality rate.

- **Dental aspects of malignant hyperthermia**

If a positive family history is obtained, dentistry can usually be safely carried out under local anaesthesia or relative analgesia. For major oral surgery, specialist anaesthetic care is needed and thiopentone or methohexitone is used. In the event of hyperthermia, surgery must be stopped and the patient cooled. Oxygen and a bicarbonate intravenous infusion (2 mEq/kg) to counteract the metabolic acidosis, should also be given. Dantrolene sodium (1–2 mg/kg i.v. every 5–10 min to a total dose of 10 mg/kg) or procainamide are effective in controlling the disease. Dantrolene given preoperatively and postoperatively for about 3 days (4–7 mg/kg/day) may prevent hyperthermia.

Dental infections should be quickly and effectively treated since they also may precipitate attacks.

NEUROLEPTIC MALIGNANT SYNDROME

A rare but potentially lethal complication of the use of certain non-anaesthetic drugs such as phenothiazines, haloperidol or flupenthixol, and other neuroleptics, and tricyclic or monoamine oxidase inhibitor antidepressives, or abrupt withdrawal of levodopa, is known as neuroleptic malignant syndrome. The salient features are hyperthermia, muscle rigidity, fluctuating consciousness and autonomic dysfunction. The last causes pallor, sweating, tachycardia, labile blood pressure and incontinence. Symptoms may persist for several days or death can result from renal failure. The relationship to malignant hyperthermia is unknown. The causative drug should be stopped and dantrolene or bromocriptine should be given.

To avoid this hazard, phenothiazines should be avoided for patients who have stopped their levodopa before a general anaesthetic. Levodopa can be given before a general anaesthetic apart from the fact that it may cause vomiting.

HYPERLIPOPROTEINAEMIA (HYPERLIPIDAEMIA)

The main plasma lipids are triglycerides, cholesterol ester and phospholipids (lecithin,

---

Table 15.3   Primary hyperlipoproteinaemias

Type		*Main manifestations*
I	Hypertriglyceridaemia (hyperchylomicronaemia)	Xanthomas Acute pancreatitis (rare)
II	Hyperbetalipoproteinaemia (hypercholesterolaemia)	Atherosclerosis Ischaemic heart disease Xanthomas and xanthelasmas (common)
III	Dysbetalipoproteinaemia (broad-beta disease)	Atherosclerosis Peripheral vascular disease Xanthomas Hyperglycaemia (rare)
IV	Endogenous hyperlipoproteinaemia	Mild glucose intolerance Hyperuricaemia Atherosclerosis Xanthomas (common)
V	Mixed hyperlipidaemia	Acute pancreatitis Xanthomas (rare)

---

sphingomyelin etc.). Non-esterified fatty acids and cholesterol are also present. Plasma lipoproteins are responsible for the transport of lipids and cholesterol within the body. The lipoproteins are divided into four groups based on their density and electrophoretic mobility.

Hyperlipoproteinaemia can be primary or secondary. Primary hyperlipoproteinaemias are often genetically determined (*Table 15.3*). Their importance is that several of them lead to accelerated atherosclerosis and premature death from ischaemic heart disease. Secondary hyperlipoproteinaemias may be caused by diabetes, hypothyroidism, nephrotic syndrome, liver disease, alcoholism and use of oral contraceptives. Pravastatin reduces blood cholesterol levels and serious cardiovascular events.

- ### Dental aspects of the hyperlipoproteinaemias

Premature coronary heart disease may result from hyperlipoproteinaemias, especially type II. Other factors such as hypertension, diabetes or smoking further increase the risk of coronary heart disease. Occasionally patients with hyperlipoproteinaemias may be recognized by the presence of cutaneous xanthomas (xanthelasmas) on the eyelids (*Fig. 15.1*). Xanthomas consist of slightly raised yellowish plaques. Although seen in familial dysbetalipoproteinaemia and then associated with accelerated atherosclerosis and heart disease, xanthelasmas are not specific to type II hyperlipoproteinaemia. A unique feature of this disorder, however, is the association of prominent xanthomas on the elbows and

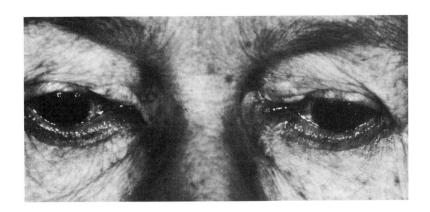

Fig. 15.1 Xanthelasma in familial hyperlipidaemia: such lesions may suggest a high risk of ischaemic heart disease

knees, especially with yellow to orange discoloration of the palmar creases.

Type IV and V hyperlipoproteinaemias may be complicated by sicca syndrome.

HYPOLIPOPROTEINAEMIAS

Pulpal calcifications and unusual odontomes may be found in high density lipoprotein deficiency (Tangier disease).

THE PORPHYRIAS

Porphyrias are inborn errors of haem metabolism. Porphyrias are divided into two main groups according to the principal site of the enzyme defect, namely in the liver (hepatic porphyrias) or the red blood cells (the erythropoietic porphyrias). Only the hepatic porphyrias, particularly variegate and acute intermittent porphyria, are important in dentistry (*Table 15.4*).

Variegate porphyria is estimated to affect 1 in 400 South Africans of Afrikaner descent. The main features are attacks of acute, severe abdominal pain accompanied by neuropsychiatric and cardiovascular disturbances. The neurological disturbance is typically a peripheral sensory and motor neuropathy but respiratory embarrassment or major convulsions can develop. Tachycardia and hypertension develop in the majority and may be followed by postural hypotension. Barbiturates, some other drugs, fasting, acute infections and pregnancy can precipitate attacks, but between attacks patients may appear normal apart from severe photosensitivity rashes which affect about 80 per cent of Afrikaner patients. These rashes typically cause hyperpigmentation of the face and hands (exposed areas).

Table 15.4   The porphyrias

- Hepatic porphyrias
  Acute intermittent porphyria (AIP)
  Hereditary coproporphyria
  Variegate porphyria
  Cutaneous porphyria
- Erythropoietic porphyrias
  Erythropoietic protoporphyria
  Congenital porphyria

Acute intermittent porphyria shows essentially the same features but the attacks may be even more severe and end in fatal respiratory failure. Rashes are not, however, a feature.

The diagnosis of the acute hepatic porphyrias is confirmed by demonstrating aminolaevulinic acid and porphobilinogen in the urine.

The essentials of treatment of attacks are, if possible, to stop the administration of the triggering drug and to give fluids, electrolytes and glucose by intravenous infusion.

• Dental aspects of porphyria

Prevention of attacks in hepatic porphyrias is by the avoidance of various drugs. Antidepressants, antihistamines, barbiturates (including the intravenous barbiturates), benzodiazepines, carbamazepine, cephalosporins, enflurane, flucloxacillin, halothane, ketoconazole, lignocaine, mefenamic acid, miconazole, pentazocine, prilocaine, sulphon-

---

Table 15.5   Drugs contraindicated and alternatives used in porphyria

	Contraindicated	Safe to use
Local anaesthetics	Lignocaine Prilocaine	Bupivacaine
General anaesthetics	Barbiturates Enflurane Halothane	
Analgesics	Diclofenac Mefenamic acid Pentazocine Opioids	Aspirin Paracetamol Codeine
Antibiotics	Doxycycline Erythromycin Sulphonamides[a]	Amoxycillin Ampicillin Penicillins Tetracyclines
Antifungals	Fluconazole Ketoconazole Miconazole	
Psychoactive drugs	Barbiturates Benzodiazepines Carbamazepine Chlordiazepoxide Dichloralphenazone Imipramine Meprobamate Monoamine oxidase inhibitors Phenytoin Tricyclics	Chlorpromazine Promazine Temazepam
Endocrine active drugs	Chlorpropamide Contraceptive pill	

[a]Co-trimoxazole contains a sulphonamide.

amides, trimethoprim and other drugs (*Table 15.5*) liable to precipitate attacks are absolutely contraindicated. Bupivacaine, penicillins (except pivampicillin), aspirin, paracetamol, codeine, dihydrocodeine, opioids and corticosteroids are safe.

One type of erythropoietic porphyria is characterized by red discoloration of the teeth (which fluoresce in ultraviolet light), hypertrichosis, severe mutilating photosensitivity rashes and haemolytic anaemia. Fewer than 100 cases have probably ever been reported, but it has been suggested that this disease might have been the source of the werewolf legend because of the red teeth (thought to be dripping with blood), the hairy distorted facial features and avoidance of daylight.

HAEMOCHROMATOSIS

Haemochromatosis is an uncommon disorder of iron metabolism characterized by high serum ferritin levels and deposition of iron, as haemosiderin, in many tissues, particularly the liver, abdominal lymph nodes, skin, adrenals, pancreas, salivary glands and heart. A sicca syndrome may be a complication. A fibrotic reaction to these deposits can result in cirrhosis, skin pigmentation, adrenocortical insufficiency, diabetes (bronze diabetes) or cardiomyopathy, any of which can affect dental management. Treatment is by venesection.

HOMOCYSTINURIA

Homocystinuria is an inborn error of methionine metabolism with an autosomal recessive inheritance. Affected patients are tall with a Marfanoid appearance, joint hypermobility, ectopia lentis and visual and mental deterioration. Blood vessel abnormalities together with increased platelet adhesiveness predispose to thromboembolism, both spontaneously and postoperatively. Dextran 40 or 70 infusion intravenously perioperatively may reduce the thromboembolic risk.

GLYCOGEN STORAGE DISEASES (GSD)

GSD are rare disorders characterized by an accumulation of glycogen due to inherited

---

Table 15.6 Causes of gingival enlargement

I Generalized

Congenital
Hereditary gingival fibromatosis and related disorders
Mucopolysaccharidosis I-H
Fucosidosis
Aspartylglycosaminuria
Leprechaunism (Donohue syndrome)
Pfeiffer syndrome
Infantile systemic hyalinosis
Primary amyloidosis
Others

Acquired
Haematological
   Acute myeloid leukaemia
   Preleukaemic leukaemia(s)
   Aplastic anaemia
   Vitamin C deficiency
Drugs: Phenytoin
      Cyclosporin
      Calcium channel blockers – nifedipine
                              diltiazem
                              nitrendipine
                              felodipine
                              verapamil
      Others – sodium valporate
                     tranexamic acid
Deposits
   Lipoid proteinosis
   Ligneous conjunctivitis
   Mucocutaneous amyloidosis

II Localized

Congenital
Fabry's syndrome (angiokeratoma corporis diffusum universale)
Cowden's syndrome (multiple hamartoma and neoplasia syndrome)
Tuberous sclerosis
Sturge–Weber angiomatosis
Congenital gingival granular cell tumour

Acquired
Heck's disease
Lymphomas
Langerhans' cell tumours
Multiple myeloma
Plasmacytomas
Other primary and
secondary neoplasms, e.g. papillomas
                    squamous cell carcinoma
                    Kaposi's sarcoma
Wegener's granulomatosis
Pregnancy epulis
Fibrous epulis
Giant cell epulis (e.g. secondary to primary hyperparathyroidism)
Sarcoidosis
Crohn's disease and related disorders

defects in degradative enzyme. Glycogen cannot therefore be mobilized to glucose. Hypoglycaemia is common, as are infections. Glycogen accumulates mainly in liver and muscle, and hepatomegaly is common. Muscle pain, weakness, respiratory muscle weakness and cardiac failure may be seen. Enlarged tongue, periodontal breakdown and masticatory muscle pain have been described. Patients with GDS type 1b have a bleeding tendency, corrected pre-operatively by 24–48 hours' glucose infusion.

GINGIVAL SWELLING DUE TO METABOLIC DEPOSITS

A few cases of gingival hyperplasia are part of an obviously systemic syndrome (*Table 15.6*). In some instances the gingival swelling is only a very minor aspect of a wider disorder caused by abnormal deposits of various materials – such as in infantile systemic hyalinosis. A variety of hyaline deposits, ranging from classical amyloid, to mixtures of immunoglobulins, fibrin, fibrinogen and albumin, or lipoid material, may be found in the gingivae and, indeed, amyloid is itself a non-specific term for a spectrum of different entities including immunoglobulin light chains, serum amyloid fibrillar proteins, beta$_2$-microglobulin, keratin, transthyretin and others. Ocular lesions are uncommonly seen in disorders associated with gingival swelling but have been recorded in primary amyloidosis, lipoid proteinosis – sometimes termed hyalinosis cutis et mucosae or Urbach–Wiethe disease, ligneous conjunctivi-tis, gingival fibromatosis with corneal dystrophy – the Rutherford syndrome, and in a newly described disorder of generalized gingival enlargement due to amyloid-like material.

Lipoid proteinosis is a rare, recessively inherited disorder characterized by hyaline infiltrates in the skin, larynx, internal organs and oral tissues. The infiltrate appears at an early age and may present with hoarseness, yellow-brown nodules on the face and lips mainly, and sometimes elsewhere such as over the elbows, in the axillae, and particularly on the margins of the eyelids. The oral mucosae may be affected with infiltrates in the tongue, fauces, lips and, occasionally, gingivae. Gingival swelling, sometimes with ulceration, has been the main oral feature described, the hyaline material staining strongly with periodic acid Schiff (PAS) and for lipid (Sudan Black), while amyloid stains are negative. Deposits in lipid proteinosis are initially around capillaries and there are changes in collagen.

Ligneous conjunctivitis is a rare idiopathic form of chronic membranous conjunctivitis often with associated lesions in the larynx, nose, cervix and gingivae. The lesions are characterized by subepithelial eosinophilic infiltrates containing fibrin, immunoglobulin and albumin. There is no staining for glycogen lipid or amyloid. In most instances ligneous conjunctivitis may represent an autosomal recessive disorder or there may be other causes of blood vessel hyperpermeability, including drugs. The gingival lesions described in ligneous conjunctivitis have been swelling with ulceration

ACQUIRED METABOLIC DISORDERS

AMYLOID DISEASE

This is discussed in Chapter 6.

DIET AND NUTRITION

These are the most important factors affecting metabolism.

Dietary disorders

The importance of diet in dental health is well reviewed elsewhere (Rugg-Gunn 1993). The importance of diet in oral health has been less well appreciated until recently but it is now clear that mucosal health is also dependent on correct nutrition (Chapters 5 and 6, and Midda and Konig 1994).

Many recent studies have implicated dietary factors as influencing the development of cancer (Chapter 5), arteriosclerosis and coronary artery disease (Chapter 3), birth defects such as facial clefts and spina bifida (Chapters 9 and 17) and cataracts. Overall the evidence suggests the following to be beneficial.

1. Minimizing the intake of fats which are saturated (especially those from dairy sources) and partially halogenated vegetable fats. Consumption of mono-unsaturated fats such as olive oil might be beneficial.
2. Eating generous amounts of vegetables and fruit daily. Such habits appear to offer protection against cancers of the stomach, colon and lung, and possibly against cancers of the mouth, larynx, cervix, bladder and breast. Fibre intake also offers some protection against hypertension and coronary heart disease. In contrast, suboptimal intake of folic acid in pregnancy predisposes the fetus to neural tube defects and facial clefts.
3. Carbohydrates are best taken as whole grain unrefined products. These offer some protection against caries, colon cancer and diverticulitis.

Obesity

Obesity rather than malnutrition is the main nutritional problem in the Western World. Although many fat people believe that they have a glandular disorder, this is hardly ever the case. Obesity simply results from eating more than the body needs. Obesity can, however, *occasionally* be the result of hypothalamic disease (Fröhlich's, Laurence–Moon–Biedl or Prader–Willi syndromes, *see* Appendix of Miscellaneous Rare Conditions) and can also be caused by endocrinopathies (hypothyroidism, Cushing's disease or insulinoma).

Obesity predisposes to or aggravates several disorders (*Table 15.7*). There is about a threefold increase in premature deaths in obese patients. Management includes calorie restriction, more exercise and possibly appetite suppressants such as fenfluramine, dexfenfluramine or phentermine for a limited period.

Table 15.7 Complications of obesity

- Cardiovascular
  Hypertension
  Ischaemic heart disease
  Varicose veins
- Orthopaedic
  Accidents
  Painful osteoarthritis
- Psychological
  Depression
- Gastrointestinal
  Hiatus hernia (and other hernias)
  Gallstones
  Colonic disease (diverticulitis/carcinoma)
- Respiratory
  Cor pulmonale
- Metabolic and endocrine
  Diabetes mellitus
  Hyperlipoproteinaemias (type II, III and IV)
- Gynaecological
  Uterine prolapse
  Polycystic ovaries
  Amenorrhoea

• Dental aspects of obesity

Dental treatment of obese patients may be complicated by diabetes or cardiovascular disease, or, rarely, by an organic cause of the obesity. Cardiac dysrhythmias may be produced by the interaction of halogenated anaesthetics and large doses of amphetamines or amphetamine-like appetite suppressants (all Controlled Drugs) which should be discontinued a week before general anaesthesia. Appetite suppressants may cause xerostomia.

The total work of breathing is increased in obese patients and even at rest obese patients need to ventilate more than normal. Respiration is further impaired in the supine position.

Some 10 per cent of grossly obese persons have hypoventilation, cor pulmonale and episodic somnolence (Pickwickian syndrome).

Jaw wiring of obese patients appears to be an effective and safe way of substantially reducing weight in those in whom simpler methods fail, but relapse frequently follows this extreme measure.

Lactovegetarianism

A prolonged lactovegetarian diet may result in dental erosion. Citrus fruits, vinegar and acidic berries are especially responsible, particularly if ingested just before retiring to sleep.

Vegetarians and vegans

Complete absence of meat products can lead to vitamin B_{12} deficiency (Chapter 5), though the latter is surprisingly rare in vegans. Vegetarians may have less caries than others.

Malnutrition

Certain types of latent malnutrition may predispose to burning mouth syndrome, mouth ulcers, glossitis and angular stomatitis (Chapter 5). Such states are relatively common in the elderly or others of low socio-economic status, and in some food fads.

Severe malnutrition can result from poverty, especially in the developing world or in war zones, where there is an obstruction to the pharynx or oesophagus, and in disorders such as anorexia nervosa or bulimia (Chapter 18). Malnutrition can cause multiple deficiencies and can result in retarded tooth eruption. Sialosis may ensue (Chapter 9). Resulting immunodeficiencies predispose to oral ulceration, angular stomatitis, necrotizing gingivitis and rarely gangrenous stomatitis (noma; cancrum oris) or sialosis.

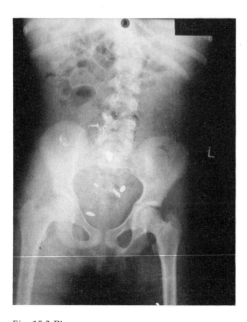

Fig. 15.2 Pica

Whether chronic malnutrition is a significant factor which underlies many oral cancers is unclear but there is a protective effect of diets rich in fresh fruits and vegetables, and in vitamins A and C, and iron deficiency is seen in the Paterson–Kelly (Plummer–Vinson) syndrome (Chapters 5 and 6).

Pica

Pica is a condition in which the appetite is perverted. This may sometimes be due to iron deficiency but is more common in persons with learning disability or psychiatric disease. A range of unusual objects and substances may be ingested, with untoward or catastrophic effect. Objects such as buttons, screws, pins, nails etc. may cause gastrointestinal obstruction or perforation (*Fig 15.2*). In the past children sometimes chewed painted objects and succumbed to lead poisoning.

BIBLIOGRAPHY

Barba M.W., Post A.C. and Duncan W.K. (1985) Dental treatment of a malignant hyperthermia susceptible child. *Pediatr. Dent.* **7**, 61–5.

Barrett A.P., Buckley D.J. and Katelaris C.H. (1990) Oral complications in type 1b glycogen storage disease. *Oral Surg. Oral Med. Oral Pathol.* **69**, 174–6.

Brownell A.K.W. and Paaruke R.T. (1986) Use of local anaesthetics in malignant hyperthermia. *Can. Med. Assoc. J.* **134**, 992–4.

Cantin R.Y., Poole A. and Ryan J.F. (1986) Malignant hyperthermia. *Oral Surg. Oral Med. Oral Pathol.* **62**, 389–92.

Carson J.M. and van Sickels J.E. (1982) Preoperative determination of susceptibility to malignant hyperthermia. *J. Maxillofac. Surg.* **40**, 432–5.

Cleary M.A., Francis D.E.M. and Kilpatrick N.M. (1997) Oral health implications in children with inborn errors of intermediary metabolism. *Int. J. Paed. Dent.* **7**, 133–41.

Dougherty N. and Gataletto M.A. (1995) Oral sequelae of chronic neutrophil defects: case report of a child with glycogen storage disease type 1b. *Pediatr Dent.* **17**, 224–9.

Douglas M.J. and McMorland G.H. (1986) The anaesthetic management of the malignant hyperthermia susceptible patient. *Can. Anaesth. Soc. J.* **33**, 371–8.

Ellis F.R. and Halsall P.J. (1980) Malignant hyperpyrexia. *Br. J. Hosp. Med.* **24**, 318–27.

Garrow J.S. and Gardiner G.T. (1981) Maintenance of weight loss in obese patients after jaw wiring. *Br. Med. J.* **282**, 858–60.

Goss A.N. (1980) Treatment of massive obesity by

prolonged jaw immobilization for edentulous patients. *Int. J. Oral Surg.* **9**, 253–8.

Keith O., Scully C. and Weidmann G.M. (1990) Orofacial features of Scheie (Hurler-Scheie) syndrome (L-iduronidase deficiency). *Oral Surg. Oral Med. Oral Pathol.* **70**, 70–4.

Linkosalo E. and Markkanen H. (1985) Dental erosions in relation to lactovegetarian diet. *Scand. J. Dent. Res.* **93**, 436–41.

Midda M. and Konig K.G. (1994) Nutrition, diet and oral health. *Int. Dent. J.* **44**, 599–612.

Porter S.R. and Scully C. (1996) *Innovations and Developments in Non-Invasive Oral Health Care.* Northwood, Science Reviews.

Porter S.R., Malamos D. and Scully C. (1986) Mouth–skin interface. 2: Connective tissue and metabolic disorders. *Dent. Update* **33**, 94–6.

Reilly S., Wolke D. and Skuse D. (1992) Tooth eruption in failure-to-thrive infants. *J. Dent. Child.* **59**, 350–2.

Rosenberg H. and Fletcher J.E. (1995) International malignant hyperthermia workshop and symposium. *Anesthesiology* **82**, 803–5.

Rugg-Gunn A.J. (1993) *Nutrition and Dental Health.* Oxford University Press, Oxford.

Scully C. (1988) *The Dental Patient.* Oxford, Heinemann.

Scully C. (1989) *The Mouth and Perioral Tissues.* Oxford, Heinemann.

Scully C. (1989) *Patient Care: a Dental Surgeon's Guide.* London, British Dental Association.

Scully C. (1995) Oral precancer: preventive and medical approaches to management. *Oral Oncol.* **31**, 16–26.

Scully C., Cawson R.A. and Griffiths M.J. (1990) *Occupational Hazards to Dental Staff.* London, British Dental Journal.

Sessler D.I. (1986) Malignant hyperthermia. *J. Pediatr.* **109**, 9–14.

Thornhill M.H. (1996) Masticatory muscle symptoms in a patient with McArdle's disease. *Oral Surg.* **81**, 544–6.

Willett W.C. (1994) Diet and health; what should we eat? *Science* **264**, 532–7.

APPENDIX TO CHAPTER 15

INBORN ERRORS OF METABOLISM

Disease	*Management problems*
Abetalipoproteinaemia	Ataxia: haemorrhage
Acatalasaemia	Gingival ulceration
Acid lipase deficiency	Mental handicap; anaemia
Acrodermatitis enteropathica	Severe oral ulceration; neuropathies
Adenosine deaminase deficiency	Immunodeficiency
α_1-antitrypsin deficiency	Hepatic disease; emphysema
Argininaemia	Spasticity; mental handicap; epilepsy
Aspartylglucosaminuria	Mental handicap
Cerebrotendinous xanthomatosis	Dementia; ataxia; paresis; cataracts
Cholinesterase deficiency	Suxamethonium sensitivity
Chronic granulomatous disease	Lymph node abscesses (cervical etc.)
	Liability to severe bacterial infections
Combined hyperlipidaemia	Atherosclerosis
Congenital adrenal hyperplasia	Hypoadrenocorticism
Crigler–Najjar syndrome	Jaundice
Cystinosis	Renal disease
Cystinuria	Renal disease
Diphosphoglycerate mutase deficiency	Anaemia
Dubin–Johnson syndrome	Jaundice
Dysbetalipoproteinaemia	Atherosclerosis
Fabry's disease	Neuropathy; thromboses; renal failure; pulmonary failure
Familial dysautonomia (Riley–Day syndrome)	Sensitive to barbiturates; dysphagia; sialorrhoea; insensitive to pain; mental handicap; epilepsy; blood pressure labile
Familial goitre	Hypothyroidism
Fanconi syndrome	Aminoaciduria; osteomalacia; oral cancer

continued

Fucosidosis	Mental handicap
Galactosaemia	Mental handicap; hepatic disease; cataracts; hypoglycaemia
Gilbert's disease	Jaundice
GM$_1$ gangliosidosis	Mental handicap; epilepsy; blindness
GM$_2$ gangliosidosis	" " " "
Tay–Sachs disease	" " " "
Sandhoff disease	" " " "
Gaucher's disease	Mental handicap; spasticity; thrombocytopenia; leucopenia
Glucose 6-phosphate dehydrogenase deficiency	Haemolytic anaemia
Glutaric aciduria	Hypoglycaemia
Glycogen storage disease:	
I	Hypoglycaemia; caries; bleeding tendency
II	Cardiomyopathy; respiratory infection; neurological abnormalities
III	Hypoglycaemia
IV	Hepatic disease; cardiac failure
VI	Mild hypoglycaemia
VIa	Mild hypoglycaemia
O	Mild hypoglycaemia
Gout	Renal disease; hypertension; atherosclerosis
Haemochromatosis	Diabetes; hepatic disease; cardiomyopathy
Hereditary angioedema	Airways obstruction
Hereditary fructose intolerance	Hepatic disease; hypoglycaemia
Hereditary oroticaciduria	Severe anaemia; leucopenia
Hereditary spherocytosis	Haemolytic anaemia
Hexokinase deficiency	Anaemia
Histidinaemia	Hearing deficit; speech deficit; infections; mental handicap
Homocystinuria	Mental handicap; epilepsy; blindness; hepatic disease; chest deformities; thrombotic disease
Hypercalcaemia	Renal disease; cardiac subaortic stenosis; mental handicap (William's syndrome)
Hypercholesterolaemia	Atherosclerosis
Hypercystinuria	Renal disease
Hyperornithinaemia	Mental handicap
Hyperoxaluria	Renal disease
Hypertriglyceridaemia	Atherosclerosis; pancreatitis
Hypophosphatasia	Skeletal abnormalities; dental hypoplasia
Krabbe disease	Mental handicap; blindness
Lecithin/cholesterol acetyltransferase deficiency	Haemolytic anaemia; atherosclerosis; renal disease
Lesch–Nyhan syndrome	Mutilation of tongue or lips; mental handicap; epilepsy; athetosis
Lipoprotein lipase deficiency	Pancreatitis
Lysinuria	Epilepsy
Mannosidosis	Mental handicap
Metachromatic leucodystrophy	Mental handicap; blindness; psychoses
Methionine malabsorption	Epilepsy
Mucolipidosis (I cell disease)	Mental handicap; blindness; valvular heart disease
Mucopolysaccharidoses (MPS)	
I Hurler syndrome	Mental handicap; blindness; cardiac disease; trismus

continued

II Hunter syndrome	As in MPS I
III Sanfilippo syndrome	Mental handicap
IV Morquio syndrome	Blindness; chest deformity; aortic valve disease; enamel hypoplasia
V Ullrich–Scheie syndrome	Blindness; valvular heart disease
VI Maroteaux–Lamy syndrome	Mental handicap; blindness
VII	Mental handicap
Myeloperoxidase deficiency	Candidosis
Niemann–Pick disease	Mental handicap; epilepsy; pancytopenia
Neuronal ceroid lipofuscinoses	Mental handicap; epilepsy; blindness
Orotic aciduria	Megaloblastic anaemia
Oxalosis	Renal disease
Phenylketonuria	Mental handicap; epilepsy
Porphyrias	Drug sensitivities; neuropathies; hypertension
Primary hypophosphataemia (vitamin D-resistant rickets)	Dwarfism; rickets; dental abscesses
Prolinaemia	Epilepsy; deafness
Purine nucleoside phosphorylase deficiency	Immunodeficiency
Pyruvate kinase deficiency	Anaemia
Renal glycosuria	Glycosuria (confusion with diabetes)
Refsum's disease	Blindness; deafness
Rotor syndrome	Jaundice
Transcobalamin II deficiency	Macrocytic anaemia; pancytopenia
Triosephosphate isomerase deficiency	Anaemia
Tyrosinaemia	Hepatic disease
Tyrosinosis	Myasthenia; epilepsy
Wilson's disease (hepatolenticular degeneration)	Hepatic disease; renal disease; spasticity; tremor
Wolman's disease	Mental handicap
Xeroderma pigmentosum	Skin cancers

16

Musculoskeletal disorders

Key points

- Osteogenesis imperfecta is a genetic disorder which presents with brittle bones and repeated fractures, and needs differentiating from child abuse.
- Osteogenesis imperfecta may be associated with dentinogenesis imperfecta, and sometimes with mitral valve prolapse or aortic incompetence.
- Cleidocranial dysplasia is mainly a genetic disorder of membrane bone formation in which there are often multiple supernumerary teeth and dentigerous cysts.
- Osteopetrosis is a genetic defect of osteoclasts that presents with dense bone (marble bone) predisposed to fracture and infection.
- Marfan's syndrome is a genetic disorder of arachnodactyly, ocular defects and cardiac valve incompetence.
- Ehlers–Danlos syndrome is a genetic disorder characterized by hyperextensible ligaments, joint hypermobility, jaw dislocation and, in some, periodontal disease.
- Rickets and osteomalacia are disorders of vitamin D which affect bones and, if severe, the developing teeth.
- In fibrous dysplasia, fibrous tissue replaces bone to form a swelling during childhood, with arrest in young adult life.
- Fibrous dysplasia may affect one bone, or can be polyostotic and then sometimes associated with precocious puberty and skin pigmentation (Albright's syndrome).
- Paget's disease may affect one or more bones, which enlarge and may compress adjacent structures, are hypervascular and occasionally transform to osteosarcoma.
- Hypercementosis and dense bone may make extractions difficult in Paget's disease, and there may be postoperative infection.
- Osteoarthritis affects mainly weight-bearing joints, with pain and stiffness. Despite views to the contrary, prosthetic joints are rarely infected with oral bacteria.
- Rheumatoid arthritis is an immunologically mediated disorder mainly of small joints. Nearly one-fifth of patients develop salivary changes of Sjögren's syndrome.
- The temporomandibular joint is often affected by rheumatoid arthritis but usually asymptomatically, except in children where joint damage can be seen.
- Cervical spine involvement in rheumatoid arthritis may predispose to spinal cord damage if the neck is extended abruptly during general anaesthesia.
- Reiter's disease often follows shigella or salmonella gut infections, or urethritis, and is seen almost exclusively in males with HLA B27.
- Mouth lesions like geographic stomatitis, ulcers, conjunctivitis, arthritis and keratoderma blenorrhagica are the typical features of Reiter's disease.
- The muscular dystrophies are genetic myopathies leading to progressive weakness, loss of lung and cardiac function, and often early death. General anaesthesia is contraindicated.

- Polymyositis is an acquired myopathy with weakness and pain, skin lesions and, in some, Raynaud's phenomenon, myocarditis, fibrosing alveolitis or malignancy.
- Giant cell arteritis is an inflammatory condition that affects mainly medium sized arteries in the head and neck, and may endanger the retinal artery and sight.
- Giant cell arteritis may also cause orofacial pain or headache. It is a medical emergency, requiring systemic corticosteroids to protect vision.

Of the three main components of the skeletal system, the joints are considerably more frequently affected by disease than the muscles or bones. The jaws and temporomandibular joints are part of this system but are rarely involved by systemic disease and few skeletal diseases affect the management of the dental patient directly. Muscle disorders are relatively uncommon and involvement of the masticatory and facial muscles is not necessarily a prominent feature. However, for patients with musculoskeletal disease, access to the dental clinic or getting into or out of the chair may be difficult.

DISEASES OF BONE

The skeleton is a highly vascular structure and bone is a dynamic tissue, constantly remodelling. The organic matrix of bone consists largely of collagen and is produced by osteoblasts rich in alkaline phosphatase. The inorganic mineral phase contains mainly calcium and phosphorus but also smaller amounts of magnesium, sodium and other ions. The mineral component is present largely as hydroxyapatite together with a smaller amount of amorphous calcium phosphate. Bone formation is influenced particularly by parathyroid hormone and vitamin D, and depends on other factors such as bone morphogenetic proteins (BMPs). The latter are now available as recombinant proteins, finding application in the repair of periodontal defects, other bone defects, and in implantology. Bone resorption is mediated mainly by osteoclasts (rich in acid phosphatases), but also by prostaglandins and some cytokines (Chapter 20), and is influenced mainly by parathyroid hormone.

GENETIC SKELETAL DISEASES

Many genetic disorders of the skeleton are rare and of little clinical importance in dentistry. Their main features are summarized in the Appendix to this chapter and only the more relevant disorders are discussed here.

Osteogenesis imperfecta (fragilitas ossium)

Osteogenesis imperfecta (brittle bone disease) is a rare inherited usually autosomal dominant, disorder with a frequency of 1 in 12 000 births. The gene for dentinogenesis imperfecta, one of the more common heritable defects of the teeth, is closely related. There are several variants (*Table 16.1*).

The underlying defect, as in Marfan's and Ehlers–Danlos syndromes, appears to be in type I collagen formation, and although osteoblasts are active the total amount of bone formed is small and mostly woven in type. The long bones are typically normal in length, with epiphyses of normal width, but slender shafts, frequently giving a trumpet-shaped appearance.

The bones are fragile and multiple fractures follow minimal trauma. Healing is rapid but usually with distortion and the ultimate effect in severe cases is gross deformity causing dwarfism. The frequency of fractures usually tends to diminish after puberty. The parietal regions of the skull may bulge outwards causing eversion of the upper part of the ear. Other defects are blue sclerae, deafness, easy bruising and weakness of tendons and ligaments causing loose-jointedness and often hernias. The severity and extent of the disease is very variable but occasionally clinical difficulties may be caused by chest deformities or cardiovascular disease such as mitral valve prolapse or aortic incompetence.

Table 16.1   Osteogenesis imperfecta: subtypes

Type	Inheritance	Bone disease	Stature	Extraskeletal involvement
I[a]	AD	Mild: fractures in childhood	Almost normal	Common. Blue sclerae: otosclerosis: thin aortic valves: hypermobile joints: Dentinogenesis imperfecta ±
II	AR	Severe: skull virtually unossified: multiple fractures: lethal	—	—
III	AR some sporadic	Progressive: few can walk unaided	Reduced	Blue sclerae. No dentinogenesis imperfecta
IV	AD	Severe	Reduced	Sclerae not blue. Dentinogenesis imperfecta common
V	Varied	Mild	Almost normal	Loose-jointedness a prominent feature

AD, Autosomal dominant.
[a]Constitutes 80 per cent of all cases.

- ## Dental aspects of osteogenesis imperfecta

In those with associated dentinogenesis imperfecta, the teeth may have the characteristic abnormal translucency and brown or purplish colour. The enamel may adhere poorly to the dentine and be progressively shed under the stress of mastication. By adolescence the teeth may be worn down to the gum margins but obliteration of the pulp chamber by dentine usually prevents exposure of the pulp. The softness of the dentine, however, makes the fitting of post crowns impractical so that extraction and replacement by dentures is the usual form of treatment in severe cases. In spite of the brittleness of most of the skeleton, the jaws rarely fracture. Dental extractions can usually therefore be safely carried out in most patients but care should obviously be taken to support the jaws and to use minimal force.

Apart from the obvious management problems related to bone fragility, there may be a risk from general anaesthesia if there are chest deformities or cardiac complications with a risk of infective endocarditis.

Care should be taken not to confuse children with brittle bone syndrome from those who have been subjected to physical abuse (Chapter 23).

Chondrodysplasias

The chondrodysplasias are heritable disorders of skeletal growth, presenting typically with dwarfism, high forehead, cleft palate and various ocular anomalies. Over 150 distinct variants have been described, but achondroplasia is the best known. Surgery is usually required for the cleft palate and other deformities.

Achondroplasia

Achondroplasia is a defect in cartilaginous bone formation, often inherited as an autosomal dominant trait. Defective long bone growth leads to dwarfism with short limbs, a normal spine length with lumbar lordosis and an apparently large head. These appearances have traditionally led to many achondroplastics becoming circus dwarfs. Nasal septal and base of skull growth is impaired so that the bridge is depressed and skull bossed. Many patients are otherwise completely normal, but spinal deformity can be severe and occasionally cause spinal cord compression.

- ## Dental aspects of achondroplasia

The only significant dental aspects are orthodontic in nature as a result of malocclusion but diabetes and kyphosis may affect management.

Cleidocranial dysplasia (cleidocranial dysostosis)

Cleidocranial dysplasia is a rare defect mainly of membrane bone formation inherited as an autosomal dominant trait related to chromosome 6, though sporadic cases may arise. The defects mainly involve the skull and clavicle.

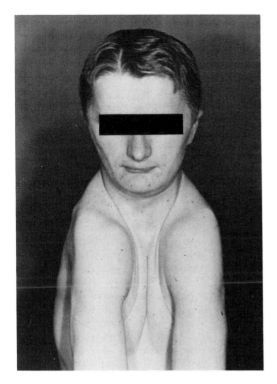

Fig. 16.1 Cleidocranial dysostosis

The head is large but brachycephalic and with bulging frontal, parietal and occipital bones and a persistent metopic (frontal) suture. The fontanelles persist and there are numerous wormian bones. There is occasionally delayed closure of the mandibular symphysis. The middle facial third is hypoplastic leading to a relative mandibular protrusion, and the nasal bridge is depressed. Abnormalities of the cranial base may be seen on lateral cephalograms, and clefts of the hard and soft palate have been recorded.

The clavicles are either absent or defective thus conferring the unusual ability to approximate the shoulders anteriorly (*Fig. 16.1*). Other skeletal defects such as kyphoscoliosis or pelvic anomalies may be associated.

• Dental aspects of cleidocranial dysplasia

Apart from the facial anomalies there may be persistence of the deciduous dentition, multiple unerupted permanent teeth and supernumeraries, twisted roots, malformed crowns and dentigerous cysts. The associated problems are dealt with in textbooks of oral and maxillofacial surgery.

Osteopetrosis (Albers–Schönberg disease)

Osteopetrosis (marble-bone disease) is a rare disorder of variable severity characterized by a general increase in bone density probably as a result of a defect in osteoclastic activity and hence of the bone remodelling mechanism. The bones, though abnormally dense, are weak.

In mild osteopetrosis there may be no symptoms and the diagnosis is made by chance by radiography. Other patients suffer bone pain, fractures or osteomyelitis. Fractures, though common, usually heal normally.

In more severe disease (malignant infantile osteopetrosis) added complications can be cranial neuropathies leading, for example, to optic atrophy. Hydrocephalus, epilepsy and mental handicap are less frequent.

The medullary cavities are filled with bone, and anaemia is common in spite of extramedullary haemopoiesis in the liver, spleen and lymph nodes. Macrophages and neutrophils are defective, resulting in susceptibility to infections. Serum levels of acid phosphatase are raised but calcium and phosphate levels are normal. Treatment is unsatisfactory. Corticosteroid therapy may be of some help but marrow transplantation may be the only hope.

• Dental aspects of osteopetrosis

Management problems may include anaemia (Chapter 5) and corticosteroid therapy (Chapter 14).

The face may be broad, with hypertelorism, snub nose and frontal bossing. There may be retarded tooth eruption. Radiography shows excessive bone density and thickness, especially obvious in the skull.

Trigeminal or facial neuropathies may complicate the disease and fracture of the jaw or osteomyelitis may complicate extractions. Once established, infection is difficult to eradicate, so that surgery should be minimally traumatic, mucoperiosteal flaps preferably not raised and antibiotic cover should be given. Eruption of posterior teeth may be complicated by osteomyelitis.

Table 16.2 Marfan's syndrome		
Skeletal defects	*Cardiovascular defects*	*Neuro-ocular defects*
Disproportionately long limbs	Dilatation of ascending aorta	Ectopia lentis
Arachnodactyly	Dissecting aneurysm	Blue sclerae in some
Loose joints	Aortic regurgitation	Mental handicap (sometimes)
Pectus excavatum	Mitral valve prolapse	
Temporomandibular joint subluxation		

Note: Marfan's syndrome shares the features of loose-jointedness, cardiac valvular defects and ocular lesions with various of the subtypes of Ehlers–Danlos syndrome. However, the most obvious distinguishing feature of Marfan's syndrome is the long, thin body habitus and long slender fingers.

Marfan's syndrome

Marfan's syndrome is an autosomal dominant disorder of connective tissue with skeletal, ocular and cardiovascular manifestations. The disease has a prevalence of about 1 in 10 000 and is of such variable expression that diagnosis may be difficult and there can be confusion with other, rare disorders, particularly homocystinuria and congenital contractural arachnodactyly (*Table 16.2*, Appendix to this chapter).

Skeletal manifestations are excessive length of tubular bones so that patients are tall with wide arm span and long spider-like fingers (arachnodactyly). Ligaments are so lax that hyperextensibility, subluxation or dislocation of joints and hernias are common. Lung cysts may lead to spontaneous pneumothorax and respiratory function can also be impaired by kyphoscoliosis.

The eyes are affected in most patients and the lens subluxes or dislocates in 80 per cent – often causing visual impairment.

Cardiovascular abnormalities affect 90 per cent of patients with Marfan's syndrome. Aortic dissection can be life-threatening. There is often severe aortic and mild mitral incompetence. Death in the fifth decade is common.

It has been suggested that Abraham Lincoln may have had Marfan's syndrome. His facial appearance and build suggest a mild case. However, casts of his hands, which were broad and strong, disprove this idea.

• Dental aspects of Marfan's syndrome

Management may be complicated by chest deformities and cardiovascular abnormalities, which may be contraindications to general anaesthesia, and there is a risk of infective endocarditis (Chapter 3).

A Marfanoid body build may also be a feature of the multiple endocrine adenoma syndrome (MEA III) (Chapter 14). The palatal vault is high and temporomandibular joint dysfunction or recurrent subluxation may be a prominent symptom.

Ehlers–Danlos syndrome

Ehlers–Danlos syndrome is a group of disorders of collagen formation (*Table 16.3*) characterized by hyperextensible skin, propensity to bruising and loose-jointedness. The most common forms are inherited as autosomal dominant traits while the remainder are recessive. There have been recent advances in the understanding of some of the molecular abnormalities of collagen in this group of diseases so that the nature of the subtypes in earlier reports of oral manifestations may be uncertain.

There is wide variation in the clinical features of the different types of Ehlers–Danlos syndrome but hypermobility of the joints is the best known manifestation. Typical features, seen in varying degrees in the whole group, are as follows.

The skin is typically soft, abnormally extensible, feels fine and thin and may appear lax in some sites. Even when it appears normal, it may be possible to pull the skin out for one or two inches. Fragility of the skin and oral mucosa may cause wounds to gape or to split after slight trauma. Slow healing may leave fragile scars with a tissue-paper texture while easy ('spontaneous') bruising may mimic purpura caused by haematological disease.

Hypermobility of the joints may be extreme (India-rubber man) but the severity varies in

Table 16.3 Ehlers–Danlos syndrome: subtypes

Types	Inheritance	Hyper-extensibility	Skin fragility and bruising	Joint hypermobility	Special features
I (gravis)	AD	++	++	++	Parrot face. Frequent musculoskeletal disorders. Mitral valve prolapse
II (mitis)	AD	+	+	+ Hands and feet only	Mitral valve prolapse. Bruising common
III (benign hypermobile)	AD	±	+	++	Dislocations, haemarthrosis, early onset arthritis. Mitral valve prolapse
IV (ecchymotic)	AR	±	+++	± Digits only	Bleeding from major arteries. Cerebrovascular accidents, severe purpura from minimal trauma, spontaneous rupture of bowel, skull defects
V (sex-linked)	X-linked	++	+	±	Frequent musculoskeletal disorders. Males only
VI (ocular or hydroxylysine deficient)	AR	++	±	++	Fragile cornea and sclera. Multiple ocular defects, deafness, often early loss of sight
VII (multiple congenital dis-location or arthro-chalasis multiplex congenita	AR	+	±	++	Early onset of multiple dislocations. Some laxity of ligaments, short stature
VIII (periodontal)	AD	±	±	±	Severe early onset periodontitis and loss of teeth. Blue sclerae
IX (skeletal and urinary tract dysplasia)	AR	–	±	±	—
X (fibronectin deficiency)	AR	±	±	±	Bleeding tendency

AD, Autosomal dominant; AR, autosomal recessive.

the different subtypes. It may be possible to hyperextend the fingers until they are at right-angles to the back of the hand and to pull the thumb back until it touches the forearm. Recurrent, semi-spontaneous dislocation may result.

Internal complications affecting the cardiovascular system (especially mitral valve prolapse or conduction defects), gastrointestinal tract, urinary tract and respiratory system also result from weakness of their connective tissue component. Mitral valve prolapse (floppy valve syndrome), which is typical of type III Ehlers–Danlos syndrome, may confer susceptibility to infective endocarditis or lead to rapid development of mitral insufficiency and heart failure. Spontaneous rupture of major arteries can cause fatal haemorrhage and internal bleeding can cause abdominal emergencies. Widespread purpura can readily be mistaken for haematological disease with haemorrhagic tendencies but is unlike any of the latter because of the combination of subcutaneous, submucosal and deep bleeding. These, though of vascular origin, may mimic a coagulation defect such as haemophilia clinically.

Haemostatic function is usually normal but platelet defects have occasionally been reported. The latter may be caused by the same defect that underlies the connective tissue disorder.

- ### Dental aspects of Ehlers–Danlos syndrome

Patients with mitral valve prolapse may develop heart failure with attendant risks during anaesthesia and there is also a risk of infective endocarditis (Chapter 3).

The most severe vascular abnormalities are seen in type IV (ecchymotic type) in which there is severe semi-spontaneous purpura with extensive ecchymoses and also weakness of arterial walls.

Severe bleeding from the gingivae, especially after toothbrushing, or from extraction sockets, may sometimes be the main complaint. Post-extraction bleeding is likely to be most severe in type IV. Hypermobility of joints is severe in types I, VI and VII and, in all of these, dislocation of the temporomandibular joint is a possibility.

In type VIII Ehlers–Danlos syndrome there is early onset of periodontal disease, which is widespread and severe with early loss of teeth. Other, incidental oddities that may be seen in Ehlers–Danlos syndrome may include the ability to touch the nose with the tip of the tongue and dental abnormalities. The teeth may be small with short or abnormally shaped roots, and large numbers of pulp stones.

Pseudoxanthoma elasticum

Pseudoxanthoma elasticum is a rare autosomal recessive disorder of connective tissue characterized by yellow papular or reticular skin lesions, visual impairment and cardiovascular abnormalities.

The skin is hyperextensible, as in Ehlers–Danlos syndrome, and there may be blue sclerae and loose-jointedness. Abnormalities in the eye include streaks beneath the retina (angioid streaks) and often haemorrhages and scarring.

Cardiovascular involvement includes calcification of elastic tissue in vessel walls leading to poor peripheral blood flow, causing intermittent claudication, and ischaemic heart disease. Hypertension is common. Some patients develop hypothyroidism; others bleed from the upper gastrointestinal tract, uterus, renal or respiratory tracts.

Some patients have a normal lifespan but others succumb to haemorrhage, cardiac disease or cerebrovascular accidents.

- ### Dental aspects of pseudoxanthoma elasticum

Skin lesions may be seen around the face and mouth and there may be nodules in the lips, or sometimes in the mouth. Dental management may be complicated particularly by cardiovascular disease.

DISEASES OF CALCIUM METABOLISM AND BONE

Localized bone diseases such as osteomyelitis or tumours are not within the remit of this text and reference should be made to oral pathology texts. Hyperparathyroidism is discussed in Chapter 14 .

The main factors controlling bone metabolism and blood calcium levels include the following:

1. Vitamin D from the diet is absorbed from the upper small intestine with other fat-soluble vitamins. Precursors are also synthesized in the skin under the influence of sunlight. The most active metabolite is produced by hepatic and then renal conversion of precursors to 1,25-dihydroxycholecalciferol (DHCC), a process enhanced by parathyroid hormone and low phosphate levels. The active metabolite controls bone metabolism, enhances calcium absorption and, incidentally, affects the proliferation of various cells other than those of bone.
2. Active vitamin D and parathyroid hormone promote intestinal transport of calcium and phosphate to maintain their normal extracellular fluid levels.
3. Parathormone (PTH) secretion is regulated by blood calcium levels: when these fall, PTH is secreted, accelerates the removal of calcium from bones to raise the blood calcium level and enhances the formation of active vitamin D.
4. Calcitonin opposes the action of parathormone and lowers the blood calcium level, mainly by increasing deposition of calcium in the bones.
5. Several other hormones, including corticosteroids, oestrogens and thyroxine, affect bone formation and metabolism to varying degrees.

Bone is a dynamic tissue which is being constantly remodelled throughout life. It is a reservoir of calcium, magnesium, phosphate and other ions necessary for many homeostatic functions.

Osteoblasts secrete osteoid which becomes mineralized during bone development by deposition of calcium phosphate, both as hydroxyapatite and amorphous calcium phosphate, in this matrix. The resorption of bone is carried out by multinucleated osteoclasts and mononuclear cells. During the growth period, bone develops by the remodelling and replacement of cartilage to form the long bones, or in the case of the flat membrane bones, by mineralization of osteoid matrix. Increase in the length of bones is dependent on epiphyseal growth whilst increase in the width and thickness is the result of periosteal deposition.

When bone is resorbed, calcium and phosphate are removed and released into the extracellular fluid. Osteoclasts are rich in acid phosphatase which may be released into the serum in significant amounts when there is widespread osteolysis. Osteoblasts, by contrast, contain alkaline phosphatase, the level of which rises in the serum when osteoblastic activity increases. Mineralization depends on the extracellular fluid calcium and phosphate levels.

Rickets and osteomalacia

Rickets is a disease of childhood characterized by defective skeletal mineralization. Osteomalacia is a disease with the same pathogenesis but affects adults in whom there is failure of mineralization of replacement bone in the normal process of bone turnover. Causes include one or more of the following:

1. Nutritional deficiency of vitamin D.
2. Failure of vitamin D synthesis in the skin because of lack of sunlight.
3. Vitamin D malabsorption.
4. Renal disease: loss of calcium, loss of phosphate, acidosis and impaired vitamin D metabolism.
5. Vitamin D-resistant rickets: an X-linked defect of renal reabsorption of phosphate (familial hypophosphataemia).
6. Prolonged treatment with drugs such as phenytoin or occasionally phenobarbitone, rifampicin or others, leading to accelerated metabolism of vitamin D.
7. Excessive calcium demands in pregnancy and lactation.
8. Liver disease leading to impaired absorption of vitamin D.
9. Isoniazid interfering with vitamin D metabolism.
10. Vitamin D-dependent rickets – a defect of the enzyme required to form 1,25-dihydroxycholecalciferol.

Vitamin D is abundant in fish liver oil and animal livers, and is synthesized in the skin under the influence of sunlight. Rickets and osteomalacia can, therefore, be a result of a dietary deficiency in poorly nourished communities, especially among immigrants from the Indian Sub-Continent living in northern Britain. In this group, contributory factors may be the lack of sunshine and eating of chapattis of wholemeal flour containing phytates, which bind calcium and impair its absorption.

Osteomalacia is most prone to develop in adult women as a result of the demands of pregnancy and lactation, in malabsorption states, or in the presence of any cause of impairment of absorption of vitamin D.

Chronic renal failure can also cause osteomalacia, because of excess calcium loss and inability of the diseased kidneys to synthesize the active metabolite of vitamin D. Similar problems may complicate vitamin D-resistant rickets, renal tubular acidosis or the Fanconi syndrome.

In rickets, the bones are weak and readily deformed. The bones also fracture easily but incompletely (greenstick or pseudofractures). Affected infants and young children are often listless and irritable, the muscles are weak and hypotonic and they suffer bone pains.

In osteomalacia the inadequate mineralization and excess formation of osteoid matrix (swellings at the costochondral junctions cause a 'rachitic rosary'), unsupported by calcium salts, weakens the bones. Deformity of weight-bearing bones is, therefore, the most obvious consequence. The plasma calcium level tends to be low, with normal or low phosphate levels (*see* Chapter 15). Alkaline phosphatase levels are raised.

- ## Management of rickets and osteomalacia

An adequate intake of vitamin D and calcium is important. Complications, such as bone deformity, must also be treated.

- ## Dental aspects of rickets and osteomalacia

The teeth escape surprisingly well from the effects of rickets. Dental defects are seen only in unusually severe cases, but eruption may be retarded. Vitamin D deficiency is not a contributory cause of dental caries. The jaws may show abnormal radiolucency.

In malabsorption syndromes there may be secondary hyperparathyroidism (Chapter 14) or vitamin K deficiency (Chapter 4), with endocrine or bleeding disorders respectively and oral manifestations of malabsorption (Chapter 9).

In vitamin D-resistant rickets (familial hypophosphataemia), the skull sutures are wide and there may be frontal bossing, but dental complaints frequently bring notice to the disease. The teeth have large pulp chambers, abnormal dentine calcification and are therefore liable to pulpitis and multiple, apparently spontaneous, dental abscesses. Since even minimal caries or attrition can lead to pulpitis, preventive care and prophylactic occlusal coverage are needed.

Osteoporosis

Osteoporosis is a deficiency of both bone matrix and calcium salts. The bone is structurally normal but there is too little of it (osteopenia). Overall, it is probably the most common disease of bone. Women after the menopause are mainly affected but while diminishing bone mass is a normal concomitant of ageing, there are several other causes (*Table 16.4*).

The chief complications are fractures, particularly of the neck of the femur or of the vertebral bodies causing gradual collapse of the spine. Low back pain is common. There are often no biochemical abnormalities but there may be increased urinary loss of calcium and hydroxyproline, and in women who lose bone particularly fast, urinary tests can be informative. Until recently there have

Table 16.4   Causes of osteoporosis
• Senile
• Post-menopausal
• Hypogonadism
• Cushing's syndrome
• Corticosteroid therapy
• Hyperthyroidism
• Alcoholism
• Immobilization

been no simple methods of quantifying bone mass and of recognizing osteoporosis before bones start to fracture. Dual X-ray absorptiometers (Dexa equipment) now allow rapid assessment but are currently available only at a limited number of specialist centres.

- ## Management of osteoporosis

The control of osteoporosis is often only partially successful and depends on the underlying cause, if it can be identified. Hormone replacement therapy (oestrogen plus progesterone) may be effective in postmenopausal women and may also help to relieve other postmenopausal symptoms such as flushing (see Chapter 15). However, oestrogens can cause vaginal bleeding and there is a slightly increased risk of breast cancer. Alternative treatments are bisphosphonates and in particular etidronate, and calcitonin. The latter, however, has to be given by injection. Additional calcium and 1 a-hydroxy vitamin D may also be helpful. There is considerable controversy as to any benefits of fluoridation on osteoporosis and consequent fractures.

- ## Dental aspects of osteoporosis

Patients with osteoporosis may have any of the problems of the elderly (Chapter 23) and may be at risk during general anaesthesia if there has been vertebral collapse and chest deformities. There are no specific oral manifestations of osteoporosis and the association of osteoporosis with excessive alveolar bone loss in the elderly has been difficult to confirm because of the lack, until recently, of objective methods of quantifying bone mass. Nevertheless, there does seem to be a correlation.

Hypercalcaemia–supravalvular aortic stenosis syndrome (William's syndrome)

This syndrome comprises, in its rare complete form, infantile hypercalcaemia, characteristic so-called elfin facies, supravalvular subaortic stenosis or other cardiovascular abnormalities and mental deficiency. Most such cases appear to be sporadic. Hypercalcaemia typically remits in infancy but leaves growth deficiency, osteosclerosis and craniostenosis. Despite the mental defect, these children may be sociable and talkative ('cocktail party manner').

- ### Dental aspects of William's syndrome

Cardiovascular lesions may contraindicate general anaesthesia. Masseter spasm has been reported in a child with William's syndrome during general anaesthesia with halothane and suxamethonium. However, malignant hyperthermia did not develop and it is not clear whether these children are particularly prone to this complication. Dental defects are varied but may include hypodontia, microdontia and hypoplastic, bud-shaped teeth. The upper arch may be disproportionately wide and overlap the lower.

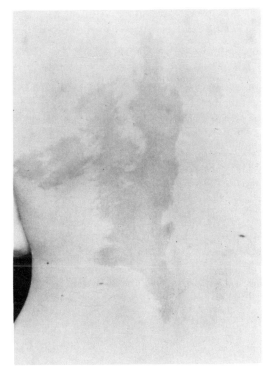

Fig. 16.2 Albright's syndrome: café-au-lait pigmentation on the back

Tumoral calcinosis

Tumoral calcinosis is a rare disease characterized by ectopic, soft tissue calcifications but normocalcaemia. Dental and periodontal changes are typical features and serve as markers of the severity of the disorder: early onset periodontitis has been reported.

Fibrous dysplasia

Fibrous dysplasia may affect a single bone (monostotic) or is less commonly multiple (polyostotic). The aetiology is unknown. The natural history of cherubism also has some features in common with fibrous dysplasia but may cause bilateral lesions of the maxilla causing the eyes to 'upturn towards heaven'.

The essential feature of the osseous lesions of fibrous dysplasia is replacement of an area of bone by fibrous tissue and production of a localized swelling. The process typically starts in childhood and, as the skeleton matures, the lesions ossify progressively and ultimately, when skeletal growth ceases, usually become stabilized.

Monostotic fibrous dysplasia is more common in females, and frequently involves the jaws, particularly the maxilla.

Polyostotic fibrous dysplasia may affect either sex and may involve over 50 per cent of the skeleton, but is uncommon. The lesions may be unilateral and 50 per cent of patients have abnormal skin hyperpigmentation of a café-au-lait type, especially over the dorsum of the trunk and limbs, usually on the same side as the bone lesions (Jaffe's syndrome).

Albright's syndrome (Fig. 16.2) is the term given when polyostotic fibrous dysplasia with pigmentation of the skin is seen with precocious puberty in females. There are episodic rises in serum oestrogen and falls in gonadotropin levels.

Radiography typically shows a ground-glass appearance with no defined margins. Serum calcium and phosphate levels are normal but, in many, the serum alkaline phosphatase level is high and urinary hydroxyproline raised.

• Management of fibrous dysplasia

Patients are usually managed by surgery and sometimes calcitonin. Testolactone is effective treatment for the precocious puberty of Albright's syndrome.

• Dental aspects of fibrous dysplasia

The facial bones are frequently involved in monostotic fibrous dysplasia and in 25 per cent of cases of polyostotic disease facial deformity is the presenting feature.

Fibrous dysplasia is typically a self-limiting condition that ceases to progress after adolescence in most cases. Surgery can then be used to correct any cosmetic defect. Radiotherapy should be avoided, as osteosarcomas have been reported after such treatment.

Monostotic fibrous dysplasia is not a medical problem but it is possible for the polyostotic type of the disease to be unrecognized when the facial lesions are the most obvious feature. Hyperthyroidism or diabetes mellitus may occasionally be associated with polyostotic fibrous dysplasia and therefore may, rarely, complicate treatment.

Mucosal pigmentation has been reported in Albright's syndrome but is rare. In the differential diagnosis, it may be confused with that of Addison's disease while the skin pigmentation may simulate that of neurofibromatosis. From the histological viewpoint the lesions of fibrous dysplasia may show small foci of giant cells, and differentiation from hyperparathyroidism or giant cell granuloma may have to be considered.

Paget's disease of bone (osteitis deformans)

Paget's disease is a common disorder characterized by progressive deformity and enlargement of bones. Radiographic evidence of its presence can be found in more than 5 per cent of those over 55 years of age in the UK. There appears to be considerable geographic variation in the prevalence of Paget's disease but there is always a male predominance.

The aetiology of Paget's disease is unknown but a slow virus and, in some, a genetic factor, may be involved. Its essential features are total disorganization of the normal orderly replacement of bone and an anarchic alternation of bone resorption and apposition. In the earlier stages resorption predominates (osteolytic phase) but later apposition takes over and, as disease activity declines, the affected bones become enlarged and dense (sclerotic stage).

Clinically, symptoms are absent in the early stages which can only be detected radiologically. The effects are most apparent in the elderly. Bone pain is the most common feature, is usually felt around the hips or knees, but is non-specific. One or many bones may be affected, and in the polyostotic type the axial skeleton is mainly involved. The hands and feet are usually spared. Other possible complications of Paget's disease are deformities or pathological fractures, and sometimes compression of cranial nerves with such effects as deafness or impairment of vision. Rarely there is brain stem compression. If the disease is widespread, hypervascularity of the bones can produce, in effect, an arteriovenous fistula and high-output cardiac failure. Development of osteosarcoma is a recognized, but uncommon, complication.

• General management of Paget's disease

Diagnosis is made on the clinical, radiographic and scintigraphic features, and chemical changes. Radiographs of affected bones show predominantly radiolucencies due to osteolysis early on but mixed areas of lysis with sclerosis later, and the affected bones are thicker. Radionuclide scanning shows increased uptake of technetium diphosphonate. The serum total alkaline phosphatase level is grossly raised when many bones are affected, but in general, there is little or no change in calcium or phosphate levels. More specific is a rise in bone-specific alkaline phosphatase There is then also increased urinary hydroxyproline and pyridinoline excretion. Currently the most effective treatment is with bisphosphonates such as disodium etidronate, pamidronate or tiludronate. Alendronate, clodronate and risendronate are also used in some countries. Calcitonin is given by injection or intranasally

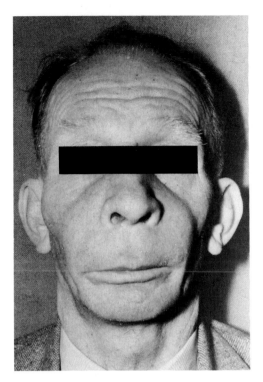

Fig. 16.3 Leontiasis ossea in Paget's disease

feature is a large irregular area of relative radiolucency (osteoporosis circumscripta). Later basilar invagination may be seen with also a 'cotton-wool' appearance of the vault of the skull on radiography.

The maxilla is occasionally and the mandible rarely involved. Typically, enlargement of the maxilla causes symmetrical bulging in the malar region (leontiasis ossea, *Fig. 16.3*). There is increased radio-opacity with loss of the normal landmarks and an irregular cotton-wool appearance. The intraoral features are gross symmetrical widening of the alveolar ridges, sometimes loss of lamina dura, root resorption and hypercementosis often forming enormous craggy masses which may become fused to the surrounding bone. Pulpal calcification may be seen.

Serious complications follow efforts to extract severely hypercementosed teeth. Attempts using forceps may fail to move the tooth, or cause fracture of the alveolar bone. Alternatively, the tooth may be mobilized but retained as if in a ball-and-socket joint. In the early stages of the disease, the highly vascular bone may bleed freely; later, the poor blood supply to the bone makes it susceptible to chronic suppurative osteomyelitis as a result of such trauma.

If hypercementosis is severe, a surgical approach with adequate exposure should be used for extractions, and prophylactic administration of an antibiotic such as penicillin (immediately before and for 3 or 4 days after the operation) may help to prevent postoperative infection.

In the edentulous patient, dentures have to be replaced as the alveolar ridge enlarges.

Osteosarcoma is particularly rare in the jaws, where no fully authenticated case appears to have been reported. Benign giant cell tumours may, however, be seen.

to relieve bone pain and deafness but may be immunogenic.

• Dental aspects of Paget's disease

If the patient is in heart failure, the usual precautions (Chapter 3) have to be taken but, since general anaesthesia may be needed for extractions, this aspect of the disease needs to be kept in mind. Chest deformity may also complicate general anaesthesia.

When the skull is affected a typical early

JOINT DISORDERS

Temporomandibular pain-dysfunction syndrome

This common affliction is discussed in Chapter 19.

Osteoarthritis

Osteoarthritis (osteoarthrosis) is a common disease, and is especially painful in weight-bearing or traumatized joints in the elderly.

Osteoarthritis has been traditionally regarded essentially as a wear-and-tear phenomenon, but excessive stress on the joints, as a result of occupation for example, does not, of itself, necessarily predispose to it. The disease has a significant systemic component which leads to disordered regulation of chondrocyte activity and failure of repair of articular cartilage. However, this may be aggravated by other kinds of disturbance of joint function or abnormal internal stresses, caused, for example, by operations such as meniscectomy.

The essential change in osteoarthritis is degeneration of articular cartilage with compensatory thickening of the underlying bone which becomes exposed. The bone is at first smooth and shiny but later the surface becomes roughened, cystic spaces form beneath and bone proliferates at the joint margins. Exposure and collapse of the cystic cavities, together with continued peripheral proliferation, cause progressive deformity.

The main clinical feature is usually pain with stiffness, progressively diminished function and deformity of one or more of the larger joints, such as the hips or knees, which are heavily stressed.

In contrast to rheumatoid arthritis, there are no systemic symptoms, clinically obvious inflammation of affected joints or serological changes. Osteophytes formed at the margins of the distal interphalangeal joints of the fingers produce Heberden's nodes, which are a hallmark of the disease (*Plate 15*).

The characteristic radiographic features of osteoarthritis include:

1. Narrowing of the joint space.
2. Marginal osteophyte formation (lipping).
3. Subchondral bone sclerosis.
4. Bone 'cysts' (rounded areas of radiolucency just beneath the joint surface).
5. Deformity.

• General management of osteoarthritis

Weight reduction, physiotherapy, heat treatment and the use of various appliances are helpful. Anti-inflammatory analgesics are usually needed and arthroplasty may prevent disablement in advanced disease. Joint replacements are now commonplace.

• Dental aspects of osteoarthritis

Dental management may be complicated by a bleeding tendency if the patient takes high doses of aspirin or when, after joint replacement, the patient is anticoagulated (Chapter 4). Age and immobility may also influence dental care (Chapter 23). The question of antibiotic prophylaxis for persons with joint replacements is discussed below.

Osteoarthritis has been described in temporomandibular joints in some elderly patients. However, patients with osteoarthritis of other joints do not appear to have significantly more involvement of the temporomandibular joints than controls. The radiographic severity of temporomandibular joint osteoarthritis does not correlate with symptoms, although palpable crepitus may be common. Patients should not therefore be made anxious by being told of such findings, since osteoarthritis of this joint is rarely of clinical significance.

A syndrome of dry mouth and osteoarthritis (sialoadenitis, osteoarthritis, xerostomia – SOX) has been described but needs confirmation.

Rheumatoid arthritis

Rheumatoid arthritis is a multi-system disease, but joint pain and damage are the most prominent features (*Table 16.5*). The disease appears to be immunologically mediated. An abnormal immunoglobulin is formed in the joint tissues and an autoantibody to the abnormal immunoglobulin (rheumatoid factor, RF) is produced in response. It is postulated that immune complex (antigen–antibody complex) formation may then lead to the activation of complement, inflammation and synovial damage.

Rheumatoid arthritis is a widespread disease which probably affects about 2 per cent of the population in Britain and the USA. Women are affected approximately three times as frequently as men.

The onset is typically between the ages of 30 and 40 and is often insidious, with increasing stiffness of the hands or feet which is worse in the morning. In the acute stage there is aching, swelling, redness, tenderness and limitation of movement of the joints.

Table 16.5	Rheumatoid arthritis: features and complications
Joints	Arthritis
	Tenosynovitis
	Laxity of ligaments
	Subluxation
	Spinal nerve root compression
Non-specific features	Fever
	Malaise
	Fatigue
Dermal, oral and para-oral	Palmar erythema
	Various rashes
	Subcutaneous nodules
	Sjögren's syndrome (dry mouth)
	Temporomandibular arthritis
	Oral drug lesions
Muscle	Weakness
	Wasting
Bone	Osteoporosis
Eyes	Sjögren's syndrome (dry eyes)
	Episcleritis, scleritis or scleromalacia
Cardiovascular	Pericarditis
	Myocarditis
	Valvulitis
	Vasculitis
Haematological	Anaemia
	Leucopenia
	Thrombocytopenia
Respiratory	Pleurisy and pleural effusion
	Nodules in lung
	Fibrosis
	Bronchiolitis
Neurological	Various neuropathies
Renal	Various nephropathies
	Amyloidosis
Hepatic	Abnormal liver function

The disease usually first affects the small joints of the hands and feet symmetrically – later the wrists, elbows, ankles and knees are commonly involved. The interphalangeal joints typically become spindle-shaped as a result of joint swelling with muscle wasting on either side (*Fig. 16.4*). The onset is sometimes acute with fever and malaise in addition to the joint pain. Other common manifestations are tenosynovitis, subcutaneous nodules, leucocytosis and anaemia. Clinically apparent effects on other systems are less common. The anaemia is typically normochromic (anaemia of chronic disease) and can be severe. Other laboratory findings are shown in *Table 16.6*.

Table 16.6	Laboratory findings in rheumatoid arthritis	
Test	*Typical findings*	
Full blood count	Normocytic hypochromic anaemia Mild leucocytosis (or leucopenia) Mild thrombocytopenia	
Erythrocyte sedimentation rate	Raised	
Protein electrophoresis	Hypergammaglobulinaemia	
Rheumatoid factor – latex agglutination	Positive	
Antinuclear antibodies	Positive in 20–60%	

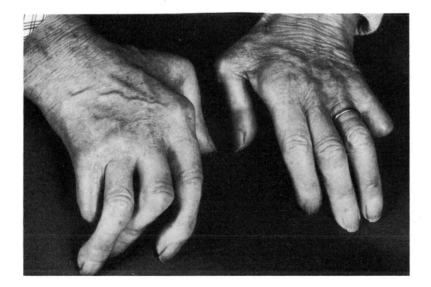

Fig. 16.4 Rheumatoid arthritis showing the characteristic deformities affecting the hands, particularly the deviation of the fingers (ulnar deviation)

- ## General management of rheumatoid arthritis

The serological marker of rheumatoid arthritis is rheumatoid factor, which is present in 60–70 per cent. It is detected by the sensitive latex agglutination test in which IgG-coated latex particles are agglutinated if the patient's serum contains IgM autoantibody to IgG. The Rose–Waaler test, using agglutination of sensitized sheep erythrocytes, is less sensitive but more specific for rheumatoid arthritis. In so-called seronegative cases, rheumatoid factor may be IgG rather than the typical IgM and is therefore not detected by these routine methods. Antinuclear antibodies are also often found but are usually in low titre (*Table 16.6*).

Radiographic features are soft tissue swelling and widening of the joint space due to accumulation of fluid in the early stages. Later there is increasing osteoporosis of the adjacent bone, cyst-like spaces and narrowing of the joint space. Ultimately there may be severe bone destruction and deformity, but ankylosis does not follow.

The main aspects of management are:

1. Rest in acute phases, but between these episodes maintenance of mobility of the affected joints.
2. Non-steroidal anti-inflammatory drugs are the safest and most effective drugs and should be given in increasing doses until the side-effects become disproportionately great in relation to the benefits.
3. Other drugs such as gold, penicillamine, methotrexate, cyclosporin or corticosteroids.
4. Haematinics in an attempt to treat anaemia.
5. Physiotherapy and psychological care. Depression may result from persistent pain and restriction of activity, so that antidepressant treatment may sometimes be needed.
6. Joint replacement is occasionally needed.

- ## Dental aspects of rheumatoid arthritis

In some patients, as a result of weakness of the ligaments of the neck, dislocation of the atlanto-axial joint or fracture of the odontoid peg can readily follow sudden jerking extension of the neck. Disastrous accidents of this sort have been known to follow adjustment of the head-rest of older types of dental chair, or sudden extension of the neck during the induction of general anaesthesia.

A few patients are treated with corticosteroids (Chapter 14). Patients with joint prostheses because of rheumatoid disease may require antibiotic cover before surgical procedures since those with rheumatoid disease are regarded as mildly immunocompromised.

The main oral complication of rheumatoid arthritis is Sjögren's syndrome (Chapter 9). Patients may also have severely restricted manual dexterity and consequent difficulty maintaining adequate oral hygiene. Despite the predilection of rheumatoid arthritis for small joints, including the temporomandibular joints (TMJ), these are often painless though there may be limitation of opening or stiffness. Radiographic changes are common in the TMJ and consist of erosions, flattening of the joint surfaces and marginal proliferation. Pain felt in the TMJ itself and tenderness on palpation is not significantly more common than in control subjects but there may be referred pain. The TMJ, therefore, shows radiographic changes of rheumatoid arthritis more frequently than is often suspected but symptoms are usually slight. Even when the disease is severe, pain from the TMJ appears to trouble only a minority (*Table 16.7*).

The drugs used in rheumatoid arthritis are a cause of oral side-effects (*Table 16.8*) and high dose aspirin may cause a bleeding tendency. Iron deficiency anaemia secondary to gastrointestinal blood loss caused by aspirin can also produce oral manifestations (Chapter 5) or, with the anaemia of rheumatoid disease, may be severe enough to affect management.

Felty's syndrome

Felty's syndrome comprises rheumatoid arthritis, splenomegaly and lymphadenopathy. These patients are at risk from infections because of leucopenia and may suffer severe oral ulceration or oropharyngeal infections, including chronic sinusitis. Management can also be complicated by anaemia and mild thrombocytopenia.

Table 16.7 Rheumatoid arthritis of the temporomandibular joint: subtypes

Type[a]	TMJ disease	TMJ symptoms	TMJ radiographic findings	Occlusal and facial features
I	Early adult	Continuous dull pain; limitation of movement; crepitus	Erosive changes	Normal
II	Advanced	Variable pain; crepitus; loss of mobility	Gross erosive changes and loss of condylar height	Open bite. Decreased ramus height. Increased anterior facial height
III	Arrested	Often none	Loss of condylar shape	Open bite. Decreased ramus height. Increased anterior facial height
IV	Idiopathic condylar resorption	Variable symptoms including subluxation or dislocation	Flattened, shortened condylar stump	Open bite. Decreased ramus height. Increased anterior facial height

[a]After Kent et al. (1986).

Table 16.8 Drugs in rheumatoid arthritis: oral side-effects

Drugs	Side-effects
Corticosteroids	Candidosis
Methotrexate	Ulceration
Gold	Lichenoid reactions
Pencillamine	Loss of taste
	Lichenoid reactions
	Severe ulceration
Antimalarials	Lichenoid reactions
Non-steroidal anti-inflammatory agents	Lichenoid reactions (rarely)
	Ulceration

Juvenile rheumatoid arthritis (childhood polyarthritis)

Although uncommon compared with adult rheumatoid arthritis, it is estimated that at least 10 000 children suffer from this distressing and often crippling group of diseases. One important form of this disease predominantly affects girls in late childhood, affects virtually any joint and is associated with rheumatoid nodules, mild fever, anaemia and malaise. Rheumatoid factor is positive in all cases and antinuclear antibodies are present in 75 per cent. Over 50 per cent develop severe arthritis and deformity. There are, however, several subtypes of juvenile chronic arthritis, of which Still's disease is one.

At its worst, juvenile arthritis is considerably more severe than the adult disease and can lead to gross deformity.

Damage to the temporomandibular joint of various types has occasionally been described. Complete bony ankylosis has been reported and it has been suggested that micrognathia may develop in 4–25 per cent. Chronic use of aspirin may occasionally cause tooth erosion.

Psoriatic arthritis

Joint disease closely resembling rheumatoid arthritis is sometimes a feature of psoriasis. However, psoriatic arthritis is usually milder, can affect the lower spine and sacro-iliac joints and there are no characteristic serological abnormalities.

When psoriatic arthritis affects the temporomandibular joint, the clinical effects are slight. In spite of the high prevalence of psoriasis (which may affect 2–3 per cent of the population), oral mucosal lesions are exceedingly rare and histologically verified oral psoriasis has been reported on few occasions. The oral lesions are not conspicuous and typically consist of pale, somewhat translucent plaques that are usually associated with pustular psoriasis. Psoriasis may occasionally be treated with methotrexate which may cause oral ulcers.

Note: Severe damage to the temporomandibular joint, including bony ankylosis, has been reported in the past in rheumatoid, psoriatic and other non-infective arthritides. However, in view of recent surveys doubt must be expressed about whether these earlier reports were of uncomplicated disease or whether the diagnoses would fulfil current strict criteria. However, even if these reports are valid, the effects they describe are quite exceptional.

Infective arthritides of the temporomandibular joint

Infective arthritides of the temporomandibular joint are very rare but may follow penetrating wounds, extension from adjacent septic areas or haematogenous dissemination. Possible causes are *Neisseria gonorrhoeae, Haemophilus influenzae, Staphylococcus aureus* or *Mycobacterium tuberculosis*. Ankylosis can be a complication.

Lyme disease

Lyme disease is caused by a spirochaete *Borrelia burgdorferi* which is mainly transmitted by ixodes ticks from deer. It is considerably more common in the USA than in Great Britain, but cases are seen in most parts of the world.

The first sign is usually a rash (erythema marginatum chronicum) which spreads outwards from the site of the insect bite. Arthritis may develop in the acute phase and be transient, or later be persistent. The knees are typically most severely affected.

Other effects include neurological involvement which may result in facial palsy, and lymphadenitis. Lyme disease of the temporomandibular joint has been reported but is rare, even in endemic areas in the USA.

Gout

Primary gout is an inborn error of metabolism which causes raised serum levels of uric acid and deposition of urates, especially in the joints. Secondary gout, which is considerably more common, is usually caused by drug treatment or radiotherapy of myeloproliferative diseases releasing large amounts of purines into the blood.

Primary gout is partly genetically determined and mainly affects adult men. Contrary to popular belief, over-eating and drinking do not *cause* gout, but food rich in purines (such as fish roe), or an alcoholic 'binge', can precipitate an attack in those with the underlying metabolic disorder.

In gout, phagocytosis of urate crystals by polymorphs results in release of lysosomal enzymes and acute inflammation.

Gouty tophi are masses of urate crystals which, in joints, interfere mechanically with function and also destroy bone and cartilage to cause a severe, deforming arthritis. Chronic tophaceous gout is often associated with renal disease.

Extra-articular tophi typically form in the helix of the ear and are conspicuous as almost white, hard, subcutaneous nodules (*Plate 16*). The overlying skin may become necrotic and allow extrusion of semi-solid masses of urates.

Clinically, an acute attack of gout (typically in a man in his forties) causes sudden and intensely severe joint pain, usually in the big toe, associated with fever, leucocytosis and raised serum uric acid levels.

Gout leads to renal disease which, unless treated, leads to fatal renal failure in up to 25 per cent of patients. Many gouty patients are obese, middle-aged males and there is a high incidence of hyperlipidaemia, hypertension, diabetes mellitus and atherosclerosis with their attendant complications.

• General management of gout

Serum should be taken for estimation of uric acid and possibly for renal function tests, especially in chronic tophaceous gout. Secondary gout should be investigated for the underlying disorder.

Colchicine and indomethacin relieve an acute attack. Colchicine, however, can cause severe side-effects so that anti-inflammatory analgesics, but not aspirin, which interferes with uricosuric agents, may be more suitable. Allopurinol can be used to decrease uric acid production. In severe cases uric acid levels can be lowered by the use of uricosuric agents such as probenecid or sulphinpyrazone.

• Dental aspects of gout

The chief importance of this disease is its important associations with hypertension, ischaemic heart disease, cerebrovascular disease, diabetes mellitus and renal disease. Aspirin is contraindicated as it interferes with the action of uricosuric agents.

Drugs used for the treatment of gout, particularly allopurinol, can also occasionally cause severe oral ulceration (*see* Appendix to Chapter 25). Gout can affect the temporo-mandibular joint but only rarely.

In Lesch–Nyhan syndrome, a rare inborn error of metabolism, hyperuricaemia is associated with mental handicap, choreo-athetosis and compulsive self-mutilation, as a result of the lips being chewed away and of self-inflicted injuries especially to the face and head, despite the pain it obviously causes.

Ankylosing spondylitis

Ankylosing spondylitis is a chronic inflammatory arthritis predominantly affecting the spine, mainly in young males. Ankylosing spondylitis is partly genetically determined and the family history is sometimes positive. The aetiology is unknown but over 90 per cent of patients are HLA-B27.

The synovial changes resemble those of rheumatoid arthritis, but inflammation involves the insertions of ligaments and tendons and is followed by ossification, forming bony bridges which fuse adjacent vertebral bodies or cause ankylosis of other joints.

The onset is usually insidious, with low back pain and stiffness followed by increasing pain and tenderness in the sacro-iliac region. The hip joints may also be involved. Over the course of years the back becomes fixed, usually in extreme flexion, with the result that chest expansion is limited and respiration impaired. About 25 per cent of patients develop ocular lesions (uveitis or iridocyclitis) and about 10 per cent develop cardiac disease – usually aortic insufficiency or conduction defects.

On radiography, the spine shows progressive squaring-off of the vertebrae which become rectangular, and then, as intervertebral ossification develops, a bamboo spine appearance is produced. The sacro-iliac joints typically become obliterated.

• General management of ankylosing spondylitis

Apart from a raised ESR, mild anaemia and the association with HLA-B27, there are no significant laboratory findings. Autoantibodies are not found. Treatment consists of anti-inflammatory analgesics to control pain and allow the back to

be kept as mobile as possible. Phenylbutazone and its analogues, or indomethacin, may be used but all can cause side-effects which are sometimes severe. Physiotherapy and exercises are also essential. Occasionally, radiotherapy to the spine is needed but this carries with it the risk of leukaemia.

• Dental aspects of ankylosing spondylitis

General anaesthesia can be hazardous because of severely restricted opening of the mouth, impaired respiratory exchange associated with severe spinal deformity, or cardiac disease with aortic insufficiency.

Ankylosing spondylitis can affect the temporomandibular joints in about 10 per cent of patients, especially those over 40 years of age with widespread disease. However, temporomandibular joint symptoms are usually mild with little pain but usually some trismus. Very occasionally the disability is severe enough to require condylectomy.

Reiter's disease

Reiter's syndrome comprises arthritis, urethritis and conjunctivitis, but there are numerous other effects and it is more common now to speak of Reiter's disease. The pathogenesis is unknown but it appears to be a post-infective response, particularly after gut infections such as *Shigella flexneri* or *Salmonella typhimurium*. The disease may also follow sexually transmitted infection but urethritis is a feature of the disease itself. Reiter's disease almost exclusively affects males between 20 and 40 years of age, about 80 per cent of whom are HLA-B27 positive. The arthritis is chronic or recurrent and migratory and affects the small joints of the hands and feet and also the weight-bearing joints in asymmetrical fashion. Fever, malaise and loss of weight may accompany the acute symptoms. The conjunctivitis is usually bilateral and iritis may sometimes develop.

Characteristic skin lesions of hyperkeratotic thickening, which can be gross, affect the palms and soles (keratoderma blenorrhagica). The penis may have circinate lesions (circinate balanitis) resembling those seen in the mouth.

Leucocytosis is common and the ESR is often raised. The urethritis is purulent but sterile on culture. Anti-inflammatory analgesics are used to control the acute phase of the disease, which usually subsides within a few months but may recur.

• **Dental aspects of Reiter's disease**

The possibility of sexually transmitted disease should be considered in the differential diagnosis.

Oral lesions are said to be very frequent but are transient and painless and often, therefore, unnoticed. The most characteristic lesion is a pattern of scalloped white lines surrounding reddish areas and closely resembling one variant of migratory glossitis (geographic tongue), but affecting any part of the mouth.

PROSTHETIC JOINT REPLACEMENTS

There is no reliable evidence of a need for antibiotic prophylaxis before dental treatment in most patients with prosthetic joints. Occasional infections of prosthetic joints have been with oral organisms such as *Streptococcus sanguis*, but most have been due to non-oral organisms such as staphylococci, and the risks from adverse reactions to antibiotics given routinely for all cases probably exceed any potential benefit. In the largest published study, a single case out of 1855 joint infections followed dental intervention, and how many of the rare, late infections of prosthetic hip joints that have been reported to follow dental treatment have been due to oral bacteria is questionable.

However, where patients are immunocompromised, such as those with diabetes or rheumatoid disease, it would seem prudent to give antibiotic prophylaxis with clindamycin 600 mg orally or intravenously, or cephradine 1 g orally or intravenously, 1–1.5 hours before dental treatment likely to initiate a bacteraemia.

DISEASES OF MUSCLES

Muscle diseases (myopathies) are uncommon and rarely either cause oral manifestations or affect dental management.

GENETIC MYOPATHIES

The genetic myopathies comprise the muscular dystrophies and the myotonic disorders.

Muscular dystrophies

Muscular dystrophies are a group of uncommon genetically determined diseases which nevertheless are now the main crippling diseases of childhood in the West. They are characterized by degeneration of muscle, leading to progressive weakness, complications such as loss of ability to walk, loss of lung and cardiac function and often early death (*Table 16.9*).

Duchenne muscular dystrophy is the most common form and is a recessive sex-linked disorder, with an incidence of about 1 in 5000 live male births, which results in lack of a muscle protein, dystrophin. The pelvic girdle is affected first and the disease appears as the infant begins to walk: there is a waddling gait and severe lumbar lordosis. The child has difficulty in standing and, after lying down, typically has to climb up his legs in order to stand (Gower's sign). The shoulder girdle is also weak, and winging of the scapulae is characteristic. Weakness spreads to all other muscles but tends to spare those of the head, neck and hands. The affected muscles enlarge (pseudohypertrophy) but the child is crippled and, before puberty, becomes confined to a wheelchair.

Cardiac disease (cardiomyopathy), respiratory impairment and intellectual deterioration complicate this disease at an early stage, and patients usually die in their twenties.

• **Dental aspects of muscular dystrophy**

Cardiomyopathies and respiratory disease are the usual causes of death in Duchenne dystrophy and are contraindications to general anaesthesia.

In those muscular dystrophies where there is facial myopathy (classically in the

Table 16.9 Muscular dystrophies

Type	Inheritance	Muscles affected	Pseudo-hypertrophy	Onset	Progress	Other features
Duchenne (pseudo-hypertrophic)	X-linked	All	Usual	Early childhood	Rapid	Cardiomyopathy Death in early adulthood
Becker	X-linked	All	Usual	Late childhood	Variable	More benign than Duchenne type
Childhood muscular	AR	All	Usual	Late childhood	Variable	More benign than Duchenne type
Limb girdle (Erb)	AR	Pelvic and shoulder girdles	Occasional	Adolescence	Variable	Severely disabling May be cardiomyopathy
Facioscapulo-humeral	AD	Starts in face and shoulder	Rare	Adolescence	Slow	Most benign type Normal life expectancy Pouting of lips with facial weakness
Scapuloperoneal	AD or X-linked	Scapular Peroneal	Occasional	Adolescence	Slow	Cardiac conduction defects Relatively bengin
Congenital muscular	AR	All	Rare	Birth	Variable	—
Distal myopathy	AD	Distal	Rare	Any age	Slow	—
Oculopharyngeal	AD	Facial and sterno-mastoid	Rare	Adult	Slow	Dysphagia may be prominent Weakness of masticatory muscles and tongue

AD, Autosomal dominant; AR, autosomal recessive.

facioscapulohumeral type) there is lack of facial expression and, often, inability to whistle. Malocclusions, especially expansion of the arches, may be seen, but there is no abnormal susceptibility to dental disease.

Myotonic disorders

Myotonic disorders are conditions characterized by abnormally slow relaxation after muscle contraction. There are four main types.

Myotonia congenita (*Thomsen's disease*) is a generalized myotonia without weakness that appears in infancy but there are no other problems.

Myotonia congenita (*Becker type*) appears later in childhood and is characterized by muscle hypertrophy. Patients may have dental management problems resulting from treatment with corticosteroids or phenytoin, or from susceptibility to malignant hyperthermia (Chapter 15).

Paramyotonia congenita causes myotonia and weakness after exposure to cold.

Dystrophia myotonica (*Steinert's myotonic dystrophy*) is the most disabling form of myotonia and can lead to ptosis, progressive facial weakness, cataracts, testicular atrophy and frontal baldness. The onset typically becomes apparent in the third decade.

There is atrophy of the temporalis, masseter and sternomastoid muscles (producing a swan neck appearance), and sometimes distal limb weakness and wasting. Myotonia in the tongue causes difficulty in speaking (dysarthria) and there may also be difficulty in masticating food.

Other complications include cardiac conduction defects, respiratory impairment, mild endocrinopathies, intellectual deterioration and personality changes.

• **Dental aspects of myotonic dystrophy**

General anaesthesia may be a risk because of:

1. Cardiac conduction defects.
2. Suxamethonium sensitivity (Chapter 15).
3. Respiratory impairment.

Table 16.10 Metabolic myopathies

- Endocrine
    Acromegaly
    Hyperthyroidism
    Hypothyroidism
    Cushing's syndrome and steroid therapy
    Hyperaldosteronism
    Diabetes mellitus
- Bone disease
    Hyperparathyroidism
    Osteomalacia
    Chronic renal failure
- Drugs
    Alcohol
    Diuretics
    Carbenoxolone
    Vincristine
    Cimetidine
    Tryptophan
- Malignant hyperthermia
- Neuromuscular disorders
    Peroneal muscular atrophy (Charcot–Marie–Tooth disease)
    Hypertrophic polyneuritis (Dejerine–Sottas disease)
    Glycogen storage diseases
    Mitochondrial myopathies

4. Behavioural problems.
5. Malignant hyperthermia (Chapter 15).

The dystonias (*see* Chapter 17)

Other genetic myopathies (*see* Table 16.10)

Atrophy of the masticatory muscles leads to an open mouth posture. There may also be dysphagia, dysarthria and increased caries.

ACQUIRED MYOPATHIES

Polymyositis and dermatomyositis

Polymyositis and dermatomyositis are rare inflammatory myopathies which are immunologically mediated. Muscle weakness and pain are the main features. Polymyositis is usually associated with a variety of systemic abnormalities, and if there are associated skin lesions the condition is known as dermatomyositis. Circulating autoantibodies of various types are frequently present: in a few cases, other connective tissue diseases or distant neoplasms are associated.

Polymyositis and dermatomyositis usually develop between the fifth and sixth decades. Women are affected twice as often as men. The onset is characteristically insidious but is occasionally acute, with weakness usually of the pelvic girdle and the proximal limb muscles, especially those of the legs. Speaking and swallowing may become difficult. In severe cases, weakness may make patients bedridden and ultimately, atrophy, contracture and calcinosis of muscles can develop.

A characteristic rash affects about 30 per cent of patients with polymyositis. It is dusky and violaceous (heliotrope) with a butterfly distribution across the bridge of the nose and adjacent cheeks but may spread to the upper part of the body. Small ulcerated skin lesions may develop over bony prominences.

Raynaud's phenomenon and features of the other connective tissue diseases, particularly scleroderma, may be associated in about 20 per cent of cases, especially those with dermatomyositis, and other complications include myocarditis and fibrosing alveolitis. Underlying malignant disease is found in up to 10 per cent and is the main cause of death.

• General management of polymyositis

Raised serum levels of the enzymes creatinine phosphokinase (CPK), aldolase and aspartate transaminase (AST) may be found and the diagnosis is confirmed by electromyography and muscle biopsy.

The most effective drugs are corticosteroids or other immunosuppressants, but these are much less effective when there is underlying malignant disease.

• Dental aspects of polymyositis

Dental management may be complicated by corticosteroid therapy or associated disorders such as other connective tissue diseases, including Sjögren's syndrome (Chapters 9 and 21).

A minority of patients have pharyngeal weakness. Oral lesions have rarely been reported in polymyositis/dermatomyositis but it has been suggested that they may be found in 10–20 per cent of patients. These oral lesions appear to be variable in character and comprise dark or purplish erythema and oedema of the oral mucosa and possibly also of the gingival margins. Small whitish patches occasionally with shallow ulceration may also develop and bear some resemblance to the oral lesions of lichen planus or lupus erythematosus.

CRANIAL ARTERITIS AND POLYMYALGIA RHEUMATICA

These disorders are vasculitides, not myopathies, but are relatively common causes of muscle pain and headache in the middle-aged and elderly.

The basic lesion, which may be immunologically mediated, is inflammation of the walls of medium-size arteries with prominent giant cells. There is obliteration of the vessel lumen and ischaemia of the part supplied.

Clinically, giant cell arteritis usually either affects the craniofacial region, and is then called cranial or temporal arteritis, or alternatively it can be more widespread, affecting particularly the shoulder and pelvic regions and is then known as polymyalgia rheumatica. The common feature of these diseases is muscle pain caused by ischaemia, but the eyes and other structures can also be affected, leading to blindness.

Cranial arteritis

The most common complaint is severe unilateral throbbing headache. Women are predominantly affected, usually after the age of 55. The headache is acute and can be mainly in the temporal region or more widespread. The temporal artery is typically prominent, tortuous and tender. Biopsy of an affected part of the vessel confirms the diagnosis. Associated features are malaise, fever and usually a greatly raised ESR and serum interleukin-6 level.

The most severe complication of cranial arteritis is ischaemia of the optic nerve causing blindness, which in the absence of treatment may develop in up to 30 per cent of patients. It is obligatory to give systemic corticosteroids (60 mg prednisone daily reducing as the ESR returns to normal) as soon as the diagnosis is made to prevent this complication. The clinical response to these drugs is rapid.

- **Dental aspects of cranial arteritis**

Ischaemic pain in the muscles of mastication can cause severe pain when eating and has been reported in 20 per cent of these patients. This is sometimes called 'claudication' of the masticatory muscles but, though they share the feature of ischaemic muscle pain, it seems unreasonable to suggest that the masticatory muscles are limping – the literal meaning of claudication.

A rare manifestation of cranial arteritis is ischaemic necrosis and gangrene of the tongue and it is probably the only cause of this unusual and unpleasant phenomenon.

The most important aspect is to differentiate the masticatory pain of cranial arteritis from temporomandibular pain-dysfunction syndrome by the later onset, greater severity of pain, the high ESR and, often, local signs of inflammation of the temporal artery. There is no diagnostic serological test. Artery biopsy is the one confirmatory diagnostic measure and even this may be negative as the lesions are patchily distributed. Accurate diagnosis is, however, essential because of the danger of blindness.

Temporal arteritis may occasionally have to be differentiated from trigeminal neuralgia where the pain can also be triggered by mastication. The pain of trigeminal neuralgia is, however, different in character and distribution, systemic symptoms are absent, the ESR is normal and there is usually a good initial response to carbamazepine.

Systemic corticosteroids may complicate dental management.

Polymyalgia rheumatica

Polymyalgia rheumatica can co-exist with cranial arteritis, or develop as a separate entity. The age and sex distribution, and associated systemic disturbances, are the same and the typical arterial changes may be found. In polymyalgia rheumatica there is pain, stiffness and weakness across the shoulders, in the upper arms and in the pelvic region radiating into the thighs. In most cases the disease is ultimately self-limiting though it frequently persists for 1–2 years. In the absence of cranial symptoms relatively small doses of corticosteroids usually give rapid relief. The dose should be adjusted to bring the ESR to – and maintained to keep it at – the normal level.

- ## Dental aspects of polymyalgia rheumatica

The main oral and perioral features have been mentioned earlier. Patients may be on treatment with systemic corticosteroids.

Eosinophilia myalgia syndrome

Tryptophan may be used as an antidepressant or for the treatment of insomnia. This syndrome, first described in 1989 in patients taking tryptophan, has an abrupt onset of myalgia with oedema of the extremities, rashes of various types and peripheral eosinophilia. About a third of patients have had to be hospitalized and some have died from an ascending polyneuropathy and respiratory failure.

The disease has mainly been seen in the US and appears to be caused by a contaminant of trytophan. It is a rare cause of facial pain but tryptophan has now been withdrawn in Britain and can only be given under exceptional circumstances to individual, named patients.

MYASTHENIA GRAVIS (*see* Chapter 17)

BIBLIOGRAPHY

Audran M. and Kumar R. (1985) The physiology and pathophysiology of vitamin D. *Mayo Clin. Proc.* **60**, 851–66.

Barrett A.W., Griffiths M.J. and Scully C. (1993) Osteoarthritis, the temporomandibular joint and Eagle's syndrome. *Oral Surg. Oral Med. Oral Pathol.* **75**, 273–5.

Bartzokas C.A., Johnson R., Jane M. *et al.* (1994) Relation between mouth and haematogenous infection in total joint replacements. *Br. Med. J.* **309**, 506–8.

Beard C.J., Key L., Newburger P.E. *et al.* (1986) Neutrophil defect associated with malignant infantile osteopetrosis. *J. Lab. Clin. Med.* **108**, 498–505.

Carette S. (1995) Fibromyalgia 20 years later: what have we really accomplished? *J. Rheumatol.* **22**, 590–4.

Cawson R. A. and Scully C. (1986) Temporomandibular joint disorders. *Medicine Int.* **2**, 140–1.

Cawson R.A., Spector R.G. and Skelly A.M. (1995) Basic *Pharmacology and Clinical Drug Use in Dentistry*, 6th edn. Edinburgh, Churchill Livingstone.

Chesley L.D. and Van Gilder J.W. (1990) Eosinophilic myalgia syndrome masquerading as facial pain. *J. Oral Maxillofac. Surg.* **48**, 980–1.

Danielson C., Lyon J.L., Egger M. *et al.* (1992). Hip fractures and fluoridation in Utah's elderly population. *J. Am. Med. Assoc.* **268**, 746–8.

Editorial (1984) Osteogenesis imperfecta 1984. *Br. Med. J.* **289**, 394–5.

Eppley B.L., Green P., Bixler D.P. *et al.* (1992) Developmental significance of delayed closure of the mandibular symphysis. *J. Oral Maxillofac. Surg.* **50**, 677–80.

Eskinazi D. (1989) Is systemic antimicrobial prophylaxis justified in dental patients with prosthetic joints? *Oral Surg. Oral Med. Oral Pathol.* **66**, 430–1.

Evans J.M., Batts K.P. and Hunder G.G. (1994). Persistent giant cell arteritis despite corticosteroid treatment. *Mayo Clin Proc.* **69**, 1060–1.

Fadavi S. and Rowold E. (1990) Familial hypophosphatemic vitamin D resistant rickets. *J. Dent. Child.* 212–15.

Feuillan P.P., Foster C.M., Pescovitz O.H. *et al.* (1986) Treatment of precocious puberty in the McCune–Albright syndrome with the aromatase inhibitor testolactone. *N. Engl. J. Med.* **315**, 1115–19.

Field E.A. and Martin M.V. (1991) Prophylactic antibiotics for patients with artificial joints undergoing oral and dental surgery : necessary or not? *Br. J. Oral Maxillofac. Surg.* **29**, 341–6.

Friedman R.D., Joe J. and Bodak G.L.Z. (1980) Myotonic dystrophy. *Oral Surg.* **50**, 229–32.

Frohberg U. and Tiner B.D. (1995). Surgical correction of facial deformities in a patient with cleidocranial dysplasia. *J. Craniofac. Surg.* **6**, 49–53.

Hazes J.M.W. and Silman A.J. (1990) Review of UK data on the rheumatic diseases: 2. Rheumatoid arthritis. *Br. J. Rheumatol.* **29**, 310–2.

Hill C.M. (1980) Death following dental clearance in a patient suffering from ankylosing spondylitis – a case report with discussion on management of such problems. *Br. J. Oral Surg.* **18**, 73–6.

Horton W.A. and Schinke R.N. (1980) Osteopetrosis: further heterogeneity. *J. Pediatr.* **97**, 580–8.

Hosking D.J. (1982) *Paget's Disease of Bone*. London, Update Publications.

Hosking D., Meunier P.J., Ringe J.D. *et al.* (1996) Paget's disease of bone: diagnosis and management. *Br. Med. J.* **312**, 491–4.

Jacobsen P.L. and Murray W. (1980) Prophylactic coverage of dental patients with artificial joints: a retrospective analysis of thirty-three infections in hip prostheses. *Oral Surg. Oral Med. Oral Pathol.* **50**, 130–3.

Jacobson J.J., Millard H.D. and Plezia R. (1986) Dental treatment and late prosthetic joint infections. *Oral Surg. Oral Med. Oral Pathol.* **61**, 413–17.

Jaspers M.T. and Little J.W. (1985) Prophylactic antibiotic coverage in patients with total arthroplasty: current practice. *J. Am. Dent. Assoc.* **111**, 943–8.

Lindholm T.S. (1996) *Bone Morphogenetic Proteins: Biology, Biochemistry and Reconstructive Surgery.* San Diego, Academic Press.

Kent J.N., Carlton D.M. and Zide M.F. (1986) Rheumatoid disease and related arthropathies. *Oral. Surg. Oral Med. Oral Pathol* **61**, 432–9.

Leading Article (1980) Learning from Ehlers–Danlos. *Lancet* **ii**, 1062–3.

Leading Article (1987) Vitamin D: new perspectives. *Lancet* **i**, 1122–3.

McGowan D.A. and Hendrey M.L. (1985) Is antibiotic prophylaxis required for dental patients with joint replacements? *Br. Dent. J.* **158**, 336–8.

Medsger T.A. (1990) Tryptophan-induced eosinophilia-myalgia syndrome. *N. Engl. J. Med.* **322**, 926–8.

Migliorisi J.A. and Blenkinsopp P.T. (1980) Oral surgical management of cleidocranial dysostosis. *Br. J. Oral Surg.* **18**, 212–20.

Morgan-Hughes J. (1980) Diseases of muscle. *Medicine (UK)* **34**, 171–31.

Mulligan R. (1980) Late infections in patients with prostheses for total replacement of joints: implications for the dental practitioner. *J. Am. Dent. Assoc.* **101**, 44–6.

Nebgen D., Wood R.S. and Shapiro R.D. (1991). Management of a mandibular fracture in a patient with cleidocranial dysplasia. *J. Oral Maxillofac. Surg.* **41**, 462–8.

Paganini-Hill A. (1995) The benefits of estrogen replacement therapy on oral health. *Arch. Intern. Med.* **155**, 2325–9.

Patterson A., Barnard N., Scully C. and Griffiths M.J. (1992) Necrosis of the tongue in a patient with intestinal infarction. *Oral Surg. Oral Med. Oral Pathol.* **74**, 582–6.

Penarrocha M., Bagan J.V., Vilchez J. *et al.* (1990) Oral alterations in Steinert's myotonic dystrophy. *Oral Surg. Oral Med. Oral Pathol.* **69**, 698–78.

Pope F.M. and Nicholls A.C. (1984) Molecular abnormalities of collagen proteins and genes. In: Malcolm A.D.B. (eds) *Molecular Medicine.* Lancaster, MTP Press, p. 117.

Porter S.R. and Scully C. (1996) *Innovations and Developments in Non-Invasive Oral Health Care.* Northwood, Science Reviews.

Prockop D.K. and Kivirikko K.I. (1981) Heritable diseases of collagen. *N. Engl. J. Med.* **311**, 376–86.

Prockop D.K. and Kuivaniemi H. (1986) Inborn errors of collagen. *Rheumatology* **10**, 246–71.

Ramsay A.N. (1986) *Post Viral Fatigue Syndrome – the Saga of Royal Free Disease.* London, Gower.

Roche N.E., Fulbright J.W., Wagner A.D. et al (1993). Correlation of interleukin-6 production and disease activity in polymyalgia rheumatica and giant cell arteritis. *Arth. Rheum.* **36**, 1286–94.

Royce P.M. and Steinmann B. (1993) *Connective Tissue and Its Heritable Disorders.* New York, Wiley-Liss.

Scully C. (1979/80) Orofacial manifestations of disease. 4: Fungal and viral infections, skeletal disorders and malignancies. *Dent. Update* **7**, 87; *Hosp. Update* **5**, 1119.

Scully C. (1988) *The Dental Patient.* Oxford, Heinemann.

Scully C. (1989) *The Mouth and Perioral Tissues.* Oxford, Heinemann.

Scully C. (1989) *Patient Care: a Dental Surgeon's Guide.* London, British Dental Association.

Scully C. and Cawson R.A. (eds) (1986) Oral medicine. *Med. Int.* **28**, 1129–51.

Scully C., Cawson R.A. and Griffiths M.J. (1990) *Occupational Hazards to Dental Staff.* London, British Dental Journal

Scully C., Eveson J.W., Barrett A.W. and Cunningham S. (1993) Necrosis of the lip in giant cell arteritis. *J. Oral Maxillofac. Surg.* **51**, 581–3.

Seow W.K. and Latham S.C. (1986) The spectrum of dental manifestations in vitamin-D-resistant rickets and implications for management. *Pediatr. Dent.* **8**, 245–50.

Simmons N.A., Ball A.P., Cawson R.A. *et al.* (1992) Case against antibiotic prophylaxis for dental treatment of patients with joint prostheses. *Lancet* **339**, 301.

Simoen O. and Laitinen O. (1985) Does fluoridation of drinking water prevent bone fragility and osteoporosis? *Lancet* **ii**, 432–4.

Singer F.R. and Wallach S. (eds) (1991) *Paget's Disease of Bone.* New York, Elsevier Press.

Smith B.J. and Eveson J.W. (1981) Paget's disease of bone with particular reference to dentistry. *J. Oral Pathol.* **10**, 233–47.

Thyne G.M. and Ferguson J.W. (1991) Antibiotic prophylaxis during dental treatment in patients with prosthetic joints. *J. Bone Joint Surg.* **73B**, 191–4.

Wenneberg B. and Kapp S. (1982) Clinical findings in the stomatognathic system in ankylosing spondylitis. *Scand. J. Dent. Res.* **90**, 373–81.

Worton R. (1995) Muscular dystrophies: diseases of the dystrophin-glycoprotein complex. *Science* **270**, 755–6.

APPENDIX TO CHAPTER 16

SOME GENETICALLY DETERMINED SKELETAL DISORDERS

Achondroplasia	(p.312)
Albers–Schönberg syndrome	(p.313)
Albright's syndrome	(p.319)
Apert's syndrome	Craniostenosis; syndactyly
Cheney syndrome	Osteoporosis; early loss of teeth
Cherubism	Familial symmetrical self-limiting soft tissue jaw lesions
Cleidocranial dysplasia	(p.312)
Congenital hyperphosphatasia	Thickened calvarium; early loss of teeth; visual or hearing defects; blue sclerae
Crouzon's syndrome	Hypoplastic midface; proptosis; craniostenosis; hearing defects
Ellis–van Creveld syndrome	Atrial septal defect; dwarfism; polydactyly
Gardner's syndrome	(p.154)
Gaucher's disease	(Appendix 15)
Goldenhar's syndrome	Same as Treacher–Collins syndrome plus epibulbar dermoids
Gorlin's syndrome	(p.246)
Hallermann–Streiff syndrome	Cataracts; mandibular retrognathism; scanty hair
Holt–Oram syndrome	Abnormalities of thumb, wrist and clavicle; atrial septal defect
Hypophosphataemia	Vitamin D-resistant rickets; dentinal anomalies leading to early pulp involvement in caries
Klippel–Feil deformity	(Appendix, p.558)
Maffuci's syndrome	(p.559)
Mucopolysaccharidoses	(Appendix 15)
Noonan's syndrome	(Appendix, p.558)
Odontomatosis	Multiple odontomas; cirrhosis; oesophageal stenosis
Ollier's disease	Multiple enchondromas
Orofacial digital syndromes	Facial anomalies; fraenal hyperplasia; tongue hamartomas; digital anomalies
Osteogenesis imperfecta	(p.311)
Pierre Robin syndrome	Micrognathia; cleft palate; glossoptosis
Rubinstein–Taybi syndrome	Broad thumbs and toes; maxillary hypoplasia; patent ductus arteriosus
TAR syndrome	Thrombocytopenia, absent radius; atrial septal defect or tetralogy of Fallot
Treacher–Collins syndrome	Hypoplastic malars and mandible; palpebral fissures slope down and out; colobomas; hearing defects
van Buchem's syndrome	Generalized cortical hyperostosis; facial palsy; optic atrophy; hearing defects

DIFFERENTIATION OF MARFAN'S SYNDROME FROM CONGENITAL CONTRACTURAL ARACHNODACTYLY (CCA) AND HOMOCYSTINURIA

	Marfan's	*CCA*	*Homocystinuria*
Inheritance	AD†	AD	AR†
Arachnodactyly	+	+	+
Loose joints	+	+ contractures	±
Pectus excavatus	+	−	+
Ectopia lentis	+	−	+
Mental handicap	±	−	+
High palate	+	+	+
Crowding of teeth	+	−	+

continued

Vascular	Dilatation of ascending aorta Dissecting aneurysm Aortic valve disease	–	Thromboses
Others	Blue sclerae Jaw cysts	Scoliosis Ear deformities Retrognathia	Malar flush Osteoporosis Prognathic mandible
Management problems	Risk of infective endocarditis	—	Postoperative thromboses

†AD, Autosomal dominant; AR, Autosomal recessive.

17

Neurological disorders

Key points

- Neurological disorders may be detected by the presence of paralyses, disorders of sensation, consciousness, speech or muscle tone or tremor or wasting.
- The neurological disorders of most relevance include cerebral palsy, facial palsy, stroke, trigeminal neuralgia, multiple sclerosis, epilepsy and Parkinsonism.
- Cerebral palsy (CP) is commonly a result of brain damage around birth, and usually presents with palsy, increased muscle tone and contractures (spasticity), and thus disability.
- CP may also be associated with malocclusions, abnormal orofacial muscle movements and tone, learning disability, epilepsy and defects of the special senses.
- Spina bifida is a neural tube defect, sometimes due to folic acid deficiency, which may result in paraplegia and urinary or faecal incontinence, and a susceptibility to meningitis.
- Patients with spina bifida are often chair-bound, may have hydrocephalus, and may develop allergy to latex.
- Huntington's chorea is a genetic, ultimately lethal, disorder with progressive involuntary movements and dementia. Dopamine receptor antagonists may help.
- Facial sensory loss is usually caused by extracranial damage to the trigeminal nerve but stroke, tumours, multiple sclerosis, infections and connective tissue diseases may be causal.
- Facial paralysis is usually caused by stroke or Bell's palsy – probably a viral infection – but other infections such as HIV and Lyme disease, tumours, sarcoidosis and other disorders may be causal.
- Blindness is a major disability resulting from a wide spectrum of causes, especially trauma, inflammatory states, diabetes and drugs.
- Epilepsy is typically idiopathic but trauma, tumours, brain disease, drug addictions and metabolic causes must be excluded. Learning disability and cerebral palsy are sometimes associated.
- Grand mal epileptics may damage themselves, especially the orofacial tissues, and need to be on long-term anticonvulsant medication, often leading to serious oral neglect.
- Drugs such as methohexitone, enflurane and others which may be epileptogenic should be avoided.
- Brain abscesses are usually secondary to middle ear sinus, or lung infection, and a few follow lung abscesses from inhalation of oral bacteria, dental restorations or other items.
- Encephalopathy is an important feature in some patients with HIV disease.
- Strokes (cerebrovascular accidents) are common and caused by haemorrhage, thrombosis or embolism, may be lethal, or may leave hemiplegia, facial palsy, speech defects or other sequelae.

- Parkinson's disease is a condition characterized by tremor, rigidity, abnormal posture and bradykinesia, often with akathisia.
- Often idiopathic, Parkinsonism may be caused by repeated trauma (boxing), drugs, toxins or infections. It is managed mainly with levodopa and antimuscarinic agents, rarely by brain surgery.
- Multiple sclerosis (MS) is a common disorder, often starting in younger adults, in which neurological lesions are disseminated in site and time.
- Transient visual, sensory or motor disturbances are common features of MS, and some patients present with trigeminal neuralgia.
- The progress of MS is tremendously variable but in some there is progressive paralysis and loss of sphincter control.
- Motor neurone disease is an uncommon but lethal disease, affecting males mainly, with progressive muscle wasting and weakness, fortunately sparing sphincters and sensation.
- Brain tumours are the second most common neoplasms in childhood. Most brain tumours in adults are metastases from cancer of the lung, breast, stomach or colon. Lymphomas are seen in AIDS.
- Myasthenia gravis (MG) is an autoimmune disease often associated with thymic hyperplasia or thymoma, where antibodies damage neuromuscular acetylcholine receptors.
- Muscle fatigue, increasing as the day progresses, and affecting the head and neck, facial and masticatory muscles is the main feature of MG, and respiration may ultimately be affected.
- General anaesthesia is contraindicated in MG, and drugs such as tetracyclines and aspirin which can accentuate the weakness are best avoided.

Orofacial pain is common and may have a neurological cause. Facial palsy and facial sensory loss are other neurological conditions with which dental staff may have to deal. Patients with maxillofacial or head injuries may have brain damage with impaired ocular movements or pupil reactions and loss of the sense of smell (anosmia). Dental staff should therefore be able to recognize abnormalities involving the cranial nerves, especially the trigeminal, facial, glossopharyngeal, vagal and hypoglossal nerves. Moreover, some disorders traditionally held to be psychiatric in origin now appear to be primary disorders of the nervous system albeit with no definable *anatomical* defect but rather a neuroendocrine-biochemical abnormality. This chapter deals with the most relevant neurological abnormalities and some other causes of oral symptoms. Facial pain is discussed in Chapter 19.

CONGENITAL NEUROLOGICAL DISORDERS

CEREBRAL PALSY

Cerebral palsy (CP) is the motor manifestation of cerebral damage or defect caused before or at birth, mainly by brain damage from hypoxia, trauma, infection or hyperbilirubinaemia. CP results in disordered movement and posture, but because of the many types of brain damage there is no uniform pattern of CP defects (*Table 17.1*). CP is the most common congenital physical handicap and patients are often loosely referred to as 'spastics'. Some patients with CP are highly intelligent but have such severely impaired speech as to appear subnormal. About 50 per cent have additional disorders such as learning impairment, epilepsy, defects of hearing, vision or speech,

Table 17.1	Types of cerebral palsy	
Type		*Involves*
Spastic	Monoplegic	Only one limb
	Paraplegic	Lower extremities
	Hemiplegic	One upper and lower limb on same side
	Double hemiplegic	All limbs, but mainly the arms
	Diplegic	All limbs, but mainly the legs
	Quadriplegic (tetraplegic)	All limbs equally
Athetoid	Athetosis	All limbs equally
	Chorea	
	Choreoathetosis	
Ataxic		
Rigid		
Mixed		

or emotional disturbances. CP in the infant usually causes poor feeding, delayed development and abnormal muscle tone.

Spastic cerebral palsy

Fifty per cent of CP patients are spastic and have excessive muscle tone, contractures, pathological reflexes and hyperactive tendon reflexes as a result of an upper motor neurone lesion (*Fig. 17.1*).

Hemiplegia is the most common form of spastic CP. Learning impairment is not usual but associated neurological disorders such as visual field defects, epilepsy or sensory deficits are common.

Quadriplegics with CP are usually more frequently mentally handicapped than hemiplegics but are less often epileptic.

Paraplegics and diplegics with CP have an IQ intermediate in level between quadriplegics and hemiplegics, but are the least likely to have epilepsy.

Athetoid cerebral palsy

From 15 to 20 per cent of CP is athetoid and caused by an extrapyramidal lesion, usually in the basal ganglia. There is increased muscle tone (of 'lead pipe' type) but normal tendon reflexes and no contractures.

Unlike most spastic CP, athetoid CP usually involves all four limbs – especially the arms. Smooth worm-like movements of the distal parts of the extremities are characteristic and become exaggerated if the patient is anxious. Learning impairment is less common than in spastic CP but epilepsy can be associated. Athetoid CP is often accompanied by high tone deafness and is caused mainly by intrauterine rubella (the rubella syndrome, Chapter 11) and by hyperbilirubinaemia (kernicterus, e.g. in Rhesus incompatibility).

Ataxic cerebral palsy

Ataxic cerebral palsy is characterized by disturbance of balance. It accounts for about

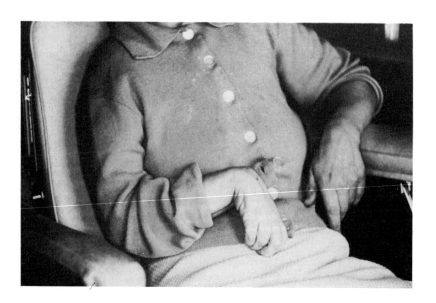

Fig. 17.1 Cerebral palsy: the limbs assume characteristic deformities, with flexion at all joints in the upper limbs and scissoring of the lower limbs if physiotherapy is neglected

10 per cent of all CP and is caused by a cerebellar lesion.

• Dental aspects of cerebral palsy

In uncomplicated CP, where oral hygiene can be maintained, routine dental procedures can be carried out. However, in some, dental management may be difficult for the following reasons:

1. Communication difficulties, which may give a misleading impression of low intelligence.
2. Epilepsy.
3. Anxiety.
4. Cooperation; concentration is often poor.
5. Posture and mobility. Manual support is often required and ataxic patients may need the chair to be tilted backwards. Many, however, become apprehensive when this is done.
6. Abnormal swallowing.
7. Drooling. Poor control of the oral tissues and of head posture often leads to drooling.
8. Learning impairment in some patients.

Anxiety may increase athetosis or spasticity, so that anxiolytic drugs such as diazepam are useful as premedication. Patients restricted to wheelchairs can sometimes be treated in their chair but it is often better to transfer them to the dental chair by carrying them or by sliding them across a board placed between the wheelchair and dental chair.

There is no dental disease unique to CP, but there may be delayed eruption of the primary dentition and enamel hypoplasia is common. Caries incidence appears normal, unless there is over-indulgence by parents, but lack of treatment frequently leads to premature loss of primary teeth, and earlier eruption of premolars and permanent canines.

Most dental disease is more common when the arms are severely involved. Periodontal disease is common, especially in the older child because soft tissue movement is abnormal and oral cleansing is impaired. Mouth breathing worsens the periodontal state. A papillary hyperplastic gingivitis may be seen, even in the absence of treatment with phenytoin.

Malocclusion is common and thought to be caused by abnormal muscle behaviour. The maxillary arch is frequently tapered or ovoid, with a high palate. The upper teeth are often labially inclined, due to the pressure of the tongue against the anterior teeth during abnormal swallowing. Most, however, have skeletal patterns within normal limits.

Bruxism, abnormal attrition and spontaneous dislocation or subluxation of the temporomandibular joint are common. Certain oral lesions are more prevalent in different types of cerebral palsy.

In cerebral palsy, preventive dental care is important. Parental counselling about diet, oral hygiene procedures and the use of fluorides should be started early. Manual dexterity is usually poor but favourable results are often achievable with an electric toothbrush or a modified handle to the normal brush.

NEURAL TUBE DEFECTS (SPINA BIFIDA)

Spina bifida is the failure of fusion of vertebral arches, of unknown aetiology, though it is now recognized that deficiency of folic acid in pregnancy may predispose. Spina bifida is an important cause of spinal cord disease and severe physical handicap in children.

Spina bifida occulta

There is rarely any obvious clinical or neurological disorder but the defect can be detected radiographically in about 50 per cent of normal children. The most obvious sign is a small naevus or tuft of hair over the lumbar spine in some patients.

Spina bifida cystica

There is an extensive vertebral defect through which the spinal cord or its coverings protrude. The incidence of this severe form of spinal bifida is about 2 per 1000 live births in the United Kingdom. There are two main types:

Meningocele is protrusion of the meninges as a sac covered by skin. Neurological defect is rare but 20 per cent have hydrocephalus.

Myelomeningocele is a protrusion of meninges and nerve tissue which are exposed and liable to infection, particularly meningitis. It is ten times more common than meningocele.

Myelomeningocele causes severe neurological defects. The usual pattern is complete paralysis of and loss of sensation and reflexes in the lower limbs. Deformities of the lower limbs follow. Patients with myelomeningocele therefore tend to suffer from paraplegia and hence they have:

1. Inability to walk.
2. Liability to develop pressure sores.
3. Urinary incontinence.
4. Faecal retention.
5. Meningitis risk.
6. Other problems such as hydrocephalus, cerebral complications (epilepsy or learning impairment), other vertebral or renal anomalies.

• **General management of spina bifida cystica**

Surgical closure of myelomeningocele and decompression of hydrocephalus is often carried out, usually in early infancy. These patients are severely handicapped and require specialist paediatric attention to manage urinary tract, bowel and locomotion disabilities.

• **Dental aspects of spina bifida cystica**

Children with spina bifida must be managed in consultation with the physician and with due regard to the possible problems outlined earlier. Bowel and bladder are best emptied before dental treatment. Care must also be taken not to traumatize the patient who is unable to respond protectively. Postural hypotension is likely, and thus the patient is best not treated supine. In any event, many are chairbound, and it is better just to tilt the wheelchair back slightly if there are facilities for this, or transfer the patient to the dental chair using a board between wheelchair and dental chair, and then treat the patient in the semi-reclined position. There is a very high prevalence of latex allergy in these patients (Chapter 25). Some patients are on anticoagulants or other appropriate medication.

SYRINGOMYELIA

Syringomyelia is of unknown aetiology and characterized by cavitation of the central part of the spinal cord, causing disruption of pain and temperature neurones of the anterior commissure of the cord. This leads to loss of pain and temperature sense, but preservation of the sense of touch.

Symptoms begin in adolescence or adult life and progress erratically. There is segmental loss of pain and temperature sense leading to painless ulcers, injuries or burns, and deranged (Charcot's) joints. Touch sensation is retained. Damage to the sympathetic neurones in the intermediolateral column of the spinal cord can cause Horner's syndrome and, late in the disease, the pyramidal tracts may be involved with signs of spasticity in the legs. Kyphoscoliosis develops at an early stage.

If the condition affects the brain stem it is known as *syringobulbia* and may cause facial or oral sensory changes or paralyses.

Syringobulbia can cause facial sensory loss with unilateral palatal and vocal cord palsies, nystagmus, weakness and atrophy of the tongue, dysphagia and dysarthria. Damage to the medulla in syringobulbia does not usually, however, significantly affect the respiratory or cardiovascular centres.

There is no effective treatment.

HUNTINGTON'S CHOREA

Huntington's chorea is an autosomal dominant condition characterized by progressive dementia and involuntary movements related to atrophy of the caudate nucleus of the basal ganglia.

Clinically, signs of Huntington's chorea usually appear in early to middle age. Irregular involuntary movements (chorea), causing gross disturbances of speech and gait, are typically associated with progressive dementia and behavioural changes. Patients can often understand what they are being told but are unable to respond, and may give a false impression of the degree of dementia. Progress of the disease is slow, but life is often ended by intercurrent infection, or sometimes suicide, since patients are often aware of the family history and prognosis. There is no effective treatment, though dopamine receptor antagonists such as butyrophenone or phenothiazines and antidepressants may help.

There may be darting movements of the tongue and head which subside if physical control is applied. Oral hygiene may be impaired and worsened by medications that impair salivation. The chorea can make the construction and wearing of prostheses difficult or impossible.

Other causes of tremor in addition to Huntington's chorea, Parkinson's disease and cerebellar disease, are shown in *Table 17.2*.

FRIEDREICH'S ATAXIA

Friedreich's ataxia, usually an autosomal recessive trait, leads to degeneration of many tracts of the spinal cord extending up to the brain stem. This causes severe ataxia, loss of reflexes and secondary deformities. Degenerative heart disease with dysrhythmias may be associated. Treatment is symptomatic only.

Table 17.2 Causes of involuntary movements

Disease	Features
Essential tremor	Worse with anxiety; better with alcohol, benzodiazepines or beta-blockers
Neurological disease	
Cerebellar disease	Ataxia and nystagmus
Parkinsonism	Rigidity and akinesia
Athetoid cerebral palsy	Writhing movements and deafness
Huntington's chorea	Chorea and dementia
Sydenham's chorea	Complication of rheumatic fever
Tardive dyskinesia	Facial grimacing and jaw clenching
Liver failure	Tremor
Wilson's disease	Tremor and cirrhosis
Alcoholism	Delirium tremens

ACQUIRED NEUROLOGICAL DISORDERS

The nervous system is evaluated by assessing the following:

1. Mental state
   Level of consciousness
   Cognition
2. Speech
3. Motor system (*Table 17.3*)
   Muscle tone
   Power
   Reflexes
   Gait
4. Sensory system
   Touch
   Pin-prick
   Joint position
   Two-point discrimination
   Vibration sense
5. Cerebrum and cerebellum (*Table 17.4*)
6. Cranial nerves

Table 17.3 Motor abnormalities

Disorder	Features	Main conditions
Akathisia	Restlessness	Neuroleptic drugs
Akinesia	Lack of movement	Parkinsonism
Athetosis	Dystonia of limbs	Athetoid cerebral palsy
Chorea	Continual flow of jerky movements	Huntington's chorea
Clonus	Rhythmic contractions	UMN lesions
Dyskinesia	Involuntary chewing or grinding	Phenothiazines
Dystonia	Sustained spasms causing abnormal posture	Phenothiazines
Fasciculation	Spontaneous contractions of muscle fibres	LMN lesions
Hemiballismus	Chorea affecting half the body	Subthalamic lesion
Rigidity	Limbs resist passive movement	Parkinsonism
Spasticity	Excess tone in arm flexors, leg extensors	Cerebral palsy; UMN lesion
Tremor	Rhythmic movements of a part:	
	at rest	Parkinsonism
		Anxiety, drugs, thyrotoxicosis, benign, or brain lesion
	on intention to move	Cerebellar disease

Table 17.4 Localizing signs of brain lesions	
Location of lesion	*Signs*
Cerebellopontine angle	Nystagmus; palsies of Vth and VIIth nerves; ipsilateral deafness; cerebellar signs
Cerebellum	Intention tremor; ataxia; nystagmus
Corpus callosum	Disturbance of intellect
Frontal	Loss of inhibitions; hemiparesis, convulsions; return of grasp reflex
Midbrain	Sleepiness; recent amnesia; unequal pupils; inability to look up or down
Occipital	Contralateral visual field defects
Parietal	Dysphasia; loss of two-point discrimination; sensory loss
Temporal	Dysphasia; memory deficit; visual field defects; hallucinations of senses

CRANIAL NERVES: EXAMINATION AND LESIONS

The history and full neurological and physical examination are the essential aspects of neurological assessment, but investigations may be useful. These may need to include

1. Full blood count.
2. Electrolytes.
3. Liver, kidney or endocrine function tests.
4. Cerebrospinal fluid (CSF) examination.
5. CNS imaging: although plain radiographs can be helpful, CT and MRI have been major advances in the delineation of neurological lesions. Positron emission tomography (PET) allows cerebral functional studies and has opened the way for advances such as single photon emission computed tomography (SPECT).
6. Electrophysiological studies, such as electroencephalography (EEG).

The olfactory nerve (Ist cranial nerve)

Unilateral anosmia is often unnoticed by the patient. Bilateral anosmia is common after head injuries, but in practice the patient may complain of loss of taste rather than sense of smell. An olfactory lesion is confirmed by inability to smell substances such as orange or peppermint oil. Ammoniacal solutions must not be used – they stimulate the trigeminal rather than the olfactory nerve.

The optic nerve (IInd cranial nerve)

Blindness or defects of visual fields are caused by ocular, optic nerve or cortical damage but the type of defect varies according to the site and extent of the lesion. If there is a complete lesion of one optic nerve that eye is totally blind, there is no direct reaction of the pupil to light (loss of constriction) and, if a light is shone into the affected eye, the pupil of the *unaffected* eye also fails to respond (loss of the consensual reflex). However, the nerves to the affected eye that are responsible for pupil constriction run in the IIIrd cranial nerve and should be intact. If, therefore, a light is shone into the unaffected eye, the pupil of the affected eye also constricts even though it is sightless. Lesions of the optic tract, chiasma, radiation or optic cortex cause various visual field defects involving both visual fields but without total field loss on either side. An ophthalmological opinion should always be obtained if there is any suggestion of a visual field defect.

The oculomotor nerve (IIIrd cranial nerve)

The oculomotor nerve supplies most of the orbital muscles that move the eye (but not the lateral rectus and superior oblique), and the muscle that raises the upper eyelid. The oculomotor also carries the nerve supply to the ciliary muscle and constrictor of the pupil. Normally the medial rectus (supplied by the IIIrd nerve) moves the eye medially (adducts). The lateral rectus (VIth nerve) abducts the eye. When the eye is abducted it is elevated by the superior rectus (IIIrd nerve) and depressed by the inferior rectus (IIIrd nerve). The adducted eye is depressed by the superior oblique muscle (IVth nerve) and elevated by the inferior oblique (IIIrd nerve). Disruption of the IIIrd nerve therefore causes:

1. Paralysis of internal, upward and downward rotation of the eye.
2. Double vision and divergent squint. The affected eye points downwards and later-

ally – 'down and out' in all directions except when looking towards the affected side.

3. Ptosis (drooping upper eyelid).
4. A dilated pupil which fails to constrict on accommodation or when light is shone either onto the affected eye (negative direct light reaction) or into the unaffected eye (negative consensual light reaction).

The trochlear nerve (IVth cranial nerve)

The trochlear nerve supplies only the superior oblique muscle which moves the eye downwards and medially towards the nose. Damage to this nerve causes serious disability, because there is diplopia maximal on looking down and the patient may have difficulty reading, going downstairs or seeing obstructions on the ground. The lesion is characterized by:

1. The head tilted away from the affected side.
2. Diplopia, maximal on looking downwards and inwards.
3. Normal pupils.

There is often damage to the IIIrd and VIth nerves as well.

The trigeminal nerve (Vth cranial nerve)

The trigeminal nerve supplies sensation over the whole face apart from the angle of the jaw, and the front of the scalp back to a line drawn across the vertex, between the ears. It also supplies sensation to most of the mucosa of the oral cavity, conjunctivae, nose, tympanic membrane and sinuses. The motor division of the trigeminal nerve supplies the muscles of mastication (masseter, pterygoids, temporalis, mylohyoid and anterior belly of the digastric). Taste fibres from the anterior two-thirds of the tongue, and secretomotor fibres to the submandibular and sublingual salivary glands and lachrymal glands, are also carried in branches of the trigeminal nerve.

Damage to a sensory branch of the trigeminal nerve causes hypoaesthesia in its area of distribution (*see* p. 346 for causes). Lesions involving the ophthalmic division also cause corneal anaesthesia: this is tested by *gently* touching the cornea with a wisp of cotton wool twisted to a point. Normally this procedure causes a blink, but not if the cornea is anaesthetic and the patient does not see the cotton wool. Lesions of the sensory part of the trigeminal nerve initially result in a diminishing response to pin-prick to the skin and, later, complete anaesthesia. It is important, with patients complaining of facial anaesthesia, to test all areas but particularly the corneal reflex, and the reaction to pin-prick over the angle of the mandible. If, however, the patient complains of complete facial or hemifacial anaesthesia, but the corneal reflex is retained or there is anaesthesia over the angle of the mandible, then the symptoms are probably functional rather than organic.

Taste can be tested with sweet, salt, sour or bitter substances carefully applied to the dorsum of the tongue, or by asking the patient to touch his tongue between the terminals of a pocket torch battery: this normally gives a tingling sensation and a characteristic metallic taste.

Damage to the motor part of the trigeminal nerve can be difficult to detect and is usually asymptomatic if unilateral but the jaw may deviate towards the affected side on opening. It is easier to detect motor weakness by asking the patient to open the jaw against resistance, rather than by trying to test the strength of closure.

The abducens nerve (VIth cranial nerve)

The abducens nerve supplies only a single eye muscle, the lateral rectus. Lesions comprise (*Fig. 17.2*):

1. Paralysis of abduction of the eye.
2. Deviation of the affected eye towards the nose, and convergent squint with diplopia maximal on looking laterally towards the affected side.
3. Normal pupils.

Lesions of the abducens can be surprisingly disabling.

The facial nerve (VIIth cranial nerve)

The facial nerve is the motor supply to the muscles of facial expression and also carries taste sensation from the anterior two-thirds of

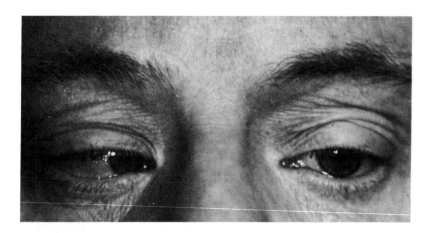

Fig. 17.2 Lesions of the abducens nerve: with the patient looking directly ahead, the affected eye deviates medially as the lateral rectus muscle is functionless

the tongue (via the chorda tympani), secretomotor fibres to the submandibular and sublingual salivary glands and to the lachrymal glands, and branches to the stapedius muscle in the middle ear.

The neurones supplying the lower face receive upper motor neurones from the contralateral motor cortex, whereas the neurones to the upper face receive bilateral upper motor neurone (UMN) innervation. An upper motor neurone lesion causes unilateral facial palsy with some sparing of the frontalis and orbicularis oculi muscles because of the bilateral cortical representation. Furthermore, although voluntary facial movements are impaired, the face may still move with emotional responses, for example on laughing. Paresis of the ipsilateral arm (monoparesis) or arm and leg (hemiparesis), or dysphasia, may be associated because of more extensive cerebrocortical damage.

Lower motor neurone (LMN) facial palsy is characterized by unilateral paralysis of all muscles of facial expression for both voluntary and emotional responses. The forehead is unfurrowed and the patient unable to close the eye on that side. Attempted closure causes the eye to roll upwards (Bell's sign). Tears tend to overflow on to the cheek (epiphora), the corner of the mouth droops and the nasolabial fold is obliterated. Saliva may dribble from the commissure and may cause angular stomatitis. Food collects in the vestibule and plaque accumulates on the teeth on the affected side. Depending on the site of the lesion, other defects such as loss of taste or hyperacusis may be associated.

Facial weakness is demonstrated by asking the patient to close the eyes against resistance, to raise the eyebrows, to whistle or to raise the lips to show his teeth. Schirmer's test for lacrimation, carried out by gently placing a strip of filter paper on the lower conjunctival sac and comparing the wetting of the paper with that on the other side, may be helpful. Lacrimation is diminished in a VIIth nerve lesion. Taste is tested by applying sugar, salt, lemon juice or vinegar on the tongue and asking the patient to identify each of them.

The vestibulocochlear nerve (VIIIth cranial nerve)

The auditory nerve has two components, the vestibular (concerned with appreciation of the movements and position of the head) and the cochlear (hearing). Lesions of this nerve may cause loss of hearing, vertigo or ringing in the ears (tinnitus). An otological opinion should be obtained if a lesion of the vestibulocochlear nerve is suspected, as special tests are needed for diagnosis.

The glossopharyngeal nerve (IXth cranial nerve)

The glossopharyngeal nerve is the sensory supply to the posterior third of the tongue and pharynx; it carries taste sensation from the posterior third of the tongue, and the motor supply to the stylopharyngeus. It also carries secretomotor fibres to the parotid. Lesions of the glossopharyngeal are usually associated with lesions of the vagus, accessory and hypoglossal nerves (bulbar palsy, p. 350). Symptoms resulting from a IXth nerve lesion include impaired pharyngeal sensation so that the gag reflex may be weakened; the two sides should always be compared.

The vagus nerve (Xth cranial nerve)

The vagus has a wide parasympathetic distribution to the viscera of the thorax and upper abdomen but is also the motor supply to some soft palate, pharyngeal and laryngeal muscles.

Lesions of the vagus are rare in isolation but have the following effects:

1. Impaired gag reflex.
2. The soft palate moves towards the unaffected side when the patient is asked to say 'aah'.
3. Hoarse voice.
4. Bovine cough.

The accessory nerve (XIth cranial nerve)

The accessory nerve is the motor supply to the sternomastoid and trapezius muscles. Lesions are often associated with damage to the IXth and Xth nerves and cause ipsilateral:

1. Weakness of the sternomastoid (weakness on turning the head away from the affected side).
2. Weakness of the trapezius on shrugging the shoulders.

Testing this nerve is useful in differentiating patients with genuine palsies from those with functional complaints. In an accessory nerve lesion there is weakness on turning the head away from the affected side. Those shamming paralysis often simulate weakness when turning the head towards the 'affected' side.

The hypoglossal nerve (XIIth cranial nerve)

The hypoglossal nerve is the motor supply to the muscles of the tongue. Lesions cause:

1. Dysarthria (difficulty in speaking) – particularly for lingual sounds.
2. Deviation of the tongue towards the affected side, on protrusion.

The hypoglossal nerve may be affected in its intra- or extracranial course. Intracranial

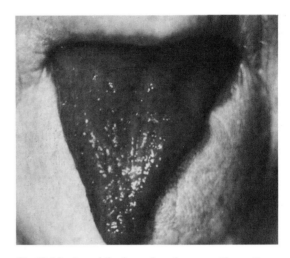

Fig. 17.3 Lesion of the hypoglossal nerve with wasting of the left side of the tongue (lower motor neurone lesion)

lesions typically cause bulbar palsy (*see below*). In an upper motor neurone lesion the tongue is spastic but not wasted; in a lower motor neurone lesion there is wasting and fibrillation of the affected side of the tongue (*Fig. 17.3*). Disease in the condylar canals, such as Paget's disease or bone tumours, and peripheral lesions, such as glomus jugulare, carotid body or other tumours, trauma or radiation damage, can cause an isolated deficit.

FACIAL SENSORY LOSS

Facial sensation is mediated through the trigeminal nerve; the skin over the angle of the mandible is supplied by cervical nerves.

Facial sensory loss may be caused by intracranial, or much more frequently by extracranial lesions of the trigeminal nerve.

Intracranial causes of facial sensory loss

Some intracranial causes of facial sensory loss are shown in *Table 17.5*. Important causes are stroke, multiple sclerosis, cerebral tumours (especially acoustic neuroma), collagen diseases and infections. Syringomyelia is a particularly rare cause.

Lesions in the cavernous sinus can affect the maxillary and ophthalmic divisions; lesions in the superior orbital fissure can affect the ophthalmic division.

Table 17.5 Causes of sensory loss in the trigeminal area

Intracranial		
Congenital	Syringobulbia	
Acquired	Inflammatory	Multiple sclerosis
		Neurosyphilis
		Sarcoidosis
		Tuberculosis
		Connective tissue diseases
		AIDS
	Neoplastic	Cerebral tumours
	Vascular	Cerebrovascular disease
		Aneurysms
	Drugs	Stilbamidine
	Occupational	Trilene (dry cleaning)
	Idiopathic	Benign trigeminal neuropathy
		Paget's disease
Extracranial		
Acquired	Trauma	To infraorbital, inferior dental, lingual or mental nerves or middle cranial fossa fracture
	Inflammatory	Osteomyelitis
	Neoplastic	Carcinoma of antrum or nasopharynx
		Metastatic tumours
		Leukaemic deposits

In posterior cranial fossa lesions, facial sensory loss predominates, but is associated with loss of the corneal reflex and other features such as:

1. Facial weakness (VIIth nerve involvement).
2. Deafness or vertigo (VIIIth nerve involvement).
3. Nystagmus and ataxia (cerebellar involvement).
4. Extensor plantar response with spastic weakness of the leg (pyramidal tract involvement).

Lesions in the middle cranial fossa, the base of skull, or in the trigeminal nerve itself, may cause sensory and motor defects. Middle cranial fossa lesions tend to cause a trigeminal sensory deficit and there may also be:

1. Weakness or atrophy of the masticatory muscles (Vth nerve). The mandible deviates on opening, towards the affected side.
2. Extraocular palsies (IIIrd, IVth or VIth nerves affected).

Extracranial causes of sensory loss

Common extracranial causes of facial sensory loss are shown in *Table 17.5*. Damage to branches of the maxillary division of the trigeminal nerve may be caused by trauma (middle-third facial fractures) or a tumour such as carcinoma of the antrum. The mandibular division may be damaged by inferior dental local anaesthetic injections, trauma in a mandibular fracture or surgery (particularly osteotomies or surgical extraction of lower third molars). Tumours at the base of the skull, in the pterygomandibular space, or deposits in the mandible (metastases or leukaemic deposits for example), may affect the mandibular nerve or branches to cause labial paraesthesia or anaesthesia. Foreign material such as an implant or endodontic material introduced into the inferior alveolar canal can damage the nerve. Osteomyelitis in the mandible may involve the inferior dental nerve. Occasionally the mental foramen lies beneath a lower denture and there is labial anaesthesia as a result of pressure on the labial nerve. Labial gland biopsies can sometimes cause limited labial anaesthesia. The lingual nerve may be damaged during lower third molar surgery.

Nasopharyngeal carcinomas may invade the pharyngeal wall to infiltrate the mandibular division of the trigeminal nerve, causing pain and sensory loss and, by occluding the Eustachian tube, deafness (Trotter's syndrome).

FACIAL PARALYSIS

The motor supply to the facial muscles is the VIIth cranial nerve and common causes of facial paralysis are strokes – cerebrovascular accidents (upper motor neurone lesion) – and Bell's palsy (lower motor neurone lesion). Other causes are shown in *Table 17.6* and include neurosarcoidosis, Lyme disease, Melkersson–Rosenthal syndrome, HIV and HTLV-1 infection, Ramsay–Hunt syndrome, and underwater barotrauma. Facial paralysis in Kawasaki's disease (Chapter 11) is rare, but particularly unusual in that it is seen in infancy (often at only 6–9 months) and is self-limiting. Features differentiating upper motor neurone from lower motor neurone lesions

Table 17.6   Facial paralysis

Site of lesion	Causes	Muscles paralysed	Lacrimation	Hyper-acusis	Taste	Other features
Upper motor neurone (UMN)	Cerebrovascular accident Cerebral tumour Trauma	Lower face	N	—	N	Emotional movement retained ± mono- or hemiparesis ± aphasia
Lower motor neurone (LMN) Facial nucleus	Cerebrovascular disease Moebius syndrome Multiple sclerosis Syphilis HIV infection Lyme disease	All facial muscles	↓	+	↓	+ VIIth nerve damage
Between nucleus and geniculate ganglion	Fractured base of skull Posterior cranial fossa tumours Sarcoidosis	All facial muscles	↓	+	↓	+ VIIIth nerve damage
Between geniculate ganglion and stylomastoid canal	Middle ear infection Cholesteatoma Ramsay–Hunt syndrome Mastoiditis	All facial muscles	N	±	N or ↓	—
In stylomastoid canal or extracranially	Bell's palsy Trauma Misplaced inferior dental anaesthetic Parotid tumour Sarcoidosis Leprosy	All facial muscles	N	—	N	—
Branch of facial nerve extracranially	Trauma Local anaesthesia	Isolated facial muscles	N	—	N	—

N, normal; ↓, reduced.

Table 17.7   Differentiation of upper from lower motor neurone lesions of the facial nerve

	UMN lesion	LMN lesion
Emotional movements of face	Retained	Lost
Blink reflex	Retained	Lost
Ability to wrinkle forehead	Retained	Lost
Drooling from commissure	Uncommon	Common
Lacrimation, taste and hearing	Unaffected	May be affected
Tongue protrusion	Normal	Deviates to unaffected side

are outlined in *Table 17.7* but the main differences are that in the upper motor neurone lesions the frontalis and orbicularis oculi muscles are less paralysed, the facial muscle may appear non-paralysed during emotional reactions, and there is usually a degree of paralysis of the ipsilateral arm and leg, or aphasia.

• Management of facial paralysis

Clinical assessment should include a full history and neurological and physical examination for possible causes, as shown in *Table 17.6*, but the first requirement is to distinguish upper from lower motor neurone lesions. The history should be directed to elicit features suggestive of stroke, traumatic episodes, underwater diving, camping or walking in areas that may contain ticks, possibility of HIV infection and – in Afro-Caribbeans especially – HTLV-1 infection. Facial nerve stimulation or needle electromyography may be useful, as may electrogustometry, serum ACE levels for sarcoidosis, HIV and HTLV-1 serology, ELISA test for Lyme disease, chest and skull radiography, CT or MRI scans or, occasionally, lumbar puncture.

Cerebrovascular accidents (*see* p. 362)

Bell's palsy

Lower motor neurone paralysis of the face where no local or systemic cause can be identi-fied is termed Bell's palsy. In this there is inflammation of the facial nerve in the stylo-mastoid canal with demyelination and oedema, further hazarding the blood supply. This may be immunologically mediated and associated with infection. Herpes simplex virus is commonly implicated but similar features may be seen after infection with HIV, VZV, CMV, EBV and influenza viruses (Chapter 11). Other infections such as Lyme disease and systemic disease such as sarcoidosis must be excluded.

The onset of paralysis in Bell's palsy is acute over a few hours, maximal within 48 hours, although pain in the region of the ear or in the jaw may precede the paralysis by a day or two. There is usually only unilateral facial palsy. Occasionally hyperacusis (loss of function of nerve to stapedius), or loss of taste (chorda tympani), are noted. Patients may complain of facial numbness, but sensation is actually intact on testing.

Incomplete paralysis in the first week is a favourable prognostic sign: 85 per cent of patients totally recover spontaneously within a few weeks but some have residual perma-nent palsy. Where paralysis is complete, only 50 per cent recover completely within one week, and few who have not recovered by two weeks will do so. A favourable prognos-tic sign is persistence of the stapedial reflex, measured by electroneurography if possible. Bad prognostic signs are hyperacusis, severe taste impairment and/or diminished lacrima-tion or salivation, especially in older, diabetic or hypertensive patients.

If paralysis persists and function remains incomplete the palpebral fissure may narrow and the nasolabial fold deepen; facial spasm may develop. Rare complications, apparently caused by anomalous regeneration of the facial nerve, include irregular or anomalous lacrimation (crocodile tears) when the facial muscles are used, such as during eating, retraction of the commissure when the eye is closed, or hemifacial spasm

• Management of Bell's palsy

Although some patients recover sponta-neously, the after-effects in the remaining 10–20 per cent can be severe and distressing. Corticosteroids result in 80–90 per cent complete recovery compared with about 50-60 per cent in the absence of such treatment. Therefore there is a strong argument for treat-ing all patients with corticosteroids. Prednisolone 20 mg four times a day for 5 days, then tailed off over the succeeding 4 days is often recommended. The combination of oral aciclovir 400 mg five times daily with oral prednisolone 1 mg/kg daily for 10 days is more frequently effective.

During the acute phase, the cornea should be protected with an eye pad. In chronic cases surgical decompression of the nerve in the stylomastoid canal may be attempted.

In progressive facial paralysis, radiographic evaluation of the internal acoustic canal, cerebellopontine angle and mastoid may be needed to exclude an organic lesion such as a tumour.

• Dental aspects of facial paralysis

Most patients with Bell's palsy are otherwise healthy and present no other management difficulties, but there are occasional (possibly coincidental) associations with diabetes melli-tus, hypertension and lymphoma. Facial paralysis is also a feature of Melkersson–Rosenthal syndrome, sarcoidosis, HIV infec-tion, Lyme disease, acoustic neuroma, Guillain–Barré syndrome, multiple sclerosis, HTLV-1 infection and a variety of other disor-ders (*Table 17.6*).

Facial palsy may result in poor soft tissue cleansing and accumulation of food debris in the vestibules and of plaque on the teeth on the affected side. Where there is residual palsy, saliva may leak from the affected side and cause angular stomatitis, and there is a cosmetic defect. Construction of a splint to support the angle of the mouth may then improve the aesthetics to some degree. A facial graft or other manoeuvres such as facial–hypoglossal nerve anastomosis may ameliorate the cosmetic deformity, but the results are not always entirely satisfactory

Ramsay–Hunt syndrome

Severe facial paralysis with vesicles in the ipsilateral pharynx and external auditory canal (Ramsay–Hunt syndrome) may be due to herpes zoster of the geniculate ganglion of the facial nerve.

Bilateral facial paralysis

Bilateral facial paralysis is rare but may be seen in acute idiopathic polyneuritis (Guillain–Barré syndrome); sarcoidosis (Heerfordt's syndrome – uveoparotid fever, Chapter 8), arachnoiditis and posterior cranial fossa tumours.

Other causes of facial weakness

An apparent facial palsy may be caused by myasthenia gravis, some myopathies (Chapter 17) or Romberg's syndrome.

Facial hemiatrophy of Romberg

This is a rare form of lipodystrophy, affecting females mainly, in which there is progressive disappearance of facial fat unilaterally and mimicking facial paralysis, starting typically in adolescence. Patients appear to be otherwise well. Plastic surgery is the only treatment.

TRIGEMINAL MOTOR NEUROPATHY

Trigeminal motor neuropathy may occasionally be seen in isolation and is possibly related to a viral infection. More frequently it is associated with trigeminal sensory neuropathy or found in lesions affecting the motor division of the trigeminal nerve when there are usually other cranial nerve deficits. Weakness and sometimes wasting of the masseter and temporalis muscles may be found.

ABNORMAL FACIAL MOVEMENTS

Dystonias are a group of uncommon diseases characterized by abnormal movements associated with muscle spasm, and are focal or generalized. *Dyskinesias* are abnormal movements of the tongue or facial muscles, sometimes with abnormal jaw movements, bruxism or dysphagia. Dystonias differ from dyskinesias mainly in that muscle spasm is more prominent, but they may be difficult to differentiate clinically.

Dystonias

An example of focal dystonia is torticollis. Despite the fact that a neurological disorder cannot always be identified (primary dystonias), it seems likely that there is usually a lesion in the basal ganglia. Support for this idea is given by the fact that many dystonias respond to antimuscarinics or levodopa. Dystonias that result from defined organic diseases affecting the brain are known as secondary dystonias.

Oromandibular dystonia refers to recurrent spasmodic episodes of lip movement, tongue protrusion and retraction, and jaw clenching or opening. This may be associated with blepharospasm and is then sometimes termed Meige's syndrome. The respiratory muscles and speech may be impaired. Over one-third of patients may suffer from depression. Treatment is difficult but benzodiazepines may be helpful.

Acute oromandibular dystonia (drug-induced parkinsonism) can also appear within a short time (hours or days) of starting treatment with neuroleptics such as phenothiazines and butyrophenones (*see* Appendix to Chapter 25). It may resolve after withdrawal of the drug or be improved with antimuscarinic drugs such as benztropine. However, it is made worse by levodopa, which can itself also cause involuntary spasmodic movements if the dose is too great.

Dyskinesias

Involuntary tongue protrusion and retraction, and facial grimacing, are common dyskinesias. *Tardive dyskinesia*, which is usually a late (hence *tardive*) complication of long-term treatment with neuroleptics such as the phenothiazines or butyrophenones, is somewhat similar to oromandibular dystonia. It rarely responds to the withdrawal of the offending drug, is usually made worse by giving antimuscarinics and indeed may be resistant to any form of treatment.

Facial tics

Common tics are blinking, grimacing, shaking the head, clearing the throat, coughing or shrugging. Most facial tics are benign spasms (habit spasms) and usually affect children. Emotion or fatigue intensify tics but the natural history is of spontaneous remission. If persistent, haloperidol may be helpful.

Gilles de la Tourette syndrome

In this familial early onset syndrome, seen mainly in males, chronic motor tics involving the head and neck especially are associated with compulsive vocal tics and sometimes swearing (coprolalia). Many of those affected have obsessive-compulsive tendencies or have attention-deficit hyperactivity. Intelligence is usually normal. Tongue thrusting and lip smacking are common and may be regarded by some observers as lewd (copropraxia). Temporomandibular or other oral pain may result. Self-mutilation such as tongue and lip biting may be associated.

The dopamine receptor blocker haloperidol is usually effective and this suggests that there is overactivity in the basal ganglia. Pimozide and/or clonidine may also be used. Many of the drugs used to treat the syndrome can cause xerostomia or tardive dyskinesia. Interactions of these drugs with general anaesthetic agents, other CNS depressants and atropine means that dental treatment for such patients is best carried out under local analgesia.

Hemifacial spasm and blepharospasm

Hemifacial spasm (clonic facial spasm) mainly affects adults, particularly the elderly. The spasm affects especially the angle of the mouth or the eyelid and worsens towards evening. Some cases herald a cerebellopontine angle lesion or other lesion irritating the facial nerve and some follow facial palsy but many are idiopathic. Occasionally facial paralysis or trigeminal neuralgia follow.

Blepharospasm is a spasm of both eyelids that may be seen in the elderly in isolation, or with hemifacial spasm.

Local injections of botulinum toxin into the affected muscles may give relief for up to 3 months but these must be given with extreme care, as there is a hazard of corneal exposure and glaucoma, and the toxin is contraindicated in pregnancy.

Facial myokymia

Facial myokymia is a rare condition in which there are continuous fine, worm-like contractions of one or more of the facial muscles – especially the perioral or periorbital muscles. Facial myokymia starts suddenly, lasts for variable periods and is unaffected by voluntary movements. Facial myokymia is frequently associated with multiple sclerosis, brain stem or posterior cranial fossa tumours or other neurological disorders. Neurological assessment is therefore crucial.

Facial myokymia must be distinguished from facial hemispasm, facial tics or blepharospasm (which involves several muscles synchronously), and from benign fasciculation and myokymia of the lower eyelid, which are quite innocuous.

MULTIPLE CRANIAL NERVE PALSIES

Several cranial nerves may be affected by the same disease process. Occasionally idiopathic, such lesions may include trauma, sarcoidosis, midline and Wegener's granulomas, Behçet's syndrome, various tumours, HIV infection and other disorders.

Bulbar palsy

Bulbar palsy is the term given to weakness or paralysis of muscles supplied by the medulla, namely the tongue, pharynx, larynx, sternomastoid and upper trapezius (cranial nerves IX–XII inclusive). Poliomyelitis or diphtheria can cause acute bulbar palsy. Chronic causes are progressive bulbar palsy, tumours or aneurysms of the posterior cranial fossa or nasopharynx, or strokes. Various other syndromes, some of which are rare, are recognized, and these are tabulated in the

Appendix to this chapter. See below for details of dental management.

BLINDNESS AND VISUAL IMPAIRMENT

Visual impairment can vary from limitations in sight for distance, colour, size, or shape, to full blindness. Impaired vision is an important disability and invariably restricts the activity of the patient to some degree. The main visual defects associated with significant systemic disorders which may complicate management are shown in *Table 17.8*. Visual defects are also among the most common genetic disorders, and congenital blindness may be associated with other handicaps such as epilepsy.

- ### Dental aspects of patients with visual defects

Clearly communication is best verbally though, for the partially sighted, writing matter can sometimes be used but must be in large bold black type on a white background. Visual defects do not, in themselves, directly affect dental management or routine oral hygiene. Many of the causes of visual impairment, such as short-sightedness, though a nuisance or worse to those afflicted, present few difficulties during dental management. However, constant gentle explanation and reassurance about every phase of dental treatment is needed to prevent a sightless patient from being frightened by unexpected noises or unpleasant sensations such as injection of a local anaesthetic.

Treatment should be verbally oriented – 'tell, then do'. Partially sighted or blind persons may have heightening of other senses and have an increased hearing and touch sensitivity; some do not like the operating light being shone on their eyes.

Maintenance of oral hygiene may be difficult when the patient is unable to see whether or not toothbrushing has been effective.

Several causes of late-onset disturbance or loss of vision are severe systemic diseases, such as diabetes mellitus or atherosclerosis, which may complicate dental treatment in various ways so that, from the dental viewpoint, the visual defects should prompt consideration of the underlying causes and consideration of their practical implications. In many cases,

Table 17.8 Causes of impaired vision

- Congenital
  Intrauterine infections (rubella, cytomegalovirus, syphilis*)
  Cerebral lipidoses
  Laurence–Moon–Biedl syndrome
  Various inborn errors of metabolism
  Marfan's syndrome*
  Ehlers–Danlos syndrome*
- Acquired
  Infections
  Herpes simplex*
  Herpes zoster*
  Cytomegalovirus*
  Toxoplasmosis*
  Inflammatory
  Behçet's syndrome*
  Reiter's syndrome*
  Stevens–Johnson syndrome*
  Multiple sclerosis*
  Temporal arteritis*
  Sjögren's syndrome*
  Mucous membrane pemphigoid*
  Ulcerative colitis*
  Glaucoma
  Trauma
  Metabolic
  Diabetes mellitus*
  Acromegaly*
  Malignant hypertension
  Drugs
  Methanol
  Quinine
  Phenothiazines*

*May be oral features.

however, damage to sight is a late complication and many such patients are edentulous.

It is also important to emphasize that visual defects or blindness can be complications of diseases which may appear to be mainly oral or mucocutaneous. Referral to an ophthalmologist may, paradoxically, therefore be the most important aspect of the investigation of a patient with oral disease, such as Sjögren's syndrome or mucous membrane pemphigoid. Patients with visual defects following maxillofacial or head injuries must be seen early by an ophthalmologist, as loss of sight is a serious handicap.

Patients with glaucoma must not be given diazepam or atropine.

Diplopia

Double vision (diplopia) is not uncommon after maxillofacial trauma but usually

Table 17.9 Diplopia

Structure involved	Site	Causes	Features that may be associated
Extraocular muscles	Orbit	Trauma	Middle-third facial fracture
		Exophthalmos	Thyrotoxicosis
		Myasthenia gravis	Myopathy elsewhere
Cranial nerves III, IV and VI	Orbit	Trauma	Middle-third facial fracture
		Tumour	
		Sarcoid	
	Superior orbital fissure	Trauma	Often several muscles paralysed
		Tumour	Involvement of ophthalmic division of trigeminal
		Sarcoid	Pupil often normal
	Cavernous sinus	Aneurysms	Similar to superior orbital fissure syndrome
		Infection	
		Fistula	
		Trauma	
	Skull base	Aneurysms	May be involvement of single nerves: may be
		Tumours	pupil dilatation
		Meningitis	
		Fractures	
Cranial nerve nuclei	Brain stem	Vascular lesions	May be involvement of trigeminal or facial nerves
		Tumours	or complicated neurological disorders
		Multiple sclerosis	

resolves spontaneously within a few days. Persistent diplopia after trauma can be caused by blow-out fractures of the floor of the orbit, entrapment of, or damage to, the orbital muscles or damage to the suspensory ligament to the frontal process or the zygomatic bone. Later fibrous adhesions between the orbital periosteum and coverings of the eye may cause permanent limitation of movement as may injury to cranial nerves III, IV and VI (*Table 17.9*). Diplopia may also be an occasional transient complication of dental local anaesthetic injections, presumably because the anaesthetic tracks to the inferior orbital fissure, where it can block orbital nerves.

Paralytic strabismus is characterized by variable deviation of the ocular axes according to the position of gaze and is the usual type of strabismus that follows maxillofacial injuries.

The eye affected can be identified by noting in which direction of gaze diplopia is maximal and then, while the patient looks in that direction, covering each eye in turn. The outermost image disappears when the affected eye is covered. Occasionally drugs such as carbamazepine are a cause.

Pupillary abnormalities

The pupils are normally equal in size and constrict on exposure to bright light and on accommodation for near objects. Light shone in one eye causes pupillary constriction in that eye (direct light reflex) and also in the unexposed eye (indirect or consensual reflex). Pupil size is determined by dilator fibres (the sympathetic supply from the superior cervical ganglion runs along the internal carotid artery and joins the ophthalmic division of the trigeminal nerve and the long ciliary nerves) and constrictor fibres (the parasympathetic supply runs with the oculomotor nerve). The sympathetic nerve supply is also partially responsible for contraction of the levator palpebrae superioris muscle (raising the upper eyelid).

Pupil constriction (miosis) can be caused by a lesion of the sympathetic supply, and dilatation (mydriasis) by a IIIrd nerve lesion. The most important cause of an abnormally dilated pupil is a rise in intracranial pressure when the pupil also becomes non-reactive owing to pressure on the oculomotor nerve. Other causes of unequal pupils are shown in *Table 17.10 (Fig. 17.4)*.

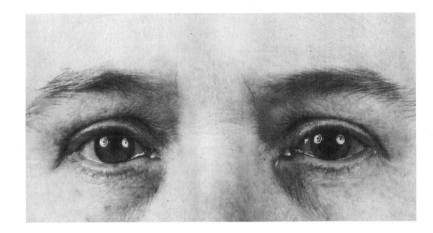

Fig. 17.4 Mydriasis: a unilateral fixed dilated pupil on the left, caused by trauma

Table 17.10 Causes of pupillary abnormalities

	Pupils	Other signs	Significance
Argyll–Robertson pupils	Small, unequal, react to accommodation but not light	—	Neurosyphilis Multiple sclerosis Diabetes mellitus
Horner's syndrome	Constricted	Ptosis Absence of facial sweating Enophthalmos sometimes	Trauma, bronchial carcinoma or other causes of damage to sympathetic fibres, usually in neck
Adie's (Holmes–Adie) pupil	One pupil dilated and reacts very slowly to light or convergence	Ankle or knee jerks may be absent	Usually benign

Adie's (Holmes–Adie) pupil

Adie's pupil is usually benign and typically affects females. One pupil is dilated and reacts only very slowly to light or convergence and there may be associated loss of knee or ankle jerks. Occasionally this condition, like the Argyll–Robertson pupil, is associated with advanced syphilis.

Argyll–Robertson pupil

This is characterized by small, irregular, unequal pupils which fail to dilate in response to light but still react, by dilating, to accommodation. An Argyll–Robertson pupil is characteristically caused by neurosyphilis, but may sometimes also be seen in other conditions affecting the Edinger–Westphal nucleus, such as diabetes mellitus, sarcoidosis, Wernicke's encephalopathy, midbrain tumours, trauma, Lyme disease, amyloidosis or multiple sclerosis.

Horner's syndrome

Horner's syndrome comprises:

1. Miosis (constricted pupil), unreactive to mydriatics.
2. Ptosis (drooping eyelid).
3. Loss of sweating of the face.
4. Enophthalmos (sometimes).

It is usually unilateral and caused by interruption of sympathetic nerve fibres peripherally, usually at the cervical sympathetic trunk, as a result, for example, of trauma to the neck, or bronchogenic or metastatic breast carcinoma infiltrating the superior cervical sympathetic ganglion. It may also be due to brain stem disease, typically in lesions affecting the medulla.

Nystagmus

A few irregular eye jerks are normal in some individuals when the eyes are deviated far to one side. However, involuntary rhythmic eye movements (nystagmus) may be a sign of disease.

Oscillating (pendular) nystagmus may result from ocular disease and is characterized by rapid oscillation of the eyes, increased on looking upwards. More common is rhythmic (jerk) nystagmus, which is usually lateral, but can be vertical or rotary, and results from:

1. Drug intoxication (e.g. barbiturates).
2. Internal ear disease.
3. Cerebellar disease.
4. Brain stem disease.

DEAFNESS AND HEARING IMPAIRMENT

Deafness is common and, in over 30 per cent of cases, is hereditary. Deafness is caused by conductive disorders involving the middle or external ear or by neural disorders such as defects of the cochlear nerve or its central connections. Dental management may be complicated by difficulty in communication, but associated medical problems are infrequent.

Deafness may occasionally be associated with congenital malformations such as first arch syndromes (Treacher–Collins syndrome, Apert's syndrome) with associated facial anomalies, or rarely with cardiac disease or learning impairment.

• Dental aspects of hearing impairment

Persons with impaired hearing or who are deaf are often lip readers, and therefore staff should face them to improve communication. Face masks should be removed. Communication is not helped by the dental staff raising their voice, but clear diction may assist. Extraneous noise should be minimized. Instruments such as the air rotor and ultrasonic scaler may interfere with a hearing aid, and the vibrations during use may be exaggerated for the person with impaired hearing.

X-rays do not damage hearing aids.

MÉNIÈRE'S DISEASE

Labyrinthine dysfunction underlies this syndrome, which comprises vertigo, tinnitus and sensorineural hearing loss, with nausea and sometimes nystagmus. Betahistine and cinnarizine have been promoted as specific treatments but phenothiazines, prochlorperazine or thiethylperazine may be required.

AUTONOMIC DYSFUNCTION

A wide range of disorders can be associated with autonomic dysfunction, many of which manifest with bladder dysfunction, impotence, anhidrosis, gastrointestinal dysfunction, orthostatic (postural) hypotension and dry mouth and eyes. Most important are diabetes mellitus, ageing, parkinsonism, amyloidosis, alcoholism, porphyria and familial dysautonomia. Such patients are sensitive to any agent causing hypotension, such as general anaesthetic agents, and to being raised quickly from the supine position. Autonomic dysfunction also appears to underlie sialosis (Chapter 9).

Riley–Day syndrome (familial dysautonomia)

Familial dysautonomia (FD) is a rare autosomal recessive disorder characterized by selective damage to the sensory, motor and autonomic peripheral nervous system. Found almost exclusively in Ashkenazi Jews, the main features are decreased pain sensation and impaired regulation of temperature and blood pressure. Aspiration pneumonias and episodes of acute abdominal pain are common.

Hypersalivation may be seen, the lingual fungiform papillae and taste sensation are reduced, and oral hygiene may be poor but the most important dental aspect is self-mutilation of hard and/or soft tissues. Splints may be used to protect the soft tissues.

EPILEPSY

Epilepsy is a group of disorders of brain function which cause episodic disturbances of consciousness and usually of motor or sensory function. It affects over 1 per cent of the general population but is more prevalent in the young and in the mentally or physically impaired. Most cases of epilepsy have

<table>
<tr><td colspan="2">**Table 17.11 Causes of fits**</td></tr>
</table>

- Idiopathic epilepsy
- Symptomatic or secondary epilepsy
  - Febrile convulsions
  - Intracranial causes: Space-occupying lesions
    - Trauma
    - Vascular defects
    - Infections
    - Cerebral palsy
    - Rubella syndrome
    - Phakomatoses
    - (neurofibromatosis, epiloia)
    - AIDS meningitis
  - Systemic causes: Anoxia
    - Hypoglycaemia
    - Inborn errors of metabolism
    - Drug withdrawal
    - (anticonvulsants, barbiturates,
    - alcohol, opioids,
    - benzodiazepines)

no identifiable cause (idiopathic epilepsy) but in a few patients it is secondary to local or generalized brain disease, drug addiction or metabolic disorders (symptomatic epilepsy) (*Table 17.11*).

Epilepsy has a variety of clinical patterns; most common are primary generalized seizures – especially tonic–clonic epilepsy.

Tonic–clonic (grand mal) epilepsy

Tonic–clonic epilepsy usually begins in the pre-school child, or sometimes at about puberty. A typical seizure consists of a defined sequence beginning with a warning (aura), followed by loss of consciousness, tonic and the clonic convulsions and finally a variably prolonged recovery. This full sequence is, however, not always completed.

The aura may consist of a mood change, irritability, brief hallucination or headache. The attack then begins suddenly with total body tonic spasm and loss of consciousness. The sufferer falls to the ground and is in danger of injury. Initially the face becomes pale and the pupils dilate, the head and spine are thrown into extension (opisthotonous) and glottic and respiratory muscle spasm may cause an initial brief cry and cyanosis. There may also be incontinence and biting of the tongue or lips.

The tonic phase passes, after less than a minute, into the clonic phase. Then there are

repetitive jerking movements of trunk, limbs, tongue and lips. Salivation is profuse with bruxism, sometimes tongue-biting and, occasionally, vomiting. There may be autonomic phenomena such as tachycardia, hypertension and flushing. Clonus is followed by a state of flaccid semi-coma for a further 10–15 minutes.

Confusion and headaches are common afterwards and the patient may sleep for up to 12 hours or more before full recovery. The attack may occasionally be followed by a transient residual paralysis (Todd's palsy) or by automatic or aggressive behaviour.

Major convulsions can cause trauma, respiratory embarrassment or brain damage, or may pass into status epilepticus, but most seizures end without mishap.

A major fit is so dramatic an event that it seems to be of longer duration than is in fact the case. If, however, it lasts more than 5 minutes (by the clock) or starts again after apparently ceasing, the patient must be regarded as being in *status epilepticus*.

Status epilepticus

In this dangerous form of epilepsy the tonic and clonic phases alternate repeatedly without consciousness being regained. Inhalation of vomit and saliva, or brain damage due to cerebral hypoxia, may result, with a mortality of up to 20 per cent.

Syndromes associated with epilepsy

Epilepsy is usually an isolated problem in otherwise normal individuals but may be associated with other diseases. Five per cent of epileptics are mentally subnormal, while more than 50 per cent of patients with cerebral palsy and 50 per cent of phenylketonurics suffer from epilepsy.

Other forms of primary generalized epilepsy

Petit mal (absence seizures) is the other common form of epilepsy and is restricted to children. It consists of sudden but usually transient arrest of movement, attention and speech, often graphically described as *absences*, and may be precipitated by overbreathing. Absence seizures can be controlled with ethosuximide or sodium valproate (*Table 17.12*).

Table 17.12 Anticonvulsant drugs: uses and adverse effects

Drug	Use	Systemic adverse effects	Oral adverse effects
Carbamazepine	TLE	Ataxia	Dry mouth
	GM	Drowsiness	Erythema multiforme
		Leucopenia	Dyskinesias
		Lupoid syndrome	
Valproate	GM	Drowsiness	
	PM	Bleeding diathesis	
Phenytoin	GM	Cerebellar damage	Gingival hyperplasia
	TLE	Hirsutes	Dental anomalies
	PM	Nephrotic syndrome	Erythema multiforme
		Hyperglycaemia	Lupoid syndrome or ulcers
			Cervical lymphadenopathy
Ethosuximide	PM	Lupoid syndrome	
		Renal damage	
		Eosinophilia	
Primidone	GM	Drowsiness	Megaloblastic anaemia
	TLE	Ataxia	
	PM	Oculomotor palsy	
Phenobarbitone	GM	Lethargy	Erythema multiforme
(virtually obsolete)	TLE	Irritability	Bullae
	PM	Depression	Fixed eruptions
		Rashes	
		Ataxia	

GM, Grand mal; TLE, temporal lobe epilepsy; PM, petit mal.

It is important not to mistake petit mal for uncooperative behaviour or for learning impairment in the affected child, and to appreciate that petit mal very occasionally precedes grand mal epilepsy.

Partial seizures

Simple partial seizures can be motor, sensory or behavioural and typically remain confined to one area. Localized motor seizures (focal motor epilepsy) may take the form of clonic movements of a limb or group of muscles, usually in the face, arm or leg. The clonus may spread (march) to adjacent muscles on the same side of the body (Jacksonian epilepsy).

Complex partial seizures, or temporal lobe epilepsy (psychomotor epilepsy) are characterized by hallucinations, illusions of taste, smell, sight and hearing, disorientation, confusion and amnesia. Lip smacking and chewing movements may be seen. It is controlled by many of the anticonvulsants used in tonic–clonic epilepsy, particularly carbamazepine.

Ictal facial pain is an unusual manifestation of sensory epilepsy. It usually affects women of late middle age and consists of a throbbing diffuse pain which may be associated with facial or masticatory muscle twitches or generalized convulsions. It is usually controllable with phenytoin.

• General management of tonic–clonic epilepsy

Major epilepsy is frequently idiopathic but it is necessary, especially if fits begin in adult life, to exclude brain disease, such as a

Table 17.13 Causes of fits at different ages of onset

Age at onset	More common causes
Young child	Birth trauma, fevers, metabolic disease, congenital disease or idiopathic
Adolescent	Idiopathic or traumatic
Young adult	Traumatic, neoplastic, idiopathic, alcoholism or barbiturate abuse, AIDS
Middle age	Neoplastic, traumatic, cerebrovascular disease, AIDS or drug abuse
Elderly	Cerebrovascular disease or neoplasm

cerebral tumour (*Table 17.13*). Most patients with major epilepsy having more than one attack in a year are maintained on prophylactic anticonvulsants. Epileptics may not drive a motor vehicle until they have been seizure-free for more than one year, or over a three-year period have only had sleep attacks. Patients with epilepsy who are drowsy from medication should not operate machinery or drive.

Anticonvulsant medication is typically started with a single drug, mainly now with carbamazepine, or valproate or occasionally phenytoin or phenobarbitone, and is of such a long-term nature that side-effects are common. Carbamazepine usually is the first choice for the management of tonic–clonic epilepsy and, though capable of causing a variety of side-effects, these are fewer than those caused by phenytoin and uncommon in relation to the scale of use. Alternatively, sodium valproate may be used, particularly when major fits are associated with absence seizures.

Lamotrigine shows similar efficacy to carbamazepine, but less adverse effects. Phenobarbitone is effective but undesirably sedating in adults and can cause behavioural disturbances in children. Newer agents such as vigabatrin, gabapentin, topiramate and piracetam are being evaluated.

Plasma anticonvulsant levels may sometimes need to be monitored, particularly with phenytoin where small changes in dosage can cause disproportionately great changes in plasma levels and toxic effects. Saliva may be used for this purpose.

Combined treatment may sometimes cause more toxic effects or interactions than a single drug in adequate doses. A second drug should only be given if a single agent in maximal dosage fails to control fits or causes undesirable toxic effects.

In pregnancy, drug treatment should follow the same principles as for non-pregnant patients but plasma levels need to be monitored as they may fall during the later stages. Antiepileptic drugs, particularly phenytoin, are potentially teratogenic, but there is a greater risk to the fetus from uncontrolled epilepsy. Antiepileptic drugs, apart from barbiturates, should also be continued during breast-feeding. Some interfere with the oral contraceptive.

- **Oro-dental complications of epilepsy or its treatment**

I. Injuries caused by the fit:
    Laceration of tongue or buccal mucosa.
    Injuries to the face from falling (lacerations, haematomas, fractures of the facial skeleton).
    Fractures, devitalization, subluxation or loss of teeth (a chest radiograph may be required).
    Subluxation of the TMJ.
2. Complications of treatment (*see also* Table 17.12):
    Phenytoin – gingival fibrous hyperplasia (of interdental papillae particularly).
    Folate deficiency (rarely) megaloblastic anaemia and recurrent aphthae.
    Dental anomalies (small, late-erupting teeth).
    Cervical lymphadenopathy.
    Phenobarbitone – bullous erythema multiforme (exceptionally rarely).

- **Dental treatment of epileptics**

It is essential to appreciate that epileptics have good and bad phases and that various factors can precipitate seizures in susceptible patients (*Table 17.14*). Dental treatment should preferably be carried out in good phases when attacks are infrequent.

Large doses of lignocaine given intravenously for severe dysrhythmias may occasionally cause convulsions. An over-enthusiastic casualty officer may therefore blame a dental local anaesthetic for causing a fit. There is no evidence that this can happen,

---

Table 17.14 Factors precipitating fits in susceptible subjects

- Withdrawal of anticonvulsant medication
- Epileptogenic drugs
    Methohexitone (and some other anaesthetics)
    Sympathomimetic amines
    Tricyclics
    Phenothiazines
    Alcohol
    Fluoxetine and other SSRIs (p. 381)
- Fatigue, starvation or stress
- Infection
- Menstruation
- Flickering lights (television; strobe lights)

especially as intravenous lignocaine has also been advocated for the *control* of status epilepticus.

Those who have infrequent seizures, or who are dependent upon others (such as those with a learning impairment), may fail to take regular medication and thus be poorly controlled.

The main problems in the dental care of epileptic patients are:

1. Convulsions and their sequelae.
2. Drug reactions.
3. Psychiatric disorders.
4. Associated handicaps (Chapter 23).
5. Bleeding tendency caused by sodium valproate.

Convulsions and their sequelae: Trauma frequently results from a grand mal attack when the patient falls unconscious or from the muscle spasm. Such injuries include fractures of the vertebrae or limbs, dislocations, or periorbital subcutaneous haematomas in the absence of facial fractures.

When carrying out dental treatment in a known epileptic, a strong mouth prop should be kept in position and the oral cavity kept as free as possible of debris. As much apparatus as possible should be kept away from the area around the patient.

Drug reactions: Methohexitone, enflurane and ketamine are epileptogenic. Chlorpromazine, alcohol, fluoxetine and tricyclic antidepressants may also be epileptogenic and should be avoided. Many of the anticonvulsants may increase the risk of hepatotoxicity from paracetamol.

Psychiatric problems in the epileptic: Temporal lobe (psychomotor) epilepsy in particular is associated with paranoid and schizophrenic features. Antisocial and psychopathic behaviour may then make dental management difficult (Chapter 18).

Management of a fit in the dental surgery: Fits in the dental surgery are usually in known epileptics but it should be remembered that fits can also result from cerebral hypoxia when, for example, a normal patient faints but is not laid flat.

When a fit starts the patient should be constantly attended and should be laid on their side in the head injury position to maintain the airway. The face is rotated down to allow vomit to be expelled from the mouth and not inhaled. It is probably impractical to hold the traditional padded spatula between the teeth; the patient must, however, be placed away from equipment or furniture so that they cannot damage themselves.

In an uncomplicated seizure no other treatment is necessary. If, however, the seizure persists or status epilepticus develops, diazepam 10 mg or lorazepam 4 mg or clonazepam 2 mg should be given slowly intravenously or intramuscularly and repeated if the episode is not terminated. Oxygen may also be needed. Intravenous 50 per cent sterile glucose may stop the seizures even where hypoglycaemia is not expected.

Febrile convulsions

Febrile convulsions result from a rise in body temperature usually caused by infection. These convulsions usually affect children, about 3 per cent of whom go on in later life to develop epilepsy. Severe febrile convulsions can cause brain damage. Those under 18 months should be admitted to hospital since the fit may be due to meningitis.

Children who develop high fevers (above 38 °C) should be put in a cool environment and bathed with tepid water and given paracetamol elixir.

SYNCOPE

Syncope is transient loss of consciousness caused by a sudden decrease in cerebral blood flow. The main causes include:

1. Vasovagal attack (fainting – *see below*).
2. Respiratory syncope (severe coughing).
3. Cardiac syncope (dysrhythmias, heart block, aortic stenosis).
4. Paralytic syncope – in the elderly, especially those taking drugs such as phenothiazines, levodopa, hypotensive agents, tricyclics or benzodiazepines.
5. Brain stem syncope. Migraine or vertebrobasilar disease, usually in the elderly.

Vasovagal syncope (fainting)

Vasovagal syncope is a reflex mediated by autonomic nerves in which there is splanchnic and skeletal muscle vasodilatation, bradycardia and loss of consciousness. Fainting can be precipitated by psychological factors such as pain, or fear at the sight of an injection needle or blood.

Fainting may also be caused by postural changes, anoxia or the carotid sinus syndrome. The latter is usually seen in elderly patients in whom mild pressure on the neck causes syncope with bradycardia or cardiac arrest – a vagal effect.

- **Management of syncope**

Syncope is dangerous if the patient is not laid flat, since cerebral anoxia can result and the patient may then have a convulsion and suffer from hypoxic encephalopathy.

RAISED INTRACRANIAL PRESSURE

Raised intracranial pressure can be a complication of head injury and be fatal. As a result of the rigidity of the cranium any expansion of its contents causes a rise of intracranial pressure which, in turn, tends to impede the venous return from the brain and further to increase the pressure. Cerebral blood flow is thus diminished even though the raised CSF pressure causes a reflex rise in systemic blood pressure in an attempt to improve cerebral blood flow. Examples of causes of raised intracranial pressure include the following:

1. Intracranial haemorrhage (after head injury).
2. Space-occupying lesions (abscess or tumour).
3. Oedema of the brain (often a consequence of trauma, malignant hypertension, vascular lesions or tumours of the brain).
4. Obstruction to the flow of CSF (blockage of the aqueduct of Sylvius or subarachnoid adhesions due to meningitis).

Intracranial haematomas are a major cause of mortality following head injuries and it is therefore essential to recognize signs of raised intracranial pressure and cerebral compression which include:

1. Papilloedema (bulging of the optic disc with engorgement of its vessels seen by ophthalmoscopy).
2. Headache (in the conscious patient).
3. Restlessness (in the unconscious patient).
4. Vomiting.
5. Decreasing consciousness.
6. Rising blood pressure and slowing of the pulse.
7. Dilatation of the pupil on the side of the lesion and diminished reaction to light.

Lumbar puncture is contraindicated if intracranial pressure is raised as it can precipitate brain herniation and death by coning of the brain stem and medullary compression.

Herniation of the brain

Herniation is the displacement of part of the brain from one dural compartment to another and is a serious consequence of raised intracranial pressure. The effects depend on the direction of displacement.

The possibility of herniation is suggested by signs of raised intracranial pressure, particularly pupil dilatation and reduced reactivity to light caused by stretching of the oculomotor nerves.

HYPOXIC ENCEPHALOPATHY

Acute cerebral hypoxia is particularly important in dental practice as it can readily follow head injuries or impaired oxygenation during general anaesthesia, particularly with intravenous barbiturates. There is often then a combination of contributory factors. The anaesthetic agent can depress respiration but there may also be partial, often unnoticed, respiratory obstruction. The patient may also have cerebrovascular disease which impairs the cerebral circulation and if there is anaemia the situation is made even worse. As a consequence, some patients can die and others can suffer brain damage. Cerebral hypoxia can remain unrecognized because the patient is already unconscious from the anaesthetic. The main causes of cerebral hypoxia include:

1. Hypoxia – airways obstruction, respiratory failure or anaesthetic accidents.
2. Severe hypotension – cardiac arrest, shock syndrome, severe bradycardia.

Cerebral hypoxia causes loss of consciousness in less than a minute but, if the circulation and oxygenation of the blood are restored within about 3 minutes, recovery should be complete.

More prolonged hypoxia causes coma with dilated pupils unresponsive to light, inert or rigid limbs, unresponsiveness to all stimuli, abolition of brain stem reflexes and no electrical activity on electroencephalography (brain death).

The most vigilant supervision of all patients with head injuries or undergoing general anaesthesia is, therefore, essential. Special care must be taken to ensure that the patient is respiring fully and effectively, that oxygen supplies are adequate and maintained, and that no signs of hypoxia, however slight, develop (Chapter 22).

INFECTIONS OF THE NERVOUS SYSTEM

Suppurative meningitis

The chief causes are *Haemophilus influenzae*, *Neisseria meningitidis* (meningococcus), *N. gonorrhoeae*, *Streptococcus pneumoniae* (pneumococcus) and less frequently *Listeria monocytogenes*. The causative organisms differ in different age groups. In adult life, the pneumococcus becomes increasingly important, particularly in those with impaired resistance as a result of such causes as alcoholism or sickle cell disease.

The meningococcus is carried in the nasopharynx and sometimes causes epidemics. Recent outbreaks have been of group B and C meningococci. Group B, type 15 meningococcus in particular causes a severe form of the disease. Spread of the bacteria to the meninges is by the bloodstream or occasionally as a result of a maxillofacial fracture involving the cribriform plate of the ethmoid (Chapter 22).

The onset of meningitis is marked by severe headache, nausea or vomiting, drowsiness, stupor or coma and occasionally, convulsions. An important clinical sign is pain and stiffness of the neck.

A purpuric rash is characteristic of meningococcal septicaema which can go on to adrenocortical failure as a result of bleeding into the adrenal cortex, with vasomotor collapse, shock and death (Waterhouse–Friedreichsen syndrome).

Diagnosis is confirmed with a Gram-stained smear and culturing the organism from a lumbar puncture specimen of CSF. However, antibiotic treatment should start before the results are available. If treatment is prompt, the overall mortality is low, but about 20 per cent of patients have permanent neurological damage such as cranial nerve injuries (blindness, deafness or palsies), epilepsy, or mental retardation.

Patients with maxillofacial injuries involving the middle third of the face should be given prophylactic antimicrobials because of the danger of meningitis (Chapter 22).

There have been rare cases of meningitis caused by viridans streptococci which may have originated from the mouth.

Brain abscess

Brain abscesses are usually secondary to chronic middle ear, sinus or pulmonary infections. Patients with congenital heart disease, particularly those with right-to-left shunts, and those with hereditary haemorrhagic telangiectasia are also at risk. Brain abscess may also be a complication of trauma to the head, or infective endocarditis.

Bacteria from periodontal pockets, particularly anaerobes, or periapical periodontitis are a recognized cause of cerebral abscess. Inhalation of a tooth fragment or materials used in dentistry can cause a lung abscess which can metastasize to the brain with serious consequences.

In immunocompetent persons, frontal lobe abscesses often result from sinusitis and contain a heavy growth of *Streptococcus milleri*. Sphenoidal sinusitis is notorious in this respect, and can be difficult to diagnose. Post-traumatic or postoperative abscesses are often related to *Staphylococcus aureus*. Temporal lobe abscesses often arise from middle ear mixed bacterial infections, with large numbers of anaerobes. In immunocompromised persons, brain abscesses may be fungal (mainly candida, aspergillus, or cryptococcus) or protozoal (toxoplasma).

An established cerebral abscess characteristically causes signs and symptoms similar to other space-occupying lesions of the brain. CT and MRI are extremely useful in the diagnosis. Immediately after the diagnosis has been confirmed, treatment is by high doses of antibiotics (usually penicillin or metronidazole) followed, where necessary, by aspiration or drainage. The mortality is still between 10 and 20 per cent.

Viral meningitis

Meningitis can be caused by several different viruses, particularly Coxsackie viruses and Echoviruses. In viral meningitis there is little involvement of brain tissue and the infections are generally mild and self-limiting. No specific treatment is available.

Herpetic encephalitis

Herpes simplex infection of the mouth or genitals is common but herpetic encephalitis is rare, though still the most frequent cause of encephalitis in temperate climates. Evidence as to whether it is a primary or reactivation infection is conflicting.

Clinical effects are highly variable. Early symptoms such as disorientation, personality changes, hallucinations and ataxia can be mistaken for drunkenness or psychosis. Other effects include stupor, fits, paralyses and sensory loss. Coma is often pre-terminal.

The disease has often been fatal, particularly because confirmation of the diagnosis by brain biopsy is slow. However, the prognosis has improved greatly as a result of treatment with aciclovir, which is frequently given now, on suspicion. The incidence of neurological damage among survivors has also been reduced.

Neurosyphilis

Syphilis can affect the nervous system in the tertiary stage but is exceedingly rare, as a result of early treatment (Chapter 11). Neurosyphilis can take any of the following forms.

Meningovascular neurosyphilis has highly variable early symptoms but late effects may be hydrocephalus or lesions of the IInd, IIIrd and VIIIth cranial nerves. Pupils are also unequal and unresponsive to light (Argyll–Robertson pupils).

Paretic neurosyphilis begins insidiously with subtle mental disturbance going on to severe personality changes, complete dementia and widespread paralyses (general paresis of the insane, GPI).

Tabes dorsalis (locomotor ataxia) is mainly characterized by atrophy of the lumbar posterior nerve roots and sometimes of the optic nerves. Clinically, tabes dorsalis is characterized by sudden attacks of lightning-like pain and paraesthesiae of the leg or trunk. There is also loss of normal pain sensation and of deep proprioceptive reflexes. These cause the peculiar tabetic gait in which the feet are slapped on to the ground as a result of loss of sense of their position. These neuropathic joints then become disorganized (Charcot's joints).

Syphilis may be associated with HIV infection and then takes an atypical, accelerated course. Progress to the tertiary stage may be rapid and gummata may develop while the secondary stage is still active. Relapse is common despite treatment or the response to penicillin may be poor. The antibody response is also atypical and unpredictable.

- **Dental aspects of neurosyphilis**

Neurosyphilis is a rare cause of atypical trigeminal neuralgia but is now of little dental significance. Its presence should, however, be suspected in a patient with a gumma or syphilitic leucoplakia, which typically involves the dorsum of the tongue.

HIV-associated neurological disease

Intracranial infections of many kinds and also brain tumours, particularly lymphomas, are common complications of HIV disease. The virus itself can also attack the brain to cause a wide variety of neurological symptoms culminating in dementia and death. These effects are not necessarily associated with the typical picture of immunodeficiency.

Neurological manifestations of HIV can be acute, subacute or chronic. Acute disease can include such features as fever, malaise, depression, fits, facial palsy and neuropathy of the extremities. Recovery usually, however, follows after several months.

Subacute encephalopathy affects about 30 per cent of AIDS patients. Typical features are gradual development of a confusional state associated with fever and depression. The patient may eventually become bedridden and incontinent.

Myelopathy or neuropathy can cause weakness of the legs, sometimes paraesthesiae and in severe cases ataxia and incontinence. Alternatively, a form of meningitis may precede more typical features of AIDS and be characterized by headache, fever, meningeal signs and cranial nerve palsies most commonly affecting nerves V, VII and VIII.

In brief, therefore, the neurological effects of HIV infection are so varied that it should be suspected in any high risk patient who develops unexpected behavioural or mood changes and neurological signs such as cranial nerve palsies.

CEREBROVASCULAR ACCIDENTS (CVA, STROKES)

Strokes are a common cause of disability and death, especially in the elderly. Strokes result from acute destruction of part of the brain caused by cerebral haemorrhage or ischaemia. The main types of stroke are:

1. Subarachnoid haemorrhage.
2. Cerebral haemorrhage, thrombosis and embolism.

Subarachnoid haemorrhage

Rupture of a congenital berry aneurysm of the circle of Willis accounts for about 10 per cent of strokes. Hypertension, atherosclerosis and acute physical or emotional stress are contributory.

Blood from the ruptured aneurysm spreads into the subarachnoid space but can burst through the brain into a cerebral ventricle causing death within a few minutes.

Clinically, subarachnoid haemorrhage can affect any age group from the twenties onwards, and is characterized by the sudden onset of excruciatingly severe headache, quickly followed by coma. In some cases slow leakage from the aneurysm causes headache or minor neurological dysfunction before the acute attack.

Unlike other types of stroke, localizing signs, such as hemiplegia, are typically absent. The prognosis is poor and about 30 per cent of patients die from the initial haemorrhage. Neurosurgery can be curative, but many of the survivors have a fatal recurrence within 6–12 months.

Cerebral haemorrhage, thrombosis and embolism

Cerebral haemorrhage is the most lethal type of stroke and mainly affects those past middle age. Predisposing factors are hypertension and atherosclerosis and, in general, the higher the blood pressure the greater the risk of cerebral haemorrhage. Bleeding into the brain destroys and tears apart the tissue, forming an expanding lesion, distorting the brain and causing gross cerebral oedema.

Cerebral thrombosis is the most common cause of stroke. Atherosclerosis is the main contributory factor to thrombosis, which then cuts off the blood supply to part of the brain.

Cerebral emboli originate from such sources as a fibrillating atrium or intracardiac thrombosis secondary to a myocardial infarct, and are relatively uncommon.

These different types of stroke may not be distinguishable clinically. Embolism, however, is typically of dramatic suddenness and may affect a younger person, in whom a source of the embolus should be identifiable. Thrombosis tends to be the least rapid in its development but, like haemorrhage, is most

---

Table 17.15 Clinical features of different types of strokes

	Haemorrhage	Thrombosis	Embolism
Prodromal signs	—	Transient ischaemic attacks	—
Onset	Rapid	Gradual	Sudden
First symptom	Headache (50%)	Ill-defined	Headache
Progression	Hemiplegia and aphasia	Gradual and intermittent	Immediate
Underlying diseases	Hypertension Atherosclerosis	Hypertension Atherosclerosis	Atrial fibrillation Infective endocarditis
Prognosis	75% die in a month	Range from minimal dysfunction to death in a week	Recurrence in 80%

frequently associated with hypertension and atherosclerosis in the middle-aged and elderly (*Table 17.15*).

Typical features of a stroke are as follows:

1. Sudden loss of consciousness, often going on to coma or death.
2. Hemiplegia (loss of voluntary movement of the opposite side of the body to the lesion).
3. Loss of speech (aphasia) is usually the result of a lesion on the left side of the brain, so that most patients are also deprived of the ability to write.

Some patients have recurrent minor features – transient ischaemic attacks (TIA).

- **General management of a cerebrovascular accident**

The airway must be protected during the acute attack and precautions must be taken in the care later of the comatose patient. These include prevention of pressure sores and care of bladder and bowel. Anticoagulation may be used only if it has been established with certainty that the stroke is thrombotic or embolic.

- **Dental aspects of stroke**

Difficulties in dental management may include:

1. Communication difficulties, since there may be cognitive and sensory defects as well as dysarthria, aphasia, confusion, memory loss and emotional distress.
2. Loss of protective reflexes, such as the swallowing and gag reflexes in brain stem lesions.
3. Impaired mobility.
4. Anticoagulation
5. Hypertension.
6. Cardiovascular disease.
7. Diabetes mellitus.
8. Old age.

Patients after a stroke may have unilateral (upper motor neurone) facial palsy. This differs from Bell's palsy in that the lower face is mainly affected and emotional facial responses may be retained. Oral hygiene tends to deteriorate on the paralysed side and impaired manual dexterity may interfere with

toothbrushing. An electric toothbrush may therefore help. Patients are best treated in the upright position, and extra care must be taken to avoid foreign bodies entering the pharynx. Good suction must be at hand.

Subarachnoid or cerebral haemorrhage can be precipitated by acute hypertension and fatal subarachnoid haemorrhage has resulted from the use of noradrenaline in local anaesthetic solutions. Cerebral haemorrhage can also result from hypertension caused by interactions of monoamine oxidase inhibitors with other drugs, particularly pethidine. On the other hand, opiates and barbiturates are best avoided in strokes as they may cause severe hypotension.

Strokes are also a possible cause of sudden loss of consciousness in the dental surgery and should be recognizable by the features already described, especially the sudden loss of consciousness and, usually, signs of one-sided paralysis. Protection of the airway and a call for an ambulance are the only useful measures.

PARKINSON'S DISEASE

Idiopathic Parkinson's disease (paralysis agitans) is a common disorder, due to degeneration of the pigmented cells of the substantia nigra, leading to deficiency of the neurotransmitter dopamine. Its prevalence increases with age and there is no sex predilection.

Parkinsonism may also be caused by cerebrovascular disease, head injury (particularly in boxers), encephalitis lethargica (von Economo's disease), some toxins (such as heavy metals or carbon monoxide) or drugs, particularly the phenothiazine and butyrophenone neuroleptics, which are dopamine receptor blockers. Severe parkinsonism has followed the use of an illicitly manufactured opioid (MPTP; methyl phenyl tetrahydropyridine); this has led to better understanding of the pathogenesis and the suggestion that many cases of apparently idiopathic disease are due to unidentified environmental toxins.

The main features of Parkinson's disease are:

1. Tremor – mainly affecting the hands (pill rolling) and arms, and worst at rest.

2. Rigidity – the arms are flexed and held stiffly at the sides. Limb movement has a so-called cog-wheel rigidity.
3. Abnormal posture – the neck and shoulders are rigid, causing a stooping posture.
4. Bradykinesia – slowness in the initiation and execution of movements and poverty of spontaneous movements. Speech and swallowing may be affected. The patient may be slow at starting to walk but then runs forwards (festinant gait) or shuffles with slow, short steps. Bradykinesia may progress to akinesia and total rigidity.
5. Akathisia – restlessness.

Complications include subtle psychiatric disorders, deformities of the hands and feet, ocular abnormalities and urinary and gastrointestinal disturbances. Autonomic dysfunction may cause mild postural hypotension, disordered respiratory control and hypersalivation which, with the movement defect, may result in drooling. The face in parkinsonism is often expressionless and there is a loss of the blink reflex as a response to gentle tapping of the bridge of the nose. Oculogyric crises may be seen in drug-induced or post-encephalitic disease.

- **General management of Parkinson's disease**

If the diagnosis can be made sufficiently early, the monoamine oxidase B inhibitor, selegiline, by decreasing the breakdown of dopamine in the basal ganglia, may delay progress of the disease slightly. Other drugs are used alone or in combination for the following main effects.

Levodopa improves akinesia and imbalance.

Other *dopaminergic drugs* (bromocriptine, lysuride, pergolide, apomorphine) help where levodopa is not effective but can have serious neuropsychiatric side-effects or cause hypotension.

Anticholinergics are most effective at reducing the tremor at rest.

Propranolol or *primidone* are best for action tremor.

For disabling idiopathic Parkinson's disease, levodopa – a precursor of dopamine – is the most effective drug but has many toxic effects, especially nausea, dysrhythmias, neuropsychiatric reactions and liver dysfunc-

tion. It is therefore usually given in combination with an inhibitor of the degradative enzyme, dopa decarboxylase such as carbidopa (co-careldopa) or benserazide (co-beneldopa), to increase the concentration of dopamine centrally. In such combinations, levodopa is effective at lower doses and adverse effects (such as nausea, vomiting and cardiovascular disorders) are lessened. Domperidone is often used to overcome the nausea. A major disadvantage of levodopa is that its major benefits persist for only a few years and then the duration of control from each dose diminishes. It may cause depression, psychoses and hallucinations and is contraindicated in glaucoma. Many combinations of drugs have been used in the attempt to overcome these problems but as yet there is no practical alternative to giving levodopa to maintain mobility but at the cost of increasing dyskinesias. Pergolide, bromocriptine, apomorphine and lysuride are direct dopamine agonists useful particularly when levodopa cannot be tolerated.

Antimuscarinic drugs such as trihexyphenidyl, benztropine, biperiden and procyclidine give some help to nearly 60 per cent of patients with mild symptoms, particularly tremor. Antimuscarinics (or selegiline) may be given with levodopa in severe cases. Antimuscarinics are also given for post-encephalitic and drug-associated parkinsonism which may be made worse by levodopa.

Stereotaxic neurosurgery of the globus pallidus is now rarely used, since medical treatment is generally safer and more effective. Experimentally, brain grafts of fetal nigral tissue have been given. The value of this procedure is as yet unclear.

- **Dental aspects of Parkinson's disease**

It is essential in patients with Parkinson's disease not to let the blankness of expression and apparent unresponsiveness be mistaken for stupidity. The parkinsonian tremor may affect the tongue and/or lips. Sympathetic handling is therefore particularly important, as anxiety increases tremor. Drooling of saliva may be troublesome, though treatment with antimuscarinic drugs reduces both the tremor and salivation to some degree. Levodopa may produce reddish saliva. Caries is *less* common than in controls, and teeth are retained longer. The main problems in parkinsonism therefore are tremor and drooling, and dysphagia. Orofacial involuntary movements (dyskinesia) such as 'flycatcher tongue' and lip pursing are side-effects of levodopa and bromocriptine (*see* Appendix to Chapter 25).

The monoamine oxidase inhibitor, selegeline, used in Parkinson's disease differs from other MAOIs in that it should not cause acute hypertensive episodes. However, a serious interaction with pethidine has been reported. Pethidine should therefore be avoided in patients receiving selegeline or other MAOIs.

MULTIPLE SCLEROSIS

Multiple (disseminated) sclerosis (MS) is the most common neurological disease affecting young adults, and is characterized by symptoms disseminated in both site and time. There is a high prevalence of multiple sclerosis particularly in Northern Europe and Northern America.

The aetiology is unknown but may perhaps be viral, possibly human herpes virus 6, with immunologically mediated damage resulting in demyelination.

Though up to 35 per cent of cases are subclinical, typical clinical features of progressive disease are as follows:

1. The onset is characteristically highly capricious: transient visual disturbance or blindness (optic neuritis), or weakness or paralysis of a limb with complete though temporary recovery, are common features.
2. Later nystagmus, ataxia, jerky (scanning) speech, tremors and loss of muscular coordination develop as a result of cerebellar involvement.
3. Ultimately, widespread paralysis and often loss of sphincter control and urinary incontinence can develop.
4. Depression can be a feature but, perhaps fortunately, euphoria also.

• General management of MS

There is no specific laboratory diagnostic aid or specific treatment. Courses of ACTH or corticosteroids may be used during acute episodes, while diazepam or other relaxants may be needed to control muscle spasm. Beta interferon may reduce relapses.

• Dental aspects of MS

Limited mobility and psychological disorders may interfere with routine dental treatment. Patients with severe MS are best not treated fully supine, as respiration may be embarrassed. Treatment is best carried out under local analgesia if possible. Some patients may have difficulty localizing orofacial pain. Some patients are on corticosteroids, with their attendant complications (Chapter 14). Dental preventive care and treatment is important since oral hygiene may be poor, as in other conditions causing disability (Chapter 23).

There are no specific oral manifestations but this diagnosis should always be considered in a young patient presenting with trigeminal neuralgia, particularly if there have been other neurological disturbances, if the pain lasts minutes or hours, or if it is bilateral. It may respond to carbamazepine. Facial palsy is occasionally caused by MS and then is usually not associated with retroaural pain or with loss of taste sensation such as may be seen in Bell's palsy. Facial myokymia or hemispasm may be seen. Abnormal perioral sensation, such as extreme hypersensitivity or facial anaesthesia, may develop especially in advanced MS, as may tremor. In addition to abnormalities of speech, cerebellar involvement may cause tremor and spasm of the muscles of the head and neck. Atropinics used in the treatment of bladder dysfunction may cause dry mouth.

GUILLAIN–BARRÉ SYNDROME (INFECTIVE OR IDIOPATHIC POLYNEURITIS)

The Guillain–Barré syndrome appears to be an immunologically mediated disorder resulting from various infections, especially viral, or vaccination.

Any age group can be affected and the clinical features are highly variable. Symptoms range from bilateral facial palsy with minor motor and sensory loss in the limbs, to fulminating disease with raised intracranial pressure, quadriplegia and respiratory paralysis. Sudden respiratory paralysis develops in 10–20 per cent of cases and is lethal unless immediate mechanical ventilation can be given, sometimes with plasmapheresis. The disease usually reaches a peak within about a week, then gradually subsides after about 3 weeks. The majority recover slowly – but between 10 and 30 per cent have severe residual disabilities after a year.

MOTOR NEURONE DISEASE

Motor neurone disease (MND) comprises a group of uncommon lethal diseases affecting motor neurones (especially anterior horn cells) at various levels in the nervous system. MND mainly affects males, especially in old age. The aetiology is unclear but may be viral. There are three subtypes:

1. *Progressive muscular atrophy* is characterized by wasting and weakness which starts in the small muscles of the hands and spreads proximally. Lesions are limited to the anterior horn below the foramen magnum.
2. *Progressive bulbar palsy* is characterized by wasting, weakness and fasciculation of the muscles of the pharynx, tongue, palate, sternomastoid and trapezius which result from involvement of cranial nerve motor neurones arising in the medulla (IX–XII inclusive). It involves anterior horn cells of the brain stem.
3. *Amyotrophic lateral sclerosis* involves lesions of the anterior horn and pyramidal tract, affecting upper and lower motor neurones with wasting and weakness of the hands and spasticity of the legs. The disease is relentless and within 5 years there is death, typically from respiratory paralysis. However, even in the late stages, sensory, bowel, bladder and cognitive functions are spared. Involvement of the brain stem leads to *pseudobulbar palsy* – bulbar palsy with emotional lability (involuntary weeping or laughing).

- **Dental aspects of motor neurone disease**

Motor neurone disease is only important in dentistry in so far as oral hygiene may be impaired as in other conditions with disability, and weakness or paralysis of the neck and head and oral musculature can lead to dysphagia. Drooling can be a problem. Protection of the airway may also be impaired but patients with this degree of disability, however, are likely to be hospitalized. Morphine or pethidine are frequently needed for terminal care.

MERCURY INTOXICATION

Mercury is neurotoxic in its metallic form and as salts, particularly methyl mercury. Mercury salts are also nephrotoxic and renal damage can be caused by the diuretic, mersalyl, which as a consequence is virtually obsolete. Metallic mercury can be absorbed by inhalation of its vapour or through the skin and mucous membranes. Mercury salts are absorbed after ingestion.

At the end of the last, and early in this century, a number of children and others suffered from acrodynia (pink disease) which appears to have been related to the use of a mercury salt, calomel, in teething powders and some gastrointestinal medications. Environmental poisoning from methyl mercury was widespread in Minimata Bay and Nigata, Japan, between 1953 and 1960, as a result of eating fish contaminated by mercury from industrial discharge. Many persons suffered neurological damage, some died, and later there was a high incidence of cerebral palsy in newborn children. It is now a problem in Brazil.

Acute poisoning by massive inhalation of mercury vapour is very rare but can cause potentially fatal pneumonitis and neurological symptoms, particularly tremor and excitability.

Chronic poisoning by inhalation of mercury vapour primarily affects the CNS. It is highly lipid-soluble, rapidly penetrates the blood–brain barrier and infiltrates neurones. However, initial symptoms include not merely lassitude, but gastrointestinal disturbances, anorexia and weight loss. More prolonged exposure can cause tremor, memory loss, timidity and excitability (*erethism*). This syndrome was well recognized, particularly in the previous century, among workers with mercury such as thermometer makers and felt hat makers – hence, 'mad as a hatter'.

Other effects of chronic mercury poisoning include hypersalivation, accelerated periodontitis and a characteristic black gingival line due to deposition of sulphides of mercury along the line of the gingival crevice. Rarely, necrosis of the jaw could follow, but such manifestations are now mainly of historical interest.

• **Dental aspects of mercury toxicity**

Apart from rare cases of poisoning there are three main considerations, namely:

1. Occupational exposure of dental staff to mercury.
2. Alleged mercury-related neurological symptoms ('mercury allergy') in patients.
3. Local effects of mercury-containing amalgam fillings.

Mercury as an occupational hazard
The metal is highly volatile and readily absorbed through the respiratory tract and skin. In addition some mercury can be absorbed from foods, particularly fish, and it is also an environmental pollutant.

Dental staff can be far more heavily exposed to mercury than the general population. On average up to 1.5 kg of mercury are used by a dental practice annually and, when little attention was paid to mercury hygiene, mercury vapour in the surgery atmosphere and its levels in the blood, hair, nails and urine in dentists were frequently above controls. Up to 45 per cent of dental personnel had higher levels of mercury in hair than controls and the median blood mercury concentration in a study of 130 Danish dentists was significantly raised. However, none of the latter's blood levels of mercury was over the recognized 'safe' limit of 35 µg/l. Levels were highest in fish eaters, indicating that at least part of the mercury burden was from non-dental sources and, as with the rest of the population, some would have come from the environment.

Recent studies of dentists and dental surgery assistants have not shown excessively high urinary mercury levels where good mercury hygiene was practised, and urinary mercury levels appear to be lower in dentists in 1996 than in 1983.

The greatest hazard is from inhalation of mercury vapour as a result of spillage, particularly when in proximity to an autoclave or other source of heat. Droplets of mercury can also accumulate in significant amounts in surgery carpeting or crevices in the floor. Mercury is also absorbed during hand trituration of amalgam or other skin contact. Removal of old amalgams from teeth with an air-rotor produces traces of mercury vapour but not if adequate water-cooling and aspiration are used.

In the past, after decades of practice, a few dental staff have suffered from chronic mercury toxicity with tremor, incoordination, polyneuropathies and accelerated senility. Rarely, deaths have been reported after prolonged heavy exposure. Autopsy studies have shown mercury deposits, particularly in the pituitary glands and occipital lobes in dentists. In another study, of female dentists and dental surgery assistants, a history of reproductive failures, menstrual disorders and spina bifida in their children appeared to be related to mercury levels in hair, but this has not been widely confirmed and other larger studies have shown no such correlation. Indeed the perinatal death and birth defects rate for infants born of dentists is *lower* than normal.

Objective investigation of neurological and psychological function, in 1982, showed evidence of a polyneuropathy in dentists with high tissue mercury levels. However, neurological defects were not evident clinically and it seems unlikely that these findings would apply now to dentists who apply adequate standards of mercury hygiene.

Mercury and its salts are also potential sensitizing agents and exposure to them can occasionally lead to contact dermatitis. As a consequence the frequency of positive patch tests increases as dental students progress through their course. Nevertheless, contact dermatitis to mercury surprisingly rarely restricts dental practice.

In summary therefore, mercury presents an occupational threat to the health of dentists and dental assistants, but provided that reasonable care is taken in its use, does not appear to represent a significant hazard. Indeed, dentists, despite exposure to mercury, have one of the lowest mortality rates of any profession (Scully *et al.* 1990).

'Mercury allergy'

A few patients have genuine contact sensitivity to mercury. Nevertheless they can tolerate the placement of amalgam restorations, provided that none is spilt onto the skin.

Another group of patients have symptoms such as headache, lassitude, a general feeling of ill-health which they ascribe to mercury toxicity or allergy. Unfortunately this belief has been encouraged by unscrupulous practitioners who carry out expensive but spurious tests to detect alleged effects of dental amalgams. However, there is no evidence that sufficient mercury is absorbed from amalgams to cause neurological damage.

It has also been shown that patients who complain of amalgam-related symptoms also suffer more frequently from other, unrelated complaints, such as chronic craniofacial pain, than controls. It was noteworthy in that in this same study, out of 20 patients who complained of amalgam-related symptoms and were offered blood tests for mercury concentrations, only 5 were willing to be tested.

Because of this concern about possible mercury toxicity from dental amalgams, the American Dental Association has carried out extensive investigation of the data available and, in 1989, their Council on Dental Therapeutics concluded that 'there is insufficient evidence to justify claims that mercury from dental amalgams has an adverse effect on the health of patients'. In view of the claims that could result from litigation if this information were shown to be incorrect, and in view of the strong financial stimulus to use more expensive materials, such a statement was certainly not lightly made.

Local effects of mercury-containing restorations (see *Chapter 12*)

TUMOURS OF THE CENTRAL NERVOUS SYSTEM

Brain tumours account for approximately 2 per cent of all cancer deaths but are second only to leukaemia as a cause of death in children.

A possible relationship between brain tumours and dental radiography has been reported but not as yet confirmed.

Cerebral tumours are usually metastatic. Most primary cerebral tumours are malignant but even histologically benign tumours have a poor prognosis because they are often not amenable to surgery. Intracranial lymphomas are a well recognized feature of HIV disease and are increasing in prevalence.

Typical features of cerebral tumours are:

1. Localizing signs dependent on the site: examples are convulsions or paralysis.
2. Signs of raised intracranial pressure: these include headache, vomiting, papilloedema, disturbance of consciousness, a rising blood pressure and slowing of the pulse.

Epileptiform fits developing for the first time in an adult are strongly suggestive of a cerebral tumour.

Metastatic tumours

Metastatic tumours are second only to cerebrovascular lesions as a cause of neurological disease. The main sources are carcinomas of the lung, breast, gastrointestinal tract and kidney, of which a cerebral tumour is sometimes the first indication.

Acoustic neuroma (neurofibroma)

This is a benign tumour arising from the neural axonal or neural sheath in the cerebellopontine angle, at the root of the vestibular part of the VIIIth cranial nerve, where it leaves the brain stem in the posterior cranial fossa. Bilateral acoustic neuromas are the characteristic feature of neurofibromatosis type II.

Clinically, an acoustic neuroma produces a highly characteristic picture as the trigeminal, facial, glossopharyngeal and vagus nerves become stretched over the growth. Typical early results are tinnitus (ringing in the ears), deafness and rotational vertigo (a sensation of spinning). Further growth of the tumour causes postauricular pain, disturbance of balance, facial twitching or weakness and paraesthesia, together with difficulty in speaking and swallowing.

The growth can be completely removed, though with difficulty, in about 60 per cent of cases.

Pituitary tumours

Adenomas are the most common pituitary tumours but their endocrine effects dominate the clinical picture and they are discussed in Chapter 14. Non-functional pituitary tumours compress the gland and can cause hypopituitarism, but can also produce signs common to other cerebral tumours. The most important non-functional tumours are adenomas and the craniopharyngioma. The latter arises from Rathke's pouch, an upgrowth from the primitive stomatodeum, and may resemble an ameloblastoma or calcifying odontogenic cyst microscopically. Most manifest in childhood with headache, vomiting and papilloedema and visual defects. Short stature, delayed sexual development and diabetes insipidus may be associated. Suprasellar calcification may be seen, especially on CT.

- **Dental aspects of cerebral tumours**

Cerebral tumours rarely have important dental implications, but an acoustic neuroma and occasionally other tumours can cause impaired sensation or motor function in the trigeminal or facial nerves, as discussed earlier. Pituitary adenomas may cause acromegaly, Cushing's disease or Nelson's syndrome (Chapter 14).

MYASTHENIA GRAVIS

Myasthenia gravis, a rare cause of muscle weakness and fatiguability, is a disorder not of the nervous system but rather a lesion at the neuromuscular junction. The response of the muscle to the neurotransmitter acetylcholine (ACh) is weak and circulating autoantibodies to ACh receptor proteins can be detected in at least 85 per cent of patients. These autoantibodies are associated in 75 per cent of cases with thymic hyperplasia and, in the remainder, a thymoma.

Women between 20 and 30 are usually affected but the diagnosis is often delayed. The main feature is rapidly developing and severe fatigue of muscles, particularly of those in most active use. Typically the extraocular muscles and the muscles of face, tongue, neck and extremities are severely affected. Facial weakness causes a snarling appearance as the

patient attempts to smile. Weakness of the masticatory muscles causing the mouth to hang open (hanging or lantern jaw sign) is a characteristic feature and patients typically tend to support the jaw with their hand. Speech may have a nasal quality. Ptosis, diplopia, squinting and difficulties in swallowing with nasal regurgitation of food and drink may also develop. Disability is worsened by fatigue of the muscles, particularly towards the end of the day. A potentially lethal complication is involvement of the respiratory muscles, particularly in the elderly. Respiratory insufficiency may result either from the disease itself (myasthenic crisis), or treatment (cholinergic crisis).

Occasional cases are associated with carcinoma elsewhere (Eaton–Lambert syndrome) or other diseases. Thymic disease can also depress immunological responses and there is an uncommon syndrome of thymoma, myasthenia gravis, depressed cell mediated immunity, chronic mucocutaneous candidosis and haematological disease (Good's syndrome, Chapter 20).

- **General management of myasthenia gravis**

The diagnosis is made from clinical features and an anticholinesterase test, sometimes supported by electrodiagnostic tests and serum antibodies to acetylcholine receptors. Thymic disease should be excluded by mediastinal CT or MRI, and autoimmune disorders should be sought. Myasthenia gravis very occasionally remits spontaneously but in those with thymomas the prognosis is poor. An anticholinesterase such as pyridostigmine, given orally, restores muscle strength in the majority of patients, but is not curative and atropine is often also required to counteract its parasympathomimetic effects such as diarrhoea or bradycardia.

Corticosteroids, preferably in combination with azathioprine or cyclosporin, are also effective. Thymectomy increasingly is used, as it typically cures the disorder.

- **Dental aspects of myasthenia gravis**

Dental treatment is best carried out during a remission. Fatigue or emotional stress may precipitate a myasthenic crisis and weakness increases during the day. Therefore, treatment is best carried out early in the day, within 1–2 hours of routine medication with anticholinesterases. Local anaesthesia is preferred but minimal doses should be given. Lignocaine, prilocaine or mepivacaine can safely be used, but the older ester types (such as procaine) are contraindicated. A small dose of a benzodiazepine may be given if the patient is anxious.

General anaesthesia or intravenous sedation must not be given in the dental surgery since bulbar or respiratory involvement impairs respiration. Many drugs used in general anaesthesia, such as opioids, barbiturates, suxamethonium, curare or anaesthetic agents, are potentiated by or aggravate the myasthenic state. Postoperative respiratory infection can result and may also cause myasthenia to worsen.

Corticosteroids, other immunosuppressants, or emotional lability may also complicate dental treatment. Other drugs to be avoided include tetracyclines, clindamycin, lincomycin, sulphonamides and aminoglycosides, since they increase weakness. Penicillin or erythromycin can safely be used. Occasionally, aspirin has produced a cholinergic crisis in those on anticholinesterases. Paracetamol and codeine do not have this potential disadvantage.

Masticatory muscle fatigue is often conspicuous; occasionally there is also furrowing, atrophy or paresis of the tongue or uvula palsy. Salivation is increased if an anticholinesterase, alone, is being taken. Occasionally, Sjögren's syndrome or other autoimmune disorders, particularly pemphigus, may be associated. If there is a thymoma there may be chronic candidosis.

PATIENTS WITH RESPIRATORY PARALYSIS

Respiratory difficulties or paralysis may result particularly from spinal cord lesions or from poliomyelitis.

Spinal cord lesions

Spinal cord damage is most frequently caused by trauma, particularly road traffic accidents, when it may be associated with maxillofacial injuries. Other causes of spinal cord disease include infarction, haemorrhage, myelitis or tumours.

Severe and permanent disablement may result, but the type of disability depends largely on the level and extent of the lesion within the spinal cord. High level lesions can be lethal, or cause respiratory paralysis and quadriplegia. Lower level lesions may result in paraplegia and many of the problems that afflict persons with spina bifida (*see above*).

Poliomyelitis

Anterior poliomyelitis (polio) is a viral infection, spread faeco-orally, that damages the lower motor neurones and sometimes motor cranial nerves. Rare in the developed world since the introduction of an effective vaccine, it is still common in the developing world, and appears in the developed world in some immigrants or where vaccine uptake is poor. Typically causing wasting and paralysis of the lower limb, it may affect other areas including the medulla oblongata when it can cause bulbar palsy and respiratory paralysis. To survive, such patients must be permanently artificially ventilated (on an 'iron lung').

- **Dental management of patients with bulbar or respiratory palsy**

Those with poliomyelitis, bulbar palsy or a high level spinal lesion may have impaired gag and cough reflexes, and thus their airway must be carefully protected. Good suction must be used. Patients with quadriplegia may benefit from the dentist constructing a mouthstick or bitestick appliance with which to operate a computer, telephone and other means of communicating or performing manual functions. Those with paraplegia require care similar to persons with spina bifida (*see above*).

PERIPHERAL NEUROPATHIES

The peripheral neuropathy of greatest relevance in dentistry is Bell's palsy. Peripheral neuropathies may also be seen in vitamin B_{12} deficiency (Chapter 5), diabetes mellitus (Chapter 14), alcoholism and abuse of nitrous oxide (Chapter 24). Less common causes are summarized in the Appendix to this chapter.

DISTURBED TASTE AND SMELL

Taste loss is mentioned in Chapter 9. Impairment can have a range of causes shown in the Appendix to this chapter.

BIBLIOGRAPHY

Ali G.N., Wallace K.L., Schwartz R. *et al.* (1996) Mechanisms of oral-pharyngeal dysphagia in patients with Parkinson's disease. *Gastroenterol.* 110, 383–92.

Baringer J.R. (1996) Herpes simplex virus and Bell's palsy. *Ann. Intern. Med.* 124, 63–5.

Brodie M.J., Richens A., Yuen A.W.C. *et al.* (1995) Double-blind comparison of lamotrigine and carbamazepine in newly diagnosed epilepsy. *Lancet* 345, 476–9.

Cawson R.A., Spector R.G. and Skelly A.M. (1995) *Basic Pharmacology and Clinical Drug Use in Dentistry,* 6th edn. Edinburgh, Churchill Livingstone.

Cawson R.A., McCracken A.W., Marcus P.B. *et al.* (1989) *Pathology: the Mechanisms of Disease,* 2nd edn. St Louis, Mosby.

Chia L.G. (1988) Pure trigeminal motor neuropathy. *Br. Med. J.* 296, 609–11.

Cloran A.J., Davies W.J. and Campbell T.M. (1983) Special design of mouthstick device for a patient with upper extremity bilateral amputations. *Spec. Care Dent.* 5, 112–13.

Cnossen M.W. (1985) Considerations in the dental treatment of patients with multiple sclerosis. *Oral Med.* 37, 62–4.

Dacso C.C. and Bortz D.L. (1989) Significance of the Argyll–Robertson pupil in clinical medicine. *Am. J. Med.* 86, 199–202.

Da Fonseca M.A. and Walker P.O. (1993) Dental management of a child with Huntington's disease. *Spec. Care Dent.* 13, 21–3.

Dios P.D. (1995) Oral care in the blind and visually impaired. In Porter S.R. and Scully C. *Oral Health Care for Those with HIV Infection and Other Special Needs.* Northwood, Science Reviews, pp. 219–21.

Fernando I.N. and Phipps J.S.K. (1988) Dangers of an uncomplicated tooth extraction: a case of *Streptococcus sanguis* meningitis. *Br. Dent. J.* 165, 220.

Flint S. and Scully C. (1990) Isolated trigeminal sensory neuropathy: a heterogeneous group of disorders. *Oral Surg. Oral Med. Oral Pathol.* 69, 153–6.

Flanders R.A. (1992) Mercury in dental amalgam – a public health concern? *J. Pub. Hlth Dent.* 52, 303–11.

Friedlander A.H. and Cummings J.L. (1992) Dental treatment of patients with Gilles de la Tourette's syndrome. *Oral Surg. Oral Med. Oral Pathol.* 73, 299–303.

Getchell T.V. (ed) (1991) *Smell and Taste in Health and Disease.* New York, Raven Press.

Graham S.H., Sharp F.R. and Dillon W. (1988) Intraoral sensation in patients with brainstem lesions: role of the rostral spinal trigeminal nuclei in pons. *Neurology* 38, 1529–33.

Hanson M. and Pleva J. (1991) The dental amalgam issue; a review. *Experientia* 47, 9–22.

James D.J. (1996) All that palsies is not Bell's. *J. R. Soc. Med.* 89, 184–7.

Jolly D.E., Paulson R.B., Paulson G.W. and Pike J.A. (1989) Parkinson's disease; a review and recommendations. *Spec. Care Dent.* 9, 74–8.

Jones A.A. *et al.* (1986) Dental X-rays found to have no effect on hearing aids. *J. Am. Dent. Assoc.* 113, 912–3.

Lamartine de Assis J., Marchion P.E. and Scaff M. (1994) Atrophy of the tongue with persistent articulation disorder in myasthenia gravis. *Auris Nasus Larynx (Tokyo)* 21, 215–18.

Larner A.J. (1986) Aetiological role of viruses in multiple sclerosis. *J. R. Soc. Med.* 79, 412–17.

Leading Article (1982) Bell's palsy. *Lancet* i, 663.

Leading Article (1989) Carbamazepine update. *Lancet* 2, 595–7.

Lowe O. (1986) Tourette's syndrome: management of oral complications. *J. Dent. Child.* 53 , 456–60.

Ludman H. (1981) Facial palsy. *Br. Med. J.* 282, 545–7.

Luker J. and Scully C. (1990) The lateral medullary syndrome. *Oral Surg. Oral Med. Oral Pathol.* 69, 322–4.

Marks P.V., Patel K.S. and Mee E.W. (1988) Multiple brain abscesses secondary to dental caries and severe periodontal disease. *Br. J. Oral Maxillofac. Surg.* 26, 244–7.

Mass E., Sarnat H., Ram D. *et al.* (1992). Dental and oral findings in patients with familial dysautonomia. *Oral Surg. Oral Med. Oral Pathol.* 74, 305–11.

Mattson R.H. (1995) Comparing antiepileptic drugs. *Lancet* 345, 467–8.

Norris F.H. (1992) Motor neurone disease. *Br. Med J.* 304, 459–60.

Persson M., Osterberg T., Granerus A-K. *et al.* (1992). Influence of Parkinson's disease on oral health. *Acta Odont Scand.* 50, 37–42.

Porter S.R. and Scully C. (1996) *Innovations and Developments in Non-invasive Oral Health Care.* Northwood, Science Reviews.

Preston-Martin S. and White S.C. (1990) Brain and salivary gland tumours related to prior dental radiography: implications for current practice. *J. Am. Dent. Assoc.* 120, 151–8.

Robinson B.B., Harris M. and Harvey W. (1983) Abnormal skeletal and dental growth in epileptic children. *Br. Dent. J.* 154, 9–13.

Rontal E. (1982) Lesions of the hypoglossal nerve – diagnosis, treatment and rehabilitation. *Laryngoscope* 92, 927.

Ruboyianes J.M., Trent C.S., Adour K.K. *et al.* (1996) Bell's palsy treatment with acyclovir and prednisone compared with prednisone alone: a double-blind, randomized, controlled trial. *Ann. Otol. Rhinol. Laryngol.* 105, 371–8.

Schiffman S.S. (1997) Taste and smell losses in normal aging and disease. *JAMA* **278**, 1357–62.

Schrader V. and Sumner A. (1996) Idiopathic (Bell's) facial palsy. In *Neurological Disorders: Course and Treatment*. New York, Academic Press, pp. 113–16.

Scully C. (1980) Orofacial manifestations of disease. 6. Neurological, psychiatric and muscular disorders. *Hosp. Update* **6**, 135; *Dent. Update* **7**, 375; **8**, 135.

Scully C. (1988) *The Dental Patient*. Oxford, Heinemann.

Scully C. (1989) *The Mouth and Perioral Tissues*. Oxford, Heinemann.

Scully C. (1989) *Patient Care: a Dental Surgeon's Guide*. London, British Dental Association.

Scully C. and Cawson R.A. (eds) (1986) Oral medicine. *Med. Int.* **28**, 1129–51.

Scully C., Cawson R.A. and Griffiths M.J. (1990) *Occupational Hazards to Dental Staff*. London, British Dental Journal.

Severn A.M. (1988) Parkinsonism and the anaesthetist. *Br. J. Anaesth.* **61**, 761–70.

Shaw D.H., Cohen D.M. and Hoffman M. (1985) Dental treatment of patients with myasthenia gravis. *J. Oral Med.* **37**, 118–20.

Stevens M.R. and Wong, M.E. (1988) Meige syndrome: an unusual cause of involuntary facial movements. *Oral Surg. Oral Med. Oral Pathol.* **66**, 427–9.

Talako A.A. and Reade, P.C. (1990) Progressive bulbar palsy. *Oral Surg. Oral Med. Oral Pathol.* **69**, 182–4.

Tolosa E.S. (1981) Clinical features of Meige's disease: idiopathic orofacial dystonia. *Arch. Neurol.* **36**, 147–51.

Williams A.C. (1995) Dopamine, dystonia, and the deficient co-factor. *Lancet* **345**, 1130.

APPENDIX TO CHAPTER 17

PERIPHERAL NEUROPATHIES

1. Hereditary
Charcot–Marie–Tooth disease
Refsum's disease
Déjérine–Sottas disease

2. Acquired

Infective:	Herpes zoster
	Guillain–Barré syndrome
	Leprosy
	Diphtheria
	Lyme disease
Neoplasms:	Various
Trauma	
Metabolic:	Diabetes mellitus
	Vitamin deficiencies, especially B_{12}
Toxic:	Alcohol
	Heavy metals
	Gold
Nitrous oxide abuse	
Idiopathic:	Bell's palsy

CRANIAL NERVE SYNDROMES*

Syndrome	Cranial nerves involved	Site of lesion	Other features
Avellis'	X	Medulla	Hemiplegia Horner's syndrome
Benedikt's	III	Midbrain	Cerebellar ataxia Tremor Hemiplegia
Cerebellopontine angle	V, Vll, VIII and sometimes IX	Posterior cranial fossa	Cerebellar ataxia
Claude's	III	Midbrain	Cerebellar ataxia Tremor

continued

Collet–Sicard	IX, X, XI, XII	Retroparotid space	–
Foix's	III, IV, V (ophthalmic), VI	Cavernous sinus	Proptosis
Gradenigo's	V, VI	Petrous temporal	Pain
Jackson's	X, XII	Medulla	Hemiplegia Horner's syndrome
Jacob's	II, III, IV, V, VI	Middle cranial fossa	–
Millard–Gubler	VII, VI	Pons	Hemiplegia
Nothnagel's	III	Midbrain	Cerebellar ataxia
Parinaud's	III, IV, VI	Midbrain	–
Sphenoid fissure (superior orbital fissure)	III, IV, V (ophthalmic), VI and sometimes II	Superior orbital fissure	Proptosis
Vernet's	IX, X, XI	Jugular foramen Nasopharynx	–
Villaret's	IX, X, XI, XII	Retroparotid space	Horner's syndrome
Wallenberg's (posterior inferior cerebellar artery, PICA)	V, IX, X, XI	Medulla	Horner's syndrome Cerebellar ataxia Loss of pain and temperature sense
Weber's	III	Midbrain	Hemiplegia

CAUSES OF TASTE LOSS

Aging
Xerostomia
Drugs
    Antihistamines
    Antihypertensives
    Antidepressants
    Cytotoxic agents
Irradiation of the oral cavity
Neurological disorders
    Alzheimer's disease
    Head trauma
    Multiple sclerosis
    Parkinson's disease
    Neoplasia
Nutritional defects
    Zinc deficiency
    Vitamin B deficiency
Endocrinopathies
    Diabetes
    Cushing's syndrome
    Hypothyroidism
Metabolic disorders
    Chronic renal failure
    Hepatic disease

*Modified from Victor M. and Adams R.D. (1980) In Isselbacher K.J. *et al.* (eds) *Principles of Internal Medicine*, 9th edn. Tokyo, McGraw-Hill Kogakusha, p. 2020.

18

Psychiatric disorders

Key points

- Psychiatric disorders are common and can significantly influence oral health care, predominantly because of behavioural abnormalities.
- Psychiatric disorders may be revealed by the history, medication, appearance, behaviour, type of speech, mood, orientation, memory and concentration.
- Particular note should be taken of the form of speech and content; abnormal beliefs and experiences; orientation in time, place and person; and memory and concentration.
- Anxiety before dental treatment is common but usually manageable with reassurance and, occasionally, mild anxiolytics such as short-acting benzodiazepines.
- Sometimes anxiety is extreme enough to warrant the term 'phobia', when there are symptoms such as terror, rapid breathing, palpitations and agitation.
- Phobics require psychiatric support, sometimes with medication such as buspirone, or a benzodiazepine. Painless dental care and the use of sedation may help.
- Neuroses are common, often remain untreated or unrecognized, but usually the person affected has insight. Psychoses are less common but more serious, and insight is typically lacking.
- Depression is characterized by lowering of mood and many aspects of activity, and is dangerous since sufferers may attempt suicide.
- Depression may underlie a variety of oral complaints, particularly atypical facial pain and dry mouth.
- Monoamine oxidase inhibitors, tricyclics and selective serotonin uptake inhibitors are the main antidepressants.
- GA is best avoided in patients taking antidepressants but local anaesthetics, provided they contain no noradrenaline, can be safely used.
- Obsessional neuroses are not uncommon and manifest by thoughts repeatedly coming into consciousness against the will of the patient, and often compelling them to undertake an action.
- Munchausen's syndrome is the term given to a disorder in which patients go to extraordinary lengths to fabricate stories and symptoms, in order to be operated upon.
- Anorexia nervosa (slimming disease) and bulimia are eating disorders with a high mortality, seen mainly in young females of higher socioeconomic class, who starve themselves into poor health.
- Anaemia is common in the eating disorders, and is a contraindication to general anaesthesia, as is hypokalaemia. Paracetamol has heightened hepatotoxicity in these conditions, and should be avoided.
- Repeated vomiting in the eating disorders may cause tooth erosion, and sialosis may also be seen.

- Hypochondriacal states are common, and underlie some patients who complain of orofacial pain, dry mouth, abnormal taste or halitosis.
- Manic depression is a psychosis characterized by phases of depression and mania (elation, hyperactivity, flight of ideas, lack of restraint), often requiring psychiatric care.
- Manic depression is often treated with lithium, which may precipitate dysrhythmias, contraindicating general anaesthesia, and can cause dry mouth.
- Schizophrenia is a common major psychosis which affects mood, thought and behaviour, often with illusions, delusions, hallucinations and sometimes paranoia.
- Schizophrenia is controlled with phenothiazines or butyrophenones mainly, and thus dry mouth and extrapyramidal features such as orofacial dyskinesias are commonly seen.
- The acutely disturbed patient may be suffering from psychiatric disease such as a psychosis, organic disease such as infections, drug intoxication, or drug withdrawal.
- Dementia, the loss of intelligence, memory and cognitive functions, usually seen in the elderly, can be caused by vascular disease, HIV, other causes, or is idiopathic (Alzheimer's disease).
- Dementia leads to general neglect of everything, including health, and thus oral hygiene deteriorates and oral disease increases. Close care is required.

Most patients who come for dental treatment are anxious – a normal reaction to an unpleasant experience. Anxiety and disturbances of mood are extremely common in the general population. It is essential, therefore, not to dismiss patients who will not accept a proposed treatment as simply being 'uncooperative'. Anxious patients may genuinely want dental care but be unable to cooperate, often are unaware of their anxiety and, as a consequence, may be hostile in their responses or behaviour.

In contrast, it is important to be aware that psychiatric disorders are exceedingly common but often under-diagnosed, and what may appear to be rather unusual behaviour may indeed be a manifestation of psychiatric disease. Drug misuse is also common, and may explain abnormal behaviour in some patients.

Some patients are difficult or even impossible to manage because of anxiety, phobia, personality disorders or psychiatric disease but age, drug use, cultural and other factors can also cause difficulties in communication and, as a consequence, require extra time and patience. Compliance with appointments or treatment is often poor. Furthermore, there may be difficulties in gaining informed consent to treatment from a person with psychiatric disease.

In addition, some of the more severely ill or neglected patients are at high risk from diseases of deprivation and lifestyle, such as tuberculosis. There may also be oral neglect with a high prevalence of caries and periodontal disease, difficulties coping with dental prostheses, and self-induced lesions or other oral symptoms caused by the psychiatric disease or its treatment. Drugs such as monoamine oxidase inhibitors, tricyclic antidepressants, phenothiazines, lithium or barbiturates cause xerostomia or other orofacial disorders, or influence dental care (Appendix to Chapter 25).

STRESS

Stress may play a greater role in health and disease than formerly supposed. There is growing evidence of neuroimmunological mechanisms that might influence immunological and inflammatory disorders and defence against infection. There is even now some data suggesting that stress might underlie some periodontal disease.

There is almost a folklore that dentistry is a stressful occupation both for dentist and ancillary staff. The evidence suggests a fair degree of dissatisfaction in general practice amongst dental nurses and hygienists in terms of working conditions, relations with other staff and management skills of the dentist, while dentists are often concerned about the business aspects of practice. In contrast, community dentists appear concerned about matters such as treating medical emergencies or difficult patients.

Whatever the truth, there is little doubt that stress in dental staff does not help interpersonal or work relationships or interactions with patients.

ANXIETY STATES

Anxiety can be generated by dental or medical appointments, or such ordeals as public speaking or solo musical performances, examinations or interviews. This is to be expected, and symptoms such as agitation, slight tachycardia and dry mouth mainly caused by sympathetic overactivity are usually controllable by reassurance and possibly a very mild anxiolytic or sedative such as a low dose of a short-acting benzodiazepine (temazepam, lorazepam or diazepam) provided the patient is not pregnant and does not drive, operate dangerous machinery or make important decisions for the following 24 hours. Temazepam 10 mg orally on the night before and 1 hour before dental treatment can be used to supplement gentle sympathetic handling and reassurance of the anxious patient. Intravenous sedation with midazolam, or relative analgesia using nitrous oxide and oxygen, are also useful.

Anxiety can, however, cause severe physical effects as a result of overwhelming sympathetic activity: thus public speakers have been shown to develop severe pre-ischaemic ECG changes, while instrumental soloists may freeze and be unable to perform. These patients may well require drugs to control the anxiety but they respond better to beta-blocking agents (for example propranolol) than to benzodiazepines and with less impairment of their performance.

Anxiety neuroses

Although fear and anxiety are normal reactions to stressful situations, excessive anxiety, often amounting to panic, characterizes the anxiety neuroses. These may develop from long-standing personality disorders. Sometimes the anxiety is centred about a specific situation such as unwelcome dental treatment and is then known as a 'phobia'. Tension and agitation amounting to terror, hypochondriasis, rapid breathing, palpitations, giddiness, tremor, sweating, flushing and dry mouth are common features of a panic attack, while hostility readily develops if the anxious patient is forced to face the perceived threat which is the focus of the phobia.

- ### General management of anxiety neuroses

As a broad generalization, anxiety can be characterized by agitation and a diffuse sense of dread. Physical signs as described earlier may be associated but are usually not the chief problem. It is important to exclude organic causes such as hyperthyroidism or hypoglycaemia. Anxiety may also develop as a consequence of withdrawal of alcohol, other drugs of abuse, benzodiazepines or other sedatives (Chapter 24), but also abuse of such drugs may, in part at least, result from an attempt to gain relief from an anxiety neurosis. Reassurance, explanation and the encouragement of family support are therefore the first lines of treatment.

Benzodiazepines are the drugs most frequently given for the relief of severe anxiety since they are safer and more effective than most. However, they should only be given for a short period because of development of tolerance and the risk of dependence. A paradoxical effect may be seen, especially in children, with hostility and aggression. Benzodiazepines should not be taken with alcohol and, as judgment is impaired, patients must not drive, operate machinery or make important decisions for 24 hours.

There are no great differences between the various benzodiazepines, apart from their duration of action, but lorazepam or oxazepam are sometimes useful for their briefer activity than diazepam. Alprazolam, bromazepam, clobazam and chlorazepate have a sustained action like diazepam. Beta-blockers are preferred if there are severe somatic symptoms (for example palpitations) and some patients benefit from low doses of phenothiazines (chlorpromazine), butyrophenones (haloperidol) or thioxanthenes (flupenthixol). Antidepressants, especially MAOI, can lessen anxiety, and have the advantage of less risk of inducing drug dependence than the benzodiazepines.

Panic attacks can be minimized by avoiding precipitating exposures, and by using tricyclics, citalopram (p. 381), antidepressants, MAOI or high potency benzodiazepines such as clonazepam or alprazolam.

• Dental aspects of anxiety states

Dental treatment is usually straightforward unless there are difficulties as a result of: (a) alcoholism or drug dependence, (b) drug treatment with major tranquillizers, MAOIs or tricyclics. Oral manifestations such as a complaint of dry mouth, lip-chewing or bruxism may be seen and sometimes cancerphobia is an indication of an anxiety state.

PHOBIAS (PHOBIC NEUROSES)

A phobia is a morbid fear or anxiety out of all proportion to the threat. Phobic neuroses differ from anxiety neuroses in that the phobic anxiety arises only in specific circumstances, whereas patients with anxiety neuroses are generally anxious. Most patients are female. Phobias may also be a minor part of a more severe disorder such as depression, obsessive neurosis, anxiety state, personality disorder or schizophrenia.

Most phobias are centred on understandable threats such as flying, anaesthetics or dental treatment and, under these circumstances, normal life is possible if such threats are avoided. Agoraphobia (fear of leaving sheltered familiar places) and claustrophobia (fear of closed spaces) are probably the most common phobic disorders. Social phobias (such as fear of performing social duties in public) can severely limit normal activities.

• General management of phobic states

Supportive or intensive psychotherapy is indicated. Behaviour therapy aims at desensitization by slow and gradual exposure to the frightening situation. Implosion is a technique where patients are asked to imagine a persistently frightening situation for 1 or 2 hours.

Phobias can also sometimes be controlled by anxiolytic drugs. Buspirone is particularly useful since it lacks the psychomotor impairment, dependency and some other features of benzodiazepine use. Diazepam, lorazepam, oxazepam or alprazolam can be used but are habituating. Antidepressants, especially tricyclics, are used if there is a significant depressive component.

• Dental aspects of phobias

Patients with a true phobic neurosis about dental treatment are uncommon, but when seen demand great patience on the part of the dental staff. The main aids are confident reassurance, patience, careful painlessly performed dental procedures and, sometimes, the use of anxiolytics such as oral diazepam, supplemented if necessary with intravenous or inhalational sedation during dental treatment. Most of the comments above, concerning anxiety states, apply to the phobic states.

PERSONALITY DISORDERS

Personality disorders are chronic peculiarities of character or maladaptation to life. These

Table 18.1   Personality disorders

Disorder	Characteristics
Antisocial	Selfish, callous, disloyal, in conflict with everyone and everything
Asthenic	Tired all the time
Cyclothymic	Rapid alternation between depression and elation
Explosive	Rage or aggression on minor provocation
Hysterical	Immature, manipulative, attention-seeking, shallow interpersonal relationships
Inadequate	Continually dependent on others, often anxious and depressed
Obsessive	Chronically worried about standards and self-image; unable to relax and often depressed
Paranoid	Suspicious, litigious, lacking humour, blames others
Passive–aggressive	Stubborn, obstructive, awkward, anti-authority
Schizoid	Secretive, isolated, lacks friends

disorders shade into neuroses or psychoses, but insight is not lost and most patients manage to pursue a fairly normal lifestyle, though they are frequently made unhappy by the fact that their inadequacies prevent them from forming satisfactory relationships or cause them to be in frequent conflict with others. Severe personality disorders can lead to grossly antisocial criminal behaviour (*Table 18.1*).

Handling patients with personality disorders requires patience and tolerance, and the exercise of tact and skills which only come with appreciation of the existence of these disorders and with experience. Even then, little progress may be possible. A dental surgeon may also have a personality disorder and find him or herself in conflict with others, including colleagues – often to the dental surgeon's disadvantage – and may find it difficult not to antagonize patients and staff.

PSYCHOSOMATIC DISEASES (PSYCHOGENIC DISORDERS)

Psychosomatic diseases are bodily (somatic) disorders thought to be initiated or aggravated by psychological factors. Chronic emotional problems such as anxiety and depression may be contributory.

Typical examples of disorders in which there is often a psychosomatic element are asthma and migraine. Disorders such as anorexia nervosa, psychogenic vomiting and, sometimes, obesity, may be psychosomatic or hysterical in nature, and depression may be responsible for oral complaints such as atypical facial pain and burning mouth.

FUNCTIONAL DISORDERS

'Functional disorders' is a term used for those that have no demonstrable organic cause. There are two broad groups, the *neuroses* and the *psychoses*. A neurosis is a disease in which contact with reality and insight are retained and there are no bizarre symptoms such as delusions or hallucinations. A psychosis, by contrast, is characterized by impairment of contact with reality and sometimes phenomena such as delusions or hallucinations. There are, however, no defects of memory, intellect or consciousness – features which suggest organic disease.

Neurotic illnesses, particularly anxiety and depressive states, are by far the most common types of psychiatric disease (*Table 18.2*), but frequently remain unrecognized or untreated. Nearly everyone becomes anxious or depressed at some time and these mood changes must be accepted as part of life. However, if the symptoms or signs are out of proportion in severity or duration, to an adverse event, they suggest psychiatric disease. Psychotic illnesses are less common

Table 18.2	Neuroses: features
Depressive	Excessive pessimism, self-criticism, low self-regard, depression of mood, sleep disturbances and physical complaints
Anxiety	Excessive diffuse anxiety, irritability and physical complaints, e.g. palpitations
Phobic	Intense irrational fears of particular situations or objects
Obsessional	Preoccupation with thoughts or acts
Hysterical	Extreme reactions; conversion type – physical symptoms; dissociative type – alteration in consciousness not associated with organic disease
Hypochondriacal	Morbid preoccupation with disease and physical complaints

but more destructive to the individual and to those with whom they come into contact. Insight is lacking. It has been said that 'neurotics build castles in the air but psychotics live in them'.

NEUROSES

DEPRESSIVE NEUROSIS

Approximately 5 per cent of adults suffer from depression at some stage in their life. There is lowering of mood (affect), ranging from complete apathy towards the normal more pleasurable aspects of life, to utter despair or misery so extreme that death is sought as a release. The features of major depressive illness are shown in *Table 18.2*, but it must be appreciated that the clinical manifestations of depression are frequently atypical.

The main effects of depression appear to relate to changes in the hypothalamic centres that govern food intake, libido, circadian rhythms and various thalamic hormones. Hypercortisolism is common. However, the immediate mechanism of depression appears to be the result of depleted cerebral amine levels, particularly of serotonin and noradrenaline. These are raised by antidepressant drugs and, more rapidly, by electroconvulsive therapy. Disturbances of bodily functions such as sleep, appetite or sexual activity and slowing of thought and action (psychomotor retardation) are frequently associated. Agitation, anxiety or crying attacks may be prominent, but symptoms often vary in severity from day to day, or in less severe cases may be relatively effectively repressed. In the latter case, drugs that have a releasing effect often allow latent depression to become apparent. Thus, the tearful drunk is a well-known phenomenon but depression following the taking of diazepam is usually ascribed, unfairly, to an effect of the drug itself. In other cases, relief from depression is sought in alcohol or other drugs and leads to dependence (Chapter 24).

Reactive depression follows some unpleasant experience, such as a bereavement, but symptoms are disproportionate in intensity or duration.

Dysthymic disorder is a chronic, less intense form of depression but may progress to major depression.

Seasonal affective disorder (SAD) is a chronic cyclic form of depression which appears as daylight hours shorten, and is characterized by winter somnolence and craving for carbohydrates.

Involutional melancholia, which is often characterized by severe anxiety and hypochondriasis, is a depressive illness beginning in later life and mainly affects women.

Myalgic encephalitis (ME) is believed by many to be largely due to depression and may respond to antidepressant drugs if patients can be persuaded to take them. A swing to a manic phase after antidepressant treatment has also been reported in a patient with ME (*see* p. 384).

Depression may also accompany other psychiatric diseases such as schizophrenia or be caused by drugs such as ibuprofen, indomethacin, prednisone, benzodiazepines, levodopa, reserpine, methyldopa, fenfluramine, corticosteroids or oral contraceptives; by withdrawal of drugs such as amphetamines or antidepressants; by parkinsonism; by a stroke; after a myocardial infarction; by endocrinopathies such as diabetes; by viral infections such as influenza, viral hepatitis or infectious mononucleosis; or by various malignant diseases.

- **General management of depressive illness (*Fig. 18.1*)**

Treatment of depression should be carried out by specialists, especially as there may be

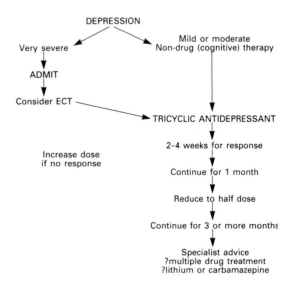

Fig. 18.1 Management of depression (ECT = electroconvulsive therapy)

a risk of suicide. Though the level of risk of suicide is frequently difficult to assess, it is generally agreed that it is high if the patient has plans for suicide or has previous attempts, is socially isolated, or abuses drugs or alcohol. If there is a risk of suicide or there are psychotic features such as delusions or hallucination, admission to hospital is desirable. However, it is frequently difficult to persuade a depressed patient of the need for psychiatric treatment.

None of the available antidepressant medications is perfect and all suffer from at least one of the following drawbacks:

1. Delayed onset of action from 7 to 28 days.
2. Anticholinergic effects.
3. Sedation.
4. Agitation.
5. Cardiotoxicity.
6. Weight gain.

Antidepressants can be divided into those with substantial sedative effects (amitriptyline, clomipramine, dothiepin, doxepin, maprotiline, mianserin, trazodone and trimipramine), and those without (amoxapine, imipramine, lofepramine, nortriptyline and viloxazine) and most fall into one of several groups: tricyclics, monoamine oxidase inhibitors (MAOIs) or selective serotonin receptor uptake inhibitors (SSRIs).

Tricyclic antidepressants
Tricyclic derivatives, despite their undesirable side-effects, are probably the most effective antidepressants and have stood the test of time. Their onset of action is, however, slow and they may take 4 weeks to exert their full effect. The action of tricyclic antidepressants is dose-dependent and lack of effect is often the result of failure to achieve adequate plasma levels. Nortriptyline has less antimuscarinic effects than some others, which therefore cause dry mouth, constipation, impaired visual accommodation and sometimes postural hypotension. Tricyclics are therefore contraindicated in patients with urinary obstruction or glaucoma. More serious side-effects include dysrhythmias and heart block, and tricyclics may be contraindicated in persons with cardiac failure and are absolutely contraindicated if the patient has had a recent myocardial infarct. Tricyclics may also be epileptogenic and some can

Table 18.3	Tricylic antidepressants
Drug	*Special comments*[a]
Amitriptyline	More sedative and antimuscarinic than many. Caution with general anaesthesia
Amoxapine	May cause tardive dyskinesia
Butriptyline	Less sedative than some
Clomipramine	Possibly less sedative
Dothiepin	Sedative
Doxepin	Sedative: less cardiac effects
Imipramine	Possibly less sedative than most but more antimuscarinic
Lofepramine	Avoid in renal or hepatic disease
Nortriptyline	Possibly less sedative and antimuscarinic effects
Protriptyline	Has a stimulant effect
Trimipramine	Photosensitive rashes

[a]Up to 4 weeks are required before symptom control can be expected. Reduce doses in the elderly. Dysrhythmias and heart block may be seen as well as drowsiness, dry mouth, urinary retention and constipation (antimuscarinic actions).

cause liver dysfunction or blood dyscrasias. Side-effects of the tricyclics are more serious in the elderly. Tricyclics should therefore only be given after a full blood count, liver function tests and, if the patient is over 45, an ECG, show the patient to be fit. They should not be used within 2 weeks of the use of MAOIs. The most commonly used tricyclic antidepressives are amitriptyline, dothiepin and imipramine. Sedation is a common side-effect, particularly with amitriptyline, but this may be an advantage if the patient is agitated (*Table 18.3*). Various other tricyclics have particular advantages: imipramine, for example, is mildly stimulating and clomipramine appears to be useful where there are obsessional or phobic problems. Doxepin (similar to imipramine) is the drug of choice if there is evidence of cardiovascular disease. Mianserin, a drug related to the tricyclics, causes less antimuscarinic effects, but frequently causes dizziness or, occasionally, marrow depression and is thought by many to be less effective.

Monoamine oxidase inhibitors
The monoamine oxidase inhibitors (MAOIs) were the first effective antidepressants and, though many newer agents have been introduced, still have a place in treatment. The MAOIs are thought by some to be particu-

larly useful in specific cases such as those where there is also anxiety or panic attacks and are used, either alone or in combination with tricyclic antidepressants, in spite of possible interactions between these two groups of drugs. The commonly used MAOIs are phenelzine and isocarboxazid.

Dry mouth and hypotension are not uncommon side-effects of MAOIs. The most serious adverse effects of the earlier and non-selective irreversible MAOIs such as phenelzine, isoniazid and tranylcypromine are, however, drug or food interactions. Hypertensive crises have resulted from inter-action of these MAOIs with foods containing tyramine, particularly cheese, and also with yeast products, chocolate, bananas, broad beans, some red wines and beer, pickled herring or caviar. Drugs such as pethidine and other opioids are potentiated (*see* Appendix to Chapter 25). Interactions of MAOIs with pethidine are the most danger-ous and have sometimes been fatal. Interactions with tricyclics are also danger-ous. Ephedrine and similar drugs often present in nasal decongestants or cold remedies may cause severe hypertension.

Selective MAOIs such as selegiline, used mainly in parkinsonism rather than depres-sion, were thought to be less likely to provoke hypertensive reactions with foods or drugs as were moclobemide, toloxatone and clorgy-line. However, reports are now appearing to suggest that the same precautions should be applied to these, as to the other MAOIs. Interactions with SSRIs have produced the serotonin syndrome (see below).

SSRIs

Fluoxetine, fluvoxamine, citalopram, sertra-line and paroxetine are drugs that are selec-tively serotonin re-uptake inhibitors (SSRIs). They appear to offer advantages over the tricyclics since they have low anticholinergic activity, weight gain or cardiac conduction effects. SSRIs can be epileptogenic and should not be used with tricyclics or within 2 weeks of MAOIs.

Though regarded by some as a valuable antidepressant, in the USA fluoxetine has allegedly been associated with aggressive behaviour, including murders. Adverse effects include anorexia, nausea, anxiety,

diarrhoea and sexual dysfunction, and rarely mania, paranoia or extrapyramidal features. It may interact with tricylics or neuroleptics to cause a rise in plasma concentration and effect of these drugs. Interactions of SSRIs with MAOIs, carbamazepine or lithium may produce the *serotonin syndrome* of CNS irritability, hyperreflexia and myoclonus. This is lethal occasionally. SSRIs may cause xeros-tomia and some cause dysrhythmia if the patient is using terfenadine.

Lithium

Lithium is useful mainly for the prophylaxis of manic–depressive illness. It affects thyroid function and ECG, and can produce nephro-genic diabetes insipidus. It is also a teratogen. It must only be used where blood levels can be monitored as overdose can cause tremor, ataxia, convulsions and renal damage. Side-effects include thirst and dry mouth, and nausea. Povidone-iodine is contraindicated in patients on lithium. Carbamazepine or valproate may also effectively control mania.

Electroconvulsive therapy (ECT) is sometimes given for severe depression, where drugs have been ineffective, or where there is strong risk of suicide. Amnesia is the main side-effect.

• Dental aspects of depression

The features aiding recognition of depression have been suggested above and dental staff should be alert to this possibility, particularly where the patient appears withdrawn, diffi-cult or aggressive, or where there are oral complaints of the types described earlier. Great tact, patience and a sympathetic but unpatronizing manner are needed in handling depressed patients. Dental treat-ment is preferably deferred until the depres-sion is under control but preventive programmes should be instituted at an early stage.

In the case of tricyclic antidepressants *intra-venous* adrenaline and noradrenaline have been shown experimentally to cause hyper-tension. Severe hypertension can also result from high concentrations (1:20 000) of *noradrenaline* in local anaesthetic agents, whether or not the patient is receiving anti-depressants. Despite reported statements to the contrary there is no clinical evidence of interactions between tricyclic antidepressants and adrenaline in local anaesthetic agents used in dentistry causing either hypertension or significant dysrhythmias. Nevertheless, aspirating syringes should always be used and the dose of adrenaline should not exceed 0.05 mg. Atropinics are potentiated by tricyclic antidepressants.

Patients on MAOIs are at risk from general anaesthesia since prolonged respiratory depression may result. Any CNS depressant, especially opioids and phenothiazines, given to patients on MAOIs (or within 21 days of their withdrawal) may precipitate coma. Pethidine is particularly dangerous (*see* Appendix to Chapter 25).

Indirectly acting sympathomimetic agents such as ephedrine or cocaine can interact with MAOIs to cause hypertension, and must therefore not be used. There is no evidence, however, of any danger to patients on MAOI from adrenaline in local anaesthetic solutions but aspirating syringes should always be used.

Tricyclics and MAOIs can cause postural hypotension and a patient should not be stood immediately upright if they have been lying flat during dental treatment; the chair should slowly be brought upright. Some depressed patients resort to drug misuse, and this must be considered (Chapter 24).

Oral symptoms associated with depression or its treatment
The most common complaint of depressed patients under treatment is of dry mouth, especially as a result of the use of tricyclic antidepressants or lithium. This may predispose to oral candidosis and increased caries, especially since taste sensation may be disturbed, and patients tend to increase the sugar content of their diet. The effect of xerostomia can occasionally result in ascending suppurative parotitis. The most effective treatment is to change the antidepressant to another which has little anticholinergic activity, but if this is not acceptable the dry mouth should be managed as in Sjögren's syndrome (Chapter 9). Smoking, and other drugs which may add to the xerostomia, such as antihistamines, hyoscine or other atropine-like drugs, or SSRIs should therefore be avoided. Both MAOIs and tricyclics have been reported occasionally to cause facial dyskinesias (*see* Appendix to Chapter 25) and prolonged use

of flupenthixol can lead to intractable tardive dyskinesia.

Bodily complaints, often related to the mouth, are common in depression and the dental surgeon should appreciate the possibility of a psychiatric basis for such oral complaints.

Depression is associated especially with the following painful disorders of the orofacial region:

1. Atypical facial pain.
2. Burning mouth or sore tongue (oral dysaesthesia).
3. Temporomandibular pain-dysfunction syndrome may occasionally be associated with depression.

Other oral complaints may be delusional and include:

- Discharges (of fluid, slime or powder coming into the mouth)
- Dry mouth or sialorrhoea despite normal salivary flow
- Spots or lumps
- Halitosis
- Disturbed taste sensation

It must be emphasized that the recognition of psychogenic symptoms is usually diagnosis by exclusion, but it is important to try to recognize them, however limited and subjective the methods may be. The symptoms cause real enough suffering to the patient and should, if possible, be relieved. Unnecessary surgery must also be avoided.

Features that may suggest that symptoms are psychogenic but not necessarily depressive may include any of the following.

1. *Absence of organic cause or physical signs:* The affected area typically appears normal and if, for example, a putatively diseased tooth is extracted, symptoms are unaffected.

2. *Character and duration of the symptoms:* Many complain of persistence of pain or other symptoms for very long periods, sometimes for years. Clearly, after such periods any organic cause would have become apparent.

3. *Character of the pain:* The symptoms may be bizarre, such as 'drawing' or 'gripping' sensations or apparently exaggerated 'unbearable' pain in spite of normal physical health or often sleep. The symptom is often also of fixed and unchanging character, often for very long periods.

4. *Distribution of the pain:* The site of the pain or other symptom is often somewhat vague and the patient may be unable to put a finger precisely upon the painful area. Alternatively, the distribution of the pain may not follow an anatomical pattern. Very frequently, however, atypical facial pain is in the general region of the maxilla.

5. *Provocation of symptoms:* Symptoms are usually not provoked by recognizable stimuli such as hot or cold foods, or mastication. However, psychogenic sore tongue is sometimes said to be aggravated by sharp flavoured foods.

6. *Use of analgesics:* In contrast to patients with severe organic pain who typically reach for analgesics, occasionally to the extent of analgesic abuse, many patients with atypical facial pain make little attempt to get relief from analgesics. Alternatively analgesics, after a brief trial, are said to be totally ineffective.

7. *Other signs or symptoms of psychiatric disturbance:* Patients' personality and manner are highly variable. Some appear obviously neurotic but few are overtly depressed. Indeed the organic symptoms can be regarded as more acceptable substitutes ('depressive equivalents') for more typical manifestations of depression. These varied clinical pictures are discussed more fully below. Patients may have several so-called psychosomatic complaints at the same time.

8. *Response to psychoactive drugs:* In some patients the response to antidepressant drugs is dramatic, with relief of symptoms and striking general improvement in mood, after the drug has had time to take effect. However, effective dosage varies widely and in the case of tricyclic antidepressants the response is generally related to the plasma levels achieved. Thus doses may sometimes have to be very large before an effect is evident. Nevertheless, it is clear that there is a hard core of patients who over the course of years go from specialist to specialist without positive results from innumerable investigations or response to any form of treatment. Indeed, the patient may seem to take a sort of perverse pride in the resistance of the pain to the challenge of medical science.

Psychogenic symptoms can generally be regarded as a plea for help or attention. This occasionally becomes distressingly apparent in a patient who at the start appears well-balanced and self-controlled – even occasionally joking about symptoms – but after a little while is crying uncontrollably. At the other extreme many patients reject the possibility of mental illness and aggressively assert that 'It is not due to nerves' (even if no such suggestion has been made) and typically also reject the idea of psychiatric help, however obliquely and sympathetically suggested.

Examples of these varied clinical pictures therefore include the following:

1. The patient may be overtly depressed and cries readily or is obviously having difficulty in restraining tears. Alternatively, initial self-control is followed by unrestrainable crying.
2. The patient may complain (in effect) of depression by saying that the pain or other symptom makes them miserable.
3. Some, when allowed to discuss their symptoms, relate them to trouble with the family or at work.
4. A few are already having, or have had, antidepressant drugs but the atypical symptoms have not been controlled.
5. A few have associated bizarre (delusional) symptoms such as 'powder' or 'slime' coming out of the sore or painful area as mentioned earlier.
6. Some, given the chance of a sympathetic hearing, gratefully expand on their problems and welcome the suggestion of psychiatric help.
7. The most difficult and relatively common group is the rejectors, who are unable to accept the idea of psychiatric disturbance and refuse to have the possibility investigated or to accept that drugs – which they equate with drugs of dependence – may be helpful.

It should not need to be emphasized that, where psychogenic symptoms are suspected, discussion with the patient must be conducted patiently, gently and sympathetically. Surprisingly, this may perhaps be the first opportunity that patients have had to unburden themselves. Unfortunately some doctors are at least as intolerant of 'neurotic' patients as many members of the public. This is not to suggest that the dentist should attempt to be an amateur psychiatrist but an

Psoriasis from head to in between toes
Perpetual scream in left ear
Spasmodic pressure above left ear
Constant ulcers in mouth and on tongue
Asthma bronchitis severe bouts of indigestion
Sore mouth due to grinding of bottom right molar
Severe pain under crutch after any exertion
Constant irritation around back passage
Spasmodic bleeding piles

Medicines taken internally
Predicalone
Ventolin
Asilone suspension
Bronchipax

Fig. 18.2 Note as presented by a patient. Such histories vary in length, detail and imagination and sometimes suggest that the patient is disturbed (*maladie du petit papier*)

effort must be made to distinguish psychogenic symptoms from organic disease. It is probably unnecessary to enquire into details of family relationships or broken homes. If a patient is depressed, the cause is often as much the patient's susceptibility to depression as the so-called life situation. In any case, amelioration of the life situation is unlikely to be feasible, and it is only too common for those so affected to be unable to overcome their difficulties without help.

Finally, it is essential to appreciate that, however neurotic a patient's manner may be, the symptoms may have an organic cause. The concurrence of emotional and physical disease is one of the most difficult problems in medicine. The organic basis of the symptoms in many cases remains undiscovered until severe manifestations become obvious later. A striking example is the transient and apparently hysterical signs and symptoms of early multiple sclerosis. The most careful investigation is therefore essential to exclude possible organic causes before the diagnosis of psychogenic disorder is made (*Fig. 18.2*).

In summary, the diagnosis of depression when manifested as orofacial symptoms is difficult, as the patients often have no typical depressive symptoms. This is often the result of repression of symptoms caused in turn by shame or guilt at the idea of mental illness.

CHRONIC FATIGUE SYNDROME ('MYALGIC ENCEPHALOMYELITIS')

Chronic fatigue syndrome is a non-specific disorder characterized by lack of energy, tiredness or muscle and joint pains after minimal effort, emotional lability, poor concentration and memory and often other symptoms. Though it is widely thought to be a new disease, this clinical picture was described in 1867 and termed 'neurasthenia'. However, the symptoms in many ways resemble those of the recovery phase of a viral infection such as influenza. In the USA in particular, a viral cause is still being sought and the complaint is termed *postviral fatigue syndrome*. Claims for EBV, herpes virus 6 and Coxsackie B having a causative role have not been substantiated and no consistent association with any virus has yet been found. Nevertheless, most patients insist that 'ME' is a viral infection, even though this is of no help to them as there is no effective treatment for most viral infections or their after-effects.

Tests showing disorders of muscle function or any other organic lesion have also not been substantiated. By contrast, those with organic neuromuscular diseases do not have the mental symptoms characteristic of 'ME'. Most authorities believe that most cases are due, as the symptoms suggest, to depression. Fifty to eighty per cent of patients, on rigorous psychiatric assessment, have been found to fulfil the criteria for psychiatric disorder and depression in particular. Though the complaint may be heterogeneous and have a variety of causes, a typical characteristic is these patients, like many patients with more obvious depression, strongly reject any suggestion that they are depressed and the idea that depression is a 'real diagnosis'. For this reason, patients prefer to be said to have the more glamorous sounding 'myalgic encephalomyelitis' ('yuppie flu'), even though there is no evidence of a neurological lesion. Most also refuse to take antidepressives, but those who have been persuaded to do so frequently improve.

Though fatigue may persist for a long period it is ultimately self-limiting. In the interim, patients need emotional support and one authority has suggested that this need is the basis for the complaint. Controversy persists as to whether exercise or rest is better for the myalgia. When assessment indicates that depression is present, patients should be persuaded to have antidepressive treatment and are likely to benefit from it.

OTHER PSYCHOGENIC SYNDROMES RELATED TO DENTISTRY

So-called chronic candidosis syndromes are discussed in Chapter 20 and mercury allergy syndrome in Chapter 17.

OBSESSIONAL NEUROSES (OBSESSIVE-COMPULSIVE NEUROSES)

Obsessional personality traits are not uncommon, especially amongst dental and medical personnel, and are often salutary. However, the obsessional neuroses can cause significant disruption of normal life – for example, the dental surgeon who felt compelled to telephone his patients late at night because he was obsessed with the notion that, having prepared the cavity, he might have forgotten to place the filling.

Obsessional thoughts are those that come repeatedly into consciousness against the patient's will, are usually unpleasant, but are always recognized as the patient's own thoughts. Such thoughts are not, however, accepted by the patients as harmless or inevitable and an internal struggle against them leads to obsessional symptoms. To counteract the thoughts, secondary ritualistic thought or behaviour patterns (compulsions) are developed (for example, continually checking that doors are locked). The obsessional thoughts may also in turn generate depression.

Typical obsessions are the repeated questioning of decisions, the fear of harm or harming, or the fear of dirtiness or contamination. Obsessional symptoms are also associated with disorders such as depression, schizophrenia or, rarely, organic brain disease.

Obsessional patients are often intelligent, many are unmarried and many have a premorbid state such as an uncertain and vacillating, or alternatively, a stubborn, rigid, morose and irritable personality.

• General management of obsessional states

Treatment is often difficult. Antidepressants, especially the tricyclics, are useful when there is also depression, and clomipramine in particular seems to be effective. The benzodiazepines may be useful when anxiety is predominant.

• Dental aspects of obsessional states

It is questionable whether true obsessions become centred on the mouth but they may, for example, result in compulsive toothbrushing or excessive use of antiseptic mouthwashes. Occasional patients become obsessed with the possibility of infections in the mouth (as for example a patient who was obsessed with the idea that his Fordyce spots were thrush) and refuse to be reassured.

HYSTERICAL STATES

Three main hysterical states exist: hysterical personality disorders, hysterical neuroses and acute hysterical psychoses.

Hysterical neuroses

Hysterical conversion neurosis is characterized by physical complaints that have no demonstrable organic basis, such as pain, anaesthesia, dysphagia, fainting, fits, paralysis or tremor. Dissociative states are characterized by disturbances of consciousness or identity (but no physical symptoms) in the absence of demonstrable organic disease. Amnesia, states of fugue (when the patient wanders aimlessly away), or (rarely) multiple personalities, are examples of dissociative states. There are, however, no basic differences between these two types of hysterical neurosis and most patients at some time exhibit both.

Hysterical neuroses mainly affect females – sometimes those working in medical or paramedical occupations. Conversion symptoms frequently result in patients being submitted to operation and may as a result have multiple scars. It is often difficult to establish that the patient is gaining something by the illness, although in compensation neurosis the nature of the potential gain is easily recognized.

Munchausen syndrome is the term given to a disorder in which patients go to considerable length to fabricate histories and simulate symptoms apparently for the sake of undergoing operations. This may be done repeatedly, even occasionally by assuming false names and travelling to many hospitals scattered about the country. Ultimately the patient may become extensively scarred and develop other complications. Munchausen syndrome is categorized as a conversion syndrome by some but may be a delusional state.

Munchausen syndrome-by-proxy is the term given to a parent or other carer who invents symptoms in and demands medical or surgical treatment for a child.

Compensation neurosis usually follows an accident (especially a head injury), or operation, and is characterized by paralysis, chronic pain (often headache) or other symptoms of obscure origin and of no obvious organic cause. Men and women are equally susceptible, there is no previous history and the lack of insight is less convincing than in hysteria. Settlement of the claim for compensation typically results in rapid disappearance of the symptoms.

Panic disorder is the term given to recurrent, unpredictable attacks of severe anxiety with physical symptoms such as palpitations, chest pain, dyspnoea, paraesthesiae and sweating. Many or most of the symptoms may result from hyperventilation (Chapter 26) but mitral valve prolapse (Chapter 3) may be found in up to 50 per cent of these patients.

EATING DISORDERS

The main eating disorders apart from obesity are *anorexia nervosa* and *bulimia*. These disorders are relatively common, particularly among white females in the higher socioeconomic groups. Obesity (Chapter 15) may be consequence of another type of eating disorder.

Anorexia nervosa

Anorexia nervosa is characterized by severe weight loss due to self-starvation and is mainly a disease of previously healthy

---

Table 18.4 Typical features of anorexia nervosa

- Females under 25 years, mainly
- Severe anorexia overriding hunger
- Weight loss
- Sometimes self-induced vomiting (especially after orgies of eating)[a]
- No other organic or psychiatric disease
- Amenorrhoea
- Bradycardia

*Regarded as a different disorder from anorexia nervosa by some (bulimia), but having the same effects.

adolescent girls. The incidence may be as high as 1 per cent of all schoolgirls in the United Kingdom.

The disorder, which is regarded as a hysterical neurosis, is associated with a preoccupation to be thin. The body image appears to be so distorted that, even when emaciated, the patient still regards herself as too fat.

Anorectic patients usually refuse to eat or, if forced to do so, often induce vomiting. Some patients cannot control their voluntary food restriction and have episodes in which they gorge food (bulimia) and then induce vomiting. Menstrual upset is an early feature. Peripheral cyanosis and coldness with bradycardia and amenorrhoea are common, as are depression which lacks the classic features of depression in adults, and obsessional features (*Table 18.4*).

Anorexia nervosa may be complicated by anaemia, endocrine disturbances, peripheral oedema and electrolyte depletion (especially hypokalaemia).

- **General management of anorexia nervosa**

Some 2–5 per cent of cases may be fatal. However, if treatment is initiated early, prognosis is usually good. Anorexia nervosa must be distinguished from nutritional disorders, depression and Turner's syndrome. There is no specific treatment. Patients are usually admitted to hospital if weight loss is rapid or persistent. Psychiatric care is required: anxiolytics may be useful.

- **Dental aspects of anorexia nervosa**

Anaemia and the possibility of hypokalaemia and consequent dysrhythmias must be remembered if a general anaesthetic is considered necessary for dental treatment. There is some evidence that repeated doses of paracetamol may be hepatotoxic in anorexia nervosa, and thus doses should be kept to the minimum necessary.

Parotid enlargement (sialosis) and angular stomatitis may develop, as in other forms of starvation. The parotid swellings tend to subside if the patient returns to a normal diet. Erosion of teeth (perimylolysis) may result from repeated vomiting. The erosion is usually most severe on lingual, palatal and occlusal surfaces. Oral ulcers or abrasions, particularly in the soft palate, may be caused by fingers or other objects used to induce vomiting. Full-coverage plastic splints may be needed to protect the teeth and it may help to fill these splints with magnesium hydroxide. Topical daily sodium fluoride applications or a 0.05 per cent sodium fluoride mouthwash combined with bicarbonate after each vomiting incident may lessen dental damage.

Bulimia ('ox-hunger')

Bulimia has been reported in up to 10 per cent of young adult women. Bulimics, in contrast to anorectics, may be of normal or near-normal weight. Uncontrolled and unpredictable ingestion of huge amounts of foods (usually soft, sweet or starchy foods) is followed by vomiting. Bulimia may be seen in isolation, or in anorexia nervosa, and appears to be stress-related. Erosion of the teeth, sore throat, angular stomatitis and painless swelling of the parotid glands may be seen and there may be severe caries. Dental care is as described above for anorexia nervosa.

HYPOCHONDRIACAL NEUROSES

Minor degrees of hypochondriasis are common, especially among the elderly. However, hypochondriacal neurosis is a morbid preoccupation with physical symptoms or bodily functions, in which minute details are related incessantly.

There is no organic disease or physiological disturbance. Most patients are depressed and some are deluded.

- **General management of hypochondriases**

Organic disease should always be excluded, as should schizophrenia. Reassurance and supportive care are then needed and antidepressant drugs may be helpful.

- **Dental aspects of hypochondriases**

The common oral hypochondriacal symptoms are dry or burning mouth, disturbed taste and oral or facial pain.

PSYCHOSES

MANIC-DEPRESSIVE PSYCHOSIS (*Table 18.5*)

Endogenous or major (psychotic) depression is characterized by severe depressive symptoms unrelated to environmental stress, but many now believe that these are artificial distinctions. A few patients with depression have repeated mood swings from depression to mania (manic-depressive psychosis) and are sometimes classified as having bipolar depression. 'Unipolar depression' is the term used when mania is absent.

Table 18.5 Psychoses: features	
Manic-depressive	Mainly severe depression but may be manic episodes for weeks, months or years
Schizophrenia	Severe disorder of thought, behaviour and affect with hallucinations, delusions and illusions
Korsakoff's syndrome	Recent amnesia and confabulation

Mania is a recurrent disorder in which most patients also have depressive (*bipolar*) episodes (manic-depression). Between attacks the patient is usually normal, but episodes last for months or years. The disorder usually appears first in young adults and its onset in the elderly may indicate organic disease such as a neoplasm, or an effect of drugs, such as corticosteroids, alcohol or another drug of dependence. The manic state is characterized by elation, irritability, belligerence, over-confidence, generalized hyperactivity, decreased sleep, flight of ideas and lack of restraint in financial matters or social behaviour.

- ### General management of manic-depression

Psychiatric care is required and lithium is the most effective drug, but blood levels must be monitored and patients with cardiovascular, renal or thyroid disorders are at risk. Lithium may induce dysrhythmias or frank myxoedema. Carbamazepine is used for patients unresponsive to lithium and appears to be particularly effective in patients with rapid cycling manic-depressive illness. In the depressive phases there is a danger of suicide, and antidepressant treatment needs to be given.

- ### Dental aspects of manic-depression

Lithium treatment should be monitored by the regular assay of plasma concentrations since dysrhythmias may be precipitated, particularly during general anaesthesia. It may be advisable to stop lithium treatment 2–3 days before general anaesthesia. Interactions with neuroleptics such as droperidol may precipitate facial dyskinesias, while lithium with diazepam may induce hypothermia. Lithium may also interact with suxamethonium and other muscle relaxants to prolong muscle relaxation. Many non-steroidal anti-inflammatory analgesics reduce the excretion of lithium and may cause toxicity but aspirin, paracetamol or codeine are safe to use. Metronidazole, carbamazepine and phenytoin use may cause toxicity.

Lithium occasionally causes a dry mouth or impaired taste, as a result of dehydration (*see* Appendix to Chapter 25) and may promote caries. Manic-depressive patients may also be treated with antidepressant drugs with oral side-effects such as xerostomia.

SCHIZOPHRENIA

Schizophrenia is a common psychosis, with its onset in early adult life, and can affect a wide range of brain functions. About 1 per cent of the population are affected. Unlike most psychiatric disorders where the complaints are recognizable exaggerations of normal emotions or related disturbances, schizophrenia corresponds with the lay idea of madness. Moods, thoughts and behaviour are, as a result, disorganized and irrational. Disorders of perception (hallucinations) and thought (delusions) are common. Intelligence is, however, unimpaired and insight may even be retained, with the result that occasionally the patient may be aware that their behaviour is bizarre and even of the consternation that such behaviour creates in others.

However, schizophrenia is not, as popularly believed, a splitting of the personality – Doctor Jekyll and Mister Hyde are the creation of a novelist of genius – but a disintegration of the personality, causing thoughts and behaviour to be totally inappropriate and incomprehensible.

Acute schizophrenia may develop in previously normal individuals and is often precipitated by organic disorders or external stress. Affective symptoms such as depression may be associated.

Chronic schizophrenia is more common and characterized by inappropriate affect, disordered thought processes, delusions and hallucinations. Some patients are strikingly paranoid, others have mainly motor symptoms (catatonia), a bizarre mixture of emotional, behavioural and thought disturbances (hebephrenia), or neuroses.

Schizophrenic thought disorder causes loss of cohesion between logical thought sequences, and speech may include non-existent words (neologisms) or be inconsequential ('word salad'). There may be disruption of the stream of speech (thought-blocking), together with inappropriate affect and withdrawal from social contact.

Delusions are often bizarre, while catatonia with abnormalities of movement, posture and speech, negativism, echolalia, mannerisms and stereotypia may also be features.

The best known schizophrenic delusion, in the past at least, was of being Napoleon, but schizophrenic delusions are highly variable in character. Hallucinations are frequently auditory, when mysterious voices constantly whisper frightening or unpleasant things to the patient. The bizarre nature of the patient's disorder may be made obvious when they shout back at the unheard voices.

Paranoia is a projection of the patient's internal disturbance which, as a consequence, is believed to be the result of the hostility of others, such as neighbours, secret agents or foreign powers who, for example, may be projecting mysterious rays to achieve their malign objectives. Abuse of PCP and amphetamines can cause a similar picture (Chapter 24).

There is considerable variation in the diagnostic criteria of schizophrenia, but auditory hallucinations and ideas of a passive or irresistible response to external influences which may control or block the patient's thoughts, dictate, or control their behaviour to conspire to do them harm, are features most suggestive of this disorder.

- ### General management of schizophrenia

Psychiatric care is essential and admission to hospital is necessary if behaviour causes disturbance in the home. Overall, about 10 per cent will remain hospitalized and a further 30 per cent remain seriously handicapped; schizophrenia can be a remarkably disturbing condition for the patient and for those in contact in any way. There is a high prevalence in the socially deprived and in penal institutions etc.

Antipsychotic medication is usually required but compliance with therapy can be very poor. Antipsychotic medications used in the treatment of schizophrenia alter the dopamine/cholinergic balance in the basal ganglia so that extrapyramidal and anticholinergic effects are common and can be disabling. Chlorpromazine was the first agent to show real benefit in schizophrenia, but drugs from five main groups are now used.

1. Phenothiazines with pronounced sedative effects, moderate antimuscarinic and extrapyramidal effects (chlorpromazine, methotrimeprazine or promazine).
2. Phenothiazines with low extrapyramidal effects, moderate sedative and antimuscarinic effects (pericyazine, pipothiazine or thioridazine). New agents such as clozapine may have advantages in not producing tardive dyskinesia but can cause agranulocytosis. Clozapine, however, has significant antimuscarinic effect.
3. Piperazine phenothiazines, with pronounced extrapyramidal effects but low sedative and antimuscarinic activity (fluphenazine, perphenazine, prochlorperazine, or trifluoroperazine).
4. Other agents, which tend to have activities as in (3) above include butyrophenones (benperidol, droperidol or haloperidol), diphenylbutylpiperidines (fluspirilene and pimozide), thioxanthines (flupenthixol and zuclopenthixol), sulpiride, oxypertine or loxapine.
5. Risperidone, a benzisoxazole with minimal extrapyramidal effects.

Phenothiazines or haloperidol or, more recently, risperidone are commonly used to control schizophrenia. Anti-parkinsonian drugs such as benztropine, benzhexol, trihexyphenidyl or orphenadrine are required to control extrapyramidal symptoms, which sometimes develop after only a few doses.

Chlorpromazine is most commonly used but parenteral fluphenazine enanthate or decanoate, pipothiazine palmitate or zuclopenthixol decanoate by bi-weekly injection overcomes compliance difficulties. If there is considerable anxiety or hyperactivity, a phenothiazine with sedative activity (for example chloropromazine) is needed. If no sedation is needed piperazine phenothiazines may be given but may worsen depression. Butyrophenones are useful mainly for violent patients.

Maintenance therapy is conveniently carried out with long-acting preparations such as fluphenazine, pipothiazine, perphenazine or flupenthixol but these can cause intractable tardive dyskinesia. ECT may be given if there is poor response to medication or if there is catatonia.

- ### Dental aspects of schizophrenia

Phenothiazines can cause dose-related hypotension and interfere with temperature regulation. They may occasionally cause obstructive jaundice, leucopenia or ECG changes which can influence dental management. General anaesthesia, especially with intravenous barbiturates, may lead to severe hypotension and should therefore be avoided if possible.

Mild schizophrenic features (which are often unrecognized) include loss of social contact, flatness of mood or inappropriate social behaviour, which may appear at first as mere tactlessness or stupidity. Thus the patient, when asked to sit down in the surgery, sits in the operator's rather than the dental chair; attempts at communication are met by a response that indicates a failure to get through, or are interrupted by totally irrelevant remarks. Such patients may have delusional oral symptoms, the treatment of which is beyond the expertise of the dental surgeon. Psychiatric help must be sought.

Schizophrenics controlled by drugs may appear quite normal and have no complaints related to their disorder or to the treatment. However, drugs used for the treatment of schizophrenia can have severe side-effects. The long-term use of neuroleptics (phenothiazines, butyrophenones, thioxanthines and others) can lead to complications such as xerostomia (with an increased susceptibility to candidosis and caries), oral pigmentation and severe extrapyramidal symptoms. Muscular rigidity or tonic spasms (facial dyskinesias: Chapters 17 and 25) frequently involve the bulbar or neck muscles, with subsequent difficulties in speech or swallowing. Alternatively, there may be uncontrollable facial grimacing (orofacial dystonia) which may start after only a few doses. This may be controlled by stopping the neuroleptic and giving anti-parkinsonian antimuscarinic drugs. Tardive dyskinesia (uncontrollable face, jaw and tongue movements) can develop, particularly after prolonged use of neuroleptics. It does not respond to withdrawal of the neuroleptic and is frequently unresponsive to any form of treatment. Haloperidol and clozapine can cause hypersalivation, and the latter has induced parotitis.

KORSAKOFF'S PSYCHOSIS

Korsakoff's psychosis is characterized by amnesia for recent events, impaired ability to learn new facts and fabricated descriptions of recent events (confabulation). Nevertheless the patient is alert, responsible and behaves in an otherwise apparently normal manner. Chronic alcoholism associated with thiamine deficiency is an important cause, though relatively few alcoholics develop the syndrome; other possible causes include cerebrovascular disease, tumours or degenerative disorders. The disease results from a symmetrical lesion in the periaqueductal area, thalamus, mammillary bodies and cerebellar vermis.

OTHER PSYCHOSES

Psychoses can complicate various endocrine disturbances, the puerperium or drugs such as alcohol, amphetamine or psychotomimetics (*see Tables 18.6–18.8*).

OTHER DISORDERS

THE ACUTELY DISTURBED OR HOSTILE PATIENT

The acutely disturbed patient can totally disrupt his or her environment and harm those with whom they come into contact. Frequently the cause is drunkenness, drug intoxication or an acute psychosis. In other cases, the disorder may be due to organic disease such as infections, or the withdrawal of drugs such as alcohol or barbiturates.

- **Management of the acutely disturbed patient**

If the patient appears unresponsive to normal reasoning, no dental treatment should be attempted but the general practitioner or psychiatrist should be contacted. If the patient becomes violent the police have to be called; ambulance personnel cannot usually manage such cases.

No attempt should be made to sedate the patient. Benzodiazepines usually worsen violently psychotic behaviour and adequate doses of phenothiazines such as chlorpromazine can cause severe hypotension. The usual treatment, once the patient has been forcibly restrained, is to give haloperidol by injection.

Patients in Britain can only be compulsorily admitted to hospital for psychiatric care if the requirements of the appropriate sections of the Mental Health Act (England and Wales 1983) or Mental Health Act (Scotland 1960) are fulfilled (*see* Appendix).

THE CONFUSED PATIENT

The confused patient has fluctuating consciousness, impaired orientation and short-term memory. Delusions or hallucinations can cause severe agitation. Patients are usually more confused at night. Confusional states need to be differentiated from dementia, in which there are similar disturbances of orientation and memory, but consciousness is not impaired. The confused patient should receive immediate medical attention since brain damage may result from many of the causes, which include:

1. Alcohol or drug intoxication (or withdrawal).
2. Head injury.
3. Cardiac, respiratory, hepatic or renal failure.
4. Fever.
5. Cerebral infection (encephalitis) and AIDS encephalopathy.
6. Other causes (*see Table 18.5*).

PSYCHIATRIC DISORDERS CAUSED BY ORGANIC BRAIN DISEASE

Relatively few patients with psychiatric disorders have recognizable organic brain disease. The clinical features of organic disease differ somewhat from those caused by non-organic mental disorders. Acute organic brain disease is characterized by disorientation and impairment of consciousness. In chronic organic brain disease, amnesia (especially for recent

| Table 18.6 | Organic causes of psychiatric disease |

Cerebral	Systemic
Infections	*Endocrine and metabolic disease*
Neurosyphilis	
AIDS	Endocrinopathies (*see Table 18.7*)
Creutzfeldt–Jakob disease	Porphyria
Neoplasms	Vitamin B_{12} deficiency
Cerebral tumours	Severe liver disease
Subdural haematoma	Wilson's disease
Degenerative disorders	Renal dialysis
Alzheimer's disease	*Connective tissue disease*
Cerebrovascular disease	Systemic lupus erythematosus
Multiple sclerosis	Giant cell arteritis
Huntington's chorea	*Drugs*
Parkinson's disease	Alcoholism
	Others (*see Table 18.8*)
	Heavy metal poisoning

events), inability to concentrate, disorientation in time, place or person and intellectual impairment (including loss of normal social awareness) are common. Other less specific symptoms include mood changes or paranoia.

Anxiety, fear, hallucinations and delusions can be features of either chronic or acute organic brain damage.

DEMENTIA

Dementia is loss of intelligence, memory and cognitive functions. Dementia is usually associated with ageing but there are many possible causes (*Table 18.6*). Dementia is frequently of unknown or untreatable causes such as Alzheimer's or vascular (multi-infarct) disease, but increasingly now in young persons is caused by HIV infection.

Alzheimer's disease

Alzheimer's disease is the most common cause of presenile and senile dementia and is estimated to affect 10–15 per cent of those over 65 and 20 per cent of those over 80. The current attention to it results from the increasing numbers of the elderly and the fact that cerebral atrophy can be recognized by MRI. The characteristic lesions are neurofibrillary tangles and neuritic plaques consisting of

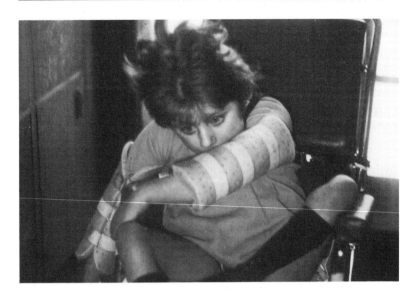

Fig. 18.3 Self-mutilation may be a manifestation of psychiatric disease, learning disability, disorders of sensation or, rarely the Lesch–Nyhan syndrome (Appendix, Chapter 10). This mentally handicapped child managed to bite through to her biceps

dying nerve fibres clustered round deposits of amyloid. Similar changes can be seen in the brains of persons over 40 with Down's syndrome and both have a defect in a gene on chromosome 21 where the amyloid protein gene is located. In Alzheimer's disease there may also be increased amounts of aluminium in the brain there is hope that the chelating agent, desferrioxamine, may delay the progress of disease.

Clinically, Alzheimer's disease is characterized by gradual, progressive loss of memory and other cognitive activity, leading to inability to recognize family or friends, or carry out the simplest tasks such as combing the hair or cleaning the teeth, general deterioration of motor skills, disorientation and grossly inappropriate or bizarre behaviour. Personality changes, delusions, mood swings or depression and disordered behaviour of many kinds, may be associated.

Diagnosis depends on evidence of progressive dementia in the absence of focal neurological deficits and exclusion of other organic dementing diseases such as hypothyroidism and vitamin B_{12} deficiency.

The anticholinesterase inhibitors donepezil and tacrine may have some benefit in Alzheimer's disease.

• Dental aspects of Alzheimer's disease

Though studies have shown that about 75 per cent of patients with Alzheimer's disease require dental attention, the chief problems of those with Alzheimer's and many other types of dementia are behavioural. In the early stages, dental appointments and instructions are forgotten. Later, there is progressive neglect of oral health as a result of forgetting the need or even how to brush the teeth or clean dentures. Dentures are also frequently lost or broken or cannot be tolerated. Finally, deterioration of dental care together with hyposalivation may lead to destruction of the dentition by caries and periodontal disease and increase the problems of management because of difficulty in eating and halitosis. Loss of taste is common. Injuries are not uncommon in demented patients. Drugs, such as phenothiazines used to manage behavioural problems, may aggravate the xerostomia and may cause dyskinesias. Attention to diet, oral hygiene and preventive care is important but after a time may no longer be practicable. Salivary substitutes may give some symptomatic relief. While it is still possible to give dental treatment, it should be planned with the knowledge that the patient will sooner or later become unmanageable for treatment under local analgesia. Treatment should, as far as possible, be carried out in the morning, when cooperation tends to be best, and with the usual carers present in a familiar environment with care to explain every procedure before it is carried out and to avoid discomfort. Preoperative sedation with haloperidol may be required.

Table 18.7   Possible endocrine causes of psychiatric disorders

Endocrine disorder	*Psychiatric complications that may result*
Acromegaly	Emotional lability
Addison's disease	Apathy, mild recent amnesia
Corticosteroid therapy, Cushing's syndrome and disease	Euphoria or depression. Psychoses with delusions or hallucinations
Hypoglycaemia (in treated diabetes mellitus)	Confusion, dementia
Hypothyroidism	Impaired concentration, amnesia, depression, paranoia, acute confusion
Hyperparathyroidism with hypercalcaemia	Apathy, depression
Thyrotoxicosis	Anxiety and agitation, depression

Table 18.8   Some drug-induced psychiatric states

	Drugs sometimes responsible	
	Used in medicine mainly	*Used in dentistry also*
Confusion	Antihypertensives Antihistamines Tricyclics	Benzodiazepines
Aggressive behaviour	Dopa derivatives	Benzodiazepines (in children)
Nightmares or hallucinations	Some antihypertensives	Pentazocine Ketamine
Mania	Levodopa	Corticosteroids
Depression	Antihypertensives Contraceptive pill	Pentazocine Corticosteroids
Delirium	Antihypertensives Antitubercular drugs Anticonvulsants Oral hypoglycaemics	Procaine penicillin Sulphonamides
Paranoia	Antihypertensives Anticonvulsants Amphetamines	Ephedrine Corticosteroids

Creutzfeldt–Jakob disease

Creutzfeldt–Jakob disease (CJD) is a rare transmissible disorder caused by a prion ('slow virus'), which produces spongiform encephalopathy and dementia. The chief risk of CJD is that it can be transmitted by transplantation of human cranial tissue, such as pituitary extracts of human growth hormone. It has also been transmitted by human dura mater which was formerly used for antral repairs and for which it is now banned. A new variant may be the result of transmission of the bovine spongiform encephalopathy (BSE; 'mad cow disease') agent.

Gerstmann–Straussler–Scheinker syndrome

This is a rare inherited autosomal dominant disorder characterized by progressive ataxia and dementia.

SEXUAL ABUSE

Sexual abuse can take a variety of forms but in addition to physical and psychological injury, the victim may acquire one or more sexually transmitted diseases, including HIV infection.

SYSTEMIC DISEASE CAUSING PSYCHIATRIC DISORDERS

Many endocrine diseases can be complicated by psychiatric disturbances (*Table 18.7*), as may alcoholism, drug abuse or therapy (*Table 18.8*).

Major trauma, surgery or severe life-threatening disease can also frequently cause emotional reactions such as anxiety or depression, or conditions such as compensation neurosis.

BIBLIOGRAPHY

Abrams R.A. and Ruff J.C. (1986) Oral signs and symptoms in the diagnosis of bulimia. *J. Am. Dent. Assoc.* **113**, 761–4.

Andreasen N.C. (1995) Symptoms, signs and diagnosis of schizophrenia. *Lancet* **346**, 477–81.

Anisman H., Baines M.G. and Berczi I. (1996) Neuroimmune mechanisms in health and disease. 2. Disease. *Canad. Med. Assoc. J.* **155**, 1075–82.

Bick P.A. (1986) Seasonal major affective disorder. *Am. J. Psychiatry* **143**, 90–1.

Brady W.F. (1980) The anorexia nervosa syndrome. *Oral Surg. Oral Med. Oral Pathol.* **50**, 509–16.

Cawson R.A. Spector R.G. and Skelly A.M. (1995) *Basic Pharmacology and Clinical Drug Use in Dentistry*, 6th edn. Edinburgh, Churchill Livingstone.

Chapman P.J. and Shaw R.M. (1991) Normative dental treatment needs of Alzheimer patients. *Aust. Dent. J.* **36**,141–4.

Clark D.C. (1985) Oral complications of anorexia nervosa and/or bulimia. *J. Oral Med.* **40**, 134–8.

Fiske J. (1990) Alzheimer's disease. *Br. Dent. J.* **169**, 188.

Freeman R.E. (1985) Dental anxiety: a multifactorial aetiology. *Br. Dent. J.* **159**, 406–8.

Freeman R. and Goss S. (1993) Stress measures as predictors of periodontal disease – a preliminary communication. *Commun. Dent. Oral Epidemiol.* **21**, 176–7.

Friedlander A.H. and Gorelick D.A. (1987) Panic disorder: its association with mitral valve prolapse and appropriate dental management. *Oral Surg. Oral Med. Oral Pathol.* **63**, 309–12.

Friedlander A.H. and Jarvik L.F. (1987) The dental management of the patient with dementia. *Oral Surg. Oral Med. Oral Pathol.* **64**, 549–53.

Friedlander A.H. and West L.J. (1991) Dental management of the patient with major depression. *Oral Surg. Oral Med. Oral Pathol.* **71**, 573–8.

Friedlander A.H., Mills M.J. and Cummings J.L. (1988) Consent for dental therapy in severely ill patients. *Oral Surg. Oral Med. Oral Pathol.* **65**, 179–82.

Goodman H.S., Ickrath M.C. and Niessen L.C. (1993) Managing patients with Alzheimer's; the primary role of dentists. *J. Am. Dent. Assoc.* **124**, 75–9.

Goodwin F.K. and Jamieson K.R. (1990) *Manic-Depressive Illness*. Oxford, Oxford University Press.

Gram L.F. (1994) Fluoxetine. *N. Engl. J. Med.* **331**, 1354–61.

Gross K.B.W., Brough K.M. and Randolph P.M. (1986) Eating disorders: anorexia and bulimia nervosa. *J. Dent. Child.* Sept, pp. 378–81.

Hamilton J.R. (1983) Mental Health Act 1983. *Br. Med. J.* **286**, 1720–5.

Harris M. and Davies G. (1990) Psychiatric disorders. In Jones J.H. and Mason D.K. (eds) *Oral Manifestations of Systemic Disease*, 2nd edn. London, Ballière Tindall Cox.

Hede B. (1995) Oral health in Danish hospitalized psychiatric patients. *Commun. Dent. Oral Epidemiol.* **23**, 44–8.

Johnson G.F.S. and Wilson P. (1989) The management of depression: a review of pharmacological and non-pharmacological treatments. *Med. J. Aust.* **151**, 397–406.

Kane J.M. and McGlashan T.H. (1995) Treatment of schizophrenia. *Lancet* **346**, 820–5.

Kiloh L.G. (1980) The diagnosis and management of depressive illness. *Medicine (UK)* **35**, 1773–6.

Kleier D.J., Aragon S.B. and Averback R.E. (1984) Dental management of the chronic vomiting patient. *J. Am. Dent. Assoc.* **108**, 618–21.

Livingstone M.G. (1995) Interactions with selective MAOIs. *Lancet* **345**, 533–4.

Marcenes W.S. and Sheiham A. (1992) The relationship between work stress and oral health status. *Soc. Sci. Med.* **35**, 1511–20.

Michels R. and Marzuk P.M. (1993) Progress in psychiatry. *N. Engl. J. Med.* **329**, 552–60, and 628–38.

Moody G.H., Drummond J.R. and Newton J.P (1990) Alzheimer's disease. *Br. Dent. J.* **169**, 45–7.

Niessen L.C., Jones J.A., Zocchi M. *et al.* (1985) Dental care for the patient with Alzheimer's disease. *J. Am. Dent. Assoc.* **110**, 207–9.

Porter S.R. and Scully C. (1996) *Innovations and Developments in Non-Invasive Oral Health Care*. Northwood, Science Reviews.

Scully C. (1982) Orofacial manifestations of the Lesch–Nyhan syndrome. *Int. J. Oral Surg.* **10**, 180–3.

Scully C. (1988) *The Dental Patient*. Oxford, Heinemann.

Scully C. (1989) *The Mouth and Perioral Tissues*. Oxford, Heinemann.

Scully C. (1989) *Patient Care: a Dental Surgeon's Guide*. London, British Dental Association.

Scully C. (1993) La maladie du petit papier. *Br. Dent. J.* **175**, 289–92.

Scully C. and Cawson R.A. (eds) (1986) Oral medicine. *Med. Int.* 1129–56.

Scully C., Cawson R.A. and Griffiths M.J. (1990) *Occupational Hazards to Dental Staff*. London, British Dental Journal.

Scully C., Eveson J.W. and Porter S.R. (1995) Munchausen's syndrome: oral presentations. *Br. Dent. J.* **178**, 65–7.

Ship J.A. (1992) Oral health of patients with Alzheimer's disease. *J. Am. Dent. Assoc.* **123**, 53–8.

Short P.W. (1981) The psychiatrically violent patient. *Br. Med. J.* **282**, 279.

Stiefel D.J., Truelove E.L., Menard T.W. *et al.* (1990) A comparison of the oral health of persons with and without chronic mental illness in community settings. *Spec. Care Dent.* **10**, 6–12.

Strauss J.S. and Carpenter W.T. (1981) *Schizophrenia.* New York, Plenum Press.

Walsh B.T., Croft C.B. and Katz J.L. (1981) Anorexia nervosa and salivary gland enlargement. *Int. Psychiatry Med.* **11**, 255–61.

Will R.G., Ironside J.W., Zeidler M. *et al.* (1996) A new variant of Creutzfeldt-Jakob disease in the UK. *Lancet* **347**, 921–5.

19

Headache and orofacial pain

> **Key points**
>
> - Most orofacial pain is caused by local disease, but psychogenic, neurological, vascular and referred pain must be excluded.
> - Local disease in the head and neck which may cause orofacial pain, ranges from trauma to odontogenic, and antral or other infections, to malignant disease.
> - Neoplasms involving branches of the trigeminal nerve can remain undetected until late, and should always be considered if an obvious local cause is not evident.
> - Although orofacial pain can lead patients to become depressed, psychogenic factors are common in atypical facial pain and oral dysaesthesia.
> - Symptoms must never be termed psychogenic until organic disease has been excluded by thorough history, examination and investigation.
> - Patients with psychogenic disease are not exempt from organic disease.
> - Atypical facial pain presents with chronic dull boring pain which does not awaken the patient from sleep, is usually in one maxilla, and has no organic cause.
> - Oral dysaesthesia is mainly felt as a burning tongue sensation. Candidosis, vitamin deficiency, diabetes and mucosal disease should be excluded.
> - Temporomandibular pain-dysfunction syndrome affects young persons mainly, with discomfort and sometimes clicking or locking of the jaw, or trismus.
> - Temporomandibular pain-dysfunction may be related to trauma, parafunction, occlusal anomalies or psychogenic factors.
> - Trigeminal neuralgia is a severe idiopathic orofacial pain, which typically responds to anticonvulsants, particularly carbamazepine.
> - Trigeminal neuralgia may occasionally arise from multiple sclerosis, a posterior cranial fossa aneurysm or tumour, neurosyphilis or other organic disease.
> - Herpes zoster (shingles) may be preceded, is accompanied, and may be followed by severe neuralgia.
> - Migraine appears to be due to vascular dilatation, sometimes in response to stress, alcohol, or tyramine-containing food or drink, and may produce neurological signs.
> - Migrainous neuralgia may be precipitated by alcohol, or high altitude, and presents with autonomic features (flushing/ sweating/conjunctival suffusion).
> - Giant cell arteritis may involve the retinal artery and threaten sight, and is thus a medical emergency requiring systemic corticosteroids.
> - Orofacial pain may be referred from the chest (e.g. lung cancer) or heart (angina) or elsewhere, or caused by meningeal irritation, or drugs (even analgesics).

Table 19.1　Causes of facial pain and headache

- Local causes
  Dental or oral disease
  Infections or tumours of paranasal sinuses and
  nasopharynx
  Neck lesions
  Ocular lesions
- Psychogenic causes
  Tension headaches
  Atypical facial pain
  Temporomandibular pain-dysfunction syndrome
- Neurological causes
  Trigeminal neuralgia
  Glossopharyngeal neuralgia
  Herpetic neuralgia
  Raeder's neuralgia
  Intracranial disease
- Vascular causes
  Migraine
  Migrainous neuralgia
  Temporal arteritis
- Other causes
  Referred pain (e.g. heart or chest)
  Raised intracranial pressure
  Meningeal irritation
  Diseases of the skull
  Medical diseases (e.g. severe hypertension)
  Trauma
  Drugs (e.g. vinca alkaloids, nitrites, dapsone,
  some analgesics)

Headache and orofacial pain are common symptoms mainly caused by local pathology, psychogenic disorders or neurological disease (*see also Tables 19.1 and 19.2*).

1. Oral or perioral lesions, or diseases of the nose, sinuses, eye, ear or neck.
2. Psychogenic causes.
3. Neurological disease.
4. Vascular causes.
5. Pain referred from a distance.
6. Drugs such as vinca alkaloids.

Most of these pains are chronic and not of sudden onset. Severe pain of sudden onset may have very serious importance, such as:

1. Subarachnoid haemorrhage.
2. Subdural or epidural haemorrhage.
3. Acute hypertension.
4. Acute glaucoma.
5. Acute lesions affecting the carotid vessels.
6. Others.

Patients with headache should be evaluated by history supplemented by physical examination, including examination of the cranium, sinuses, ears and eyes, and mental and neurological status. Investigations should include a full blood picture, basic blood chemistry and possibly endocrinological examination, as well as urinalysis. CT or MRI are often indicated and occasionally lumbar puncture, electroencephalography, electrocardiography or arteriography are indicated.

LOCAL CAUSES OF FACIAL PAIN

The mouth

The oral causes of facial pain such as pulpitis and apical periodontitis, periodontal abscesses, pericoronitis and various intraosseous lesions are fully discussed in other texts.

Table 19.2　Differentiation of headaches of different cause

	TMJ pain-dysfunction	Psychogenic	Idiopathic trigeminal neuralgia	Migraine
Age (yr)	20–30	35–60	50+	Any
Sex	F>M	F>M	F>M	F>M
Site	Temple, ear, jaws, teeth Usually unilateral	Diffuse, deep, sometimes across midline	Mandible or maxilla Unilateral	Any
Associated features	Click in TMJ, trismus	Life events Back pain etc.	—	±Photophobia ±Nausea ±Vomiting
Character	Dull, continuous	Dull, boring, continuous Stress, fatigue	Lancinating	Throbbing
Duration of episode	Weeks to years	Weeks to years	Brief (seconds)	Hours (or usually days)

The sinuses and nasopharynx

Sinusitis can cause localized pain. In acute maxillary or frontal sinusitis local pain and tenderness (but not swelling), and radio-opacity of the affected sinuses, usually follow a cold.

With maxillary sinusitis pain may be felt in related upper molars, several of which may be tender to percussion. The pain of ethmoidal or sphenoidal sinusitis is felt deeply in the nose, but may cause headache, while frontal sinusitis causes an anterior headache.

Tumours of the sinuses or nasopharynx can also cause facial pain. These tumours are often carcinomas which involve various branches of the trigeminal nerve and can remain undetected until late. Some may cause pain simulating pain-dysfunction syndrome.

Eagle's syndrome, a rare disorder associated with an elongated styloid process, due to calcification of the stylohyoid ligament, may cause pain on chewing, swallowing or turning the head. The elongated styloid process may be visualized radiographically, and palpation of it in the wall of the pharynx causes intense pain.

The elongated stylohyoid process can be shortened surgically, but regrowth and relapse are common.

The eyes

Disorders of refraction can cause frontal headaches. Retrobulbar neuritis (for example in multiple sclerosis), or glaucoma (raised intraocular pressure), may cause pain in and around the orbit.

The ears

Pharyngeal or middle ear disease may cause headaches. Oral disease can also cause pain referred to the ear. A classic picture is that of the elderly person with cancer of the tongue who complains of earache.

The neck

Cervical vertebral disease, especially cervical spondylosis, occasionally causes pain referred to the face. Tension headaches may be aggravated by cervical spine disease. Headache may rarely arise from upper cervical spine disease such as rheumatoid or osteoarthritis, and is then typically precipitated or aggravated by neck movements. Nerve block with local anaesthesia may relieve this pain.

PSYCHOGENIC CAUSES OF FACIAL PAIN

Atypical facial pain (psychogenic facial pain) (*see* p. 379)

Headache and facial pain are common symptoms most frequently caused by dental or other local infections (Chapter 9). However, there is a group of patients, mainly women, who have continuous pain, particularly in the maxillary region, in the absence of any detectable organic cause. The pain is usually a dull ache, albeit with intermittent episodic exacerbations. The pain has no obvious precipitating factors, although it may be attributed to dental disease or treatment, and is rarely completely relieved by analgesics. The pain may waken the patient in the early morning. *Organic causes for the pain must be excluded; patients may have genuine atypical facial pain along with some other disease.*

The International Headache Society has defined atypical facial pain as

> 'persistent facial pain that does not have the characteristics of the cranial neuralgias and is not associated with physical signs or demonstrable organic causes. It is present daily and persists for most or all of the day. It is confined at onset to a limited area on one side of the face and may spread to the upper and lower jaws or other areas of the face or neck. It is deep and poorly localized. The pain is not associated with sensory loss or other physical signs. Laboratory investigations including X-ray of face and jaws do not demonstrate relevant abnormalities.'

Since many of these patients have already rejected the idea of mental illness, it may be difficult to persuade them of the need for psychiatric help. In some cases it is helpful to make it clear that depression is both common and is an illness like any other – indeed worse than many – and, like other illnesses, can also cause physical symptoms. Psychiatric assistance and antidepressant treatment are then needed. Sometimes the pain may appear as a hysterical conversion neurosis and many patients have obsessional personality traits. Tricyclic antidepressants such as nortriptyline, imipramine, amitriptyline or dothiepin may be effective, but monoamine oxidase inhibitors or SSRIs may be needed. Nortriptyline 10 to 30 mg, dothiepin from 25 mg or fluoxetine from 20 mg at night are common regimens used.

Idiopathic odontalgia is a variant of atypical facial pain and is characterized by complaint of severe throbbing pain in one or several teeth which are hypersensitive to any stimulus. Extractions typically lead to transference of the symptoms to adjacent teeth.

Oral dysaesthesia (*see* p. 379)

A complaint of a burning tongue or mouth is the common type of oral dysaesthesia, although any part of the mouth may be involved. This is commonly termed the 'burning mouth syndrome'. Patients are mostly middle-aged or elderly women who have a burning sensation that comes on after waking and increases in intensity during the day. The symptoms may sometimes be relieved by chewing or drinking.

Dry mouth, disturbed taste sensations or delusions of halitosis are other dysaesthesias and are often also manifestations of a depressive neurosis. There is sometimes cancerphobia, or anxiety about the possibility, for example, of venereal disease or HIV.

Organic causes, particularly deficiency states, candidosis and diabetes, must be excluded by investigation. Once this has been done, antidepressants may be helpful, as above. Initial studies suggesting that vitamin B might help have not been confirmed.

Temporomandibular pain-dysfunction syndrome

This syndrome (with its many synonyms, such as *facial pain-dysfunction*, *myofascial pain-dysfunction* or *facial arthromyalgia*) is a common problem predominantly affecting young women. Some believe that depression may be a contributory factor and there may be a greater frequency of migraine, rhinitis, peptic ulcer and irritable bowel syndrome associated.

There is typically dull pain, usually in front of the temporomandibular joint, and sometimes joint clicking, alone or in various combinations. The pain tends to radiate over the masseter and temporalis muscles and sometimes occipitally or cervically, and there may be tenderness in the masticatory muscles including the pterygoids. The mandible often deviates towards the affected side on opening and there may be trismus ('locking'). There may be an audible click or palpable crepitus in the joint but radiography shows no significant abnormality. Nevertheless, organic disease must be excluded.

Patients frequently grind or clench their teeth or develop various (parafunctional) habits, such as pencil chewing, and there is often faceting on the teeth, ridging of the tongue margins and buccal mucosa at the occlusal line, and sometimes signs of lip-chewing. Some occupations or hobbies, such as scuba-diving, may predispose to abnormal habits and pain-dysfunction. Occlusal anomalies, especially loss of molars, may be present, as in persons without pain.

The psychiatric basis of the temporomandibular pain-dysfunction syndrome is controversial, but it may be seen in ambitious obsessional personalities, in anxiety states, or in agitated depression. Treatment consists of reassurance and use of a bite-raising appliance to provide a free, sliding occlusion. Mild anxiolytics such as diazepam (which is also a muscle relaxant) may be helpful but should only be given for a limited period and may need to be supplemented with analgesics. If there is evidence of depression, tricyclic antidepressants may be of more use. Overall, however, a temporary bite guard, providing free, sliding occlusion, alone is likely to relieve symptoms effectively. In any case, symptoms appear eventually to resolve spontaneously, and degenerative joint disease is *not* a consequence.

Tension headaches

Bilateral tension headaches are very common, especially in young adults. The pain, which is caused by muscle tension, affects the frontal, occipital or temporal muscles, and is felt as a constant ache or band-like pressure. The pain is experienced more than 15 days monthly to be classified as tension headache, is often worse in the evening and at night, lasts a few hours, but does not waken the patient. The pericranial muscles are tender on palpation.

Patients with tension headaches are frequently adamant that they suffer from migraine, as migraine is a more important-sounding diagnosis, is supposed to affect highly intelligent people, and has fewer neurotic connotations. Sometimes the two conditions do co-exist. The possibility of associated depression should also be considered. Diseases such as hypertension and hyperthyroidism should be excluded, as must drug-associated headache, such as that caused by some analgesics, antihistamines, anticonvulsants, ergotamine, steroids and antibiotics.

Reassurance may be effective but may be helped by a short course of diazepam 2–5 mg, three times daily, as this is both anxiolytic and a mild muscle relaxant. Failing this, amitriptyline is usually effective.

NEUROLOGICAL CAUSES OF FACIAL PAIN

Sensory innervation of the face and scalp depends on the trigeminal nerve, so that lesions of this nerve at any stage from its nuclei along its course from the pons can cause facial pain or sensory loss – sometimes with serious implications.

Idiopathic trigeminal neuralgia (tic douloureux)

Trigeminal neuralgia usually afflicts patients over the age of 50. The incidence is less than 0.2 per cent in those under 40 years but rises to 9 per cent in the 50–60 age group and up to 25 per cent in those over 70. It is usually a sporadic event. The pain has the following characteristics:

1. It is usually confined to the trigeminal area of one side, usually the maxillary or mandibular division or occasionally both. Infraorbital or lower lip/lower jaw pain is thus common.
2. It is severe and sharply stabbing (lancinating). It is of only a few seconds' duration, but paroxysms may follow in quick succession. The pain of trigeminal

neuralgia is typically remarkably severe and a patient seen crying with pain during an attack is not easily forgotten.
3. Mild stimuli, such as touch or cold, applied to trigger zones within the trigeminal area typically provoke an attack. Characteristic trigger zones are near the ala nasae, near the commissure or on the gingivae, and are not necessarily situated in the sensory area where the pain is felt. Touching, washing, toothbrushing or chewing may trigger an attack.
4. There is no objective sensory loss in the area, or other defined neurological deficit. Patients with idiopathic trigeminal neuralgia show no abnormal neurological signs. Neurological assessment is needed because similar pain may be secondary to multiple sclerosis, to posterior cerebral fossa lesions (particularly tumours or aneurysms), to neurosyphilis or to other lesions. Over 2 per cent of patients with neuralgia have multiple sclerosis; conversely, 1.5 per cent of persons with multiple sclerosis have trigeminal neuralgia. Severe facial pain suggestive of trigeminal neuralgia but with physical signs such as facial sensory or motor impairment can also result from brain stem ischaemia or infarction in cerebrovascular disease. Involvement of the posterior inferior cerebellar artery is often responsible. The combination of neuralgia with hemifacial spasm also suggests a posterior cranial fossa lesion.

Classic trigeminal neuralgia has been described and some purists dispute the existence of atypical variants. However, patients occasionally complain of unusual symptoms such as more continuous rather than lightning attacks of pain, or triggering by warmth rather than cold. The response of many such cases to carbamazepine strongly suggests that trigeminal neuralgia may produce a slightly variable clinical picture. Spontaneous remissions of a month or two are relatively common and may make the assessment of treatment difficult.

The cause of trigeminal neuralgia is unclear. Some believe it is caused by demyelination from pressure on the nerve caused by a tortuous blood vessel in the posterior cranial fossa involved arteriosclerotically.

Despite little evidence for this, some operations are based on the hypothesis.

The main differential diagnoses are from glossopharyngeal neuralgia (the two can co-exist), atypical facial pain, Raeder's para-trigeminal syndrome and Frey's syndrome.

- ## Management of trigeminal neuralgia

Absence of abnormal neurological signs, particularly facial anaesthesia, and conditions such as neurosyphilis must be confirmed before treatment is started. Some advise investigations, and these are warranted especially if there are any neurological features. Skull radiographs, CT scans, MRI, CSF and neurophysiological tests, such as trigeminal evoked potentials, and corneal reflex latency may be indicated.

Treatment is with anticonvulsants, which also cause a fall in gamma amino butyric acid (GABA) levels in the central pain-inhibiting systems. Carbamazepine is the main treatment for trigeminal neuralgia. Starting with 100 mg once or twice daily with food, the dose should be increased with increments of 100–200 mg every 2 weeks until symptoms are controlled or adverse effects become excessive. Though about 80 per cent obtain pain relief within 24 hours, about 20 days are required before the full effect is noted. Most patients require 200 mg three times daily but a few do not respond until doses as high as 400 mg four times daily are given. Ataxia and drowsiness are dose-related and may interfere with driving and be dose-limiting.

Monitoring of blood levels is helpful. There are many other possible toxic effects but these are uncommon: gastrointestinal upsets, rashes and leucopenia have been reported but the last is exceedingly rare. Reactions such as erythema multiforme, toxic epidermal necrolysis, thrombocytopenia, liver dysfunction or atrioventricular block are recognized, though rare, complications. In high dosage, carbamazepine, which is sometimes also used for the treatment of diabetes insipidus, may cause the syndrome of inappropriate antidiuretic hormone secretion (Chapter 14), fluid retention and hyponatraemia, particularly in the elderly or those with heart failure. Blood pressure, blood urea and electrolytes, liver function, platelet and white cell counts should therefore be established at the outset, and

monitored if there is concern. Drugs such as erythromycin, cimetidine and isoniazid can increase serum levels. Carbamazepine is contraindicated in pregnancy and porphyria, and should be used with caution in persons with hepatic, renal, cardiac or bone marrow disease. It may interfere with the effectiveness of the contraceptive pill, though most patients are beyond the age of concern in that respect. It may predispose to liver damage from paracetamol.

It is essential to appreciate that carbamazepine is not an analgesic and, if given when an attack starts, will not relieve the pain. Absorption is slow and its antineuralgic activity depends on its metabolites. Carbamazepine must therefore be given continuously for long periods. It is also important to note that if a patient has pain suggestive of trigeminal neuralgia, but has no benefit from carbamazepine, it is essential to ask the nature of the dosage regimen, as the drug is often taken intermittently under the impression that it is an analgesic. Carbamazepine will control up to 90 per cent of patients over the first few months, but this falls to about 25 per cent by one year.

Should carbamazepine in tolerated dosage fail to control neuralgia then phenytoin (starting with 100 mg three times daily) or baclofen (starting with 5 mg three times daily) can be given in addition, or pimozide (starting with 4 mg daily), oxcarbazine, valproate or clonazepam tried. If medical therapy fails, surgery may be indicated. Unfortunately, all destructive surgical procedures result in a sensory deficit in about 20 per cent of patients, and the more peripheral the procedure, the greater the recurrence of neuralgia.

Surgery (surgical division, cryosurgery, injections of alcohol or phenol) to the trigeminal nerve branches involved is usually carried out under open operation by local analgesia. Local cryosurgery can produce pain relief without permanent anaesthesia. Unfortunately the benefit of all procedures may only be temporary and relapse is common beyond 2 years.

If this treatment fails intracranial neurosurgery may be needed. Percutaneous radiofrequency retrogasserian rhizotomy is the most widely used technique but is not without morbidity and some mortality. Anaesthesia also results, with danger of damage to the cornea. Microvascular decompression via a suboccipital craniotomy may be effective but occasionally results in damage to the VIIth or VIIIth cranial nerves and also carries a small mortality. Postganglionic glycerol instillation and microvascular decompression are also used. These neurosurgical techniques can occasionally be followed by continuous facial pain (anaesthesia dolorosa) that responds very poorly to attempts at treatment with tricyclics or phenothiazines.

Glossopharyngeal neuralgia

Glossopharyngeal neuralgia (Collet–Sicard syndrome) is rare and usually idiopathic, possibly caused by an abnormal intracranial blood vessel, as in trigeminal neuralgia. The pain is equally severe, but affects the throat, especially the tonsillar region, often on the left side, and is typically triggered by swallowing or coughing. Pain may also be felt in the ipsilateral ear (Vago–Collet–Sicard syndrome) and this may simulate neuralgia of the nervus intermedius (Hunt's neuralgia). A cocaine or other anaesthetic throat spray will cause temporary pain relief which is diagnostic. There are no sensory or motor defects but in 10 per cent there is an associated bradycardia and fall in blood pressure, sometimes with syncope, especially when the neuralgia is secondary to a throat tumour. Therapy is as for trigeminal neuralgia, though carbamazepine is usually less effective than for trigeminal neuralgia and adequate relief of pain can be difficult. Neurosurgery is then indicated.

Occasionally glossopharyngeal neuralgia is secondary to herpes zoster. Lesions (often tumours) in the posterior cranial fossa or jugular foramen (jugular foramen syndrome) can cause similar pain together with lesions of the vagus (X) and accessory (XI) nerves (*see* Appendix to this chapter). Hoarseness, dysphagia, palatal deviation to the intact side, anaesthesia of the posterior pharyngeal wall, and weakness of the sternomastoid and upper trapezius are then seen.

Herpetic and post-herpetic facial neuralgia

Herpes zoster (shingles) is often preceded and usually accompanied by neuralgia (Chapter 11). Neuralgia may also persist after the rash has resolved in up to 70 per cent of cases, mainly in the elderly, but antivirals may help prevent this. Post-herpetic neuralgia is said to be present when there is still pain a month after the eruption of zoster. This neuralgia (unlike trigeminal neuralgia) causes continuous burning pain, worse with movement and thermal change, and there may be sensory changes in the affected area. It mainly affects elderly patients and may be so intolerable that suicide can become a risk.

Treatment is difficult. NSAIDs are generally ineffective but topical lignocaine or capsaicin as a cream may help. Tricyclic antidepressants, particularly desipramine or amitryptyline, may relieve the pain better than do valproate or carbamazepine. Transcutaneous electrical stimulation or neurosurgery may sometimes help if antidepressants are not effective. However, spontaneous improvement may follow after about 18 months in some patients.

Raeder's paratrigeminal neuralgia

Severe, persistent pain in and around the eye, with an associated Horner's syndrome, is often caused by a lesion at the base of the skull and requires neurological attention. This is now regarded as a migraine variant similar to migrainous neuralgia.

Facial pain caused by intracranial tumours or other lesions

Any lesion affecting the trigeminal nerve from its nuclei to the pons, through the posterior and middle cranial fossae, to the foramen ovale and rotundum, and to the superior orbital fissure, can cause facial pain. The clinical features vary with the site and extent of the lesion. Commonly, there is facial pain associated with a facial sensory deficit and impaired corneal reflex on the affected side. Anatomically closely related cranial nerves are frequently involved (*see* Appendix to Chapter 17).

Pontine infarction
Pontine ischaemia may be due to bilateral ventral pontine infarction and has been reported to cause burning orofacial pain. This needs to be recognized, as it may be an early symptom of bilateral ventral pontine infarction causing the syndrome of quadriplegia, lower cranial nerve palsies but preservation

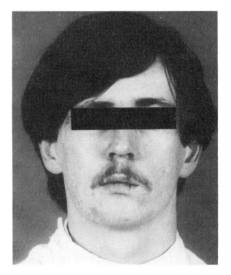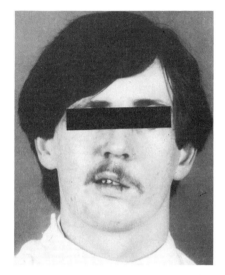

Fig. 19.1 Bell's palsy: the left side of the face is completely paralysed, as demonstrated well when the patient tries to smile

of movement of the upper eyelids and vertical gaze. This constellation of effects is termed the *locked-in syndrome* because the patient, though able to understand what is being said or what is happening, is imprisoned by their inability to speak or move anything apart from their eyes. The prognosis is poor. Lateral medullary infarction may cause a similar but unilateral burning sensation.

Cerebellopontine angle tumours
Lesions in the posterior cranial fossa, such as cerebellopontine angle tumours (acoustic neuroma or meningioma), can cause facial pain associated with an absent corneal reflex (Vth nerve), deafness, tinnitus and vertigo (from involvement of the VIIIth nerve), facial palsy (VIIth nerve involvement), ataxia, intention tremor and nystagmus (cerebellar involvement) and spasticity of the leg (pyramidal tract involvement).

Middle cranial fossa lesions
Middle cranial fossa lesions can involve the Vth and VIth nerves, causing also lateral rectus palsy. Carotid aneurysms, especially those in the cavernous sinus, or cavernous sinus thrombosis, may also cause facial pain and associated cranial nerve lesions (IIIrd, IVth and VIth nerves).
Cavernous sinus thrombosis is a life-threatening complication that may rarely result from

infection spreading back through the emissary veins from the maxillary or nasal region, or upper teeth. Infected thrombi in the anterior facial vein or less commonly the pterygoid plexus can reach the cavernous sinus via either the ophthalmic veins or the foramen ovale.

Clinically, cavernous sinus thrombosis causes gross oedema of the eyelids, ipsilateral pulsatile exophthalmos and cyanosis due to venous obstruction. The superior orbital fissure syndrome (proptosis, fixed dilated pupil and limitation of eye movements) rapidly develops. Rigors and a high swinging pyrexia are associated. In the absence of effective treatment, similar signs rapidly develop on the opposite side.

Vigorous use of anticoagulants, antibiotics, drainage and elimination of the source of infection are essential. There is a mortality of up to 50 per cent and a further 50 per cent of those that survive are likely to lose the sight of one or both eyes.

Bell's palsy (*see also* Chapter 17)

Bell's (facial) palsy is preceded or accompanied by pain in the region of the ear, spreading down the jaw in about half the cases. However, the appearance of the typical facial paralysis leaves little doubt as to the diagnosis (*Fig. 19.1*).

Table 19.3 Migraine variants

Type	Clinical features
Classic migraine	Unilateral headache preceded by an aura[a]
Migrainous neuralgia	Pain typically around the eye, often with visible effects of vasodilatation
Facial migraine	Variant of migrainous neuralgia, but affects lower face (lower-half migraine)
Hemiplegic migraine	Rare
	Often familial; hemiparesis may outlast headache by several days; may rarely cause facial palsy
Ophthalmoplegic migraine	Rare
	Affects children (boys) mainly; pain around eye with impaired eye movement
Vertebrobasilar migraine	Affects adolescent girls mainly
	Similar to classic migraine but aura associated with ataxia, vertigo, diplopia; headache usually occipital; may be loss of consciousness at the onset
Complicated migraine	Term applied to any form of migraine complicated by residual neurological defect after attack

[a]Migraine frequently lacks the 'classic' features and may not be strictly unilateral or there may be no aura – it is then difficult to distinguish from non-migrainous headache.

Facial pain caused by extracranial lesions

Branches of the trigeminal nerve may be affected by inflammatory, traumatic or neoplastic lesions causing pain or sensory loss in their distribution.

VASCULAR CAUSES OF FACIAL PAIN

Migraine

Migraine is a recurrent headache combined with autonomic disturbances. Affecting over 14 per cent of women and 7 per cent of men, the number, frequency, intensity and duration of attacks vary widely but they tend to diminish in frequency and intensity with increasing age. Spontaneous remissions are not uncommon and migraine tends to improve during pregnancy.

Migraine appears to be related to arterial dilatation. Attacks may be precipitated by alcohol, drugs such as nitroglycerin, or various foods containing tyramine or nitrites, such as ripe bananas, citrus fruits, nuts, beer, red wine or chocolate, aspartame, mono-sodium glutamate, the menstrual cycle, pregnancy or the contraceptive pill. Stress and environmental factors (noise, smoke etc.) often seems to be precipitating factors in migraine as in many other disorders. The fact that attacks are more frequent at weekends, for example, should not be interpreted as excluding stress, as there is no doubt that some find the company and demands of their families more stressful than their work. Going away on holiday (Freud's *reise fieber* – 'travel fever') is also highly stressful for many. The belief by some that migraine is caused by occlusal dysharmony is unsubstantiated.

Several types of migraine are recognized (*Table 19.3*). *Migraine without aura* is the most frequent type, presenting with unilateral headache, together with nausea, vomiting, photophobia and phonophobia. *Classic migraine with aura* is the most readily recognized type of migraine by neurological symptoms and deficits and the following features:

1. The headache is preceded by warning symptoms (an aura). The aura may last about 15 minutes and consists of visual, sensory, motor or speech disturbances. The patient may complain of photophobia and nausea. Visual phenomena are typically of zig-zag flickering light (fortification spectra) or transient visual defects. Sensory phenomena include paraesthesia or anaesthesia – usually of the contralateral upper limb, or face and mouth. Motor symptoms are mainly weakness – again of the contralateral upper limb. Epilepsy is slightly more common in migraine sufferers than in the general population. Obvious vascular phenomena may be associated but are

variable in character, and range from flushing and oedema of the face on the affected side to temporary hemiplegia.
2. The headache is severe, usually unilateral (hemicrania) and lasts for hours or days. The headache often becomes throbbing and generalized and may be associated with facial pallor.

Complicated migraine is where neurological deficits are present 7 days after an attack. Ischaemic lesions may be seen on CT brain scan.

• Management of migraine

Migraine is usually managed with drugs and avoidance of precipitating factors. In acute attacks, patients usually prefer to lie in a quiet, dark room.

There is a very significant placebo factor in the therapy of migraine. Aspirin, paracetamol or ibuprofen can be effective, and can be given with an anti-emetic such as buclizine or metoclopramide. Antiemetics such as metoclopramide (10 mg) or domperidone (10 mg) should be given orally early on to overcome the autonomic dysfunction preventing gastric emptying. In severe cases of vomiting, an antiemetic such as metoclopramide or prochlorperazine by suppository may also be required.

Sumatriptan, a 5-HT receptor agonist, is considerably effective within 1 hour if given in a dose of 100 mg orally or by injection, but this is restricted for use in severe or resistant migraine, or the patient cannot swallow tablets. Sumatriptan can cause coronary artery constriction and is contraindicated in cardiac disease, pregnancy, liver and renal disease, and may cause drowsiness and impair driving. It should not be repeated during the same attack, and the drug should not be given with other migraine treatments or antidepressants.

If these are not effective, ergotamine (1–2 mg) given orally may abort an attack, but in many cases absorption by mouth is too slow to be effective and a better alternative therefore is to use it by inhalation from a Medihaler. Even so, ergotamine must not be used within 6 hours of sumitriptan. The maximum dose of ergotamine is 4 mg in 24 hours; this must not be exceeded and treat-

ment must not be repeated at intervals of less than 4 days. Ergotamine may cause peripheral vasospasm and gangrene (ergotism) and may itself cause abdominal pain, nausea and vomiting. Ergotamine can also be given with caffeine, or as a suppository, which overcomes the problem of poor absorption if the patient is vomiting.

Intranasal lignocaine can give pain relief within 5 minutes in over half those suffering from migraine, but the pain returns after about an hour in half of the responders.

If attacks of migraine are more frequent than two a month, prophylaxis with propranolol or another beta-blocker (metoprolol, nadolol, timolol) is the treatment of choice but sometimes a serotonin antagonist (pizotifen or cyproheptadine) or amitriptyline are used. Pizotifen may cause drowsiness, and should be used with caution in renal disease, pregnancy, glaucoma or urinary retention. Low-dose aspirin (300 mg on alternate days) may reduce attacks by 20 per cent, probably by blocking prostaglandin production in response to stimulation of a 5-HT (serotonin) receptor. More recent evidence suggests that calcium-channel blockers such as verapamil or nifedipine may be useful alternatives. Methysergide has dangerous toxic effects, in particular, retroperitoneal fibrosis and fibrosis of the heart valves and pleura. It is only therefore given for refractory cases under specialist supervision. Clonidine has been found to be of little value in the prophylaxis of migraine.

Dental procedures such as tooth extraction, amalgam removal or the use of occlusal splints are of no proven value in the management of migraine.

Migrainous neuralgia

Synonyms include periodic migrainous neuralgia, cluster headaches, Horton's neuralgia, superficial petrosal neuralgia, histamine cephalgia and others.

Migrainous neuralgia is usually idiopathic, less common than migraine and causes pain localized usually around the eye, forehead, cheek and temple, with ipsilateral autonomic features (*Table 19.4*). Pain may occasionally be occipital, cervical or scapular. Males are mainly affected and typical features are the onset of severe pain at night, or the clustering of attacks at the same time, night or day,

Table 19.4 Differentiation between migraine and migrainous neuralgia

Migraine	*Migrainous neuralgia*	
Sex mainly affected	Females	Males
Family history	+ve often	–ve
Pain unilateral	Usually	Always
Frequency of attacks	Less than 3 per week	May be daily
Time of attacks	Usually daytime	Often at night
Duration of attacks	Hours to days	Minutes to a few hours
Other features	May be aura, nausea and vomiting	May be nasal congestion and lacrimation

Adapted from Greenhall R.C.D. (1980) p. 1606.

for several weeks. Episodes last from 15 to 180 minutes, and may recur from one to eight times daily. Flushing and/or sweating of the affected side of the face and features such as lacrimation, conjunctival injection and nasal congestion, and Horner's syndrome, may be associated.

Occasional cases of pain mimicking migrainous neuralgia are due to ocular disease, lesions of the trigeminal nerve, lesions of the brain stem, or lesions in the middle cranial fossa near the midline, such as lesions involving the cavernous sinus, circle of Willis, or pituitary, but then are usually atypical in presentation. A neurological opinion is indicated. Migrainous neuralgia should be differentiated from migraine, chronic paroxysmal hemicrania and nasociliaris neuralgia (Charlin's neuralgia; pain at the inner canthus with nasal and conjunctival injection, relieved by topical cocaine and adrenaline applied to the ipsilateral nasal mucosae).

Attacks of migrainous neuralgia are sometimes precipitated by alcohol and, if so, it should be avoided. Nitroglycerin and high altitude may also trigger attacks.

Migrainous neuralgia attacks are managed effectively with oxygen inhalation. Subcutaneous sumatriptan or aerosolled ergotamine are also effective, as sometimes is ipsilaterally applied intranasal lignocaine (*see above*). Corticosteroids, calcium channel blockers, verapamil or lithium are used prophylactically. Pizotifen, beta-blockers, valproate or, rarely, methysergide can also be used.

Chronic paroxysmal hemicrania

This presents in very similar fashion to migrainous neuralgia, but only sometimes at

night and rarely triggered by alcohol. In 20 per cent it follows head injury or whiplash injury, and invariably responds well to indomethacin.

Cranial arteritis (*see* Chapter 16)

OTHER CAUSES OF HEADACHE AND FACIAL PAIN (*see* Table 19.2)

Orofacial pain may be *referred* from the chest, particularly in ischaemic heart disease but occasionally in lung cancer.

Raised intracranial pressure is one of the most serious but also the least common cause of headache. It may be caused by malignant hypertension, a tumour, abscess or haematoma. The headache is severe and often worse on waking, but improves during the day. Nausea and vomiting are common and the headache is aggravated by straining, coughing, sneezing or lying down. Neurological attention is essential.

Meningeal irritation provokes severe headache with nausea, vomiting, neck pain or stiffness (inability to kiss the knees) or pain on raising the straightened legs (Kernig's sign). It is seen in meningitis or subarachnoid haemorrhage. Urgent neurological attention is needed.

Headaches are common after most *head injuries*. These headaches do not normally persist, but if they do, neurological advice must be sought to exclude intracranial haemorrhage. In the absence of neurological complications, persistent post-traumatic headaches may be due to compensation neurosis (Chapters 18 and 22).

Headache is occasionally the presenting feature of *diseases of the skull* such as bony metastases or Paget's disease (Chapter 16).

Headache can be a feature of *systemic disease*, such as any fever, hypertension, chronic obstructive airways disease or some endocrinopathies. Epstein–Barr virus appears to be associated with some headaches in young adults that recur daily but resolve spontaneously within a year (new daily persistent headache). Facial pain may occasionally be drug-induced, for example by vinca alkaloids, phenothiazines or even analgesics (*see* Appendix to Chapter 25).

BIBLIOGRAPHY

Baillie S., Woodhouse K. and Scully C. (1994) Medical aspects of ageing: facial and oral pain. In Barnes I.E. and Walls A. (eds) *Gerodontology*. Oxford, Wright–Butterworths, Oxford, pp. 7–16.

Brandt T. and Peatfield R.C. (1996) Cluster headache and chronic paroxysmal hemicrania. In Brandt T. *Neurological Disorders: Course and Treatment*. New York, Academic Press, pp. 17–27.

Brandt T., Illingworth R.D. and Peatfield R.C. (1996) Trigeminal and glossopharyngeal neuralgia. In Brandt T. *Neurological Disorders: Course and Treatment*. New York, Academic Press, pp. 49–58.

Caplan L. and Gorelick P. (1983) 'Salt and pepper on the face': pain in acute brainstem ischemia. *Ann. Neurol.* **13**, 334–44

Dalessio D.J. (1990) Aspirin prophylaxis for migraine. *J. Am. Med. Assoc.* **264**, 1721.

Diaz-Mitoma F., Vanast W.J. and Tyrrell D.L.J. (1987) Increased frequency of Epstein–Barr virus excretion in patients with new daily persistent headaches. *Lancet* **i**, 411–15.

Diener H.C. and Peatfield R.C. (1996) Migraine. In Brandt T. *Neurological Disorders: Course and Treatment*. New York, Academic Press, pp. 1–15.

Dieterich M. and Pfaffenrath V. (1996) Atypical facial pain. In Brandt T. *Neurological Disorders: Course and Treatment*. New York, Academic Press, pp. 43–7.

Feinmann C. and Harris M. (1984) Psychogenic facial pain. *Br. Dent. J.* **156**, 165–9, 205–9.

Greenhall R.C.D. (1980) Headache and facial pain. *Medicine (UK)* **31**, 1606–10.

Heloe B. and Heiberg A.N. (1980) A follow-up study of a group of female patients with myofascial-pain-dysfunction syndrome. *Acta Odont. Scand.* **38**, 129–34.

Hugoson A. and Thorstensson B. (1991) Vitamin B status and response to replacement therapy in patients with burning mouth syndrome. *Acta Odont. Scand.* **49**, 367–75.

Kittrelle J., Grouse D. and Seybold M. (1985) Cluster headaches; local anesthetic abortive agents. *Arch. Neurol.* **42**, 496–8.

Kost R.G. and Straus S.E. (1996) Postherpetic neuralgia-pathogenesis, treatment, and prevention. *N. Engl. J. Med.* **335**, 32–42.

Lamey P.J., Hammond A., Allam B.F. and McIntosh W.B. (1986) Vitamin status of patients with burning mouth syndrome. *Br. Dent. J.* **160**, 81–4.

Lazar M.L., Greenlee R.G. and Naarden A.L. (1980) Facial pain of neurologic origin mimicking oral pathologic conditions; some current concepts and treatment. *J. Am. Dent. Assoc.* **100**, 884–8.

Maizels M., Scott B., Cohen W. and Chen W. (1996) Intranasal lidocaine for treatment of migraine. *J. Am. Med. Assoc.* **276**, 319–21.

Olesen J. (1988) Classification and diagnostic criteria of headache disorders, cranial neuralgia and facial pain. *Cephalgia* **8**, 1–96.

Olesen J. and Diener H.C. (1996) Tension-type and cervicogenic headache. In Brandt T. *Neurological Disorders: Course and Treatment*. New York, Academic Press, pp. 29–35.

Porter S.R. and Scully C. (1996) *Innovations and Developments in Non-Invasive Oral Health Care*. Northwood, Science Reviews.

Reutens, D.C. (1990) Burning oral and mid-facial pain in ventral pontine infarction. *Aust. NZ Med. J.* **20**, 249.

Schott G.D. (1995) An unsympathetic view of pain. *Lancet* **345**, 634–6.

Scully C. (1982) The mouth in general practice. 3. Oral and facial pain. *Dermatol. Pract.* **1**, 16–18.

Scully C. (1988) *The Dental Patient*. Oxford, Heinemann.

Scully C. (1989) *The Mouth and Perioral Tissues*. Oxford, Heinemann.

Scully C. (1989) *Patient Care: a Dental Surgeon's Guide*. London, British Dental Association.

Scully C. (1990) Oral medicine: pain and neurological disease. In Bell C.J. (ed) *Heinemann Dental Handbook*. Oxford, Heinemann, pp. 426–32.

Scully C., Cawson R.A. and Griffiths M.J. (1990) *Occupational Hazards to Dental Staff*. London, British Dental Journal.

Van der Waal I. (1990) *The Burning Mouth Syndrome*. Copenhagen, Munksgaard.

20

Immunodeficiencies

Key points

- Primary immunodeficiencies are rare genetic disorders of leucocytes. Most common is IgA deficiency, with many affected persons appearing symptomless. Others have recurrent infections.
- Most primary immunodeficiencies present with recurrent often severe infections, often affecting the respiratory tract and skin. Mouth ulcers and sinusitis are common.
- Periodontal breakdown is a fairly common feature in many primary immune defects, particularly those affecting neutrophils (polymorphonuclear leucocytes).
- Iatrogenic immunosuppression is seen in patients on corticosteroids, azathioprine or other immunosuppressive agents, but patients after organ transplants are the most severely immunocompromised.
- Iatrogenically immunocompromised patients have depressed T-lymphocyte responses and are liable mainly to viral and fungal infections, and mycobacterioses.
- Aciclovir by slow i.v. infusion or orally is indicated for severe herpes virus infections in immunocompromised patients.
- Antifungals may be indicated for candidosis and less common mycoses in immunocompromised patients. Fluconazole orally is now frequently the agent of choice.
- Prophylactic antivirals and antifungals may be indicated in profoundly immunosuppressed persons.
- Odontogenic infections are potentially life-threatening in the immunosuppressed patient, and broad-spectrum cover is needed (such as penicillin plus gentamicin).
- Human immunodeficiency viruses (HIV) are retroviruses that infect lymphocytes and brain cells.
- HIV damages CD4 T-lymphocytes.
- Eventually the result of HIV infection is a clinically significant immune defect predisposing to fungal, viral and mycobacterial infections.
- When the CD4 count falls below 200/μl in HIV infection, or when certain marker diseases appear, the diagnosis of AIDS is given.
- In the developed world, HIV predominantly affects male homosexuals, injecting drug users and, to a much lesser extent, haemophiliacs, and children and consorts of HIV-positive patients.
- Heterosexual spread of HIV is increasing, and in the developing world, where the infection is now widespread, is the main route of transmission.
- Diagnosis of HIV disease is from clinical features, confirmed by lymphopenia and a severe T-helper lymphocyte defect (diminished CD4+ cells) and HIV antibodies.
- The main diseases in HIV infection include oral candidosis, *Pneumocystis carinii* pneumonia and disseminated cytomegalovirus infection, and *tumours*, notably Kaposi's sarcoma and lymphomas.

- Oral lesions in HIV disease may be seen at any stage but become more common as the CD4 count falls.
- Most common in HIV disease are candidosis and hairy leukoplakia, and progressive generalized lymph node enlargement.
- Antiretroviral treatment with nucleoside analogues such as zidovudine, dideoxyinosine, dideoxycytidine, stavudine and lamivudine has been the main therapy for HIV.
- Protease inhibitors such as saquinavir, ritonavir, indinavir and nelfinavir now offer additional hope.
- Dental treatment in HIV disease may carry a risk of cross-infection and patients may have problems, including bleeding tendencies, and may be immunocompromised.

Immunodeficiencies are states that result from a defect in the immune response. They are usually acquired, but may have a genetic basis and manifest with recurrent infections.

THE NORMAL IMMUNE RESPONSE

The main activity of the immune response is protection against infections. Leucocytes are central to immune responses. These are dependent on lymphocytes and macrophages and may be *humoral* (antibody) or *cell-mediated*, or often both, while complement and polymorphonuclear leucocytes are essential to phagocytosis. Non-lymphoid cells are central to inflammatory responses.

An enormous spectrum of leucocytes, now more than 70 types, is recognized, defined by their cluster of differentiation (CD) antigens, recognized by monoclonal antibodies and in large part regulated by a range of soluble proteins – cytokines – produced by a variety of cells. Cytokines produced by lymphocytes are termed lymphokines, and those that act between leucocytes are called interleukins.

The movement of leucocytes between the blood and tissues is dependent on a spectrum of leucocyte-endothelial cell adhesion molecules known as selectins, integrins, immunoglobulin gene superfamily (CD2, intercellular adhesion molecules – ICAM – and lymphocyte function antigen 3), and cartilage link protein family (CD44). The activity of leucocytes in the tissues is largely modulated by cytokines such as interleukins, discussed below (*see* Appendix to this chapter).

Humoral immunity

Antibodies are immunoglobulins (Ig) produced by plasma cells derived from B- (bursa-equivalent) lymphocytes. B-cells carry surface immunoglobulins and also receptors for IgG (CD32), and complement activated components C3d (CD21) and C3b (CD35). Antibody production is modulated by T- (thymus-derived) lymphocytes, which either assist (T-helper cells), or moderate (T-suppressor cells). A range of cytokines is involved, at least interleukins (IL) 1 to 7 and B-cell growth factor (BCGF).

Antibodies are immunoglobulins. IgA is secreted by exocrine glands and helps to protect mucosal surfaces. IgG and IgM are essential for protection against bacterial infections, by such functions as neutralizing toxins, activating complement, or promoting phagocytosis (opsonization). Recovery from infections rarely, however, depends on antibodies alone: cell-mediated responses are usually also involved. IgE is important in the mediation of atopic allergy but has a role in defence against parasites. The function of IgD is unclear.

Cell-mediated immunity

Cell-mediated immunity depends on T-lymphocytes which originate in bone marrow but differentiate within, and are under the control of the thymus (hence T). Immunological competence is normally acquired within the thymus and requires the normal functioning of purine metabolism. T-cell proliferation and differentiation is regulated by many cytokines, including interleukins (IL), tumour necrosis factors (TNF), interferons (IFN) and transforming growth factors (TGF) and T-cells can produce lymphokines.

More than 18 interleukins have been identified, most originating from T-cells, some from macrophages, mast cells, B- or other cells. IL-1, IL-6 and IL-8 are pro-inflammatory; IL-2 and IL-9 promote lymphocyte growth; IL-4 and IL-5 are involved in the switching between immunoglobulin isotype production; and IL-10 causes suppression of other cytokine production. IFN-alpha and IFN-beta are antiproliferative for a number of cell types and virally infected cells. IFN-gamma is antagonistic to IL-4, activates macrophages and induces the expression of class II major histocompatibility complex (MHC) antigens.

Circulating T-cells contain T-cell receptor (TCR) genes. Most differentiate into CD4 or CD8 cells. The CD4 cells are mainly helper cells that can induce B-cell differentiation, induce CD8 cytotoxic T-cell proliferation, produce various soluble mediators (lymphokines) and regulate erythropoiesis, but some CD4 are cytotoxic. CD4 helper cells are either TH1 (secrete IL-2 and gamma IFN) and provide help for generation of cytotoxic T-cells involved in type IV immune responses, or TH2 (secrete IL-4,5,6 and 10), which both help B-cells and regulate the production of other cytokines – and thereby the immune response. The CD8 cells are one type of cytotoxic or suppressor T-cells.

Antigens are processed by antigen presenting cells such as Langerhans' cells in epithelia and presented in the context of class I or II major histocompatibility complex (MHC) molecules to T-cells. When activated by antigens, T-lymphocytes produce lymphokines which can modulate the activity of nearby cells, particularly macrophages, and have a variety of other activities. Cell-mediated immunity is particularly important in defence against some intracellular bacteria such as mycobacteria, viruses and fungi, in graft rejection, in graft-versus-host reaction and in delayed hypersensitivity.

Complement

The complement system comprises at least nine plasma proteins, which are activated in sequence (comparable to the blood clotting cascade) by a variety of triggering agents, especially immune (antigen/antibody) complexes. Many biologically active products, including important mediators of inflammation, compounds capable of attracting leucocytes, and others causing cell membrane damage, are liberated. Complement activation is controlled by a variety of inhibitors.

Polymorphonuclear leucocytes and macrophages

These are the dedicated phagocytes which are attracted towards antigens by activated complement following an antigen–antibody reaction. They can ingest and often kill microorganisms coated by specific antibody and activated complement components. Macrophages are intimately involved in antigen-processing and the transference of information to lymphocytes. Polymorphs and macrophages may discharge degradative enzymes (lysosomal enzymes) during phagocytosis or attempted phagocytosis of, for example, immune complexes. Lysosomal enzymes may then cause local tissue damage.

Large granular lymphocytes (null cells)

Large granular lymphocytes (LGL) are non-phagocytic cells which share some of the functions of the phagocytes, by mediating natural killer (NK) cell activity and antibody-dependent cellular cytotoxicity (ADCC). NK cells recognize malignant or foreign cells by a non-immune mechanism. ADCC is the binding and lysis of antibody coated target cells by LGL.

INVESTIGATIONS OF IMMUNODEFICIENCIES

An adequate history together with the physical findings will frequently suggest the nature of disease. Recurrent infections are particularly suggestive of immunodeficiency which may result from a primary abnormality of the immune system or be iatrogenic or secondary to lymphoproliferative HIV, or other diseases.

Preliminary screening comprises:

1. Full blood picture including a differential leucocyte and platelet count.
2. Total serum protein levels.

These are straightforward, routine investigations which can identify gross abnormalities such as neutropenia or leukaemia and show whether total immunoglobulin levels are depressed. More specific investigation may include the following.

1. *Serum levels of individual immunoglobulins*, iso-agglutinin titres (anti-A, anti-B) and antibodies (diphtheria, tetanus, pneumococcal) and electrophoresis.

2. *Lymphocyte count:* total numbers of circulating B- and T-lymphocytes and the helper to suppressor T-cell ratio (CD4:CD8 cell ratio).

3. *Skin testing for delayed hypersensitivity* (cell-mediated immunity) in response to natural antigens (such as tuberculin or *Candida albicans*). Skin testing for delayed hypersensitivity measures not only T-lymphocyte responses but also the afferent (receptor) arc of the cell-mediated immune response. Thus, the majority of adults show delayed hypersensitivity to tuberculin in the tuberculin (Mantoux) test, since they have had previous contact with *Mycobacterium tuberculosis* or BCG. A positive response is generally an index of immunity to the disease and certainly does not mean that mycobacteria are actively causing cell-mediated tissue damage. By contrast, a negative reaction to tuberculin indicates susceptibility to infection or occasionally that there is overwhelming infection.

4. *In vitro tests of cell-mediated immunity:* these include the following.

Lymphocyte transformation is a blastogenic response of sensitized lymphocytes to specific antigens of interest, which include antigens of common micro-organisms such as *Mycobacterium tuberculosis* or *Candida albicans*. Greater numbers of lymphocytes are stimulated by non-specific plant substances known as 'mitogens' (phytohaemagglutinin, PHA; poke-weed mitogen, PWM; concanavalin A, con-A) which can be selected to examine B- or T-lymphocyte responses. The ability of lymphocytes to transform to lymphoblasts (to become activated) when exposed to an antigen is a normal and essential immune response. Lymphocyte transformation does not mean that an antigen is provoking immunologically mediated disease; thus penicillin provokes lymphocyte transformation in over 50 per cent of patients to whom the drug has been given, but only a few of the latter are prone to adverse reactions. Failure of lymphocyte transformation or absence of delayed hypersensitivity reactions after sensitization with appropriate antigens are typical features of immunodeficiency states.

Macrophage migration inhibition factor (MIF) is a lymphokine produced by T-lymphocytes and is used as an *in vitro* test of one aspect of cell-mediated immune function. As with lymphocyte transformation and delayed hypersensitivity, MIF production is a normal response to certain antigens. Failure of MIF production, on the other hand, is significant as it may indicate an immunological deficiency. For example, isolated failure of MIF production to *Candida albicans* is a recognized but rare limited immune defect found in a few patients with chronic mucocutaneous candidosis.

Cell-mediated immune mechanisms are, however, responsible for rejection of organ grafts, contact dermatitis and possibly for tissue damage in some other diseases. The basic problem is therefore to distinguish between cell-mediated 'immunity' (resistance to infection) and cell-mediated 'hypersensitivity' (tissue damage), since both are dependent on the same mechanism. This complex problem remains largely unresolved and the two terms tend to be used interchangeably.

5. *Assays of complement components* (mainly CH50 assay). Primary complement component deficiencies are so rare as to come low in the order of priorities, but a broad idea of the integrity of the complement system is provided by the haemolytic complement level (CH_{50}).

6. *Assessment of polymorph function*, such as assay of chemotaxis, phagocytosis, bactericidal activity and ability to reduce the dye nitroblue tetrazolium (NBT test). The value of *in vitro* neutrophil function tests is limited and mainly of value for uncommon but well-defined disorders such as chronic granulomatous disease.

7. *HIV antibody test.*

IMMUNODEFICIENCY DISEASES

A patient with immunodeficiency is often somewhat grandiloquently referred to as an 'immunocompromised host', but the diseases can be of quite different aetiology:

1. primary (genetically determined or the result of developmental anomalies), which are uncommon or rare; or
2. secondary and caused by disease or immunosuppressive treatment – by far the most common.

Human immunodeficiency virus (HIV) disease and the resultant acquired immune deficiency syndrome (AIDS) is an increasing public health problem worldwide and will soon be a more important cause of immuno-deficiency than malnutrition.

Immune defects can be caused by intrinsic leucocyte defects, disorders affecting leuco-cytes, serum inhibitors of leucocyte function or immunoregulatory cell defects or disor-ders. Immunodeficiency diseases can affect any component of the immune system but often do not produce clinical pictures precisely predictable from the immune defect. Thus in T-cell disorders, cell-mediated immunity is affected but antibody production may also be impaired.

The most important effect of any immuno-deficiency is increased susceptibility to infec-tions, frequently caused by organisms of such low pathogenicity as rarely to affect the normal individual (opportunistic infections). Infections vary in character (*Table 20.1*) as a consequence of:

1. The nature of the immune defect.
2. The kinds of micro-organisms to which the patient is exposed.

Table 20.1	Important causes of opportunistic infections in immunodeficient or immunosuppressed patients

- Viral
  Herpes simplex viruses
  Varicella zoster virus
  Cytomegalovirus
  Epstein–Barr virus
  Human herpes virus 6
  Human herpes virus 8
  Hepatitis viruses
  Human papillomaviruses
  Molluscum contagiosum
- Bacterial
  Mycobacteria
  Staphylococci (especially *S. epidermidis*)
  Pseudomonas spp.
  Klebsiella spp.
  Escherichia coli
  Serratia spp.
  Nocardia
  Bartonella (Rochilimaea)
- Fungal
  Candida albicans and other species
  Aspergillus spp.
  Zygomycosis (mucormycosis)
  Histoplasma capsulatum
  Cryptococcus neoformans
  Blastomyces
- Parasitic
  Pneumocystis carinii
  Toxoplasma gondii
  Leishmanii spp.

3. Attempts at treatment; thus for example, broad-spectrum antibiotics used to control bacterial infections increase the hazard of fungal infections.

PRIMARY (CONGENITAL) IMMUNODEFICIENCY DISEASES

Congenital immunodeficiency diseases can be categorized according to the main type of immune defect, as shown in *Tables 20.2* and *20.3*. The more severe congenital immune defects are all rare and often cause early death, so that they are not relevant to dental practice, except in so far as some are now treated by bone marrow transplantation. Their main features are summarized in *Table 20.4*.

IgA deficiency is considerably more preva-lent than most other immunodeficiency disor-ders and is considered in some detail. Defective

mucociliary function is also important in that it predisposes to sinusitis. Immune defects are also common in some chromosomal anomalies, including Down's syndrome (Chapter 23), Fanconi's anaemia and Bloom's syndrome, and in various rare hereditary metabolic defects.

SELECTIVE IgA DEFICIENCY

Selective IgA deficiency is the most common congenital immunodeficiency disorder and

<table>
<tr><td>

Table 20.2 Main categories of primary (genetically determined) lymphocyte immunodeficiencies

</td></tr>
</table>

- B-cell defects predominantly
  X-linked infantile hypogammaglobulinaemia
  IgA deficiency
  Other Ig deficiencies
  Common variable immunodeficiency
  Transient hypogammaglobulinaemia of infancy
  Hypogammaglobulinaemia after intrauterine infection
- T-cell defects predominantly
  Congenital thymic aplasia (Di George's syndrome)
  Late onset immunodeficiency (thymoma syndrome)[a]
- Combined B- and T-cell defects
  Severe combined immunodeficiency syndromes
  X-linked hyper IgM syndrome
  Ataxia-telangiectasia
  Immunodeficiency with thrombocytopenia and eczema (Wiskott–Aldrich syndrome)
- Complement component deficiencies
- Phagocyte defects
  Congenital neutropenias
  Chronic granulomatous disease
  Chediak–Higashi syndrome
  Leucocyte adhesion defects
  Myeloperoxidase deficiency
  Shwachman syndrome
  Interferon receptor deficiency

[a]Variable type of immunological defect but usually T-cell predominantly.

the prevalence in the normal population may be about 1 in 600. IgA is deficient in both serum and secretions; the levels of other classes of immunoglobulin are often normal or raised when IgA deficiency is compatible with normal health.

In others IgA deficiency may be associated with deficiency of IgG_2 and this appears to predispose to any of the following types of disease:

1. Recurrent bacterial or viral respiratory infections.
2. Atopic disease.
3. Autoimmune disease: coeliac disease, lupus erythematosus, rheumatoid arthritis and Sjögren's syndrome are significantly more common. Autoantibodies frequently form against IgA when blood transfusions or immune globulins are given, and can sometimes cause anaphylactic reactions.

- ## Dental aspects of IgA deficiency

Despite the fact that IgA is the main salivary antibody, reported effects of IgA deficiency

Table 20.3 Conditions exhibiting neutrophil disorders with oral manifestations

Condition	Neutrophil disorder	Oral manifestations
Chediak–Higashi disease	Chemotaxis Phagocytosis	Severe periodontal disease Ulcers
Papillon–Lefevre syndrome	Chemotaxis	Severe periodontal disease
Cyclic neutropenia	Number	Gingival inflammation Ulcers
Benign chronic neutropenia	Number	Gingival inflammation Ulcers
Down's syndrome	Chemotaxis	Periodontal disease
Diabetes mellitus	Chemotaxis	Periodontal disease
Job's syndrome (hyperimmunoglobulin E)	Chemotaxis	Gingival inflammation Ulcers
Chronic granulomatous disease	Cell killing	Gingival inflammation Ulcers
Juvenile periodontitis	Chemotaxis	Periodontal disease
Crohn's disease	Number Chemotaxis	Ulcers
Glycogen storage disease type 1b	Number Chemotaxis	Severe periodontal disease Ulcers
Shwachman (lazy leucocyte) syndrome	Chemotaxis	Periodontal disease Ulcers
Leucocyte adhesion defects[a]	Adhesion	Periodontal disease Ulcers

[a]LAD defect 1 (deficiency of CD18 of LFA-1, Mac 1, p150, 95)
LAD defect 2 (failure to convert mannose to fucose).

Table 20.4   Main features of primary (genetically determined) immunodeficiency diseases

Type or name of syndrome	Immunological function	Clinical effects	Possible oral features
X-linked infantile hypogammaglobulinaemia (Bruton syndrome)	Immunoglobulins of all classes deficient or absent	Recurrent pyogenic infections Hepatitis, CNS viral infections	Sinusitis, absent tonsils, cervical lymph node enlargement, ulcers
Non-X-linked hyper IgM syndrome	IgA and IgE reduced	Neutropenia, thrombocytopenia, liver disease	NR
Common variable immunodeficiency	Variable deficiency of different immunoglobulins	Respiratory infections starting in childhood	Sinusitis, hyperplastic tonsils, cervical lymph node enlargement, oral ulceration
Wiskott–Aldrich syndrome	Deficiency mainly of IgM, IgA and IgE may be increased	Recurrent infections especially by pneumococci, meningococci and *H. influenzae*	Purpura, candidosis, herpetic infections
Transient hypogammaglobulinaemia of infancy	Hypogammaglobulinaemia in early childhood only	Thrombocytopenia, eczema Eczema, food allergies	NR
Hypogammaglobulinaemia after intrauterine viral infections, e.g. rubella	Deficiency usually of only one Ig class (e.g. IgA)	Occasionally increased susceptibility to infection	Enamel hypoplasia
Congenital thymic aplasia (Di George syndrome)	Defective cell-mediated immunity. Ig production also impaired	Viral and fungal infections starting in infancy Cardiovascular defects Hypoparathyroidism	Abnormal facies, bifid uvula Candidosis, herpetic infections
Severe combined immunodeficiency[a]	Defective cell-mediated immunity and hypogammaglobulinaemia	Lack of resistance to all types of infection	Candidosis, viral infections Oral ulceration
Deficiencies of[b] MHC class II CD3, ZAP-70 or TAP-2	Decreased CD4 cells, CD8 cells	Recurrent infections	NR
Immunodeficiency with ataxia telangiectasia	Defective cell-mediated immunity. Ig production impaired	Respiratory infections starting in infancy Ataxia telangiectasia, mental handicap	Sinusitis, oral ulceration
Late onset immunodeficiency	Defective cell-mediated or hypogammaglobulinaemia	Susceptibility to various infections starting late in life Myasthenia gravis, anaemia	Chronic candidosis
IgA deficiency	Variable. Deficient IgA and sometimes IgE or IgG$_2$	Recurrent respiratory infections or atopic allergy or autoimmune disease or normal health	Tonsillar hyperplasia, possibly oral ulceration, herpetic infections
IgG$_2$ subclass deficiency	Defective humoral immunity	Recurrent respiratory infections	Sinusitis
Complement deficiencies C1, C2 or C4	Defects in complement pathways	Tend to be associated with autoimmune disease, especially lupus erythematosus	Possibly oral lesions of lupus erythematosus
C1, C3 or C5 deficiencies		Increased susceptibility to infection	NR
C1 esterase inhibitor deficiency	Abnormal complement activation	Swelling of face and neck Airway obstruction	Swellings
Cyclical neutropenia	Depression of neutrophil count at 21-day intervals	Periodic infections – especially bacterial	Recurrent oral ulceration Periodontitis
Chronic granulomatous disease	Leucocyte killing defect	Infections with catalase-positive bacteria. Lymph node abscesses	Cervical lymph node enlargement and suppuration, enamel hypoplasia

Table 20.4   continued

Type or name of syndrome	Immunological function	Clinical effects	Possible oral features
		Candidosis	Candidosis
Myeloperoxidase deficiency	Leucocyte killing defect	Albinism, recurrent infections, hepatosplenomegaly, thrombocytopenia	Cervical lymph node enlargement, oral ulceration, periodontitis
Chediak–Higashi syndrome	Leucocyte defect of chemotaxis and phagocytosis	Recurrent infection	Periodontitis
Leukocyte adhesion	Adhesion defect		

NR, Not recorded.
[a]Subtypes are caused by deficiencies of enzymes adenosine deaminase or purine nucleoside phosphorylase, involved in purine metabolism.
[b]ZAP-70 is a tyrosine kinase; TAP is a peptide transporter.

on dental caries are conflicting and there is no convincing evidence that caries or periodontal disease are more frequent or severe. Part of the reason for this apparently anomalous situation is that other immunoglobulins may be secreted in saliva. IgA deficiency may be occasionally associated with oral ulcers and herpes labialis.

MUCOCILIARY SYNDROMES

Cilia in the respiratory tract normally clear mucus and act as a defence mechanism. Impairment of this mechanism in some genetic and acquired disorders may lead to chronic sinusitis or other respiratory infections. Examples are Kartagener's syndrome (mucociliary disease and dextrocardia) and intolerance of non-steroidal anti-inflammatory drugs in the Fernand–Widal syndrome.

LEUCOPENIAS

Neutropenia from any cause is also an important determinant of abnormal susceptibility to infection (*Table 20.5*) and is sometimes famil-

Table 20.5   Some causes of leucopenia

- Bone marrow disease
  Leukaemia, other marrow infiltrations and myelofibrosis
  Aplastic anaemia (*Table 5.9*)
  Cyclic neutropenia
- Drugs
  Phenylbutazone
  Co-trimoxazole
  Sulphonamides
  Chloramphenicol
  Cephalothin
  Phenothiazines
  Anti-thyroid drugs
  Phenytoin
  Cytotoxic agents (*Table 17.1*)
- Autoimmune
  Systemic lupus erythematosus
  Felty's syndrome
  Others
- Viral infections
  HIV infection
  Others

ial or congenital. Cyclic neutropenia is a very rare form of leucopenia, which can cause oral manifestations, particularly recurrent oral ulcers.

ACQUIRED IMMUNODEFICIENCIES

Malnutrition is, worldwide, the most common cause of immunodeficiency, but immunosuppressive and other drugs, other iatrogenic problems, various chronic diseases, and HIV and other infections are increasingly important.

IMMUNOSUPPRESSIVE THERAPY

Immunosuppressive therapy is widely used, especially to suppress rejection in organ transplant recipients (bone marrow, kidney, liver, pancreas, heart and heart–lung), to treat autoimmune disorders, to treat connective tissue diseases and to control some tumours, especially lymphoproliferative neoplasms. A variety of drugs are used for immunosuppression, especially corticosteroids, cyclosporin and tacrolimus, while others such as azathioprine, cyclophosphamide and chlorambucil are cytotoxic to a range of cells, including some immunocytes. The actions of immunosuppressive drugs are complex and by no means fully understood but most of them predominantly affect cell-mediated responses and autoantibody production more strongly than normal antibody production. Patients on these agents are clearly immunocompromised and at risk from infections which may spread rapidly and which may be opportunistic (involving micro-organisms that are normally commensal) and may be clinically silent or atypical. Viral, fungal, mycobacterial and protozoal infections are a particular problem though the infections experienced are also influenced by exposure to organisms in the environment and, to an extent, by other treatments. Immunosuppressed patients are also liable to neoplasia, at least some of which is virally related; Kaposi's sarcoma (*Plate 17*), lymphomas and squamous cell carcinomas of the skin and of the lip are more frequent in these patients.

ASPLENIC PATIENTS

The spleen is essential for controlling the quality of erythrocytes in the circulation, being the site of sequestration of effete cells.

It also has an important function in the phagocytosis of micro-organisms and antibody production. Opsonins are produced in the spleen and two in particular, properdin and tuftsin, are protective against certain bacteria such as pneumococci. Splenectomy is carried out after serious splenic injuries, in some haemolytic anaemias, in idiopathic thrombocytopenic purpura, and some lymphomas. The spleen may also become hypofunctional in sickle cell disease and other disorders.

Asplenia predisposes to sepsis in up to 3 per cent, and for many years after the procedure. Children are ten times more likely than adults to develop sepsis. The infection is almost invariably pneumococcal, and rarely emanates from the oral flora. Splenectomized patients are also predisposed to hepatitis C, and tuberculosis, and to some malignant neoplasms.

- **Dental aspects of acquired immunodeficiencies other than HIV disease**

In immunosuppressed patients oral infections can be painful and a potential source of metastatic infections or septicaemia, sometimes fatal. Oral infections can be caused by a variety of organisms but can usually be controlled with topical or systemic antibiotic therapy or sometimes with antiseptics such as chlorhexidine. Mixed infections can often be controlled by a broad-spectrum antibiotic such as topical tetracycline, but this should be given together with an antifungal drug because of the risk of superinfection. Failure to respond to such treatment indicates that the causative bacteria are not sensitive and bacteriological investigation may show infection by bacteroides species, for example. Clindamycin may then be a more suitable choice.

In patients where the main defect is of cell-mediated immunity, mucosal infections by viruses or fungi are particularly common. In the immunodeficient patient, bacteria can produce plaques that clinically resemble thrush. Hairy leukoplakia can be a complication of immunosuppressive treatment. Oral Kaposi's sarcoma and lymphoma are also rare, but squamous carcinoma of the lip is a recognized complication of immunosuppression, especially if there is exposure to strong sunlight.

Dental surgical procedures should therefore be covered with an antibiotic and particular attention should be paid to the possibility of thrombocytopenia with haemorrhagic tendencies and to the risks associated with corticosteroid treatment (Chapter 14).

An oral manifestation of particular note in patients on cyclosporin is gingival hyperplasia.

In patients with a non-functional spleen, or after splenectomy, there is no indication for antimicrobial prophylaxis before dental procedures and, in any event, such prophylaxis might fail. It is important, however, to exclude thrombocytopenia and corticosteroid therapy and, in patients who are iatrogenically immunosupressed as well, there may be a need for antimicrobial prophylaxis

CHRONIC DISEASES

The most common disease associated with weakened resistance to infection is diabetes mellitus, where defective phagocytosis is probably a main factor. Immune responses can also be impaired in a wide range of diseases but particularly in cancers of lymphoid or haemopoietic tissues, as shown in *Table 20.6*, especially as a consequence of their treatment. In some of these diseases, infections such as herpes zoster or candidosis may be the first sign of the underlying immunodeficiency. Many infections cause a degree of immune defect themselves. In other diseases, the immune defect is demonstrable only by specific tests. Thus in active tuberculosis the tuberculin test may become negative (anergy).

NEUTROPENIA, LEUCOPENIA AND AGRANULOCYTOSIS

Leucopenia – low levels of circulating functional leucocytes, either in absolute numbers or as functionally effective cells – is a feature of cytotoxic drug therapy and many

Table 20.6 Secondary immunodeficiencies			
	Main defect		
Disease	*T-cell*	*B-cell*	*Phago-cyte*
• Deficiency states			
Malnutrition	+	–	+
Iron deficiency	+	–	–
Protein loss	–	+	–
• Malignant disease			
Hodgkin's disease	+	–	–
Acute leukaemia	+	±	+
Non-lymphoid cancers	+	–	–
Thymoma	+	+	–
• Infections			
HIV and AIDS	+	–	–
Severe tuberculosis	+	–	–
Leprosy (lepromatous type)	+	–	–
Congenital viral infections	+	–	–
Acute severe viral infections	+	–	–
• Autoimmune disease			
Systemic lupus erythematosus			
Rheumatoid arthritis	+	–	–
Chronic autoimmune hepatitis			
• Miscellaneous			
Drugs	+	–	–
Neutropenia	–	–	+
Diabetes mellitus	–	–	+
Chronic renal failure	+	–	–
Sickle cell disease	–	–	+
Severe burns	+	+	–

diseases (*Table 20.5*). *Agranulocytosis*, the name given to the clinical syndrome resulting from leucopenia, is characterized by abnormal susceptibility to infection and oropharyngeal ulceration. Co-trimoxazole is a relatively common cause of agranulocytosis, although overall this has been an uncommon complication in relation to the scale of use of the drug. Marrow suppression, often irreversible, was an uncommon (but frequently lethal) complication of treatment with chloramphenicol, which should therefore only be given for life-threatening infections where no other antibiotic is effective.

Clinically, agranulocytosis is often sudden in onset and characterized by fever, weakness or prostration and sore throat. Gingival, oral and pharyngeal ulceration with pseudomembrane formation are common features but ulceration can affect any mucous membrane. Lymphadenopathy and sometimes rashes are also features. Later, haemorrhagic necrosis of mucous membranes and respiratory infection may go on to septicaemia as the terminal event. Although infections may be an early feature of acute leukaemia or aplastic anaemia, their clinical picture is more variable and bleeding as a result of thrombocytopenia may be the first manifestation.

Neutropenia can develop in isolation or be associated with other effects of depressed marrow function, notably anaemia and bleeding tendencies, as in acute leukaemia and aplastic anaemia.

The diagnosis is confirmed by blood examination and marrow biopsy and treatment depends on the underlying cause. In the case of drugs the triggering agent must be stopped and this may sometimes allow marrow function to recover. Granulocyte colony stimulating factors (filgrastim, lenograstim, malogramostim) are now available and may be of benefit. The main treatment measure is to control infections, particularly by Gram-negative bacteria, with antibiotics such as ticarcillin, mecillinam or one of the third generation cephalosporins such as cefotaxime.

- **Dental aspects of leucopenias**

Septicaemia is a hazard of leucopenia, particularly in neonates and in patients treated with cytotoxic chemotherapy. Gram-positive oral micro-organisms such as viridans streptococci, mainly *S. mitis* and *S. sanguis II* are increasingly implicated and may lead to serious morbidity and mortality. Predisposing factors appear to be the presence of mucositis, the use of high doses of cytosine arabinoside, and the failure to use intravenous antibiotics at the time of bacteraemia. Infections and ulcers are the main oral manifestations and the management of such patients is similar to that of those with leukaemia. Periodontal disease may be accelerated and minor oral infections may result in gangrenous stomatitis in severe cases.

Complications of septicaemia include adult respiratory distress syndrome, pneumonia, shock or endocarditis, and mortality rates have been as high as 30 per cent. Patients should therefore be nursed in laminar-airflow rooms, and surgical procedures should be carried out under antibiotic cover. Viridans streptococci are usually sensitive to beta-lactams, vancomycin, rifampicin, macrolides, teicoplanin, lincosamides and aminoglycosides but there is increasing resistance to penicillin after prolonged exposure. Penicillin, vancomycin or roxithromycin are usually effective in decreasing the incidence of viridans streptococcus bacteraemia but co-trimoxazole is not.

INFECTION WITH HIV, AND THE ACQUIRED IMMUNE DEFICIENCY SYNDROME (AIDS)

About 20 years into the epidemic of infection with human immunodeficiency viruses (HIV), the virus has spread worldwide to create a global pandemic with the most devastating consequences ever known to mankind. No one is spared some implication, and HIV has transformed life in virtually all aspects, including especially health care, and will continue to do so. Without an effective vaccine or curative treatment, HIV infection will spread everywhere, into all communities, and will wreak havoc, especially for the socially deprived.

AIDS (Acquired Immune Deficiency syndrome) was first recognized in 1981 in young male homosexuals in the USA, though there is now evidence that sporadic cases existed well before that. Cases have been revealed as long ago as 1959 in Africa and the UK. Human immunodeficiency viruses (HIV) are almost certainly the causal agent and infect many cells, especially lymphocytes. HIV antibodies are found in high-risk groups and patients with AIDS. The virus can be transmitted with subsequent disease by blood transfusions containing HIV and the virus can be isolated from most patients with AIDS. Recent controversy suggesting that HIV is not the cause of AIDS is not borne out by detailed epidemiological data and evidence of a tremendously high turnover of HIV and HIV-infected lymphocytes.

HIV damages the immune and the nervous systems and thus presents with opportunistic infections, particularly *Pneumocystis carinii* pneumonia and oral candidosis, and neoplasms, especially Kaposi's sarcoma. After infection with HIV there is usually a long asymptomatic period but the risk of development of severe immunodeficiency, and symptoms of disease, increases with time. Damage to the CD4+ T-lymphocytes produces a profound immunological defect, mainly in cell-mediated immune reactivity, which predisposes to viral, mycobacterial, fungal and parasitic infections. The clinical features of HIV infection, therefore, range from asymptomatic infection through to severe clinical illness and immunodeficiency. Clinical disease is clearly most likely to appear when the CD4 counts fall to low levels, where the infected person has reduced defences for other reasons (such as malnutrition), and where there is exposure to potential pathogens.

A number of definitions of AIDS have been employed. The Centers for Disease Control revised their classification system in 1993 and expanded the surveillance case definition for AIDS among adolescents and adults (Centers for Disease Control, 1993). The new CDC definition includes all patients with CD4 cell counts of less than 200 per microlitre. This simplifies classification, reflects current standards of medical care for HIV-infected persons and enables a more accurate assessment of HIV-related morbidity. Unfortunately it is not universally used.

Virology and immunology

HIV is an RNA virus containing an enzyme which can transcribe nucleic acids in the reverse direction, i.e. DNA from RNA and thus termed 'reverse transcriptase'. The virus therefore is known as a 'retrovirus'. The causal virus originally identified and called HTLV-III/LAV (human T-lymphotropic virus III/lymphadenopathy associated virus) is now termed HIV-1. This virus has now spread to all continents, and a further virus, originally called LAV-2 or HTLV-IV, and now termed HIV-2, which originated in, and is the predominant HIV in, West Africa, has also now spread to Central Africa, Europe, USA, South America and the UK, though at present there are few HIV-2-infected persons reported in developed countries. HIV-1 can be classified into two major groups: M, which contains ten genetically distinct subtypes (A–J), and O, which contains several very heterogeneous viruses. The B virus is found in USA and Europe, E in Central Africa. HIV-2 contains at least five subtypes. Any effective vaccine will need to act against all HIV subtypes.

The HIV viruses are transmitted similarly and have similar biological properties, but differ in antigens and nucleic acids. Both are equally capable of causing disease. HIV-1/HIV-2 co-infection can occasionally arise. However, the remaining discussion relates to HIV-1.

HIV contains several so-called 'core' proteins and is surrounded by an envelope containing 'coat' proteins which can act as antigens. Of the three core proteins, p24 is particularly antigenic and antibodies to this form the basis for most serological testing (the HIV test). The coat proteins are subject to not inconsiderable variability and this has obvious implications for vaccine development. One coat protein, *env*, recognizes the host cell CD4 receptor. HIV binds to, and later damages, host cells bearing the T4 or CD4 receptor. Various chemokines such as CC CKR-5 are also involved in virus-cell attachment. A few patients appear to resist HIV infection, because of altered CC CKR-5 expression.

After primary infection with HIV, acute viraemia results in widespread dissemination of the virus. The virus is trapped in follicular dendritic cells in lymphoid tissue germinal centres and there is expansion of a VB19 subset of CD8 cells that are precursors of HIV-specific cytotoxic T-cells. A range of proinflammatory cytokines including interleukin-6, tumour necrosis factor, gamma-interferon and interleukin-10 are also over-expressed and may represent a protective response against HIV. Dendritic cells are involved in the initiation and propagation of HIV infection in CD4 cells. Cells with the CD4 receptor mainly are helper-inducer T-lymphocytes, monocytes and macrophages, Langerhans' cells, brain glial cells and some colonic cells. Brain tissue, in particular the cells of monocyte-macrophage lineage, can also become infected with HIV and neurological damage may also be mediated by the production by HIV-infected macrophages of factors that affect neuronal cell function or neural transmitters.

HIV damages CD4 cells and thereby predisposes the host to infections. The reduction in CD4+ lymphocytes leads to lymphopenia and a fall in the ratio of helper

(CD4+) to suppressor (CD8+) lymphocytes. The time for the onset of symptoms of AIDS varies from about 6 months to 10 years and may be influenced by titre of HIV infection, patient age, gender, drug habits, immunogenetics and other factors. The average time to development of AIDS is 10–11 years in most adults in the developed world but about 20 per cent develop AIDS within 5 years and a very few (about 2 per cent) appear not to develop AIDS over periods as long as 15 years, mostly because they retain active cytotoxic T-cells.

Transmission

The two main routes of transmission of HIV are by blood and blood products, and by intimate sexual contact.

Blood and blood products

HIV can be transmitted by infected blood or blood products, including plasma, or tissues, such as in transplantation. In developed countries, screening of blood and plasma for HIV antibody, and heat-treatment of clotting factor concentrates, has substantially reduced the risk but some seronegative but infected blood (collected during the incubation period) can still rarely transmit HIV. All HIV antibody-positive individuals are potentially infective and must not be allowed to donate blood, organs for transplantation or semen for artificial insemination. Transmission by contaminated needles and syringes is an important route in injecting drug users and transmission by needlestick injury is an occasional risk for health care workers (*see below*).

HIV can also be transmitted by blood and blood products and tissues; intravenous drug abusers are an increasing risk group (*Table 20.7*). Fortunately, haemophiliacs form only a small proportion of HIV patients; blood for transfusions is now routinely screened for HIV antibody as an indicator of possible infectivity. Children can contract HIV intrapartum or via breast milk.

Intimate sexual contact

HIV is transmitted sexually, particularly by receptive anal intercourse. Semen, saliva and breast milk may also contain HIV. Semen can transmit the infection, but transmission via the orogenital route is not common. The

Table 20.7 Major risk groups in the developed world for HIV infection and other blood-borne viruses

Risk group	Percentage of patients[a]
Men having sex with men	80.5
Intravenous drug abusers	14.3[b]
Transfusion recipients	1.0
Haemophiliacs	0.6
Heterosexual contacts of above groups	0.5
Others (such as immigrants from tropical Africa)	0.2

[a]UK figures (1997).
[b]May also be homo-/bisexual.

major risk groups in developed countries are still promiscuous homosexual or bisexual men – men who have sex with men. Heterosexual intercourse is an important route in Africa and Asia, and is an increasingly important mode of transmission in the developed world.

The epidemiology of HIV infection is similar to that of hepatitis B. Persons infected with HIV, especially those who abuse drugs intravenously or who are sexually promiscuous, may also be co-infected with other agents, including viruses such as human T-lymphotropic viruses I and II (HTLV-1 and HTLV-2), hepatitis viruses and other sexually transmitted diseases.

Homosexual or bisexual men are still the major risk groups for HIV infection in the Western world, but the risk to heterosexuals is growing. In Africa the disease appears to be transmitted *mainly* by promiscuous heterosexual activity. Both female and, particularly, male prostitutes in several areas are frequently HIV-positive. In the developed world, many of the heterosexual cases have been infections contracted on holiday, especially in Africa. Condoms lessen the risk of transmission of HIV, but are by no means completely protective.

Reports that HIV virions were present in a cell-free state in saliva have not been confirmed and saliva contains some inhibitory factors. There is as yet *no* reliable evidence for transmission by saliva (except by bites) or by normal social contact.

Epidemiology

The number of individuals infected with HIV and developing severe disease (i.e. AIDS) continues to rise worldwide. There is an annual increase worldwide approaching 20 per cent but dramatic regional variations. In the Americas the annual increase is about 11 per cent, in Europe it is about 22 per cent, in Africa it is about 26 per cent, but in Asia it is 167 per cent – evidence of the explosion of the epidemic in that region. There is evidence for very high rates of infection in areas such as Thailand. Thus, within the global pandemic are many different epidemics, each with its own dynamics, and each influenced by a range of factors – especially social and cultural issues.

The World Health Organisation (WHO) has estimated that over 3 million HIV cases had occurred worldwide by late 1997, about 1 in every 100 sexually active adults. The difference between numbers estimated and reported is due to under-diagnosis (especially in the developing world), under-reporting and delayed reporting. The WHO has estimated that, by the year 2000, there will be a worldwide prevalence of HIV infection of 40 000 000 of which 90 per cent will be in developing countries, especially Africa and Asia. By 1996, in parts of Africa 1 in 5 adults were already infected with HIV; in the Ivory Coast, AIDS was the leading cause of death of adults; and in Uganda, more than 80 per cent of deaths in adults aged 20–39 years were already caused by HIV. South and South-East Asia are now appearing as a new epicentre for HIV infection; it has been estimated that 18 per cent of adults in the region are HIV-infected (WHO 1995). India, Thailand and Myanmar (Burma) are areas of especially high prevalence. Probably 75 per cent of cases worldwide are located in Africa, about 10 per cent are in Latin America, about 7 per cent in the USA, about 5 per cent in Asia and slightly less in Europe (WHO 1995). Thus, by 1998 worldwide, Africa was the major area of HIV infection, followed by the Americas and Asia. By 2000, Asia is likely to be the major region for HIV infection.

The heterosexual spread of HIV infection continues relentlessly in many countries and is spreading from cities into rural communities. Worldwide, 75 per cent of all infection has been acquired through sexual intercourse, mostly transmitted *heterosexually*, and there is currently a male:female ratio of 3:2. There has been a gradual plateauing of new cases in homosexual males and injecting drug users, at least in Western communities but it appears now that safe sex practices in homosexual males in many countries are not being maintained. About 42 per cent of US cases are still in men who have sex with men. Only about 10 per cent of the global HIV infections have been linked to injecting drug use (IDU), 10 per cent were transmitted perinatally and the remaining 5 per cent were transmitted through blood, principally by transfusion. In the USA, about 26 per cent of cases are in injecting drug users, only 1 per cent in persons receiving blood or blood products.

HIV is thus no longer solely a problem of male homosexuals, is uncommon in recipients of blood or blood products, but is a problem for intravenous drug abusers, and is a rising problem among heterosexuals, particularly those who have unprotected sexual intercourse.

By 1998, well over half a million cases of AIDS had been reported in the USA. It is currently estimated that 60 000–70 000 persons are diagnosed per year as having AIDS in the USA and that HIV infection will continue to spread into the rural communities of the USA. Currently, HIV infection is the commonest cause of death in US men aged 25–44 years, and the third commonest cause of death in women of this age group. UK figures were 29 540 reported cases of HIV by 1997. In the UK, by 1994, HIV infection was already the fourth most common cause of death in men aged 25–44 years.

HIV infection and disease

The common manifestations of HIV infection are mainly infection (particularly fungal, viral, mycobacterial), neoplasms (especially Kaposi's sarcoma and lymphomas – which may be virally induced) and autoimmune disorders. Recent evidence suggests that Kaposi's sarcoma is sexually transmissible, and related to a newly identified virus, human herpes virus 8. The pattern of disease associated with HIV infection varies, not least geographically. For example, histoplasmosis is seen mainly in AIDS patients from endemic areas of the USA. Tuberculosis has been seen mainly in AIDS in Africa. These patterns are changing as a result of the emergence of new pathogens such as multi-drug resistant tuberculosis, and increasing air travel, exotic infections now appearing in temperate zones.

Infection by HIV is initially of CD4 cells, especially T-cells, macrophages, dendritic cells and brain microglial cells. There may be a recognized acute HIV syndrome 3–6 weeks later, with features similar to glandular fever, sometimes with neurological involvement or with a rash or mouth ulcers. Infection may then remain asymptomatic for some time (though patients may be able to transmit the disease), but then persistent generalized lymphadenopathy becomes evident. This latent stage lasts a median time of about 10 years. Finally, as the CD4 count falls to about 500/μl, a variety of clinical syndromes appears, any of which can culminate in AIDS. Oral lesions are common at this stage, including candidosis, hairy leukoplakia and aphthous-like ulcers. Shingles, wart, molluscum contagiosum and thrombocytopenia may also be seen.

With the fall in the CD4 cell count, susceptibility to an enormous variety of infections, mainly with viruses and fungi, otherwise rare tumours and neurological disease becomes evident. The constellation of opportunistic infections, particularly by *Pneumocystis carinii*, and/or Kaposi's sarcoma or other tumours (particularly lymphomas), with severe immunodeficiency is the common pattern (*Table 20.8*).

The current definition of AIDS is any HIV-infected person with a CD4 count below 200/μl as well as any HIV-infected individual with pulmonary TB, recurrent episodes of pneumonia or invasive cervical carcinoma.

Infections
Opportunistic infections with protozoa, mycobacteria, fungi and viruses are common and resistant to treatment. *Pneumocystis carinii* pneumonia (PCP), toxoplasmosis, cryptosporidiosis, tuberculosis, candidosis and cryptococcosis are common.

PCP is a protozoal infection seen in up to 80 per cent of patients and is the immediate cause of death in up to 20 per cent of patients dying with AIDS. Toxoplasmosis, infection

---

Table 20.8   Some opportunistic infections, neoplasms and other complications of HIV disease

- Opportunistic infections

Mucocutaneous[a]	Herpes simplex*
	Herpes zoster
	Cytomegalovirus
	Epstein–Barr virus (EBV)
	Human herpesvirus 8
	Human papillomaviruses
	Molluscum contagiosum
	Non-tuberculous mycobacteria
	Candida albicans
	Staphylococcus aureus
	Histoplasmosis
Gastrointestinal	Cryptosporidiosis
	Microsporidiosis
	Isosporiasis
	Giardiasis
Respiratory	*Pneumocystis carinii*
	Aspergillosis
	Candidosis
	Cryptococcosis*
	Histoplasmosis*
	Zygomycosis (mucormycosis)
	Strongyloidosis
	Tuberculosis*
	Non-tuberculous mycobacterioses*
	Legionellosis
	Pseudomonas aeruginosa
	Staphylococcus aureus
	Streptococcus pneumoniae
	Haemophilus influenzae
	Toxoplasmosis*
	Cytomegalovirus* (CMV)
Meningitis; encephalitis	Creutzfeldt–Jakob agent
	Papova viruses
	Cryptococcus neoformans
	Toxoplasma gondii

- Neoplasms
  Kaposi's sarcoma
  Lymphoma (especially of the central nervous system)
  Squamous cell carcinoma (of anus, cervix and rectum)
  Leukaemia
- Other complications
  Encephalopathy[b]
  Thrombocytopenic purpura[b]
  Lupus erythematosus
  Seborrhoeic dermatitis

---
*May be disseminated.
[a]See Chapter 11 for oral infections.
[b]These are common clinical features of AIDS; up to 60 per cent of patients may manifest symptoms of encephalopathy.

---

with the protozoon *Toxoplasma gondii*, is seen in about 15 per cent of AIDS patients, affecting particularly the CNS. Gastrointestinal infection with other protozoa (cryptosporidia, microsporidia, *Isospora belli*) often produces intractable diarrhoea.

Atypical mycobacteria are found in about 40 per cent of AIDS patients in the West, though double that number are actually infected. Over 95 per cent of these are *Mycobacterium avium* complex (MAC) infections – *M. avium* and *M. intracellulare*. Others may include *M. kansasii*, *M. fortuitum*, *M. marinum*, *M. hemophilum*, *M. gordonae* and *M. xenopi*. In contrast, tuberculosis is particularly common in Africa and is increasing in the West where some 5 per cent of patients are now infected with *M. tuberculosis*. This is increasingly multi-drug resistant (MDR). Since TB can spread by droplets, this is becoming a major public health problem.

Candidosis is extremely common in the mouth (*Plate 18*) and vagina in HIV disease and virtually all patients experience it. *Cryptococcus neoformans* is the main cause of meningitis in AIDS and is especially common in Africa, where 20 per cent of AIDS patients are affected, double the number in the West. Histoplasmosis is seen, usually as disseminated disease, mainly in persons from endemic areas in the Americas. The same applies to coccidioidomycosis.

Herpes virus infections are common in AIDS. Herpes simplex can produce severe erosive lesions around the mouth, genitals, anus or other orifices and may be seen intraorally and in the oesophagus. It can involve the skin and eyes. Herpes zoster can be severe, painful and incapacitating. Cytomegalovirus (CMV), however, is the most dangerous viral infection, capable of widespread lesions, especially ulceration throughout the gastrointestinal tract, and retinitis. EBV is associated with oral hairy leukoplakia (*Plate 19*) and with lymphomas. Patients with HIV infection are also often infected with hepatitis B, C and/or D.

Neoplasms
Kaposi's sarcoma (an otherwise exceedingly rare tumour of endothelial cells among elderly persons) is seen almost exclusively in sexually transmitted HIV infection and is common mainly in male homosexuals with AIDS, but atypical in its early age of onset, distribution (particularly in the head and neck area) and greater malignancy (*Plate 20*).

Lymphomas are also common in AIDS and frequently affect the brain. The incidence of carcinoma of the cervix and carcinoma of the anus is also increased in HIV disease.

Neurological disorders
HIV attacks the brain and nervous system. Patients can develop increasing encephalopathy and ultimately dementia, sometimes in the absence of significant immunodeficiency. CNS opportunistic infections and neoplasms may also be seen.

Up to two-thirds of AIDS patients develop a dementia complex, with dementia, personality changes, ataxia and convulsions. About 15 per cent of AIDS patients develop CNS toxoplasmosis, and 10 per cent cryptococcal meningitis. Some develop lymphomas. Spinal cord disease is seen in about 20 per cent and may progress to bladder and bowel dysfunction. Peripheral neuropathies and myopathy can be seen.

Autoimmune disorders
Autoimmune disease such as thrombocytopenic purpura is relatively common. Drug reactions are common, especially to co-trimoxazole, and may produce erythema multiforme

Paediatric and neonatal AIDS

Children may acquire HIV from exposure to blood or blood products, or occasionally in utero even as early as 20 weeks of intra-uterine life. Later they may be infected by intrapartum transmission from infected mothers.

HIV infection in children causes them to appear ill, stunts their growth and promotes staphylococcal and streptococcal infections such as otitis media, rashes and bouts of diarrhoea as well as fungal and viral infections. AIDS in young children differs from the adult disease in such respects as the following:

1. Humoral immunity is more severely affected. Hypergammaglobulinaemia is also severe and 13 per cent of children have thrombocytopenic purpura.
2. Normal CD4/CD8 ratios may persist late in the disease and lymphopenia is uncommon.

3. Bacterial infections are relatively more common because of depressed humoral immunity and may long precede changes in T-lymphocyte subsets.
4. Asymptomatic infection is less common.
5. Generalized lymphadenopathy and hepatosplenomegaly are often the first signs.
6. Neurological disease develops in the great majority.
7. Interstitial lymphoid pneumonitis is particularly characteristic.
8. B-cell lymphomas are the most common AIDS-associated tumours. Kaposi's sarcoma is rare and particularly rarely affects the skin.
9. Other systemic effects of HIV infection in children include renal disease and cardiomyopathy.
10. Chronic parotitis is a more frequent clinical manifestation than in adults.

Diagnosis of HIV infection

Apart from the history and clinical criteria, laboratory investigations are indicated after appropriate professional counselling. There may be a lymphopenia, reduced CD4 counts in the blood and a reduced CD4/CD8 ratio from a normal of about 2 to about 0.5 in AIDS, but these are not specific findings and HIV infection must be confirmed carefully by testing for HIV. Tests for HIV antibodies or virus (antigens or nucleic acid or virus culture) are available but the 'AIDS test' is for serum antibodies. These tests are affected by even minor variations in technical procedures, and thus great care is called for. In the meantime, indiscriminate screening is discouraged. Testing for HIV antibody is useful for the screening of blood and tissue donors or women in high-risk groups who are contemplating pregnancy, but in other instances any potential advantages should be weighed carefully (with appropriate counselling of patients) against the potential psychological sequelae to patients on learning that they have a potentially life-threatening infection which they can transmit to others. Patients must be counselled before testing and all results must be kept confidential.
The ELISA or agglutination screening tests for serum antibodies to HIV are the first step in sero-diagnosis. Antibodies are usually

detectable from about 6–8 weeks after infection, and most persist for life. The ELISA test has a sensitivity of about 98 per cent and a specificity of about 99 per cent under optimal conditions. It is rapid and easy to use, *but there may be false-positive or -negative results* and therefore a positive ELISA result must be re-tested in duplicate samples and, if two or more of these three ELISA results are positive, a supplemental (confirmatory) test such as Western blotting (immunoblotting) *must* be used. A positive ELISA result with an indeterminate Western blot result is not uncommon, and should be explored using nucleic acid assays. False-positives in both ELISA and Western blotting are seen in only about 1 in 100 000 tests. Indirect immunofluorescence assay (IFA) can allow detection of HIV-specific IgM antibodies as soon as 5 days after the onset of acute HIV illness, but while it is as sensitive and specific as Western blot, IFA does not permit precise delineation of specific patterns of antibody reactivity.
HIV antigens can be detected in the blood earlier than can antibodies, and assays for the p24 and other antigens are now available. However, antigen assays do not offer great benefits in the initial diagnosis of HIV infection and even antigen assays are occasionally negative in HIV-infected persons. Nevertheless, estimation of p24 levels may be a useful surrogate test of antiviral therapy.
Techniques are now also available to detect HIV nucleic acid and can be used to clarify indeterminate Western blot results. For example, the polymerase chain reaction (PCR) is very sensitive and able to detect HIV in HIV-infected but seronegative persons.
HIV can also be detected by *viral culture* or testing for HIV reverse transcriptase but these are not simple tests and lack the sensitivity and reproducibility needed for clinical work. However, they can reveal HIV-1/HIV-2 dual infection.
It is important for diagnosis to:

1. apply at least two methodologically different assays for HIV infection; and
2. repeat the test 2–3 months later.

Absence of HIV antibody usually but not invariably excludes HIV infection. Some patients are infected with HIV but do not appear to produce detectable antibody to it, or lose it as AIDS develops. Therefore, presence of antibody to HIV means that the patient has been infected with the virus; it implies a carrier state but does *not* indicate immunity to HIV. Conversely, the absence of antibody to HIV clearly does not always mean that infection is absent. There are reliable tests for HIV antigen and RNA, but their routine use does not appear to be justified as seronegative HIV-infected patients are so infrequent.

*There **must** be confidentiality regarding the results of any of these tests and the diagnosis of HIV infection or AIDS. No patient with features of HIV infection should be discharged as uninfected solely on the basis of one negative HIV test result, and no patient should be told that they are HIV-infected without the knowledge that the laboratory has confirmed the result of the test using the above criteria.*

• Management of HIV infection

Considerable care is needed regarding the social and psychological consequences of HIV infection. There is no effective treatment yet for the underlying immune defect in HIV disease.

Strategies to attack HIV itself include the use of nucleoside analogues, protease (proteinase) inhibitors and non-nucleoside reverse-transcriptase inhibitors. There is suggestive evidence that early intervention may be of benefit. Current recommendations are that nucleosides should be used in combination as the preferred therapy; protease inhibitors are best reserved for patients with high risk of disease progression. Patients are usually monitored by CD4 counts since these correlate well with clinical progress; at counts below $200/\mu l$ patients are at high risk of *Pneumocystis carinii* infection, and at counts below $100/\mu l$ CMV and *Mycobacterium avium–intracellulare* are risks. Other disease markers include beta$_2$-microglobulin, neopterin and tumour necrosis factor.

Nucleoside analogues
Several nucleoside analogues active against retroviruses have been developed. Unfortunately, HIV has an inherent tendency to develop drug-resistant variants and

adverse effects from drug therapy are not uncommon. Cost is also high.

Zidovudine: The most promising management of HIV infection was thought to have been inhibition of HIV using agents such as zidovudine – a dideoxynucleoside analogue that inhibits the reverse transcriptase enzyme. Zidovudine is inactive until phosphorylated intracellularly, when it interferes with viral replication. Zidovudine was thought to decrease the frequency of opportunistic infections, increase the medial survival after diagnosis of AIDS, slow the progression of HIV-infected patients to AIDS and reduce the frequency of opportunistic infections, neural disease and malignancies. Of concern has been the conclusion of a detailed European (Concorde) study that zidovudine offered no significant clinical advantage in symptomless HIV-infected patients. A further study also confirmed this lack of benefit. It is possible, however, that zidovudine may be of benefit if given very early in the course of HIV infection and it appears to reduce the transmission of HIV to the fetus in HIV-infected mothers.

The main adverse effect from zidovudine is bone marrow suppression but nausea, vomiting, headache, fatigue, confusion, malaise and myopathy can also be serious adverse effects. Furthermore, with continued use of zidovudine, HIV develops increasing *in vitro* resistance and this is associated with clinical deterioration. Resistant strains particularly appear after more than 6 months of zidovudine therapy and are seen in more than 90 per cent of patients who have received zidovudine for more than 18 months. Fortunately, HIV may regain susceptibility to zidovudine after a period of discontinuing the drug.

Didanosine: Didanosine (dideoxyinosine, ddI) is another nucleoside analogue inhibitor of HIV with an action activity similar to that of zidovudine. It can improve cognitive function in HIV-induced cognitive impairment, promote weight gain, reduce p24 antigenaemia and increase CD4+ lymphocyte counts. The most frequent adverse effects of ddI are abdominal cramps and diarrhoea due to the osmotic effects of the drug vehicle. Other major treatment-limiting toxicities have included painful peripheral neuropathy, acute pancreatitis and hepatotoxicity. *In vitro* HIV resistance to didanosine may emerge but emergence of resistance to didanosine may be accompanied by renewed susceptibility to zidovudine. Patients with asymptomatic HIV infection or AIDS-related complex and receiving didanosine have significantly fewer opportunistic infections than patients receiving zidovudine, and the length of time to the development of a new opportunistic infection is significantly longer.

Zalcitabine: Dideoxycytidine (ddC) (zalcitabine) is another nucleoside analogue inhibitor of HIV reverse transcriptase, available for patients refractory or intolerant to zidovudine. Adverse effects include rash, oral ulceration, fever, peripheral neuropathy and, rarely, pancreatitis.

Other nucleoside analogues and regimens: Stavudine (D4T) and lamivudine (3TC) are newer analogues. The clinical benefits of dideoxynucleoside analogues in combination have been demonstrated. The ACTG 175 trial in North America, and the Delta trial in Europe and Australia, have shown the superiority over zidovudine monotherapy of both zidovudine/didanosine and zidovudine/zalcitabine. Also superior is zidovudine/lamivudine combination.

Protease (proteinase) inhibitors

HIV protease inhibitors proved to be a major advance in therapy against HIV. Two of the protein products of HIV are known to be precursor proteins that are cleaved by a proteinase enzyme to produce proteins essential to virus replication, such as reverse transcriptase, integrase and structural proteins of HIV. Inhibitors of this proteinase are active at interfering with HIV replication, resulting in immature HIV, incapable of infecting new cells. All must be used with a nucleoside analogue inhibitor of HIV, since otherwise resistance arises within 12 weeks. Drug costs are high. All can cause dysrhythmias in patients using terfenadine and can exacerbate diabetes.

The first developed, saquinavir, is very active *in vitro* but less so *in vivo* because of poor gut absorption, and rapid liver metabolism. Newer protease inhibitors including ritonavir, indinavir and nelfinavir, are more actively antiretroviral than saquinavir, but have adverse effects. Ritonavir has been associated with gastrointestinal symptoms and may cause peripheral neuropathy. Indinavir may produce nephrolithiasis.

Non-nucleoside reverse-transcriptase inhibitors

Preliminary studies suggest benefit from these newer agents, which include nevirapine, atevirdine and phosphonylmethoxypropyladenine.

Antimicrobial prophylaxis, therapeutic and supportive treatment may prolong and improve the quality of life. Co-trimoxazole is used for prophylaxis and treatment of PCP, alternatives being pentamidine isethionate, atovoquone or clindamycin/pyrimethamine. Rifabutin is used as prophylaxis against MAC infection, isoniazid against TB. Fluconazole is often used as prophylaxis against fungal infections. Aciclovir may be used against herpes simplex and zoster infections.

Attempts are being made to produce a vaccine against HIV but, even if it can be made, it is unlikely to become available within at least the next 5 years. The main problems in the development of a safe and effective vaccine are that HIV is within lymphocytes and other cells and thus protected from immune defences, and that the proteins of HIV can undergo changes. A number of candidate vaccines are currently in the initial phases of testing in man to assess their immunogenicity and toxicity and to date, while toxicity has not been a problem, the potential immunogenicity of the various vaccines is still unclear. Post-exposure vaccination (e.g. with killed virus, envelope subunits or recombinant vaccinia vectors in combination with viral subunits) may have produced some clinical benefit, but long-term detailed trials are still required before it is known if such vaccines can provide reliable control of HIV.

As yet the only reliably effective prophylaxis is avoidance of sexual promiscuity (particularly in high-risk countries such as Africa) and dangerous practices such as unprotected intercourse, especially anal intercourse. Also important is to avoid, if possible, transfusions or invasive surgical procedures in high-risk countries. Giving zidovudine prophylactically after exposure to the virus may be beneficial.

• Dental aspects of HIV infection

Dental treatment should be carried out with the precautions outlined in Chapter 11 and

Table 20.9   Oral manifestations in HIV disease

Common	Less common	Rare
Cervical lymphadenopathy	Herpes viruses	Mycobacterial, cryptococcal or histoplasmal ulcers
	Herpes simplex	Addisonian pigmentation
Candidosis	Herpes zoster	Osteomyelitis
Hairy leukoplakia	Cytomegalovirus	Cranial neuropathies
Kaposi's sarcoma	Human papillomavirus	
	Periodontitis and gingivitis	Other infections
	Recurrent ulcers	
	Lymphomas	
	Parotitis	
	Xerostomia	

additional attention given to the possibility, though small, of postoperative infection and prolonged haemorrhage. Patients with profound immunodeficiency may require an antibiotic cover before surgery or after maxillofacial injuries. Aspirin should be avoided as it may aggravate the bleeding tendency.

Based on current evidence, casual person-to-person contact appears to pose no risk of transmission of HIV. Sexual intercourse appears to be the only type of interpersonal contact likely to lead to transmission of HIV infection, and there are now several studies that have failed to demonstrate HIV transmission from infected patients to family members through normal social contact.

Therefore, from the viewpoint of dental practice, the chief occupational risk of acquiring the infection is as a result of injury by a sharp instrument, particularly a local anaesthetic needle which can contain a significant amount of contaminated fluid. However, though needle-stick injuries can transmit the virus, infection among health personnel caring for HIV-infected patients is rare despite reports of many such injuries. In most health care workers who have acquired HIV, the infection has been sexually transmitted.

The risk of transmission of HIV occupationally (less than 1 per cent) appears to be far lower than the nearly 26 per cent of persons who develop hepatitis B infection or the 10 per cent who contract hepatitis C infection after a contaminated needle-stick injury. There have been, as yet (1998), only two reports of dental staff contracting HIV as a consequence of occupation, even in endemic areas.

HIV does appear to have been transmitted within health care facilities on rare occasions. One dentist with HIV infection in the USA appears to have transmitted it to at least 6 patients as a consequence of invasive dental procedures. That the dentist was the source of the infection was suggested by the fact that the strain of the virus was the same. The precise mode of transmission remains uncertain as the dentist has since died. Many other studies, however, have shown *no* evidence of any transmission of HIV from HIV-infected dentists to patients.

Oral manifestations: The majority of patients with HIV disease have head and neck and oral manifestations at some time (*Tables 20.9, 20.10*).

Cervical lymph node enlargement: Lymphadenopathy is an almost invariable feature of HIV disease and AIDS.

Infections: Oral candidosis (usually thrush or erythematous candidosis) is common in HIV disease and AIDS, is often the initial manifestation, and is seen in 50 per cent of patients (*see Plate 18*). Oral candidosis is frequently associated with oesophageal candidosis and is also a predictor of liability to systemic opportunistic infections. Conventional antifungal treatment is indicated initially, although fluconazole may be required, especially if there is oesophageal infection. Azole resistance is an increasing problem.

Infections with herpesviruses – herpes simplex virus, varicella zoster virus, cytomegalovirus, Epstein–Barr virus, human herpes virus 6 (HHV-6) and a new herpes virus associated with Kaposi's sarcoma (KSHV or herpes virus 8) – are also common

Table 20.10   The more common oral manifestations of HIV infection

Condition	Features	Diagnosis	Management
Candidosis	White removable lesions or red lesions, typically in the palate, but anywhere	Clinical plus investigations; smear, culture, rinse, or biopsy	Antifungals
Hairy leukoplakia	White non-removable lesions almost invariably bilaterally on the tongue	Clinical plus investigations; cytology or biopsy	None usually
Periodontal disease	Linear gingival erythema, necrotizing gingivitis or periodontitis	Clinical	Oral hygiene, plaque removal, chlorhexidine, metronidazole
Herpesvirus ulcers	Chronic ulcers anywhere but often on tongue, hard palate or gingivae	Clinical plus investigations; cytology, EM, or biopsy	Antivirals
Aphthous-like ulcers	Recurrent ulcers anywhere but especially on mobile mucosae	Clinical plus investigations; possibly biopsy	Corticosteroids or thalidomide or granulocyte colony stimulating factor
Papillomavirus infections	Warty lesions	Clinical plus investigations; possibly biopsy	Excise or remove with heat, laser, or cryoprobe, or podophyllin
Salivary gland disease	Xerostomia and sometimes salivary gland enlargement	Clinical plus investigations; sialometry, possibly biopsy	Salivary substitutes and/or pilocarpine
Kaposi's sarcoma	Purple macules leading to nodules, seen mainly in the palate	Clinical plus investigations; biopsy	Chemotherapy, usually vinblastine
Lymphomas	Lump or ulcer in fauces or gingivae	Clinical plus investigations; biopsy	Chemotherapy or radiation or both

in HIV disease and AIDS. Saliva from affected patients usually contains CMV, HSV, HHV-6 and EBV, and sometimes hepatitis viruses as in other immunocompromised patients.

Herpes simplex infections are usually intra-oral, sometimes severe and persistent but rarely disseminate: they usually respond well to aciclovir. Severe herpes zoster may be seen. CMV may cause mouth ulcers. EBV has been implicated in hairy leukoplakia and some lymphomas (*see below*). Hairy leukoplakia, though characteristic of HIV, can be seen rarely in other patients, mainly in other immunocompromised persons. It derives its name from the raised white areas of thickening, usually on the lateral borders of the tongue (*see Plate 19*). It appears not to be premalignant.

Less common oral and perioral infections include venereal warts, mycobacterial oral ulcers and oral histoplasmosis or cryptococcosis, as well as sinusitis, gingivitis or periodontitis. Chronic parotitis is common

mainly in children with HIV infection and may be associated with xerostomia. Aphthous-like ulcers may be seen. Post-extraction infections, osteomyelitis after jaw fractures and cancrum oris (noma) have been seen in severely immunocompromised persons.

Neoplasms: Kaposi's sarcoma, an endothelial cell tumour, is the characteristic malignant neoplasm found in AIDS and in 50 per cent of patients is oral or peri-oral. Kaposi's sarcoma is often an early oral manifestation, presenting as a red or purple macule or a nodule, usually on the palate (*see Plate 20*).

Oral and salivary gland lymphomas also develop more frequently in patients with AIDS than in a normal population; EBV is implicated.

Oral features of childhood HIV disease
Parotitis: As mentioned above, chronic parotitis is common in affected children and virtually pathognomonic of AIDS.

Table 20.11 Possible drug interactions in HIV-infected patients (*see also* Chapter 25)		
Drug used in oral health care	*May interact with*	*Possible consequence*
Azoles (flu-, itra-, keto- or mi- conazole)	Astemizole Cisapride Terfenadine	All produce dysrhythmias and cardiotoxicity
Benzodiazepines	Azoles Indinavir Ritonavir	All increase sedation
Fluconazole*	Rifabutin	Uveitis from rifabutin toxicity
Itraconazole*	Antacids	
Ketoconazole*	DDI H$_2$-antagonists Omeprazole	All decrease absorption of the azole
Metronidazole	Ritonavir liquid	Disulphiram reaction

*All may potentiate anticoagulants.

Candidosis: Chronic oral candidosis is present in 75 per cent and is the single most common mucocutaneous manifestation of HIV infection in children. Most types of oral candidosis may be seen but most frequently it is in the form of persistent thrush. Difficulties in swallowing usually indicate involvement of the oesophagus.

Herpetic stomatitis: Unlike normal children, those with AIDS are frequently subject to recurrent intraoral as well as labial herpetic infection. Initially the infection responds to intravenous aciclovir but becomes more resistant as AIDS progresses.

Herpes zoster: Shingles is rare in normal children, but can be an early sign of AIDS in a child, and tends to be more severe and painful.

Drug interactions.
Interactions that can occur with drugs used in oral health care are shown in *Table 20.11*.

IDIOPATHIC CD4 T-LYMPHOCYTOPENIA (ICL)

ICL is a rare syndrome associated with CD4 counts around 300/μl, in the absence of any infection with HIV, other known retroviruses, or other recognized causes of immune defect. Patients usually also have decreased numbers of CD8 and B-cells with normal or decreased immunoglobulin levels. There is no evidence for transmissibility and many patients remain asymptomatic. In others, opportunistic infections may be seen. ICL does not progress and may even improve spontaneously.

CANDIDOSIS

Thrush was aptly described in the nineteenth century as a 'disease of the diseased' and candidosis can certainly be a reflection of impaired immune responses. The importance of candidosis has become particularly evident since AIDS was first recognized. However, the most common form of candidosis (denture-induced stomatitis) is seen in patients who are usually otherwise healthy.

Oral candidosis can produce a variety of clinical pictures and can sometimes be secondary to an underlying disorder. The main types that may be seen in dental practice are as follows.

1. Thrush.
2. Erythematous candidosis.
3. Angular stomatitis.
4. Denture-induced stomatitis.
5. Candidal leukoplakia (chronic hyperplastic candidosis).
6. Rare mucocutaneous candidosis syndromes.

Thrush
Thrush is the best-known type of candidosis and produces the highly characteristic picture of soft, creamy-coloured, slightly raised patches which can be wiped off the mucosa leaving red areas. These lesions may form

isolated flecks or large confluent areas. Typical sites are the buccal mucosa or the soft palate.

Thrush is common in the newborn, in whom it may resolve spontaneously or in response to topical antifungal treatment. In adults, unless known to be having immuno-suppressive treatment, thrush is rare and should prompt investigation for an underlying cause. Thrush in a young or middle-aged adult, particularly a male homosexual, must be regarded as a sign of HIV infection until proved otherwise. The other main possibilities are antibiotic treatment, anaemia, diabetes mellitus or an immunological defect, as shown in *Table 20.6*.

The diagnosis can be readily confirmed by taking a Gram-stained smear which shows long tangled masses of candidal hyphae.

In addition to treatment of any underlying disorder the local infection should be manageable with topical antifungal drugs such as nystatin lozenges (500 000 U), nystatin pastilles (100 000 U) or amphotericin lozenges (10 mg) allowed to dissolve slowly in the mouth four times daily for a week or longer if necessary. Alternatively, a nystatin suspension (100 000 U/ml) or systemic fluconazole may be indicated.

Occasionally patches of thrush are present under a denture in association with denture stomatitis, but if not unusually severe or widespread are unlikely to be the result of any underlying systemic disorder.

Erythematous candidosis
Mucosal erythema due to candidal infection can result from antibiotic treatment, xerostomia or coverage of the mucosa with a denture. It is sometimes seen on the palate or tongue in HIV infection.

Antibiotic stomatitis occasionally follows the use of broad-spectrum antibiotics, particularly tetracycline used topically in the mouth. The whole of the oral mucosa is then typically red, oedematous and sore. One or two flecks of thrush may be found in protected situations, such as the posterior upper buccal sulcus. As with any other type of candidosis, angular stomatitis may be associated.

The treatment is to stop the use of the antibiotic, if feasible, or alternatively to give topical antifungal drugs as described earlier.

A similar picture of generalized redness and soreness of the oral mucosa is the typical manifestation of candidosis associated with xerostomia.

Angular stomatitis (angular cheilitis)
This is most frequently seen in dental practice as a complication of denture-induced stomatitis. However, angular stomatitis can be seen in association with any type of intraoral candidosis and is the only feature which they all share in common. In addition, angular stomatitis is a 'classic' sign of iron deficiency anaemia, though, in practice, this is infrequently found in patients with denture stomatitis. However, angular stomatitis is very occasionally an isolated initial sign of anaemia, such as vitamin B_{12} deficiency. Angular stomatitis is very occasionally seen in isolation, when it may be staphylococcal rather than candidal.

It is important to consider the possibility of underlying systemic disease, and treat it where possible. Clearance of intraoral candidosis with adequate antifungal treatment typically leads to healing of the lesions at the angles of the mouth without any local treatment but miconazole cream applied to the lesion may be useful. Occasionally, bacteriological examination may be necessary, but imidazoles such as miconazole or clotrimazole also have antibacterial activity and may be effective.

Denture-induced stomatitis
Denture-induced stomatitis (denture sore mouth) is a common candidal infection secondary to long-standing occlusion of part of the oral mucosa by a denture. There is no convincing evidence that trauma is a factor. Denture stomatitis is seen only rarely under a lower denture, in spite of the fact that the latter is a common cause of trauma. Denture-induced stomatitis typically develops beneath a well-fitting upper denture which effectively cuts off the mucous membrane from the normal oral defence mechanisms.

The characteristic feature is uniform bright erythema of the whole of the upper denture-bearing area and limited by the denture margin. Occasionally the erythema is patchy or there may be flecks of thrush. Symptoms are typically absent but occasionally there is associated soreness.

Angular stomatitis is frequently associated but may be intermittent and absent when the patient is first seen. In patients with deep folds at the angles of the mouth as a result of ageing, inflammation may spread for a centimetre or so along the fold, producing a conspicuous line of erythema. In other cases there may be cracking, bleeding or prominent crusting. In such cases there may be a mixed staphylococcal and candidal infection.

The vast majority of patients with denture stomatitis are healthy, as local factors determine the pathogenesis. Occasionally, patients may be anaemic but less frequently than might be expected from the fact that angular stomatitis is often regarded as a typical sign of iron deficiency. Other occasional underlying factors are dry mouth, diabetes mellitus or immune defects. It is, however, unjustifiable to screen all patients with denture stomatitis but investigation should be considered if the patient has any other complaints suggestive of such disorders or if the infection is particularly severe or intractable.

Treatment includes leaving dentures out of the mouth at night and storing them in hypochlorite to clear the fungus from the denture surface. Topical antifungals should also be used, as suggested above.

Candidal leukoplakia (chronic hyperplastic candidosis)

This appears as white plaques sometimes clinically indistinguishable from other types of keratotic lesions though they may be speckled. These candidal plaques appear quite different from those of thrush in that they are tough and firmly adherent. Most patients are men of middle age or over, and many are heavy smokers. Typical sites are the buccal mucosa just within the commissures, or the dorsum or edges of the tongue. Long-standing angular stomatitis and occasionally also denture stomatitis may be associated. Patients are usually otherwise well.

Diagnosis of candidal leukoplakia depends on biopsy when hyphae of *Candida albicans* and a characteristic inflammatory reaction can be seen in the superficial epithelial plaque. Investigation should include a family history, haematological examination and, possibly, tests for cell-mediated responses to *C. albicans*. In the great majority of cases no

abnormality is detectable but such investigations may be needed to exclude one of the rare mucocutaneous candidosis syndromes which show similar oral lesions as described below. Treatment is difficult as the response to topical antifungal drugs such as nystatin or amphotericin is poor. Excision is also followed by recurrence, but antifungals such as miconazole topically or ketoconazole or fluconazole systemically appear to be more effective.

These lesions may account for up to 10 per cent of leukoplakias and several reports of apparent malignant transformation have appeared. However, the prevalence of candidal leukoplakia and its potentialities remain uncertain.

Candidosis in immune deficiency states

Persistent oral candidosis is a well-recognized complication of defective cell-mediated immunity and may be seen in the following circumstances.

1. As a complication of primary immunodeficiencies, especially severe combined (Swiss) type or Di George's syndrome. In these conditions candidosis is not the main feature of the disease and is only one of many complications. Such patients are unlikely to be seen in dental practice.
2. As a common complication of intense immunosuppression, particularly for organ grafts. Both thrush and herpetic infection may be present together and produce confluent lesions. In most cases, the candidal infection responds eventually to antifungal drugs but sometimes immunosuppressive treatment has to be moderated for a time. Patients on long-term corticosteroid treatment for any of the immunologically mediated diseases are also susceptible to oral candidosis, but not often as a serious problem.
3. HIV infection (*Table 20.8*)
4. Chronic mucocutaneous candidosis (CMCC). In this group of disorders candidosis is the main or a prominent feature (*Fig. 20.1*). Various types of defects of cell-mediated immunity may be detected, particularly in the more severe cases, as discussed later, but are not, however, invariably present.

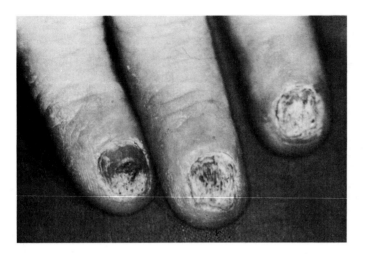

Fig. 20.1 Chronic candidosis affecting the nails in a patient with chronic mucocutaneous candidosis

The main types of these rare disorders and their salient features are summarized in *Table 20.12*. In all of them, candidosis, even if relatively mild, is persistent and responds poorly to topical treatment with nystatin or amphotericin but may respond to ketoconazole or fluconazole. In general, the more severe the infection, the greater the likelihood that immunological defects (particularly of cell-mediated immunity) will be found. However, in some cases these defects are secondary to the infection and so-called antigenic overload.

Early onset chronic mucocutaneous candidosis
The early onset forms of CMCC (types 1–3) typically have the following features in common.

1. Onset in infancy, often as persistent thrush.
2. Candidosis is mainly or entirely oral.
3. Immunological defects sometimes associated.

In the *diffuse type*, candidosis is particularly severe and can give rise to gross, proliferative and disfiguring lesions of the skin (so-called granulomas) as well as widespread oral lesions. Immunological defects are frequently found and there is also susceptibility to bacterial infections of the respiratory tract or elsewhere. Even in this unusually severe form of the disease, candidosis remains superficial and does not progress to candidal septicaemia or other types of disseminated infection.

Table 20.12	Chronic mucocutaneous candidosis (CMCC) syndromes
Type	*Clinical features*
Familial	Persistent oral candidosis Often iron deficiency
Diffuse (Candida granuloma)	Severe chronic candidosis Susceptibility to bacterial infections
Candidosis-endocrinopathy syndrome	Mild chronic oral candidosis Hypoparathyroidism Hypoadrenocorticism
Candidosis-thymoma syndrome	Chronic oral candidosis Myasthenia gravis Haematological disorders

There is also the possibility – though small – that a patient with chronic candidosis has one of the rare disorders such as the candidosis-endocrinopathy syndrome. In these diseases candidosis (when present) probably invariably involves the mouth, which is often the most severely affected site.

Candidosis-endocrinopathy syndrome has been the source of considerable misunderstanding. Candidosis is typically the initial feature and is usually mild but persistent. Endocrine disorders may not appear until 10 or 15 years later, but occasionally this sequence is reversed. There is no evidence that candidosis causes the endocrine disorders or vice versa. Hypoparathyroidism or Addison's disease or both are the most commonly associated endocrinopathies.

Table 20.13 Orofacial lesions in important deep mycoses

Disease	Organism	Source	Main endemic areas	Orofacial lesions	Clinical forms	Pathology	Prognosis
Aspergillosis	Aspergillus fumigatus, A. flavus, A. niger and other Aspergillus spp.	Ubiquitous	Worldwide	Aspergilloma in paranasal sinuses. Invasive rhinocerebral type may invade palate	Allergic bronchopulmonary Pulmonary Disseminated Aspergilloma	Invasion of blood vessels causing infarcts	Variable Poor in invasive pulmonary or disseminated types or in the immunocompromised
Blastomycosis	Blastomyces dermatitidis	Soil	Mississippi and Ohio valleys in USA, Canada, North Africa and Venezuela	Ulcers	Cavitary pulmonary Disseminated Others	Granulomatous inflammation Chronic suppuration, especially of skin lesions	Often good except in disseminated form
Coccidioidomycosis	Coccidioides immitis	Soil	Southwestern USA, Mexico, Latin America	Ulcers	Acute pulmonary Disseminated Chronic pulmonary Meningitis	Granulomatous inflammation Chronic suppuration	Often good except in meningeal forms or the immunouncompromised
Cryptococcosis	Cryptococcus neoformans	Soil, pigeon droppings	Worldwide	Ulcers	Pneumonia Meningitis Disseminated Cryptococcoma	Granulomatous inflammation	Poor especially in meningeal forms or the immunocompromised
Histoplasmosis	Histoplasma capsulatum	Soil, bird and bat droppings	Mississippi and Ohio valleys in USA,Latin America, Africa, India, Far East, Australia	Ulcers or lumps	Benign pulmonary Disseminated Chronic pulmonary Cutaneous	Granulomatous inflammation Yeast cells in macrophages	Usually good except in disseminated form or the immunocompromised
Mucormycosis	Mucor, Rhizopus and Absidia	Ubiquitous	Worldwide	Rhinocerebral form may cause swelling, necrosis, or destruction of palate Ulcers	Rhinocerebral Pulmonary Gastrointestinal	Invasion of blood vessels to cause thrombosis and infarction	Variable
Paracoccidioidomycosis (South American blastomycosis)	Paracoccidioides brasiliensis	Soil	South America, esp. Brazil		Pulmonary Disseminated	Granulomatous inflammation	Usually good in young patients
Sporotrichosis	Sporothrix schenkii	Associated with thorny plants, wood, sphagnum moss	Worldwide, especially in tropical countries	Rare	Lymphocutaneous Localized cutaneous Pulmonary Disseminated	Granulomatous inflammation and chronic suppuration	Good

This coincidental association between chronic candidosis and hypoparathyroidism (type I polyendocrinopathy syndrome), also seen in the Di George syndrome, has given rise to the myth that hypoparathyroidism predisposes to candidosis. However, treatment of hypoparathyroidism has no effect on candidosis and hypoparathyroidism from any other cause is not associated with candidosis. Branchial arch defects in DiGeorge syndrome affect both thymus (and thymocytes) and parathyroids.

The endocrine disorders in candidosis-endocrinopathy syndrome are associated with multiple organ-specific autoantibodies both in patients and unaffected relatives (Chapter 21).

Patients may for long appear to be quite well apart from chronic oral candidosis. If, therefore, a patient, particularly a child or adolescent with chronic oral candidosis, has a family history of any of the associated disorders, and autoantibodies (particularly to glandular tissues) are found, then it is probable that endocrine disease will develop in the future. The candidosis can be treated with topical antifungal agents such as miconazole, or systemically with oral ketoconazole or fluconazole.

An adult with chronic oral candidosis may have the familial form of the disease, which can escape diagnosis until middle age unless enquiry is made as to whether siblings are affected and whether there was any parental consanguinity, as the disease appears to be autosomal recessive. In familial candidosis investigation for iron deficiency should be carried out, since treatment with iron may improve the response to antifungal drugs.

Late onset chronic mucocutaneous candidosis
Chronic candidosis in the older patient can be the first manifestation of a thymic disorder. Evidence of impaired cell-mediated immunity, particularly to *C. albicans*, may then be found. In such a case investigation for a thymoma should be carried out, as early excision may improve the prognosis.

In summary therefore, it may be helpful to know whether any patient with chronic candidosis has any immunological defect, as the latter may sometimes be indicative of underlying disease. However, isolated unresponsiveness to antigens of *C. albicans* seems also to be a specific, limited immunological deficiency compatible with otherwise normal health.

'Chronic candidosis syndrome'

Many normal persons harbour *Candida albicans* as part of their normal microflora. This finding has been exploited, particularly in the USA, as a supposed explanation of such symptoms as headaches, fatigue and lassitude, rashes and gastrointestinal symptoms. This so-called syndrome has absolutely *no* scientific basis. There is no evidence that antifungal treatment is warranted and a controlled trial has shown that it has no effect on the symptoms.

OTHER ORAL FUNGAL INFECTIONS IN IMMUNOCOMPROMISED PATIENTS (*Table 20.13*; Chapter 26)

Aspergillus spp. may infect the paranasal sinuses, palate or other sites. Infection spreads by direct extension and haematogenously. Diagnosis is by serology, biopsy and demonstration of hyphae in a smear. Intravenous amphotericin may be effective.

Mucormycosis (*zygomycosis; phycomycosis*) is infection by Mucor or Rhizopus species, mainly of the paranasal sinuses and nose of poorly controlled diabetic or leukaemic patients. Diagnosis is by biopsy and culture: treatment is by control of diabetes or other underlying disease, debridement and intravenous amphotericin.

Cryptococcosis and *histoplasmosis* are the other main deep mycoses, and they present in the mouth mainly as ulcers. These are discussed in Chapter 26.

BIBLIOGRAPHY

Almeida O.P and Scully C. (1991) Oral lesions in the systemic mycoses. *Curr. Opin. Dent.* **1**, 423–8.
Axell T., Azul A.M., Challacombe S., Ficarra G., Flint S. *et al.* (1993) Classification and diagnostic criteria for oral lesions in HIV infection. *J. Oral Pathol. Med.* **22**, 289–91.

Axell T., Baert A.E., Brocheriou C., Challacombe S., Greenspan D. *et al.* (1991) An update of the classification and diagnostic criteria of oral lesions in HIV infection. *J. Oral Pathol. Med.* **20**, 97–100.

Axell T., Baert A.E., Brocheriou C., Challacombe S., Greenspan D. *et al.* (1991) Revised classification of HIV-associated oral lesions. *Br. Dent. J.* **170**: 305–6.

Buckley R.H. (1992) Immunodeficiency diseases. *J. Am. Med. Assoc.* **268**, 2797–806.

Centers for Disease Control (1993) Revised classification system for HIV infection and expanded surveillance case definition for AIDS among adolescents and adults. *MMWR*, **41** (RR17), 1–19.

Clayman H.N. (1992) The biology of the immune response. *J. Am. Med. Assoc.* **268**, 2790–6.

Cleveland J.L., Kent J., Gooch B.F. *et al.* (1995) Multidrug-resistant *Mycobacterium tuberculosis* in an HIV dental clinic. *Infect. Control Hosp. Epidemiol.* **16**, 7–11.

Cullingford G.L., Watkins D.N., Watts A.D.J. and Mallon D.F. (1991) Severe late postsplenectomy infection. *Br. J. Surg.* **78**, 716–21.

De Rossi S.S. and Glick M. (1996) Dental considerations in asplenic patients. *J. Am. Dent. Assoc.* **127**, 1357–63.

Epstein J.B. and Scully C. (1991) HIV infection: clinical features and treatment of thirty-three homosexual men with Kaposi's sarcoma. *Oral Surg. Oral Med. Oral Pathol.* **71**, 38–41.

Epstein J. and Scully C. (1992) Neoplastic disease in the head and neck of patients with AIDS. *Int. J. Oral Maxillofac. Surg.* **2**, 219–26.

Epstein J.B. and Scully C. (1993) Oral adverse effects of medical management in patients with HIV infection. *AIDS Patient Care* December, pp. 304–11.

Filho F.J.S., Lopes M., Almeida O.P.D. and Scully C. (1995) Mucocutaneous histoplasmosis in AIDS. *Br. J. Dermatol.* **133**, 472–4.

Greenspan D., Greenspan J.S., Schiodt M. *et al.* (1990) *AIDS and the Mouth.* Copenhagen, Munksgaard.

Johnson E.M., Warnock D.W., Luker J., Porter S.R. and Scully C. (1995) Emergence of azole drug resistance in Candida species among HIV-infected patients receiving prolonged fluconazole therapy for oral candidosis. *Antimicrob. Agents Chemother.* **35**, 103–14.

Laskaris G., Stergiou C., Kittas C. and Scully C. (1992) Hodgkin's disease in the gingiva in AIDS. *Oral Oncol. Eur. J. Cancer* **28B**, 39–41.

Libre J., Cucurull J., Aloy A. and Hernandez J.A. (1991) Antimicrobial prophylaxis for dental extractions after splenectomy. *Lancet* **337**, 1485–6.

Mathe G. and Abitol J. (1988) From Fernand–Widal rhinitis syndrome and chronic sinusitis to total mucociliary disease. *Biomed. Pharmacother.* **42**, 489–92.

Mellemkjaer L., Olsen J.H., Linet M.S., Gridley G. and McLaughlin J.K. (1995) Cancer risk after splenectomy. *Cancer* **75**, 577–83.

Oxelius V.A., Laurell A.B., Lindquist B. *et al.* (1981) IgG subclasses in selective IgA deficiency. *N. Engl. J. Med.* **304**, 1476.

Pascale R., Valle G.A.D., Moreau P., Milpied N., Felice M.P. *et al.* (1995) Viridans streptococcal bacteraemia in patients with neutropenia. *Lancet* **345**, 1607–9.

Porter S.R. and Scully C. (1990) Chronic mucocutaneous candidosis and related syndromes. In Samaranayke L.P. and MacFarlane T.W. (eds), *Oral Candidosis.* Bristol, Wright, pp. 200–12.

Porter S.R. and Scully C. (1990) Primary immunodeficiency. In Jones J.H. and Mason D.K. (eds), *Oral Manifestations of Systemic Disease*, 2nd edn. London, Baillière Tindall, pp. 112–61.

Porter S.R. and Scully C. (1993) Orofacial manifestations in primary immunodeficiencies involving IgA deficiency. *J. Oral Pathol. Med.* **22**, 117–19.

Porter S.R. and Scully C. (1993) Orofacial manifestations in primary immunodeficiencies: T lymphocyte defects. *J. Oral Pathol. Med.* **22**, 308–9.

Porter S.R. and Scully C. (1993) Orofacial manifestations in primary immunodeficiencies: polymorphonuclear leukocyte defects. *J. Oral Pathol. Med.* **22**, 310–11.

Porter S.R. and Scully C. (1994) HIV: the surgeon's perspective. 1: Update of pathogenesis, epidemiology, management and risk of nosocomial transmission. *Br. J. Oral Maxillofac. Surg.* **32**, 222–30.

Porter S.R. and Scully C. (1994) HIV: The surgeon's perspective. 2: Diagnosis and management of non-malignant oral manifestations. *Br. J. Oral Maxillofac. Surg.* **32**, 231–40.

Porter S.R. and Scully C. (1994) HIV: The surgeon's perspective. 3: Diagnosis and management of malignant neoplasms. *Br. J. Oral Maxillofac. Surg.* **32**, 241–7.

Porter S.R. and Scully C. (1994) Orofacial manifestations in the primary immunodeficiency disorders. *Oral Surg. Oral Med. Oral Pathol.* **78**, 4–13.

Porter S.R. and Scully C. (eds) (1995) *Oral Health Care for Those with HIV and Other Special Needs.* Northwood, Science Reviews.

Porter S.R. and Scully C. (1996) *Innovations and Developments in Non-Invasive Oral Health Care.* Northwood, Science Reviews.

Porter S.R., Cox M. and Scully C. (1986) Immunology for dental hygienists. *Dent. Health* **25**, 4–9.

Porter S.R., Scully C. and Cawson R.A. (1987) AIDS: update and guidelines for general dental practice. *Dent. Update* **14**, 9–17.

Porter S.R., Scully C. and Luker J. (1993) Complications of dental surgery in persons with HIV disease. *Oral Surg. Oral Med. Oral Pathol.* **75**, 165–7.

Porter S.R., Scully C., Luker J. and Glover S. (1990) Oral manifestations of HIV infection. *Dent. Update* **40**, 1173–80.

Porter S.R., Scully C. and Standen G. (1994) Autoimmune neutropenia manifesting as recurrent oral ulceration. *Oral Surg. Oral Med. Oral Pathol.* **78**, 178–80.

Porter S.R., Sugerman P.B., Scully C., Luker J. and Oakhill A. (1994) Orofacial manifestations in the Wiskott–Aldrich syndrome. *J. Dent. Child.* **61**, 404–7.

Reichart P.A. (1996) Oral pathology of acquired immune deficiency syndrome and oro-facial Kaposi's sarcoma. *Curr. Topics Pathol.* **90**, 98–121.

Rosen F.S., Wedgewood R.J. and Auiti F. (1983) Primary immunodeficiency diseases – report prepared for WHO by a scientific group on immunodeficiency. *Clin. Immunol. Immunopathol.* **28**, 450–75.

Schreiber R.A. and Walker W.A. (1989) Food allergy; facts and fiction. *Mayo Clin. Proc.* **64**, 1381–91.

Scully C. (1981) Orofacial manifestations in chronic granulomatous disease of childhood. *Oral Surg. Oral Med. Oral Pathol.* **15**, 148.

Scully C. (1986) Chronic atrophic candidosis. *Lancet* **ii**, 437–8.

Scully C. (1988) Is AIDS a problem in dentistry? *Microbial. Ecol.* **1**, 142–4.

Scully C. (1988) *The Dental Patient.* Oxford, Heinemann.

Scully C. (1989) *Patient Care: a Dental Surgeon's Guide.* London, British Dental Association.

Scully C. (1989) *The Mouth and Perioral Tissues.* Oxford, Heinemann.

Scully C. (1992) Oral infections in the immunocompromised patient. *Br. Dent. J.* **172**, 401–7.

Scully C. (1995) HIV: Viral infections. In Porter S.R. and Scully C. (eds), *Oral Health Care for Those with HIV and Other Special Needs.* Northwood, Science Reviews, pp. 31–42.

Scully C. (1997) The dental profession. In Collins J. and Kennedy D.A. (eds), *Occupational Blood-Borne Infections.* CAB International, pp. 133–58.

Scully C. (1997) The HIV global pandemic: the development and emerging implications. *Oral Dis.* **3** (Suppl. 1), S1–S6.

Scully C. and McCarthy G. (1992) Management of oral health in persons with HIV infection. *Oral Surg. Oral Med. Oral Pathol.* **73**, 215–25.

Scully C. and Peterson D.E. (1995) Oral infections in immunocompromised hosts. In Millard H.D. and Mason D.K. (eds), *1993 World Workshop on Oral Medicine.* Ann Arbor, University of Michigan, pp. 7–16.

Scully C. and Porter S.R. (1986) Immunodeficiency. In Ivanyi L. (ed), *Immunology of Oral Diseases.* Lancaster, MTP Press, pp. 235–56.

Scully C. and Porter S.R. (1991) The level of risk of transmission of human immunodeficiency virus (HIV) between patients and dental staff. *Br. Dent. J.* **170**, 97–100.

Scully C. and Porter S.R. (1991) An ABC of oral health care in patients with HIV infection. *Br. Dent. J.* **170**, 149–50.

Scully C. and Porter S.R. (1993) Orofacial manifestations in primary immunodeficiencies: common variable immunodeficiencies. *J. Oral Pathol. Med.* **22**, 157–8.

Scully C. and Porter S.R. (1993) Can HIV be transmitted from dental personnel to patients by dentistry? *Br. Dent. J.* **175**, 381–2.

Scully C. and Samaranayke L.P. (1992) *Clinical Virology in Oral Medicine and Dentistry.* Cambridge, Cambridge University Press.

Scully C. and Spittle M. (1995) Malignant tumours of the oral cavity in HIV disease. In Langdon J. and Henk J.M. (eds), *Malignant Tumours of the Mouth, Jaws and Salivary Glands*, 2nd edn. London, Edward Arnold, pp. 246–57.

Scully C., Almeida O.D.P. and Sposto M.R. (1997) Deep mycoses in HIV infection. *Oral Dis.* **3** (Suppl. 1), 200–7.

Scully C., Almeida O.P.D., Warnakulasuriya K.A.A.S. and Johnson N.W. (1995) Orofacial involvement by systemic mycoses in HIV infection. *Oral Dis.* **1**, 61–2.

Scully C., Davies R., Porter S., Eveson J. and Luker J. (1993) HIV-salivary gland disease: salivary scintiscanning with technetium pertechnetate. *Oral Surg. Oral Med. Oral Pathol.* **76**, 120–3.

Scully C., Cawson R.A. and Griffiths M.J. (1990) *Occupational Hazards to Dental Staff.* London, British Dental Journal.

Scully C., Epstein J.B., Porter S.R. and Luker J. (1990) Recognition of oral lesions of HIV infection. 1. Candidosis. *Br. Dent. J.* **169**, 295–6.

Scully C., Epstein J.B., Porter S. and Luker J. (1990) Recognition of oral lesions of HIV infection. 2. Hairy leukoplakia and Kaposi's sarcoma. *Br. Dent. J.* **169**, 332–3.

Scully C., Epstein J.B., Porter S. and Luker J. (1990) Recognition of oral lesions of HIV infection. 3. Gingival and periodontal disease and less common lesions. *Br. Dent. J.* **169**, 370–2.

Scully C., El-Kabir M. and Samaranayake L.P. (1994) Candida and oral candidosis. *Crit. Rev. Oral Biol. Med.* **5**, 124–58.

Scully C., Laskaris G., Pindborg J., Porter S.R. and Reichart P. (1991) Oral manifestations of HIV infection and their management. 1. More common lesions. *Oral Surg. Oral Med. Oral Pathol.* **71**, 158–66.

Scully C., Laskaris G., Pindborg J., Porter S.R. and Reichart P. (1991) Oral manifestations of HIV infection and their management. 2. Less common lesions. *Oral Surg. Oral Med. Oral Pathol.* **71**, 167–71.

Scully C., MacFadyen E. and Campbell A. (1982) Orofacial manifestations in cyclic neutropenia. *Br. J. Oral Surg.* **20**, 96–101.

Scully C., Porter S.R. and Greenspan D. (1990) Secondary immunodeficiency. In Jones J.H. and Mason D.K. (eds), *Oral Manifestations of Systemic Disease*, 2nd edn. London, Baillière Tindall, pp. 162–82.

Scully C., Porter S.R. and Luker J. (1991) An ABC of oral health care in patients with HIV infection. *Br. Dent. J.* **170**, 149–50.

Scully C., Samaranayake L.P. and Martin M. (1993) HIV: answers to common questions on transmission, disinfection and antisepsis in clinical dentistry. *Br. Dent. J.* **175**, 175–8.

Sim T.C. and Grant J.A. (1990) Hereditary angioedema: its diagnosis and management perspectives. *Am. J. Med.* **88**, 656–65.

Strains S.E. (1982) Aciclovir for chronic mucocutaneous herpes simplex virus infection in immunosuppressed patients. *Ann. Intern. Med.* **96**, 270–7.

Strains S.E. (1984) Oral aciclovir to suppress recurring herpes simplex virus infections in immunodeficient patients. *Ann. Intern. Med.* **100**, 522–1.

Tsang P.C.S., Samaranayake L.P., Philipsen H.P., McCullough M., Reichart P.A. *et al.* (1995) Biotypes of oral *Candida albicans* isolates in human immunodeficiency virus-infected patients from diverse geographic locations. *J. Oral Pathol. Med.* **24**, 32–6.

Umetsu D.T., Ambrosino D.M. and Quinti I. (1985) Recurrent sinopulmonary infection and impaired antibody response to bacterial capsular polysaccharide antigen in children with selective IgG-subclass deficiency. *N. Engl. J. Med.* **313**, 1247–51.

Weinert M., Grimes R.M. and Lynch D.P. (1996) Oral manifestations of HIV infection. *Ann. Intern. Med.* **125**, 485–96.

WHO (1997) Primary immunodeficiency diseases. *Clin. Exp. Immunol.* **109** (Suppl. 1), 1–28.

APPENDIX TO CHAPTER 20

Interleukin	Produced mainly by	Main functions
1	Monocytes	Activates T cells. Induces IL-6. Generates prostaglandins
2	T cells	T cell growth and apoptosis
3	T cells	Haematopoietic cell growth
4	T cells. Mast cells	B cell activation. Mast cell growth
5	T cells	B cell and eosinophil differentiation
6	Monocytes	Induces inflammation. Activates many cells
7	Marrow stromal cells	B cell growth
8	Monocytes	Neutrophil chemotaxis
9	T cells	T cell and mast cell growth
10	Monocytes	T cell and mast cell growth
11	T cells	Plasma cell growth
12	T cells	Induces interferon γ
13	T cells	Induces IgE
14	T cells	B cell growth
15	T cells	T cell, B cell and NK cell growth
16	T cells	CD4 cell chemoattractant
17	T cells	Induces IL-6, IL-8 and GCSF
18	Liver	Induces interferon γ

21

Immunologically mediated disease

Key points

- Immunologically mediated diseases may be allergic, autoimmune, immune complex-mediated or due to a type IV hypersensitivity or other reaction.
- Anaphylaxis in response to drugs is one of the most important immediate type 1 reactions but atopy is more common.
- Atopy includes asthma, eczema and hay fever, mediated by mast cell degranulation in a type I response to various allergens.
- Antihistamines used to control atopic features may cause dry mouth and can be a contraindication to use of various drugs.
- Allergic angio-oedema is an acute type I response which is potentially lethal as oedema affects the face, and may spread to the tongue and upper airway.
- An oral allergy syndrome has been described in which patients develop swelling orofacially mainly in response to allergens in fresh fruits and vegetables.
- Hereditary angio-oedema presents similarly to acute angio-oedema, but in response to trauma such as dental treatment, and is caused by an enzyme defect.
- Autoimmune disorders are typically familial, may be associated with HLA-B8 and DR3 and autoantibodies, are seen mainly in older females, and may be multiple.
- Pemphigus, the best example of an autoimmune disease, and pemphigoid may present with mucosal lesions.
- The connective tissue diseases (CTD) may present with Sjögren's syndrome (SS).
- Systemic lupus erythematosus is a multi-system CTD with antibodies against DNA, and often SS, mouth ulcers, renal, cardiac and CNS disease.
- Systemic sclerosis, where there are anticentromere antibodies, may present with SS, dysphagia, trismus, microstomia and cardiac, renal or pulmonary disease.
- Behçet's syndrome is a multi-system disorder with recurrent aphthae, and often genital and ocular lesions.
- Behçet's syndrome may be lethal from thromboses or CNS disease.
- Polyarteritis nodosa is a multi-system disease with vasculitis usually related to HBV or drugs, causing hypertension, angina or renal disease.
- Midline granuloma syndrome, which presents with nasal stuffiness or discharge, or ulceration, may be due to lymphoma or Wegener's granulomatosis.
- Wegener's granulomatosis is a vasculitis affecting mainly the respiratory tract, later the kidneys, and sometimes associated with nasal carriage of *Staphylococcus aureus*.

Important immunologically mediated diseases are shown in *Table 21.1* and the mechanisms of hypersensitivity reactions in *Table 21.2*. Anaphylaxis, and allergies to dental materials and drugs, are discussed in Chapter 25.

<table>
<tr><td>

Table 21.1   Examples of immunologically mediated diseases

</td></tr>
</table>

- Reactions to foreign antigens
    - Allergic rhinitis (hayfever)
    - Asthma
    - Eczema
    - Urticaria and angio-oedema (angioneurotic oedema)*
    - Drug and food allergies
    - Anaphylaxis
    - Contact dermatitis
- Disorders with an autoimmune basis
    - Rheumatoid (collagen) diseases
        - Systemic lupus erythematosus*
        - Rheumatoid arthritis*
        - Sjögren's syndrome*
        - Systemic sclerosis*
        - Polymyositis-dermatomyositis
        - Polyarteritis nodosa*
    - Haematological disease
        - Pernicious anaemia*
        - Autoimmune haemolytic anaemia
        - Idiopathic and drug-associated thrombocytopenic purpura*
        - Drug-induced neutropenia*
        - Aplastic anaemia (some cases)*
    - Gastrointestinal and liver diseases
        - Chronic atrophic gastritis and pernicious anaemia*
        - Gluten-sensitive enteropathy (coeliac disease)*
        - Chronic autoimmune hepatitis
        - Primary biliary cirrhosis
    - Cardiac diseases
        - Acute rheumatic fever
    - Renal diseases
        - Glomerulonephritis (various types)
        - Goodpasture's syndrome
    - Mucocutaneous disease
        - Pemphigus*
        - Pemphigoid*
        - Dermatitis herpetiformis*
    - Endocrine diseases
        - Chronic (Hashimoto's) thyroiditis
        - Hyperthyroidism
        - Idiopathic adrenocortical insufficiency*
        - Idiopathic hypoparathyroidism*
    - Neurological diseases
        - Guillain-Barré syndrome
        - Myasthenia gravis
    - Eye diseases
        - Sympathetic ophthalmia
        - Sjögren's syndrome*
        - Pemphigus vulgaris*
        - Mucous membrane pemphigoid*

*Also affect oral tissues.

ATOPIC DISEASE

Atopic disease is the term given to the group of allergic conditions (asthma, eczema, hay fever and others) which are by far the most common type of immunologically mediated disease and affect about 10 per cent of the population. Susceptibility is usually genetically determined. IgA deficiency (which is also common) is frequently associated with allergic disease.

Atopic disease depends on production of specific IgE antibody which binds to mast cells. Degranulation of mast cells, with release of mediators such as histamine, follows further exposure to the allergen. Cell-bound IgE is present, particularly in the bronchial tree, nasal mucosa, dermis and intestinal wall. The clinical types of atopic disease are therefore asthma, hay fever, urticaria, angio-oedema, eczema and food allergies. Common allergens are grass pollens, mites in house dust, fungal spores and milk and egg proteins, but in many cases the allergen cannot be reliably identified. Patients with atopy were also thought to be more prone to develop allergy or anaphylaxis in response to drugs such as penicillin or intravenous anaesthetic agents, but this does not appear to have been confirmed.

Normal individuals also produce IgE antibodies but without ill-effect and the reasons for the abnormal response of allergic individuals is unknown.

Diagnosis of atopic disorders

A history of 'allergy' to a variety of substances is common but may need to be confirmed by objective tests. True food allergy is rare while systemic 'allergy' to amalgam restorations and phenomena such as 'total allergy syndrome' are myths. The history should, however, indicate whether the allergy takes any of the recognized forms mentioned earlier and whether there is a positive family history. Confirmatory tests include the following.

Skin tests for allergens
Allergy to individual substances may be detected by skin testing. This can be done either by pricking the allergen into the skin (intradermal or prick testing) or, less

Table 21.2   Hypersensitivity reactions

Type of reaction[a]	Mechanism	Examples
I. Immediate (anaphylactic)	Free Ag binds to IgE fixed on mast cells and basophils, causing release of histamine etc.	Anaphylaxis Asthma Hay fever
II. Cytotoxic	Free IgG or IgM Ab binds to Ag on cell membranes to cause complement activation, cell damage or phagocytosis	Pemphigus Idiopathic thrombocytopenic
III. Immune-complex	Persistence of Ag/Ab complexes may lead to activation of complement, inflammation and tissue damage, particularly vasculitis and arthritis	Rheumatoid arthritis Serum sickness Lupus erythematosus
IV. Cell-mediated	Ag activates sensitized T-cells to become cytotoxic and to release factors (lymphokines) that stimulate other leucocytes	Contact dermatitis Graft rejection

Ag, Antigen; Ab, antibody.
[a]Some recognize type V (immunostimulatory IgG), e.g. Graves' disease.

efficiently, by applying it in an absorbent dressing taped onto the skin (patch testing). A positive reaction is shown by a wheal and erythema which starts to appear within about 20 minutes. Adequate controls must be used. A complication of skin testing is that it can induce sensitivity to the test compound. Anaphylactic reactions can occasionally follow intradermal skin test doses of penicillin.

Laboratory tests
These include:

1. Serum IgE levels (PRIST test; paper radio-immunosorbent test).
2. Radioallergosorbent test (RAST) for IgE antibodies to specific antigens.

IgE is present in very low concentration in the serum and its quantification depends on sensitive radio-immunoassay. In many cases of allergy, also, serum IgE levels are within the normal range.

In the RAST test, purified extracts of a wide range of allergens are coupled to cellulose or paper discs to which the patient's serum is applied. Its ability to react with one or more of these allergens is tested by adding rabbit anti-IgE labelled with radioactive iodine. The level of radioactivity then indicates the levels of specific IgE antibodies.

• **Management of atopic patients**

Known allergens should be avoided. This is easier said than done, since allergens can be present in the most unexpected places. In general, allergens are more likely to be unknown in commercially prepared foods and drinks however, than in natural products. No tests will reliably predict the possibility of anaphylactic reactions and the history of the response to previous exposure is the main precaution.

Desensitization of patients is attempted by administering the allergen initially in minute but in progressively increasing doses. However, there is little objective evidence of the value of this procedure and there is a risk of fatal anaphylaxis or other severe reactions during the process. Since safe and effective prophylactic drugs such as sodium cromoglycate or topically active corticosteroids are available, desensitization has few useful applications and is regarded as obsolete by many authorities.

Drugs used in the treatment of allergic disease: Antihistamines, sympathomimetic agents, sodium cromoglycate (Intal; Rynacrom) and corticosteroids are used.

FOOD INTOLERANCE

Allergy to foods is an emotive subject but far less common than the lay public believes. Adverse effects to foods may be due to intolerance, coeliac disease, reactions to food additives such as azo dyes or benzoic acid, or may be purely imaginary. Mothers have been known so to restrict the diet of their children because of alleged food allergy as to cause severe malnutrition.

Some children are hypersensitive to cow's milk protein, for example, and this may cause diarrhoea. The effects of true food allergies are varied, and in addition to gastrointestinal disturbances, can cause rhinorrhoea, bronchospasm, urticaria or angio-oedema. The last can be dangerous to those sensitive to egg protein, as discussed below, if they are given a vaccine derived from viruses grown on chick embryo.

ACUTE ALLERGIC ANGIO-OEDEMA

Angio-oedema (unjustifiably also called 'angioneurotic oedema') is characterized by rapid development of oedematous swelling, particularly of the head and neck region. The facial oedema, even though temporary, can cause embarrassment (*Plate 21*), but when oedema involves the neck and extends to the larynx, it can cause rapidly fatal respiratory obstruction. Acute allergic oedema of this type can develop alone or may be associated with anaphylactic reactions as described earlier. Since minute amounts of allergen can trigger the reaction its nature may not be recognized. Thus patients sensitive to egg proteins have had dangerous reactions to viral vaccines when the virus had been grown on chick embryo tissues.

Mild angio-oedema may respond to antihistamines or to a sympathomimetic agent such as ephedrine which can be taken by mouth. In more severe cases, especially if there is a threat to the airway, the emergency should be managed in the same way as for an anaphylactic reaction. For intractable chronic cases corticosteroids may be required.

• Dental aspects of allergic disease

The main clinical implications of atopic disease in dental practice are as follows:

1. Possibly an increased risk of sensitization or of acute allergic reactions to drugs used in dentistry (Chapter 25).
2. Problems caused by drugs, particularly corticosteroids.
3. Anaesthetic hazards in asthma (Chapter 8).
4. Management of severe asthma or anaphylaxis in the dental surgery (Chapter 26).
5. Dry mouth and drowsiness in patients taking antihistamines.

Antihistamines are useful only for minor manifestations of allergies, such as hay fever. Sedation usually accompanies effective doses, unless some of the newer agents, such as terfenadine, are used. Antihistamines can also cause dry mouth. Azole antifungals, erythromycin, various other drugs and grapefruit juice can cause dysrhythmias in patients using terfenadine.

Sympathomimetic agents such as ephedrine may be used as nasal drops to relieve congestion of the mucosa in hay fever or sinusitis, while others such as salbutamol or terbutaline are given by mouth or inhaler for the control of asthma. Sodium cromoglycate is widely used by inhalation for the long-term prophylaxis of asthma and hay fever. These drugs are unlikely to complicate dental treatment.

Corticosteroids used systemically for otherwise uncontrollable asthma can cause severe complications, but are usually now administered in aerosol form. Examples are beclomethasone dipropionate and betamethasone valerate inhalers. The doses are often of only 300–400 μg. The only significant side-effect is to cause oropharyngeal thrush in a minority of patients and there is little evidence of systemic effects. Corticosteroids absorbed from ointments used for eczema can, however, cause adrenal suppression (Chapter 14).

Apart from peri-oral and oral swelling, there is no evidence that immediate type hypersensitivity affects the oral mucosa and there is no oral counterpart of eczema. Denture stomatitis, for example, has been shown *not* to be caused by allergy to polymethylacrylate.

Other dental materials which accidentally come into contact with the patient's skin can very occasionally provoke an acute eczematous reaction or contact dermatitis.

No oral diseases have been proved to have any significant direct association with atopic disease, although patients with allergic rhinitis may be mouth-breathers and develop gingival hyperplasia.

In a few patients with aphthous stomatitis, ulceration appears to be precipitated by certain foods – especially walnuts, chocolate or citrus fruits. Although there may be a slightly greater prevalence of allergic diseases associated with aphthous stomatitis, there is little evidence for an allergic mechanism.

ORAL ALLERGY SYNDROME

The combination of oral pruritus, irritation and swelling of the lips, tongue, palate and throat, sometimes associated with other allergic features such as rhinoconjunctivitis, asthma, urticaria-angio-oedema, and anaphylactic shock have been termed the oral allergy syndrome. It appears to be precipitated mainly by fresh foods such as fruits and vegetables, sometimes by pollens because of cross-reacting allergens. Cooking often destroys the allergens.

OROFACIAL GRANULOMATOSIS (*see* Chapter 9)

NON-ALLERGIC IMMUNOLOGICALLY MEDIATED DISEASE

The clinical features are often suggestive of immunologically mediated diseases such as autoimmune or connective tissue disease, but preliminary screening comprises the following:

(a) *Full blood picture*, including erythrocyte sedimentation rate (ESR) or plasma viscosity. The blood picture will show haematological abnormalities such as haemolytic anaemia, thrombocytopenia or leucopenia that may result from autoantibody production. Alternatively, there may be leucocytosis associated with inflammatory processes. The ESR, a non-specific test, is raised as a result of hypergammaglobulinaemia or secondary to inflammation.

(b) *Serum protein levels:* These are typically raised in autoimmune diseases as a result of over-production of immunoglobulins

The following are more specific tests for auto-immune disease.

1. *Autoantibody profile:* These usually include the most commonly found abnormalities, namely rheumatoid and antinuclear factors and thyroid microsomal, gastric parietal cell, mitochondrial, smooth muscle and reticulin antibodies. Other specific autoantibodies can be identified by special tests.

2. *Biopsy and tissue immunostaining:* Immunofluorescence or immunoperoxidase showing immunoglobulin or complement deposits suggests an autoimmune pathogenesis. Vasculitis with deposits of immunoglobulins and complement in the damaged vessel walls strongly suggests immune complex injury.

3. *Serum complement levels:* Complement is consumed when the cascade is activated by antigen/antibody reactions or other triggering factors and thus levels (CH_{50}) are often depressed.

4. *Immune complexes:* Many tests, such as detection of cryoglobulins, have been used for detecting circulating immune complexes but there is no consensus yet as to which is most useful. The mere presence of circulating immune complexes alone does not establish that there is immune complex-mediated tissue damage.

HLA typing and disease

Compatible blood transfusion depends mainly on ensuring that donors' and recipients' blood are of compatible ABO groups. Tissue transplantation, by contrast, involves a much more complex system of antigens, namely the HLA (human lymphocyte antigen) system. The genes for these histocompatibility antigens are identified by a letter (A to D) and a number.

A genetically determined susceptibility to many immunologically mediated diseases is often suggested by a positive family history, and also by the finding that there is a significant association between certain histocompatibility antigens and several immunologically mediated diseases.

It is often assumed that HLA specificities determine the pattern of susceptibility to disease, particularly to autoimmune disease, and further that since the HLA specificities are determined by the appropriate genes, such diseases must be genetically determined. However, the strongest associations are between HLA-D2 and narcolepsy and HLA-B27 and ankylosing spondylitis, which are not known to be immunologically mediated. Rheumatoid arthritis, by contrast, has some association with HLA-DR4, but any genetic predisposition is controversial. Many of the organ-specific autoimmune diseases are associated with HLA-B8 and DR3, but the association is not sufficiently strong to help in the diagnosis. In contrast, HLA associations are rare in immunodeficiency states.

The significance of the association of different HLA specificities with particular diseases is, therefore, as yet unknown. HLA specificities are also of little value in diagnosis because of the inconstancy of their association with individual diseases, apart from narcolepsy and ankylosing spondylitis.

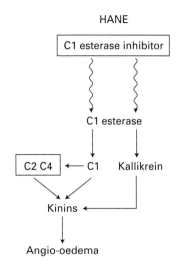

Fig. 21.1 Hereditary angio-oedema C1 esterase inhibitor is defective

HEREDITARY ANGIO-OEDEMA (C1 ESTERASE INHIBITOR DEFICIENCY)

Hereditary angio-oedema (HANE) is sometimes classified as an immune defect, mimics allergic angio-oedema, though it produces a more severe reaction. It is caused by continued complement activation resulting from a genetically determined deficiency of an inhibitor of the enzyme C1 esterase rather than an allergic reaction (*Fig. 21.1*). In this reaction C4 is consumed and its plasma level falls. The level of C3, however, is usually normal. Activation of kinin-like substances is the probable cause of the sudden increase in capillary permeability. Despite its hereditary nature, usually as an autosomal dominant trait, the disease may not present until later childhood or adolescence and nearly 20 per cent of cases are caused by spontaneous mutation. Rare cases are acquired.

Oedema typically affects the mouth, face and neck region, the extremities and gastrointestinal tract and may persist for up to 4 days. Abdominal pain, nausea or vomiting, diarrhoea, rashes and peripheral oedema sometimes herald an attack. Involvement of the airway is a constant threat. The mortality has been estimated to be as high as 30 per cent in some families but the disease is compatible with prolonged survival if

emergencies are effectively treated. Blunt injury is the most consistent precipitating event. The trauma of dental treatment is a potent trigger of attacks, and some attacks follow emotional stress.

In 85 per cent of cases the C1 esterase levels are reduced (type 1 HANE) but in 15 per cent the enzyme is present but dysfunctional (type 2 HANE); in both types the C4 level falls. Plasminogen inhibitors such as tranexamic acid have been used to mitigate attacks but currently the most effective agents are the androgenic steroids, danazol and, more recently, stanazolol, which raise plasma C1 esterase inhibitor levels to normal. The usual dose of stanazolol for an adult is 2.5–10 mg daily. However, it needs to be given for 5 days to be effective, it should not be given during pregnancy, oligomenorrhoea may be induced in women and there may be acne, hirsutism, hypercalcaemia or headache. Fortunately, C1 esterase concentrates are now becoming available for replacement of the missing factor.

AUTOIMMUNE DISEASE

Autoimmune disease can be broadly divided into two main groups (*Table 21.3*). There are, first, diseases such as pemphigus where there are tissue or organ-specific autoantibodies

Table 21.3 Types of autoimmune disease	
Organ or cell-specific autoantibodies	Non organ-specific autoantibodies: the collagen or connective tissue diseases[a]
Hashimoto's thyroiditis	Lupus erythematosus
Chronic atrophic gastritis (pernicious anaemia)[b]	Rheumatoid arthritis
	Sjögren's syndrome
Idiopathic Addison's disease	Systemic sclerosis
Idiopathic hypoparathyroidism	Dermatomyositis
Pemphigus vulgaris	Mixed connective
Pemphigoid	tissue disease
Idiopathic thrombocytopenic purpura	
Autoimmune haemolytic anaemia	

[a]Probably mediated by immune complex reactions.
[b]Not all chronic atrophic gastritis.
Note: Only the more important and typical examples are given.
 Even in the collagen diseases, cell-specific autoantibodies may also
 be produced but are incidental to the main disease processes.

Table 21.4 Typical features of autoimmune disease
• *Female predisposition*
• *Hypergammaglobulinaemia*
• *Autoantibodies* specific to tissue under attack sometimes present in the circulation. Multiple autoantibodies frequently detectable but often without clinical effect
• *Immunoglobulin and complement deposits* sometimes detectable by immunofluorescence microscopy at sites of tissue damage, e.g. damaged blood vessels
• *Associations with HLA-B8 and DR3* in some
• *Response to immunosuppressive treatment* in many
• *Family history positive* often. Circulating autoantibodies often detectable in apparently unaffected relatives

which appear to mediate the damage to the tissues. Second, there are the so-called connective tissue diseases, which are not caused by tissue-specific autoantibodies but probably mediated by immune complex reactions. The latter may be precipitated by other autoantibodies, such as antinuclear antibodies in systemic lupus erythematosus. These two groups of diseases are not entirely as clear-cut as this may imply and both types of phenomenon may be present, especially in the connective tissue diseases. Patients with one autoimmune disease are especially liable to develop further autoimmune diseases; a few develop polyglandular autoimmune diseases. Features suggestive of autoimmune disease are shown in *Table 21.4* and important examples are shown in *Table 21.3*. Several, such as pemphigus, pemphigoid, rheumatoid arthritis or endocrine disorders are described in other, appropriate chapters. Only the remaining relevant diseases are therefore discussed here, mainly the connective tissue (collagen) diseases.

The connective tissue diseases

This uninformative term is used to include a variety of disorders of which rheumatoid arthritis is the most common. Alternative terms are 'rheumatoid' diseases, 'collagen vascular' diseases or simply, and most confusingly, 'collagen diseases'. Most of these disorders share, to a variable degree, multiple autoantibodies, and immune complex reactions probably form the basis of the pathological changes. Another feature in common is that Raynaud's phenomenon and Sjögren's syndrome may develop in association with any of them. Cancer may be a late complication.

The connective tissue diseases are generally regarded as including:

1. Rheumatoid arthritis (Chapter 16).
2. Sjögren's syndrome (Chapter 9).
3. Lupus erythematosus.
4. Systemic sclerosis (scleroderma).
5. Mixed connective tissue disease.
6. Polymyositis and dermatomyositis .

Polyarteritis nodosa and a few other diseases are sometimes also included in this group but the justification is questionable.

Raynaud's disease and Raynaud's phenomenon

These disorders are characterized by change of colour of the fingers to white or blue, which is usually worst at the tips caused by cold. Discomfort, aching pain or numbness and stiffness of the fingers or toes, accompany an attack. Recovery is accompanied by redness, tingling and slight oedema of the digits.

The underlying cause is vasomotor instability. Cooling, or sometimes emotional disturbances, precipitate vasoconstriction at

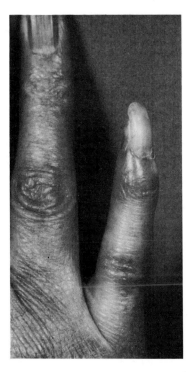

Fig. 21.2 Atrophy of the distal phalanx in severe Raynaud's syndrome in a patient with scleroderma

Table 21.5	Manifestations of systemic lupus erythematosus
Joints	Polyarthralgia
	Arthritis
Skin and mucous membranes	Rashes
	Stomatitis
Serous membranes	Pleurisy
	Pericarditis
Cardiovascular	Raynaud's syndrome
	Myocarditis
	Endocarditis (Libman–Sacks)
Lungs	Pneumonitis
Kidney	Nephritis
Neurological	Neuroses
	Psychoses
	Strokes
	Cranial nerve palsies
Eye	Conjunctivitis
	Retinal damage
Gastrointestinal	Sjögren's syndrome
	Pancreatitis
	Hepatomegaly
Blood	Anaemia
	Purpura

the extremities. The disease tends to be slowly progressive with more frequent and prolonged episodes of spasm and, in its most severe form, ischaemia can cause atrophy of the fat pads or ulceration at the tips of the fingers or toes (*Fig. 21.2*).

Raynaud's *phenomenon* is a common feature of many of the connective tissue diseases and other causes but is also seen in otherwise normal persons, when it is termed Raynaud's *disease*. In Raynaud's phenomenon only a few fingers of each hand are usually affected but Raynaud's disease spares only the thumb.

The main management measure is to stay in the warm, wear warm clothing and particularly protect the wrists and hands from chilling.

Systemic lupus erythematosus (SLE)

Lupus erythematosus is regarded as the archetypal autoimmune disease. The cause is unknown but it is believed that genetic factors are contributory and, possibly, a viral infection may initiate the disease. Some drugs (particularly hydralazine and procainamide) can also precipitate a lupus-like disease.

The main immunological feature of SLE is the formation of antibodies to DNA which may initiate immune complex reactions, in particular vasculitis (*Table 21.5*), resulting in a multi-system disease. Lupus erythematosus can thus produce a wide variety of clinical pictures depending on the organs which are predominantly affected.

The classic picture is that of a young woman with fever, malaise, anaemia, joint pains and a rash. The well-known rash with a butterfly pattern extending over both cheeks and the bridge of the nose is relatively uncommon, however, and not specific to lupus erythematosus. The rashes are variable in character but the butterfly rash is erythematous, often with raised margins and scaling, and photosensitivity rashes are common.

Renal involvement is present in about 75 per cent of cases coming to autopsy. Clinically, proteinuria and haematuria, often associated with hypertension, are common. Renal disease usually responds to immunosuppressive treatment but membranous glomerulonephritis produces a nephrotic syndrome with gradual progress to renal failure.

Ocular lesions may affect 20–25 per cent of patients, while involvement of the central nervous system is potentially lethal. Relatively minor disturbances of mood and depressive or hysterical behaviour are more common.

Serositis can cause pleurisy or occasionally pericarditis and peritonitis (polyserositis). About 40 per cent of patients with SLE also have antibodies directed against phospholipid, and about 15 per cent of patients have an antiphospholipid syndrome (APS, *see below*).

Cardiac lesions in SLE typically cause myocarditis which leads to cardiac failure. A characteristic (Libman–Sacks) endocarditis can also develop and renders the patient susceptible to infective endocarditis. Otherwise it is frequently not recognized until autopsy. Murmurs are more often caused by anaemia.

- **General management of systemic lupus erythematosus**

Haematological investigation shows a normochromic anaemia in most patients and often leucopenia, also caused by marrow depression.

Immunological abnormalities are shown in *Table 21.6*. Autoantibodies may cause thrombocytopenia and purpura or, less often, haemolytic anaemia. The titre of anti-DNA antibodies correlates well with the severity of the disease but only anti-double-stranded DNA is peculiar to SLE. About 70 per cent of patients with SLE also form antibodies against double-stranded RNA (anti-dsRNA), which is relatively specific to SLE, or against hybrid RNA/DNA molecules.

Corticosteroids and other immunosuppressive agents have been for some time the mainstay of treatment but there is increasing doubt as to their value for long-term management. Corticosteroids are probably most useful to control early acute manifestations and, together with immunosuppressive agents such as azathioprine, for the potentially lethal complications such as renal involvement. Otherwise most patients appear to do well in the long term either with non-steroidal anti-inflammatory agents or, if these are ineffective, on very low doses of corticosteroids taken on alternate days. Antimalarials

Table 21.6 Immunological findings in systemic lupus erythematosus

- Antinuclear antibodies (90 per cent)
- Anti-DNA antibodies, especially anti-double-stranded DNA (Crithidial)
- Anti-RNA antibodies
- Hypergammaglobulinaemia and raised ESR
- Hypocomplementaemia
- Rheumatoid factor (30 per cent)
- LE cell phenomenon
- False-positive serology for syphilis
- Circulating antibodies to platelets and other blood cells

such as chloroquine also appear to be effective, especially for skin and joint lesions.

The prognosis for SLE is less gloomy than was at one time thought and a 5-year survival rate of more than 90 per cent should be expected.

- **Dental aspects of systemic lupus erythematosus**

The chief problems of management include:

1. Anaemia.
2. Bleeding tendencies caused by thrombocytopenia: circulating anticoagulants rarely cause a bleeding tendency – they predispose to thrombosis.
3. Cardiac disease: cardiac failure and susceptibility to infective endocarditis if there is Libman–Sacks endocarditis.
4. Renal disease.
5. Corticosteroid or other immunosuppressive therapy.
6. Drug reactions: tetracyclines may cause photosensitivity rashes; sulphonamides or penicillins may cause deterioration in SLE.

Oral lesions, which typically consist of erythematous areas, erosions or white patches fairly symmetrically distributed, may be seen in 10–20 per cent of patients with SLE but are rarely an early feature. The lesions often resemble those of oral lichen planus. Slit-like ulcers may also be seen near the gingival margins. SLE may also be complicated by Sjögren's syndrome in 10–30 per cent of cases. Antimalarials sometimes used to control SLE can cause lichenoid oral lesions or occasionally oral hyper-pigmentation.

Erosive lesions of SLE in the oral mucosa can be difficult to manage. The best management is uncertain but corticosteroids, often in unacceptably high doses, may be the only effective treatment.

Biopsies of oral lesions show irregular epithelial thinning and acanthosis, basement membrane thickening, liquefaction degeneration of the basal cell layer and an irregularly distributed chronic inflammatory infiltrate. Vasculitis is inconstant. Immunofluorescent staining shows lumpy deposits of immunoglobulins and complement perivascularly and along the basement membrane of lesions, and under normal skin or mucosa in up to 90 per cent of patients with SLE.

Discoid lupus erythematosus

Discoid lupus erythematosus is essentially a mucocutaneous disorder in which the rashes may be indistinguishable from those of SLE but serological abnormalities are typically absent or minor, and there are no significant systemic effects. It has been suggested that discoid and systemic lupus erythematosus are different diseases but occasionally discoid disease may transform into SLE.

Oral mucosal lesions can be a feature of discoid LE and may also simulate lichen planus. In discoid LE, however, the lesions are less often symmetrically distributed and the pattern of striae is typically less well defined or conspicuous. Nevertheless, differentiation can be difficult and biopsy is essential. Even this may not be diagnostic and occasionally, histological appearances intermediate between lichen planus and lupus erythematosus are seen. Management is as for the oral lesions of SLE.

Antiphospholipid syndrome

Antiphospholipid syndrome (APS) may be seen in isolation or associated with SLE. Autoantibodies to phospholipid are present in the serum and may be deposited in small vessels, leading to intimal hyperplasia and acute thromboses, especially in cerebral, renal, pulmonary, cutaneous and cardiac arteries. Livedo reticularis, transient ischaemic attacks, Raynaud's syndrome and migrainous headaches are common. Warfarin is the most effective treatment known.

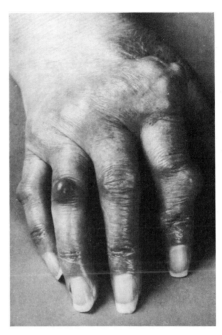

Fig. 21.3 CRST syndrome: calcinosis is shown here

Thromboses or a bleeding tendency because of anticoagulation, pulmonary and systemic hypertension are the main factors complicating dental care.

Systemic sclerosis (scleroderma)

Systemic sclerosis is an uncommon disease characterized by fibrosis of the subcutaneous tissues and viscera, and has a poor prognosis. In systemic sclerosis, the most obvious feature is Raynaud's phenomenon and the progressive stiffening of the skin, but the gastrointestinal tract, lungs, heart and kidneys are frequently also affected.

However, it is a heterogeneous disease with two main subsets – one a diffuse cutaneous form with early onset of pulmonary, cardiac and renal complications and associated in 30 per cent with anti-topoisomerase antibodies, the other a limited cutaneous form of disease with somewhat similar features but with sclerosis limited to the skin, such as CRST (calcinosis, Raynaud's, sclerodactyly and telangiectasia), with late visceral complications, but often (70 per cent) associated with anti-centromere antibodies (*Fig. 21.3*).

The pathogenesis of systemic sclerosis is unknown and the immunological abnormalities consist mainly of the topoisomerase or centromere circulating antinuclear antibodies in about 50 per cent of patients. The role of these and other autoantibodies in the disease process is unknown. Other laboratory findings are a normochromic anaemia and a raised ESR, and abnormal nailfold capillaroscopy.

Clinically, women are predominantly affected and Raynaud's phenomenon is the most common manifestation, often associated with joint pains (polyarthralgia). Visceral disease sometimes, however, causes the initial symptoms. The skin becomes thinned, stiff, tethered, pigmented and marked by prominent fine blood vessels (telangiectases or spider naevi). Eventually movement becomes limited. Involvement of the face causes characteristic changes in appearance, notably narrowing of the eyes and mask-like restriction of facial movement (Mona Lisa face).

Dysphagia and reflux oesophagitis are common. Pulmonary involvement leads to impaired respiratory exchange and, eventually, dyspnoea and pulmonary hypertension which is the main cause of serious cardiac disease. Renal damage secondary to vascular disease is typically a late feature leading to hypertension and is an important cause of death. No specific treatment is available. Penicillamine may be used but immunosuppressive drugs are not reliably effective. Calcium-channel blockers, ACE inhibitors and other drugs may be helpful but symptomatic measures are important and complications such as renal failure are managed along conventional lines. The 5-year survival rate in severe forms is about 50 per cent.

• Dental aspects of systemic sclerosis

Occasionally, involvement of the peri-articular tissues of the temporomandibular joint together with the microstomia so limit access to the mouth as to make dental treatment more or less impracticable. Otherwise, the main problems of systemic sclerosis are caused by dysphagia and pulmonary, cardiac or renal disease as potential contraindications for general anaesthesia.

Some 80 per cent of patients have manifestations in the head and neck region; in 30 per cent the symptoms start there. Constriction of the oral orifice can cause progressively limited opening of the mouth (fish-mouth). The submucosal connective tissue may also be affected and the tongue may become stiff and less mobile (chicken tongue). Despite essentially the same histological changes as those in the skin, the clinical effects on the mouth are typically relatively slight though telangiectasia may be seen.

A recognized but uncommon feature seen in fewer than 10 per cent of cases of systemic sclerosis is widening of the periodontal membrane space without tooth mobility. There is often an increase in the number of decayed, missing or filled teeth. The mandibular angle may be resorbed or rarely there is gross extensive resorption of the jaw. Sjögren's syndrome also develops in a significant minority, but very frequently when systemic sclerosis is associated with primary biliary cirrhosis.

Penicillamine therapy may cause loss of taste, oral ulceration, lichenoid reactions and other complications.

Localized scleroderma (morphoea)

Morphoea is characterized by the tissue changes of scleroderma, but localized to a single area of skin and without visceral disease or systemic effects. It was for long regarded as a variant of systemic sclerosis but more probably is a distinct entity. A typical manifestation is involvement of the side of the face causing an area of scar-like contraction aptly described as *coup de sabre*. Morphoea in childhood is believed to be a cause of facial hemiatrophy.

Mixed connective tissue disease

Mixed connective tissue disease (MCTD) is a multi-system disorder with two or more of the following features: SLE, scleroderma and polymyositis. Sjögren's syndrome is the main complication of dental interest.

Autoimmune thrombocytopenia

Acute autoimmune thrombocytopenia (idiopathic thrombocytopenic purpura: ITP) is relatively common in childhood, especially between 2 and 5 years of age. It usually follows a viral infection, and subsides spontaneously within about 3 weeks. Chronic autoimmune thrombocytopenia is mainly seen in females aged 20–50 years (*see* Chapter 4) and in HIV/AIDS.

DISEASES OF POSSIBLE IMMUNOPATHOGENESIS

Many disorders described in previous chapters have associated immunological changes but their role is often unclear. Recurrent aphthous stomatitis is discussed in Chapter 9; Behçet's syndrome (disease) may be related.

BEHÇET'S SYNDROME

Behçet described a clinical triad of oral and genital ulceration, and uveitis. The oral ulceration of Behçet's syndrome is indistinguishable from the common types of recurrent aphthae (Chapter 9) and is the most constant feature. A clinical diagnosis is usually made on the presence of any two of these features, but similar oral ulceration may also develop in other diseases which have multi-system involvement and which must be excluded when making the diagnosis (*see below*).

Behçet's syndrome is a multi-system disease with a wide variety of manifestations apart from oral, ocular and genital lesions. These may include rashes, arthritis, thrombophlebitis, cardiovascular disease and CNS involvement (*Table 21.7*). In contrast, patients with Behçet's syndrome appear not to be predisposed to connective tissue diseases, or to malignancy. Recently recognized variants of Behçet's syndrome include the MAGIC syndrome (Mouth And Genital ulcers and Interstitial Chondritis).

Behçet's syndrome is most common in persons of Mediterranean or Japanese ancestry, mainly affects young adult males, and there may be a positive family history. Features such as arthralgia and vasculitis suggest an immune-complex mediated disease, which is supported by finding circulating immune complexes. The antigen responsible for immune complex formation is unidentified but there is some evidence for a viral aetiology.

Behçet's syndrome is sometimes associated with HLA-B5, at least in some ethnic groups.

Table 21.7	Behçet's syndrome: clinical features and possible complications

- Oral
  - Aphthous stomatitis
- Ocular
  - Uveitis and hypopyon
  - Retinal vasculitis
  - Optic atrophy
  - Blindness
- Genital
  - Ulcers
- Cutaneous
  - Pustules
  - Erythema nodosum
- Joints
  - Arthralgia (large joints)
- Vascular
  - Aneurysms
  - Thromboses of vena cava
- Renal
  - Proteinuria
  - Haematuria
- Neuropsychiatric
  - Syndromes resembling multiple sclerosis
  - Syndromes resembling pseudobulbar palsy
  - Benign intracranial hypertension
  - Brainstem lesions
  - Depression

Findings such as raised serum immunoglobulin levels (especially IgA), heat shock protein and, in the acute stages, a raised ESR and mild leucocytosis, provide little information about the immunopathogenesis, which remains speculative. Indeed, since the clinical manifestations are so protean and diagnostic criteria are lacking, it is by no means certain that the many different laboratory findings that have been reported necessarily refer to the same disease.

• Management of Behçet's syndrome

Behçet's syndrome must enter into the differential diagnosis of recurrent aphthae but the diagnosis may be difficult to confirm for reasons given earlier. Oral and genital ulceration may also result from folate deficiency, when other features characteristic of Behçet's syndrome are lacking. Recurrent oral, ocular and genital lesions may also be seen in erythema multiforme and sometimes in ulcerative colitis and other conditions.

Reliable diagnostic tests for Behçet's syndrome are not available but the possibility should be considered, particularly if aphthae are associated with genital lesions and uveitis. Skin hyper-reactivity after venepuncture (pathergy) may be detectable. Patients should be screened similarly to those with aphthae to exclude underlying deficiencies and, if Behçet's syndrome is suspected, HLA typing may be of value since ocular involvement in particular is associated with HLA-B5 (B5101). An ophthalmological opinion should be obtained since ocular involvement often culminates in impaired sight. All patients should also be examined by a physician.

Oral lesions can be symptomatically managed like common aphthae. A variety of treatments, including immunosuppressive drugs such as cyclosporin and dapsone, have been tried for those with multi-system lesions, but results have been inconclusive, especially as the disease is subject to spontaneous transient remissions. Colchicine may be of value and thalidomide may be the most effective treatment for otherwise intractable oral ulceration.

SWEET'S SYNDROME

Sweet's syndrome, or acute neutrophilic dermatosis, consists of a persistent high fever, raised ESR and neutrophilia, and dull red skin nodules or plaques on the neck and forearms especially. These may become pustular. Sweet's syndrome may also include oral ulceration, conjunctivitis, episcleritis and arthralgia.

The aetiology is unclear but some cases are associated with malignancy (especially acute myeloid leukaemia), and some have followed infections – especially upper respiratory tract infections. Treatment is with systemic steroids.

POLYARTERITIS NODOSA

Polyarteritis nodosa (periarteritis nodosa, PAN) is a multi-system disease characterized by necrotizing vasculitis affecting mainly small and medium-sized arteries. It most frequently affects middle-aged men.

PAN appears to be an immune-complex disorder. Circulating immune complexes are found which, in up to 40 per cent of patients, contain hepatitis B antigens. In some cases drugs may be responsible (especially thiouracil, iodides and sulphonamides), but in many patients no precipitating factor can be identified.

Polyarteritis has protean manifestations as a result of the capricious distribution of the lesions. Fever, anorexia, weight loss, myalgia, arthralgia and peripheral neuropathies are common but non-specific. Over 60 per cent have abdominal involvement, with pain, nausea, vomiting or diarrhoea. Hypertension and angina (coronary artery disease) are common and 50 per cent have renal disease.

A closely related disease (allergic granulomatosis) is characterized by fever, asthma and eosinophilia.

• General management of PAN

There are no specific laboratory investigations for PAN: histological examination of clinically involved tissue is needed to confirm the diagnosis. Leucocytosis, eosinophilia, raised ESR, hypergammaglobulinaemia and sometimes a false-positive test for rheumatoid factor may be found. Albuminuria or haematuria is common and angiography is useful to demonstrate arterial aneurysms (early PAN) or vascular occlusions (late PAN).

The prognosis is poor in untreated disease: up to 60 per cent die within a year. Systemic corticosteroids are the drugs of choice, giving a 5-year survival of over 40 per cent. Cyclophosphamide may also be of value.

• Dental aspects of PAN

Dental management may be complicated by:

1. Corticosteroid therapy and immunosuppression.
2. Hepatitis B antigen carriage.
3. Hypertension.
4. Renal disease.
5. Cardiac disease.

Submucosal nodules, haemorrhage or oral ulcers are rare manifestations. Occasionally facial palsy or other cranial neuropathies may be complications.

Table 21.8   Polyglandular autoimmune disease[a] type I and type II

Entity	Type I	Type II
Addison's disease	100%	100%
Hypoparathyroidism	76%	—
Chronic mucocutaneous candidosis	73%	—
Alopecia	32%	0.5%
Malabsorption syndromes	22%	—
Gonadal failure	17%	3.6%
Pernicious anaemia	13%	0.5%
Chronic active hepatitis	13%	—
Insulin-dependent diabetes	4%	52%
Autoimmune thyroiditis	11%	69%
Female: male ratio	1.5:1	1.8:1
HLA associations	No constant findings	B8 (A1)

[a]Polyendocrine deficiency syndromes.

POLYENDOCRINOPATHY SYNDROMES (*see* Chapter 20)

Multiple autoimmune disorders with multiple endocrinopathies and immunodeficiency are rare syndromes that may present with oral candidosis (*Table 21.8*)

MIDLINE GRANULOMA SYNDROME (LETHAL MIDLINE GRANULOMA)

This group of diseases has been given a variety of names as a result of the different clinical pictures presented and the varied

Table 21.9   Important causes of midline granuloma syndrome

- Infections
  Tuberculosis[a]
  Syphilis[a]
  Deep mycoses
- Idiopathic
  Wegener's granulomatosis
  Peripheral T-cell lymphomas[b]
  B-cell lymphomas (rarely)

[a]Unlikely to be seen as a cause of this syndrome now.
[b]Previously called lymphomatoid granulomatosis, polymorphic reticulosis, midline malignant reticulosis, Stewart-type granuloma etc.

microscopic appearances. However, the term is best reserved for diseases of, or starting in, the nasal or paranasal tissues and resulting in midfacial destruction, sometimes of hideously disfiguring degree (so-called Stewart-type granuloma) and often with a fatal systemic involvement. More readily definable diseases such as tuberculosis, deep mycoses or neoplasms of this region should be excluded. Nevertheless, it has become apparent that these 'idiopathic' diseases are, in most cases, Wegener's granulomatosis or nasopharyngeal T-cell lymphomas (the so-called Stewart-type granuloma). The latter can produce microscopic pictures which are highly pleomorphic and not obviously lymphomatous. The causes of midline granuloma syndrome are shown in *Table 21.9* but are not reliably distinguishable clinically (*Table 21.10*). They mainly affect adults

Table 21.10   Features of the main types of idiopathic midline granuloma syndrome

	Wegener's granulomatosis	Peripheral T-cell lymphomas
Destruction of facial skeleton and soft tissues	±	+++
Systemic involvement	Pulmonary cavitation Glomerulonephritis	Predominantly lymphatic spread Liver, kidneys or other viscera may become involved
Biopsy findings	Necrotizing vasculitis, fibrinoid necrosis, multiple giant cells, ill-formed granulomas	Highly pleomorphic cellular picture, T-cells recognizable by immunocytochemistry Sometimes angiocentric and angiodestructive changes
Suggested treatment	Cyclophosphamide or azathioprine + prednisolone[a]	Radiotherapy? + cytotoxic chemotherapy

[a]Or co-trimoxazole.

between 40 and 50 years of age, and males more than females. The most common upper respiratory tract symptoms are nasal stuffiness and crusting, and often discharge, which can be bloody.

Wegener's granulomatosis

Wegener's granulomatosis is an uncommon disease characterized by granulomatous lesions in the respiratory tract and widespread vasculitis associated with giant cells. It typically terminates in a focal necrotizing glomerulonephritis and may be an immune-complex disease. Biopsy shows inflammatory changes with characteristic giant cells, though these may be few and difficult to find. A necrotizing vasculitis is the main pathological feature but is not seen in gingival biopsies where small arteries are lacking. This arteritis may, however, be seen in palatal lesions arising as a result of downward spread of the disease from the nasopharynx. Many patients are nasal carriers of *Staphylococcus aureus*.

Wegener's granulomatosis can occasionally produce a characteristic and apparently pathognomonic form of gingivitis as its initial manifestation. The gingivae are swollen, red and have a strawberry-like texture. Mucosal ulceration or delayed healing of extraction sockets are complications of the later stages of disease, particularly if renal failure develops.

The chief importance of the gingival lesions of Wegener's granulomatosis is that they may allow exceptionally early recognition of the disease, when early cytotoxic treatment may be successful. The finding of circulating antibodies to leucocyte cytoplasmic proteinase 3 (anti-neutrophil cytoplasmic antibodies, ANCA) may assist the diagnosis.

Before corticosteroids and cyclophosphamide were available, the average survival was about 6 months but these agents are effective, though they can have adverse effects. Alternatively, methotrexate with prednisolone can be used in such patients. It is now evident that trimethoprim-sulphamethoxazole may be effective treatment used alone in disease restricted to the upper aerodigestive tract, and in others can minimize some of the adverse effects of cytotoxic agents, and can minimize relapse.

Dental management may be complicated by:

1. Renal failure.
2. Respiratory disease.
3. Corticosteroid, other immunosuppressive, or cytotoxic, therapy.

Nasopharyngeal (peripheral) T-cell lymphomas

These, if allowed to progress, can cause midfacial destruction which may be so severe as to open the cranial cavity to the exterior, though this is unlikely to be seen now. In such cases death from intercurrent infection is likely to follow. Downward spread of the disease from the nasal cavity can lead to palatal necrosis and ulceration. In such cases, superimposed infection from the oral cavity can seriously confuse the microscopic picture and make diagnosis even more difficult.

In uncomplicated cases the microscopic picture is highly pleomorphic but typically characterized by angiocentric and angiodestructive changes, which mimic vasculitis. Wide dissemination follows sooner or later. Such changes are characteristic of diseases known as *lymphomatoid granulomatosis* and *polymorphic reticulosis*, but increasing evidence suggests that these are also T-cell lymphomas.

From the viewpoint of treatment and prognosis, T-cell lymphomas can have a highly variable course, sometimes with prolonged survival or even apparently spontaneous remissions. The optimal form of treatment is therefore uncertain but there have been reports of successful treatment with radiotherapy and cytotoxic chemotherapy if the disease is not advanced and too widely disseminated.

BIBLIOGRAPHY

Asherson R.A. (1992) The catastrophic antiphospholipid syndrome. *J. Rheumatol.* **19**, 508–12.

Benamour S., Zeroual B., Bennis R., Amraoui A. and Bettal S. (1990) Behcet's disease: 316 cases. *Presse Med.* **19**, 1485–9.

Bruijnzeel-Koomen C. *et al.* (1995) Adverse reactions to food. *Allergy* **50**, 623–35.

Callen J.P. (1997) Oral manifestations of collagen vascular disease. *Sem. Cut. Med. Surg.* **16**, 323–7.

Celik I., Barista I., Tekuzman G., Kansu E., Kiraz S. and Calguneri M. (1996) Behçet disease: advantageous against development of neoplasia? *Ann. Rheum. Dis.* **55**, 648.

Cicardi M. and Agostoni A. (1996) Hereditary angioedema. *N. Engl. J. Med.* **334**, 1666–7.

Condemi J.J. (1996) Update in allergy and immunology. *Ann. Intern. Med.* **125**, 744–50.

Crosher R. (1987) Intravenous tranexamic acid in the management of hereditary angio-oedema. *Br. J Oral Maxillofac. Surg.* **25**, 500–6.

Greenspan J.S. and Chisholm D.M. (1980) Connective tissue disease of doubtful origins. In Jones J.H. and Mason D.K. (eds), *Oral Manifestations of Systemic Disease*. Philadelphia, Saunders, pp. 191–210.

Jankittivong A. and Langlais R.P. (1994) Allergic stomatitis. *Semin. Dermatol.* **13**, 91–101.

Kallenberg C.G.M. (1996) Treatment of Wegener's granulomatosis: new horizons? *Clin. Exp. Rheumatol.* **14**, 1–4.

Kemmett D. and Hunter J.A.A. (1990) Sweet's syndrome; a clinicopathologic review of twenty nine cases. *J. Am. Acad. Dermatol.* **23**, 503–7.

Leading Article (1985) Cyclosporin in autoimmune disease. *Lancet* **i**, 909–11.

Liccardi G. and D'Amato G. (1996) Oral allergy syndrome after ingestion of salami in a subject with monosensitisation to mite allergens. *J. Allergy Clin. Immunol.* **98**, 850–2.

Lichtenstein L.M. and Fauci A.S. (1985) *Current Therapy in Allergy Immunology and Rheumatology*. Burlington, Ont., B.C. Decker.

Luce E.B., Montgomery M.T. and Redding S.W. (1990) The prevalence of cardiac pathosis in patients with systemic lupus erythematosus. *Oral Surg. Oral Med. Oral Pathol.* **70**, 590–2.

McCarthy N.R. (1985) Diagnosis and management of hereditary angio-oedema. *Br. J. Oral Maxillofac. Surg.* **23**, 123–7.

Mutlu S., Porter S.R., Richards A., Scully C. and Maddison P. (1993) Gingival and periodontal health in Sjögren's syndrome and other connective tissue disorders. *Clin. Exper. Rheumatol.* **11**, 95–6.

Mutlu S., Richards A., Maddison P. and Scully C. (1993) Gingival and periodontal health in systemic lupus erythematosus. *Commun. Dent. Oral Epidemiol.* **21**, 158–61.

Peterson D.S. and Klein D.R. (1980) Dental implications for systemic lupus erythematosus. *J. Oral Med.* **35**, 72–5.

Porter S.R. and Scully C. (1996) *Innovations and Developments in Non-Invasive Oral Health Care*. Northwood, Science Reviews.

Schumacher H.R., Klippel J.H. and Robinson D.R. (eds) (1988). *Primer on the Rheumatic Diseases*, 9th edn. Atlanta, Arthritis Foundation.

Scully C. (1988) *The Dental Patient*. Oxford, Heinemann.

Scully C. (1989) *Patient Care: a Dental Surgeon's Guide*. London, British Dental Association.

Scully C. (1989) *The Mouth and Perioral Tissues*. Oxford, Heinemann.

Scully C. and Porter S.R. (1990) Immunologically mediated disease. In Jones J.H. and Mason D.K. (eds), *Oral Manifestations of Systemic Disease*, 2nd edn. London, Baillière Tindall, pp. 183–270.

Scully C. and Porter S.R. (1990) Disorders of immunity. In Jones J.H. and Mason D.K. (eds), *Oral Manifestations of Systemic Disease*, 2nd edn. Philadelphia, Saunders.

Scully C., Cawson R.A. and Griffiths M.J. (1990) *Occupational Hazards to Dental Staff*. London, British Dental Journal.

Waytes A.T., Rosen F.S. and Frank M.M. (1996) Treatment of hereditary angioedema with a vapor-heated C1 inhibitor concentrate. *N. Engl. J. Med.* **334**, 1630–4.

22

Maxillofacial trauma and head injury

Key points

- Deaths due to trauma usually come within the first seconds to minutes. After that, the first hour is the time of greatest mortality.
- Airway, spine, breathing and circulatory control are essential; airway obstruction, inadequate ventilation and profound hypovolaemia must be treated immediately.
- *Primary survey* and simultaneous resuscitation of vital functions of traumatized patients is essential and should include:
    - **A**irway and cervical spine control
    - **B**reathing and ventilation
    - **C**irculation and control of haemorrhage
    - **D**isability and neurological status
    - **E**xposure and environmental control
- It is important as soon as the patient is seen, thereby to establish the vital signs of:
    - Pulse
    - Blood pressure
    - Respiratory rate
    - Pupil size
    - Conscious state; **a**lert, responding to **v**ocal stimuli, to **p**ainful stimuli, or **u**nresponsive (AVPU).
- A *secondary survey* is then necessary to:
    - Establish a baseline Glasgow Coma Scale score
    - Reassess the ABCs
    - Look for:
        - other life-threatening injuries, particularly to the cervical spine; a sturdy cervical collar or spinal board with head strap (Hines splint) should be used to prevent damage
        - thorax and abdomen injuries
        - fractures of other bones
        - leakage of cerebrospinal fluid
        - injuries to the eyes
    - Reduce and immobilize airway-threatening fractures. (Delay definitive treatment until the patient is out of danger.)
- *The primary survey must be repeated at regular intervals.*
- Further treatment includes debridement and suturing of facial lacerations and the provision of antibiotic and tetanus prophylaxis.
- Patients who should be admitted to hospital for observation after head injury include:

> children, and those with psychiatric disease or learning disability
> patients living without a responsible adult companion
> persons with a coma scale of less than 15
> those with a skull fracture
> where there is post-traumatic amnesia
> if there are other serious injuries.
> - Medical complications of head injury may include hypertension, dysrhythmias, deep vein thromboses, embolism, pulmonary oedema, coagulopathy, gastritis, infections and ADH changes.
> - Later complications of head injury may include intracranial haematomas, epilepsy, mental or physical disability, infections, endocrine or psychogenic problems.
> - Spinal cord injuries should always be ruled out, especially involving C1–2, C4–7 and T11–12.
> - Paraplegia limits access and there are hazards from pressure sores, postural hypotension, muscle contractures, urinary and bowel dysfunction, and psychological sequelae.

Accidents are the most common cause of death in children and in men under the age of 35. Head injuries are seen in about 70 per cent of them. Up to a third of these deaths are, theoretically at least, preventable. The reader should consult *The Advanced Trauma Life Support* manual for physicians (ACS 1989) and similar guides for full details on this important topic (*see* Bibliography).

Most head and maxillofacial injuries are in previously fit young men, usually from road accidents, assaults or fights. Alcohol is a frequent factor. Violence is increasing but trauma from road accidents is not (*Plate 22*). Industrial accidents, sport and epilepsy are other causes.

About 20 per cent of patients admitted with multiple injuries also have a maxillofacial injury, and about 70 per cent have a head injury. Medical complications in multiply injured patients can include hazards to the airway, and damage to the chest, spine, liver, spleen, kidneys or bladder. Shock is most unusual in uncomplicated maxillofacial injuries or head injuries and its presence is often an indication of internal haemorrhage. Nevertheless, the severity of maxillofacial injuries is often underestimated. The possibility of pre-existing disease must always also be considered.

Major complications with maxillofacial injuries apart from the obvious hazard to the airway, may therefore include:

1. Head and neck injuries.
2. Chest injuries.
3. Ruptured viscera with internal haemorrhage.
4. Eye injuries.
5. Fractures of the thoracolumbar spine.
6. Long bone fractures.

- **Management**

The management of these injuries and their complications takes precedence; *the most urgent attention is needed to maintain the airway* and control bleeding, and to prevent spinal damage by using a firm cervical collar in case there are cervical fractures. Severe maxillofacial injuries are often seen by the oral or maxillofacial surgeon after the patient has been examined and major injuries treated by other specialists, but this is not invariable and dental surgeons may find themselves in charge of the whole initial care of such patients.

INITIAL MANAGEMENT OF THE PATIENT WITH MAXILLOFACIAL INJURIES (*Table 22.1*)

The priorities of early management of a patient with maxillofacial and other injuries, especially if in coma, are as follows:

1. Ensure a clear airway.

Table 22.1 Maxillofacial trauma: early management

- Immediate care (ABC)
    Airway and cervical spine
    Breathing and bleeding
    Conscious state and chest injury
- General assessment
    State of consciousness
    Pulse
    Blood pressure
    Respiratory rate
    Pupil size and reaction
- Assessment of head injury
    Skull examination
    Examination for cerebrospinal fluid leak
    Neurological assessment
    Skull radiography
    Blood analyses
- Assessment for other injuries
    Chest
    Neck
    Spine
    Abdomen
    Perineum
    Limbs

2. Look for and control bleeding, whether intra- or extracranial.
3. Look for other serious injuries, particularly to the cervical spine, and use a collar to prevent spinal injury.
4. Look for injuries to the thorax and abdomen.
5. Look for fractures of other bones.
6. Look for leakage of cerebrospinal fluid; tell the patient not to blow the nose.
7. Look for injuries to the eyes.
8. Establish a neurological base-line from the history, conscious level, examination and pupil reactions for future reference.
9. Reduce and immobilize a fracture if it threatens the airway. There is also evidence that early stabilization of grossly displaced or comminuted facial bone fragments facilitates later management and reduces facial deformity. Definitive treatment must be delayed until the patient is out of danger.
10. Debride and suture facial lacerations.
11. Give prophylactic antibiotics and tetanus prophylaxis, and arrange investigations and admission as necessary.

In the general assessment of the patient the 'five Bs' may serve as a reminder of the practical sequence of the main investigations of the seriously injured or comatose patient. These comprise attention to:

1. **B**reathing.
2. **B**leeding.
3. **B**lood pressure.
4. **B**rain function.
5. **B**lood analyses.

Injured patients can be assessed using the Revised Trauma Score (RTS), calculated mainly from the Glasgow Coma Scale (GCS; described below), the blood pressure and the respiratory rate. Injuries can be categorized using the Abbreviated Injury Scale (AIS), which scores from minor (1) to fatal (6) injuries. The Injury Severity Score (ISS) is calculated by the addition of the AIS for the three most severely injured areas of the body.

Airway and breathing

Respiratory obstruction is the most important preventable cause of early death after maxillofacial trauma. Many patients have died from neglect of the airway before admission to hospital. Foreign bodies or the tongue can easily fall back to obstruct respiration, especially if there are bilateral fractures or comminution of the mandible, and the patient is unconscious.

Severely injured patients must be laid semi-prone on their sides, face towards the ground, to allow any potential obstruction to fall forwards. The mouth and pharynx must be quickly cleared of debris and sucked out. In the case of bilateral mandibular body fractures, a traction suture through the tongue will hold it forward, but frequently, medial displacement of the posterior fragments prevents the anterior fragment from falling backwards unless the bone is comminuted. Posterior displacement of the maxilla in middle third injuries may cause the soft palate to occlude the airway. Obstruction can then be overcome by manual disimpaction of the maxilla and insertion of a nasopharyngeal tube. In the unconscious patient a cuffed endotracheal tube is more satisfactory, but in gross trauma tracheostomy may be needed. All unconscious patients should also have a gastric tube passed to aid stomach aspiration and feeding.

Table 22.2 Indications for tracheostomy

- Obstruction of the airway by
  Gross retroposition of the middle third of the face
  Pharyngeal oedema
  Uncontrollable nasal haemorrhage
  Loss of tongue control
- Where positive pressure ventilation is needed
  e.g. crushed or flail chest
- Where tracheobronchial suction is needed
  e.g. chronic obstructive airways disease

If there is supraglottic airways obstruction an airway can be established by laryngotomy using a wide-bore (2–3 mm) needle inserted through the cricothyroid membrane. Tracheostomy can then be carried out. Indications for tracheostomy are summarized in *Table 22.2*.

There is special danger to the airway if there has been trauma to and oedema of the tongue, fauces, pharynx or larynx, or uncontrollable nasal haemorrhage. Chest injuries, particularly those causing tension pneumothorax or flail chest, or inhalation of toxic or hot gases further impair respiration (*see* Burns).

Flail chest can be recognized by extreme difficulty in breathing, associated with paradoxical movements of the chest and cyanosis. Intermittent positive-pressure ventilation must be given via an endotracheal tube.

Haemorrhage

Severe haemorrhage or shock very rarely results from maxillofacial injuries alone, unless caused by gunshot wounds. Even a ruptured inferior dental artery usually stops bleeding spontaneously.

If bleeding recurs, the damaged vessel must be ligated, at open operation if necessary, and an intravenous infusion line should be set up in case blood transfusion is needed.

Severe nose bleeds, that do not cease spontaneously after pressure or after packing with 1/2 inch ribbon gauze, may be controlled using a Foley balloon catheter passed through the nose into the nasopharynx, softly inflated and then pulled gently forwards against the posterior nasal choanae.

It is essential to remember that bleeding may be concealed, or occasionally aggravated by disseminated intravascular coagulation (Chapter 4) secondary to the head injury. Internal haemorrhage, for example into the abdomen from a ruptured viscus, or into the thigh from a fractured femur, can cause life-threatening hypotension. Haemorrhage into the pleural cavity from fractured ribs can also embarrass respiration. Latent haemorrhage may be recognized by the following:

1. Rising pulse rate.
2. Falling blood pressure.
3. Increasing pallor.
4. Air hunger.
5. Restlessness.

Severe haemorrhage can lead to cardiac or renal failure or cause fatal cerebral hypoxia.

If haemorrhage is suspected a surgical opinion should be sought and the following quarter- or half-hourly observations should be recorded:

1. Pulse rate.
2. Blood pressure.
3. Respiratory rate.
4. Urine output and fluid balance (usually hourly).

A falling blood pressure with rising pulse rate suggests hypotension because of bleeding. If haemorrhage is persistent blood should be taken for grouping and cross-matching. If, however, the blood pressure is found to be rising then cerebral oedema and increasing intracranial pressure must be suspected, as discussed later.

Blood transfusion
In view of the risks of infection with HIV and other agents, blood transfusion should be given only where the clinical condition genuinely warrants it. Blood may be needed to replace loss from acute haemorrhage. Blood transfusion is not needed to replace loss of less than 500 ml in an adult, unless there was pre-existing anaemia or deterioration of the general condition warrants transfusion. Since time is needed to obtain correctly cross-matched blood, normal saline, plasma or a plasma expander such as dextran 70 or 110 may be given initially, and dextrans or other plasma expanders such as hydroxyethyl starch together with tranexamic acid or desmopressin may be the only possibility in Jehovah's witnesses. Dextran can interfere

with blood-grouping and cross-matching so that blood samples should be collected before a dextran infusion is started (*see* Chapter 4).

HEAD INJURY

Head injuries are common, accounting for up to 20 per cent of acute surgical admissions, and are a major cause of death in patients with maxillofacial injuries. Almost 50 per cent of deaths from head injury happen before the patient reaches hospital and most of the remainder follow within the first few days. Of those with brain damage, 12 per cent die within 2 days, while approximately 50 per cent have permanent after-effects such as paralyses, loss of speech, impaired vision, epilepsy, disturbances of personality or severe mental defects, rendering them disabled for life. Delayed effects may result from ischaemia, hypoxia, cerebral oedema, intracranial hypertension, and/or abnormalities of cerebral blood flow. The underlying mechanisms are unclear but may include tissue acidosis, free radicals, prostaglandin and electrolyte changes, and a number of novel medical therapies have been tried in order to modulate these changes.

Even mild head injuries carry the risk of life-threatening complications such as intracranial haematoma or infection, or of post-traumatic epilepsy, and it is important to appreciate that the brain can be fatally damaged without fracture of the skull or even a blemish on the scalp. The presence of a skull fracture, however, greatly increases the statistical risk of an intracranial haematoma and significant intracranial lesions are found in two-thirds of those with a skull fracture. Skull fractures can also cause cranial nerve damage, and provide an entry to the CSF for leakage, infection or air (pneumocephalus). About 80 per cent of fractures are linear, and many are associated with sub- or epidural haematomas. Basal skull fractures are usually uncomplicated and may not show on routine radiography but may be revealed by bleeding which may show as haemotympanum (behind the ear drum), as ecchymosis over the mastoid process (Battle's sign), or as periorbital ecchymosis (racoon sign), by CSF rhinorrhoea or otorrhoea, or by cranial nerve lesions involving the olfactory nerve (cribriform plate fracture), optic nerve (sphenoid), facial nerve (petrous), or abducens and facial nerve (sella fracture) though there can be causes of these nerve lesions other than fractures.

Intracranial haematomas may be of three types. *Intracerebral* haematomas are within the brain and, unless they act as an enlarging mass, are usually not amenable to treatment. *Epidural* or extradural (between dura mater and skull) haematomas are usually arterial – due to tearing of the middle meningeal artery after a fracture of the temporal bone – evolve rapidly and are a neurosurgical emergency. The haematoma forms a tumour-like mass which compresses part of the brain and causes increasing intracranial pressure as it expands.

Clinically the typical story is of a heavy blow followed by loss of consciousness. There is usually then a period of apparent recovery (lucid interval) followed by signs of increasing intracranial pressure. If the clot is not removed, death from respiratory arrest follows.

A radiograph showing a fracture line crossing the line of the middle meningeal artery strongly suggests extradural haemorrhage. CT scanning will confirm the diagnosis. The neurosurgical treatment is to drill bur holes through the skull to drain the clot and ligate the bleeding vessel.

Subdural haematomas are between the dura and leptomeninges, are venous and associated with contusion of the underlying brain. They may be acute or chronic but in any event, early removal improves survival. *Acute* subdural haematoma is often the result of an injury causing a tear in the arachnoid and may be associated with laceration or contusion of the brain.

Clinically, there is a latent interval after the injury, followed by progressive deterioration of consciousness and development of symptoms somewhat similar to those of an extradural haematoma. Once coma has developed, up to 50 per cent of patients die.

Chronic subdural haematoma can be caused by very mild injury. Nevertheless, the veins between the pia and the dura mater are torn. Leakage of blood into the subdural space is very slow. There is a fibroblastic response and eventually the haematoma becomes enclosed in scar tissue or, occasionally, resorbed.

Clinically, the head injury, especially in an elderly person, may be so slight as to have been forgotten but, after several weeks, or even months, symptoms such as headache, dizziness, slowness of thinking, or confusion and disturbance of consciousness, develop. There may be localizing signs such as hemiparesis or aphasia; the patient may have ptosis and be unable to look upwards (pressure on the IIIrd nerve).

The main principles of management of a subdural haematoma are to localize the lesion and to evacuate the clot through bur holes. The results are variable and depend on the degree of cerebral damage.

The goals are therefore to prevent or reverse secondary insults to the damaged brain, such as from hypoxaemia, hypotension and haematoma, and to allow recovery of as much damaged brain tissue as possible. It is important to recognize and to treat factors that can contribute to the morbidity and mortality and which include the following:

1. Airway obstruction.
2. Hypotension.
3. Intracranial haematoma.
4. Meningitis.
5. Uncontrolled epilepsy.
6. Stress-induced gastric bleeding (Cushing's ulcer).

History

Many patients are brought in confused, concussed or in coma and as good a history as possible must therefore be obtained from witnesses. Consciousness is almost invariably impaired after diffuse brain damage, although the patient may lose consciousness only transiently. However, there is usually amnesia for the traumatic event, and afterwards (post-traumatic amnesia) for a period far exceeding that of coma. Consciousness is not, however, always lost if brain damage is local – when, for example, the skull is penetrated by a sharp object. Maintenance of consciousness does not therefore imply the absence of brain damage. Thirty per cent of patients with ultimately fatal head injuries may talk after injury and some are completely lucid for a time. Concussion, an immediate but transient loss of consciousness, is always associated with a short period of amnesia,

Table 22.3	Some causes of coma

- Local disease of the central nervous system
  Trauma
  Haemorrhage (subarachnoid, epidural or subdural)
  Infarction (thrombosis or embolism)
  Infections (abscess, meningitis or meningo-encephalitis)
  Tumours (metastatic or primary)
  Epilepsy
  Raised intracranial pressure from any cause
- Systemic causes (toxic and metabolic)
  Intoxication (alcohol, barbiturates, opiates etc.)
  Metabolic disorders (diabetic hypo- or hyperglycaemia, Addisonian crisis, hypothyroidism, hypoglycaemia from any cause, uraemia, hepatic coma)
  Severe systemic infections (pneumonia, typhoid fever, malaria)
  Hypoxia
  Acute hypotension (circulatory collapse from any cause)
  Hypertensive encephalopathy
  Hypo- or hyperthermia
  Reye's syndrome

and there is some brain damage even if after-effects are not detectable on neurological testing, CSF examination, or CT or MRI. About 3 per cent will, however, have intracranial haemorrhage. The extent of retrograde amnesia is a rough measure of the severity of injury.

The brain is, therefore, invariably damaged in those who have lost consciousness, for however brief a period, and sometimes in those who have not. Prolonged unconsciousness, when there are no complications such as haematomas and where there are no focal signs, is caused by severe brain damage or other unrelated disease (*see Table 22.3*).

Reports of nausea, vomiting or headache must be noted, as well as the medical history, especially use of drugs including anticoagulants, or any previous history of epilepsy. Family or friends may be able to provide information about the patient's medical background.

Examination

The most essential examination is to assess *the level of consciousness* by the Glasgow Coma Scale (*Table 22.4*), scoring points related to three features:

	Score
Table 22.4 Glasgow Coma or Responsiveness Scale	

	Score
Eye opening	
spontaneous	E4
to speech	3
to pain	2
nil	1
Motor response	
obeys	M6
localizes	5
withdraws	4
abnormal flexion	3
extends	2
nil	1
Verbal response	
orientated	V5
confused conversation	4
inappropriate words	3
incomprehensible sounds	2
nil	1
EMV score or responsiveness sum	3–15

7 or less = coma in 100 per cent; 9 or more = absence of coma.

1. Eye opening, spontaneously (4 points), in response to command (3), in response to pain (2), not at all (1).
2. Motor responses, with *any movement of limbs in response to command* (6 points), *movement precisely in response to command* (5), flex to painful stimuli (4), abnormally flex to pain (3), extend to painful stimuli (nail-bed pressure) (2), or fail to respond (1).
3. Verbal response, which may be oriented (5 points), confused or disoriented (4), inappropriate words (3), incomprehensible sounds (2), or lacking (1).

The degree of brain damage is assessed by the level of consciousness and, later, by the duration of coma and of post-traumatic amnesia. A fully alert and otherwise well patient with a full score of 15 and no neurological signs or symptoms and no skull fracture or intracranial haemorrhage on CT scan may not need hospital admission for observation but all patients who score less than the full 15 points should be admitted to hospital for observation, even if drugs or alcohol are the suspected causes of depressed consciousness. Those with a score of less than 8 require immediate neurosurgical attention, as do patients with major skull fractures,

deteriorating consciousness, neurological lateralization (pupillary inequality and hemiparesis) or uncontrollable bleeding from scalp, bone or brain. About 85 per cent of those with a score of 3 or 4 succumb within 24 hours.

Up to 60 per cent of all patients admitted in coma are alcoholics who have often had a head injury. Toxic and metabolic disorders cause no focal or localizing neurological signs. However, when there is disease of the CNS itself, sensory or motor disturbances may indicate the site of the lesion. In some of these diseases white cells, bacteria or blood may also appear in the CSF.

Intoxications, whether the result of exogenous agents or disorders of metabolism and severe infections, all have essentially similar effects and will not be discussed further here.

Estimation of blood urea and electrolyte levels are needed in case there has been renal failure secondary to loss of blood, and as a baseline to monitor progress and the effects of intravenous fluid replacement. A full blood picture is also needed as a baseline for possible effects of transfusion and for any coincidental haematological disease. As described above (Chapter 4), early haemoglobin levels give no useful indication of the amount of blood lost.

Admission of conscious patients to hospital

Ideally, every patient who has a head injury should be admitted for observation but this is impractical. However, the following categories of patients should be admitted:

1. Children, those with psychiatric disease, or those with learning disability.
2. Patients living alone or without a responsible adult companion.
3. If the Coma Scale score is less than 15.
4. If there is fracture of the skull. If there is evidence of a depressed skull fracture, debridement and elevation of the fracture is needed within 24 hours.
5. If there is post-traumatic amnesia.
6. If there are other serious injuries.

Patients with severe head injuries fall into three main groups:

1. Most are stable neurologically with gradual improvement in consciousness.

2. Rising intracranial pressure causing progressive deterioration in the level of consciousness in the absence of localizing signs. Cerebral oedema may be reduced by ensuring adequate oxygenation and by giving mannitol, frusemide and/or dexamethasone.
3. Progressive deterioration in the level of consciousness with localizing signs. However, localized intracranial bleeding with or without cerebral oedema, contusions or lacerations may be manageable, if the bleeding can be evacuated by craniotomy.

The level of consciousness is depressed further by sedatives and many analgesics. Alcohol must be prohibited. Benzodiazepines should not be given for such purposes as controlling fits or to allow suturing of head wounds. They cause respiratory depression which can be fatal, unless ventilation is given. If there are repeated fits, phenytoin by intravenous infusion is less likely to depress respiration.

Analgesia

Morphine and its analogues are especially dangerous because they both depress respiration and disguise eye signs of rising intracranial pressure by causing pupillary constriction. Pentazocine is also contraindicated. If analgesia is essential, codeine, diclofenac or buprenorphine can be used.

Clinical examination

Neurological function
Pupil size and reaction must be checked for localizing signs of neurological damage. A dilated fixed (unreactive to light) pupil often indicates rising intracranial pressure and is usually a serious sign. Severe facial oedema may, however, make examination of the eyes difficult and the eyelids should then be prised open. A fixed dilated pupil may also be caused by local damage to the optic or oculomotor nerves and must be differentiated by clinical examination, radiographs (including, if necessary, tomography) and by the absence of signs associated with brain damage or of rising intracranial pressure.

Rising intracranial pressure is typically associated with bradycardia and rising blood pressure, but these may sometimes be absent. Limb reflexes should be tested. Convulsions early on considerably increase the likelihood of late epilepsy.

Blood pressure
Regular monitoring of the blood pressure is essential. A low or falling blood pressure with rising pulse rate is indicative of haemorrhage or shock which can lead to fatal cerebral anoxia or renal failure. A systolic blood pressure lower than 60 mmHg brings with it a risk of brain damage. A high or rising blood pressure with bradycardia, by contrast, is indicative of raised intracranial pressure secondary to cerebral oedema or haemorrhage as a result of the injury.

Scalp lacerations and compound fractures
Lacerations of the scalp can cause severe loss of blood and provide a pathway for infection into the cranial cavity. They may also be associated with a depressed fracture, which may be palpable.

Leakage of cerebrospinal fluid
Particular care must be taken to look for cerebrospinal rhinorrhoea or otorrhoea, and signs of orbital or retromastoid haematomas (which may indicate fractures with dural tears), in all of which there is the risk of meningitis because of skull fracture. The mortality may ultimately reach 20 per cent. CSF rhinorrhoea is found in about 2 per cent of all head injuries, but is seen in 25 per cent of fractures of the middle facial third and of the nasoethmoidal complex. The leak usually persists for about a week and the risk of meningitis is greatest within the first fortnight. Occasionally the fistula may be occluded by herniated brain but the dural tear fails to heal. Meningitis may follow after some months or years and dural repair is desirable. A neurosurgical opinion should therefore be obtained.

In the early stages leakage of CSF may be obscured by haemorrhage, but any clear watery discharge from the nose is suspect. CSF contains sugar but little protein – which differentiates it from a serous nasal discharge. Lacrimal fluid, however, also contains small amounts of glucose and CSF must therefore be positively identified by protein electrophoresis and by accurate measurement of the glucose. Prophylactic antimicrobials are needed if there is a risk of meningitis and should therefore be given to all patients with a middle third injury, penetrating brain injury, or compound depressed skull fracture. Penicillin does not adequately enter the cerebrospinal fluid. Co-trimoxazole 960 mg, 12 hourly for 5–7 days, may be a suitable regimen. Because of the danger of sulphonamide crystalluria, extra fluids may need to be given.

Many bacteria causing post-traumatic meningitis, such as meningococci, *Staphylococcus aureus* or *Streptococcus pneumoniae* are resistant to sulphonamides. Effective alternatives are rifampicin 600 mg b.d. for 4 days or minocycline 100 mg b.d. for 5 days: they readily reach the CSF and are well absorbed when given orally. Rifampicin is effective against *Neisseria meningitidis*, *S. aureus* and *S. pneumoniae* and may possibly be a more suitable drug than sulphonamides for prophylaxis of post-traumatic intracranial infection.

The main toxic effects of rifampicin are influenzal, abdominal and respiratory symptoms or, rarely, renal failure or thrombocytopenia after prolonged treatment. Serious toxic effects are unlikely to complicate the short-term prophylaxis of meningitis. However, patients should be warned that their saliva and urine will turn orange.

Rifampicin may be contraindicated in those with liver disease and alcoholics – unfortunately a well-represented group amongst head injury cases.

Radiography

Radiography (typically AP, lateral and Towne's views) and CT scans are essential to exclude fractures of the skull and brain lesions. They should be carried out early before infection can reach the cranial cavity. MRI can provide better images but cannot always be used. Radiography may also reveal a depressed fracture involving the paranasal sinuses; this suggests a meningeal tear which is occasionally confirmed by seeing intracranial air (aerocele).

A linear fracture indicates the possibility of intracranial haematoma but even normal radiographs do not exclude brain damage. About 50 per cent of patients with intracranial injuries have no skull fracture, but approximately 90 per cent of patients with fractures of the skull have no resulting intracranial injury. CT signs such as compression or obliteration of mesencephalic cisterns, midline hemisphere shift, or one or more surgical masses correlate with raised intracranial pressure – and decreased survival.

Blood analyses

Some of the many causes of coma are listed in *Table 22.3*. Coma from various causes differs in the nature of the associated signs, which are discussed in more detail in this and other chapters. More than one cause may be operative. Blood and urine samples should therefore be collected for analysis for alcohol, drugs and metabolic disorders, particularly diabetes. Transient glycosuria unrelated to diabetes may, however, follow the stress of head injuries.

Observation

Patients must be carefully and regularly observed to detect the development of complications, especially intracranial haematomas which need immediate neurosurgical attention. The level of consciousness should be charted regularly half-hourly, or even more frequently, along with the pulse, blood pressure, respiration and pupil reactivity. The most important sign is deterioration of consciousness, sometimes with increasing restlessness, headache and vomiting. Dilatation of the pupil on the side of the fracture and decerebrate rigidity – late signs caused by raised intracranial pressure and brain shift – are soon followed by bilateral pupil dilatation, periodic respiration, respiratory arrest and death, unless there is immediate neurosurgical intervention.

Focal signs such as hemiparesis, dysphasia or focal epilepsy however, are uncommon. In deep coma there are no verbal or motor responses but in less severe cases the eyes may open transiently from time to time and there may be vague or weak responses to stimuli.

Medical complications of head injuries

The brain controls many organs and processes via neurological and hormonal influences, and thus injury can result in a range of medical complications, including:

1. Cardiovascular: neurogenic hypertension, myocardial dysfunction, dysrhythmias or deep vein thrombosis.
2. Respiratory: neurogenic pulmonary oedema – a form of adult respiratory distress syndrome, infections, embolism.
3. Coagulopathy: disseminated intravascular coagulopathy.
4. Electrolyte imbalance: hyponatraemia, hypernatraemia or hypokalaemia.
5. Endocrine: inadequate or inappropriate secretion of ADH.
6. Gastrointestinal: stress gastritis and haemorrhage.
7. Fat embolism, mainly where there have been fractures of long bones.
8. Neuropsychological sequelae (Chapters 17 and 18).
9. Infections: of wounds, foreign bodies, CSF, intravenous lines, intracranial pressure monitoring devices, sinuses and lungs.

Late sequelae of head injury

Late sequelae that may complicate head injuries include the following:

1. Chronic extra- or subdural haematomas.
2. Post-traumatic syndrome.
3. Epilepsy (Chapter 17).
4. Infection (*see above*).
5. Diabetes insipidus (Chapter 14).
6. Mental handicap.
7. Physical disability.
8. Compensation neurosis (Chapter 18).

Post-traumatic syndrome

The post-traumatic syndrome may be caused by mild brain damage or damage to the cochlear–vestibular apparatus and frequently follows severe head injuries. Complaints include temporary headache, irritability, inability to concentrate, short temper, loss of confidence, vertigo and hyperacusis. If symptoms persist, psychiatric advice should be sought.

Diabetes insipidus

Diabetes insipidus may follow a head injury as a result of traction on the pituitary stalk,

especially where there is a basal skull fracture (*see* Chapter 14).

Syndrome of inappropriate ADH secretion (*see* Chapter 14)

COMPLICATIONS OF MAXILLOFACIAL INJURIES

Cranial nerve injuries

Cranial nerve lesions in patients with head injuries may indicate a basal skull fracture or other lesion. Cranial nerves I, II, III, V, VII and VIII are most vulnerable to damage (*Table 22.5* and Chapter 17). Sense of smell is disturbed or lost (anosmia) in 5–10 per cent of patients with head injuries. The olfactory nerves can be damaged in frontal bone injuries and fractures involving the cribriform plate of the ethmoid. There is often also cerebrospinal fluid rhinorrhoea.

Traumatic anosmia improves in only about 10 per cent of cases and perversion of the sense of smell may develop during recovery. These effects are remarkably troublesome or even disabling, but untreatable.

Orbital injuries

Ocular or orbital injuries may need the attention of an ophthalmological surgeon. Zygomatic fractures or isolated orbital injuries may hazard vision. Diplopia (double vision) is often present early because of oedema and haemorrhage within the confined space of the orbit; circumorbital and subconjunctival ecchymoses are usually associated (*Plate 23*). Occasionally periorbital emphysema is present.

Diplopia can also result from enophthalmos associated with orbital floor or wall fractures, from muscle or nerve injury, or from muscle entrapment. Orbital blowout fractures also depress the level of the eye and limit ocular movement, especially upwards.

Disruption of the bony margins of the superior orbital fissure, haematoma or traumatic aneurysm at this site may cause the superior orbital fissure syndrome of ophthalmoplegia, ptosis, exophthalmos, a fixed dilated pupil or absence of consensual reflex,

Table 22.5 Cranial nerve lesions complicating head injuries

Nerve lesion	Usual site of injury	Comments
I (Olfactory)	Ethmoidal complex (may be no fracture)	Anosmia (usually permanent); apparent loss of taste
II (Optic)	Orbit* or sphenoid	Pupil dilated, unreactive to light, but consensual reflex retained;[a] partial or complete blindness
III (Oculomotor)	Orbit*	Affected eye looks down and out. Pupil dilated, unreactive to light. No consensual reflex. Loss of medial and vertical movement of eye. Divergent squint
IV (Trochlear)	Orbit*	Diplopia only on looking down. Similar features result if superior oblique muscle is entrapped. Pupil; normal reactivity
V (Trigeminal)	Middle fossa, orbit,* maxilla or mandible	Commonly extracranially. Anaesthesia or paraesthesia in sensory area
VI (Abducens)	Orbit* or petrous temporal	Diplopia. Loss or lateral movement of eye. Convergent squint. Pupil reacts normally
VII (Facial)	Direct trauma to nerve or basal skull fracture	Facial paralysis, which may be delayed for a few days (*see* Facial paralysis)
VIII (Vestibulocochlear)	Petrous temporal	Deafness, vertigo and nystagmus alone or together. Deafness after head injury may also be caused by ruptured ear drum or blood in middle ear
IX–XII		Uncommon as a result of head injuries

*May be damage to orbital contents with or without fracture. These nerves are often injured together and urgent neurosurgery may be indicated since nerve dysfunction, if caused by haemorrhage or oedema within the optic canal or other confined space, may be reversible.
[a]Consensual reflex is the constriction of the pupil as a normal response when a light is shone into the other eye.

and some sensory loss over the distribution of the ophthalmic division of the trigeminal nerve. These signs are caused by injury to cranial nerves III, IV, V and VI, where they pass through the orbital fissure.

The diagnosis of diplopia is discussed in Chapter 17.

OTHER INJURIES AND COMPLICATIONS

Burns

Burns can be serious injuries, especially where more than 10 per cent of the body surface area is involved. First-aid care includes maintenance of an adequate airway, the administration of oxygen if there has been exposure to hot air or smoke, and lessening pain by cooling the burn and giving analgesics. Morphine 5–15 mg for an adult may be indicated. Subsequent treatment should be in a Burns or Plastic Surgery Unit.

After receiving burns in a closed or confined space, a change in voice, hoarseness, dysphonia, stridor or the coughing of sooty sputum are all danger signs suggesting inhalation injury. Endotracheal intubation or tracheostomy may be indicated. The reader is referred to Wachtel, Frank and Frank (1981) for further details.

Adult respiratory distress syndrome (ARDS)

This is a sequel to burns and other pulmonary injury. It is characterized by diffuse alveolar damage, pulmonary oedema and hyaline membrane formation. It may culminate in respiratory failure and mortality is high. Patients showing the suggestive signs of dyspnoea, increased respiratory rate, abnormal breath sounds (râles) with bilateral diffuse interstitial and intra-alveolar oedema on radiography, should be admitted to an Intensive Care unit.

Injuries to the spinal cord

Spinal cord injuries can accompany maxillofacial injuries and are an all too common result of road traffic or sports injuries. Cord injury is usually the result of vertical

Table 22.6 Spinal cord damage	
Level of damage	*Features*
C1–C5	Quadriplegia (tetraplegia) or death
C5–C6	Paraplegia
	Arms paralysed except for abduction and flexion
C6–C7	Paraplegia
	Hands, but not arms, paralysed
T11–T12	Paraplegia
	Sensory loss T12 and below
T12–L1	Legs paralysed below knees

compression, sometimes with flexion or extension of the neck, or violent sudden extension of the neck (whiplash injury), as when a vehicle is hit from behind.

Most vertebral injuries affect the C1–2, C4–7 and T11–L2 vertebrae. The clinical effects are determined largely by the level of the cord damage (*Tables 22.6 and 22.7*). The resulting disability can be appallingly severe.

Atlanto-axial subluxation

Dislocation at the atlanto-axial joint or fracture of the odontoid peg may follow trauma or other factors such as congenital anomalies of the odontoid process (as in Down's syndrome), rheumatoid arthritis or ankylosing spondylitis.

Traumatic dislocation may be lethal. If not, there may only be weakness of the legs or even no immediate neurological sequelae. Transient blackouts, weakness of the limbs, sensory loss, facial paraesthesia, nystagmus, ataxia and dysarthria may be complaints. The possibility of such damage should always be considered in patients involved in road traffic accidents since movement of the neck may then cause serious cord damage, spastic quadriplegia or death. The neck should not be extended or rotated, and a support collar should be used prophylactically. Decompression by reduction of any vertebral dislocations should be carried out by the neurosurgeon within 2 hours of injury. *Patients should therefore be moved with great care not to extend the neck after maxillofacial injuries to avoid this complication.*

The clinical effects of spinal cord injury develop in two main stages: *spinal shock* and *reflex activity* (*Table 22.7*). If movement can be elicited or any sensation is retained during the first 2–3 days, the prognosis is more favourable. Paraplegia is common but high doses of methylprednisolone given within 8 hours of the injury may minimize cord damage. Any symptoms persisting after 6 months are likely to be permanent.

• General management of paraplegics

Treatment in general is supportive and symptomatic, and is mainly directed toward the prevention of complications such as:

1. Muscle wasting or contractures.
2. Pressure sores.
3. Postural hypotension.
4. Urinary infections.
5. Constipation.
6. Psychological problems.

Physiotherapy is essential to limit muscle wasting and to maintain function in unparalysed or partly paralysed muscles. Joints must be regularly passively moved and the

Table 22.7 Effects of spinal cord damage	
Early (spinal shock): losses of	*Delayed (after 2–3 weeks): losses of*
Motor function	Motor function
quadriplegia if damage in cervical cord	may improve if cord not completely transected
paraplegia if damage in thoracic cord	
Sensation	Sensation
below lesion, leading to skin pressure ulcers	may improve if cord not completely transected
Reflexes	Reflexes
below lesion, with muscle flaccidity	involuntary flexor, then extensor spasms below level of lesion
Bladder and bowel sphincter paralysis leading to	Bladder and bowel sphincter control
urinary or faecal retention	irregular reflex micturition and defaecation

position of the patient carefully checked, to prevent soft tissue contractures and pressure sores.

Postural hypotension and autonomic dysreflexia can complicate high level spinal cord lesions. Intense vasoconstriction below the level of the cord injury follows certain stimuli such as bladder contraction. The vasoconstriction is associated with rapid onset of hypertension, facial sweating and headache.

Urinary retention invariably complicates acute spinal cord lesions, and aseptic catheterization is needed. Infections must be treated promptly – recurrent urinary infections were previously the main factor in renal disease and amyloidosis complicating paraplegia. Latex allergy commonly arises in such patients.

- **Dental management of paraplegics**

Access to care is the main problem since patients are chairbound. Dental management may be uncomplicated, although postural hypotension in the early stages may necessitate treatment in the supine position and latex allergy should be considered (Chapter 25). Quadriplegics are at risk from respiratory infections, and general anaesthesia should be avoided if possible and never carried out in the dental surgery. Other problems are dealt with in Chapter 23.

STAB WOUNDS

A small entrance wound may well hide injuries to deeper structures. Wounds caused by stabbing or glass fragments must always be explored carefully before closure.

GUNSHOT WOUNDS

Hand guns usually inflict low velocity bullet wounds that damage only the tissues they hit and such wounds can be managed by conventional surgical methods. In contrast, high velocity missiles (explosive blast fragments or rifle bullets) produce extensive tissue damage and contamination, though the entrance wounds may be minute. To avoid

gas gangrene, necrotic tissue should be excised and antibiotics given (*see below*).

PREVENTION OF INFECTION

Four main infective problems can complicate maxillofacial injuries:

1. Meningitis.
2. Local wound infection and osteomyelitis.
3. Tetanus.
4. Actinomycosis (rarely).

Meningitis

Meningitis is an important complication of opening the cranial cavity (shown by leakage of CSF), as discussed earlier. It is by far the most important infective complication of maxillofacial injuries and can also result from lacerations of the scalp when infection can reach the brain via the emissary veins.

Wound infection

The risk of infection of lacerated or contused soft tissues, or osteomyelitis, is increased when there is:

1. Inadequate wound toilet.
2. Foreign bodies in the wound or teeth in the fracture line.
3. Gross delay in treatment.
4. Systemic disease with diminished resistance to infection, particularly alcoholism.

Intramuscular benzyl penicillin 600 mg 6-hourly or cephazolin is usually an effective prophylactic for compound fractures. Gross debris, broken teeth, detached bone and foreign bodies should be removed.

Extreme care must be taken to identify foreign material within the tissues. Some types of glass and plastic are radiolucent and may be missed unless the wound is systematically probed. After preliminary wound toilet, lacerations can usually be sutured under local anaesthesia, but larger lacerations can be covered with tulle gras and dry dressings for closure as soon as possible under general anaesthesia.

Teeth in the fracture line may need to be extracted unless required for stabilization of a bone fragment.

Table 22.8   Management of wounded patients at risk from tetanus

	Immune status of patient	*Course of action*[a]
Superficial wound or abrasion	Immune[b]	—
	Not known to be immune	Active immunization with toxoid. Full 3-dose course or, if partially immune, a reinforcing dose
Deep wounds, puncture wounds or bites or burns	Immune	Give toxoid booster[c]
	Not known to be immune	Give antibiotics and start immunization with toxoid and (*a*) if seen after 4 h give 250 units HTIG i.m.; (*b*) if seen after 24 h give 500 units HTIG i.m.

HTIG, Human tetanus immunoglobulin.
[a]Wound debridement in all.
[b]Last of 3-dose course or reinforcing dose within past 10 years.
[c]Human tetanus immunoglobulin if *highly* contaminated wound.

Tetanus

Tetanus is a dangerous infection with a mortality still between 10 and 60 per cent. Tetanus is an uncommon, non-communicable disease caused by contamination of wounds by the sporing bacterium *Clostridium tetani*. Spores are ubiquitous in soil or dust, particularly where there is faecal contamination, for example in agricultural land. Tetanus is most likely to follow contaminated deep wounds, such as puncture wounds, especially if there is necrosis, but it may also follow trivial wounds, or even complicate burns. The elderly, particularly women are at greatest risk. Neonates may develop tetanus from contamination of the umbilical stump, a condition only found in the developing world.

The incubation period of tetanus is between 4 and 21 days, commonly about 10. Immunization is usually carried out in childhood and active immunization should also be part of the routine management of wounds (*Table 22.8*). Most cases in the developed world are now seen in those who were never immunised, or in those whose immunity has declined, hence the risk in the elderly.

C. tetani produces tetanospasmin, a neurotoxin, responsible for the violent muscular spasms characteristic of the disease. Trismus (lockjaw) due to masseteric spasm is the single most common early sign. Spasm of spinal muscles causes arching of the back (opisthotonos), while laryngeal spasm leads to asphyxiation. Autonomic dysfunction can cause cardiac dysrhythmias and fluctuations in blood pressure. Facial spasm produces a so-called sardonic smile (risus sardonicus) where the eyebrows are raised with eyes closed and the lips are drawn back over clenched teeth.

Death may follow within 10 days of the onset of tetanus, usually from asphyxia, bronchopneumonia or autonomic dysfunction.

Prophylaxis: Active immunization in childhood is given as triple vaccine (diphtheria, pertussis and tetanus antigens) starting at the age of 12 weeks, followed by further injections 6–8 weeks later and then after a further 4–6 months. Booster immunization (diphtheria plus tetanus) is given on starting primary school and at 15–19 years (Appendix to Chapter 11).

The duration of immunity after such an immunization schedule is not known but current practice is to boost it every 10 years. Groups at risk, for example farm workers, should be given boosters every 5 years. It is not, however, good practice always to give tetanus toxoid after every minor injury, as severe allergic reactions can occasionally follow.

• Management of the wounded patient

Patients who have contaminated wounds, such as those associated with maxillofacial injuries caused by road traffic or riding accidents, are at risk from tetanus. The following are considered tetanus-prone wounds.

1.   Any wound or burn sustained more than 6 hours before surgical treatment of the injury.

2. Any wound or burn at any interval after injury that shows any of the following:
a significant degree of devitalized tissue
a puncture type wound
contact with manure or soil
clinical sepsis.

An outline for the management of patients with such injuries is shown in *Table 22.8*.

Treatment of tetanus: The patient should be admitted to an Intensive Care Unit. The main principles are as follows:

1. Protection of the airway.
2. Antitetanus immunoglobulin injection.
3. Control of muscle spasms.
4. Wound debridement.

The airway: Tracheostomy should be carried out if the airway is endangered and to facilitate artificial respiration should it become necessary.

Antiserum: Antiserum must be given early as it is ineffective after the toxin has become bound to nervous tissue. Human antitetanus immunoglobulin (ATG, Humotet, 500 or more units) should be given. If this is not available animal antitetanus serum (ATS) can be given after testing for hypersensitivity and with adrenaline and corticosteroids available in case a severe reaction develops.

Control of muscle spasms: Spasms are controlled by heavy sedation or, in severe cases, with general anaesthesia, muscle relaxants and mechanical ventilation.

Wound debridement: The purpose of wound debridement is to remove the source of toxin as antibiotics alone are ineffective.

Survivors recover completely but should have active immunization with toxoid. The mortality is high, especially among the elderly.

- **Dental aspects of tetanus**

Trismus is usually caused by local irritation such as pericoronitis or temporomandibular pain-dysfunction syndrome. Tetanus must always, however, be considered in the differential diagnosis of trismus in the absence of a local cause. Such patients should therefore be asked whether they have had any recent wounds, particularly if farm workers or gardeners.

Dyskinesias due to phenothiazines include facial grimacing but rarely trismus – the mouth is usually forcefully opened.

Actinomycosis

Actinomycosis is rare. It usually affects the soft tissues at the angle of the mandible. The reader is referred to textbooks of oral surgery.

SPORTS INJURIES

Injuries to the teeth and oral soft tissues are common, particularly in football, ice hockey, basketball and boxing. Those involved in these sports, as well as wrestling, karate, judo and gymnastics, should wear a mouth shield. These are usually made of vinyl or acrylic and three types are available:

1. Stock protectors. These are cheap and easily adjusted but less comfortable.
2. Mouth-formed protectors moulded onto the teeth.
3. Custom-made protectors.

CHILD ABUSE (*see* Chapter 23)

BIBLIOGRAPHY

American College of Surgeons, Committee on Trauma (1989) *Advanced Trauma Life Support*. Chicago, IL, ACS.

American Heart Association (1986) American Heart Association 1985 National Conference Standards and Guidelines for Cardiopulmonary Resuscitation (CPR) and Emergency Cardiac Care (ECC). *J. Am. Med. Assoc.* **255** (Suppl).

American Heart Foundation (1986) *Advanced Cardiac Life Support Manual*. Dallas, American Heart Foundation.

Association for the Advancement of Automotive Medicine (1990). *Abbreviated Injury Scale Booklet (AIS 90) revision*. Des Plaines, Illinois, AAAM.

Backay L. and Glassauer F.E. (1980) *Head Injury*. Boston, Little, Brown.

Baskett P.J.F. and Weller R.M. (eds) (1988) *Medicine for Disasters*. London, Butterworths.

Bowie C. (1996) Tetanus toxoid for adults – too much of a good thing. *Lancet* **348**, 1185–6.

Brockehurst G., Gooding M. and James J. (1987) Comprehensive care of patients with head injuries. *Br. Med. J.* **294**, 345–7.

Cannell H., Paterson A. and Loukota R. (1996) Maxillofacial injuries in multiply injured patients. *Br. J. Oral Maxillofac. Surg.* **34**, 303–8.

Cannell H., Silvester K.C. and O'Regan M.B. (1993) Early management of multiply injured patients with maxillo-facial injuries transferred to hospital by helicopter. *Br. J. Oral Maxillofac Surg.* **31**, 207–12.

Cawson R.A., McCracken A.W., Marcus P.B. *et al.* (1989) *Pathology: the Mechanisms of Disease*, 2nd edn. St Louis, Mosby.

Cawson R.A. Spector, R.G. and Skelly A.M. (1995) *Basic Pharmacology and Clinical Drug Use in Dentistry*, 6th edn. Edinburgh, Churchill Livingstone.

Commission on the Provision of Surgical Services (1988) *Response of the Working Party on the Management of Patients with Major Injuries*. London, Royal College of Surgeons.

Council of the Royal College of Surgeons of England (1996) *Code of Practice for the Surgical Management of Jehovah's Witnesses*. London, Royal College of Surgeons.

Gentleman D., Teasdale G. and Murray L. (1986) Causes of severe head injury and risk of complications. *Br. Med. J.* **292**, 449.

Horton J.M. (1980) Care of the unconscious. *Br. Med. J.* **28**, 638–40.

Jennett B. (1980) Medical aspects of head injury. *Medicine (UK)* **1**, 641–8.

Kaufman H.H., Timberlake G., Voekler J. and Pait T.G. (1993) Medical complications of head injury. *Med. Clin. North Amer.* **77**, 43–60.

Kerr L. (1983) Dental problems in athletes. *Clin. Sports Med.* **2**, 115–22.

Leading Article (1980) CSF rhinorrhoea. *Lancet* **i**, 408–9.

Leading Article (1989) Abnormal blood clotting after head injury. *Lancet* **ii**, 957

Lewis A.F. (1983) *The Management of Acute Head Injury*. London, HMSO.

Masters S.J., McLean P.M., Arcarese J.S. *et al.* (1987) Skull x-ray examinations after head trauma. *N. Engl. J. Med.* **316**, 84–91.

McDermott P.J.C. (1992) Jehovah's witness: a management dilemma in severe maxillofacial trauma. *Br. J. Oral Maxillofac. Surg.* **30**, 331–4.

Miller J.D. (1990) Assessing patients with head injuries. *Br. J. Surg.* **77**, 241–2.

Resuscitation Council UK (1989) *Basic and Advanced Life Support Guidelines of the Resuscitation Council UK 1989*. Hammersmith Hospital, London, Department of Anaesthesia.

Ruff R.M., Marshall L.F., Crouch J. *et al.* (1993) Predictors of outcome following severe head trauma; follow-up data from the Traumatic Coma Data Bank. *Brain Inj.* **7**, 101–7.

Schultz R.C. and de Camera D.L. (1984) Athletic facial injuries. *J. Am. Med. Assoc.* **252**, 3395–8.

Scully C. (1988) *The Dental Patient*. Oxford, Heinemann.

Scully C. (1989) *The Mouth and Perioral Tissues*. Oxford, Heinemann.

Scully C. (1989) *Patient Care: a Dental Surgeon's Guide*. London, British Dental Association.

Scully C., Cawson R.A. and Griffiths M.J. (1990) *Occupational Hazards to Dental Staff*. London, British Dental Journal.

Sheffield F.W. (1985) To give or not to give; guidelines for tetanus vaccine. *Commun. View* **33**, 8–9.

Shepherd J.P., Al-Kotany M.Y., Subadan C. and Scully C. (1987) Assault and facial soft tissue injuries. *Br. J. Plast. Surg.* **40**, 614–19.

Shepherd J.P., Gayford J.J., Leslie I.J. and Scully C. (1988) Female victims of assault: a study of hospital attenders. *J. Cranio-maxillofac. Surg.* **16**, 233–7.

Shepherd J., Irish M., Scully C. and Leslie I. (1988) Alcohol intoxication and severity of injury in victims of assault. *Br. Med. J.* **296**, 1299.

Shepherd J., Irish M., Scully C. and Leslie I. (1989) Alcohol consumption, intoxication among victims of violence and comparable UK populations. *Br. J. Addiction* **84**, 1045–51.

Shepherd J.P., Shapland M., Irish M., Scully C. and Leslie I.J. (1988) Assault: characteristics of victims attending an inner city hospital. *Injury* **19**, 185–90.

Shepherd J.P., Shapland M., Pearce N.X. and Scully C. (1990) Pattern, severity and aetiology of injuries in victims of assault. *J. R. Soc. Med.* **83**, 75–8.

Wachtel T.L., Frank D.H. and Frank H.A. (1981) Management of burns of the head and neck. *Head Neck Surg.* **3**, 458–74.

Wald S.L. (1995) Advances in the early management of patients with head injury. *Surg. Clin. North Am.* **75**, 225–42.

Zook E.G. (1980) *The Primary Care of Facial Injuries*. Littleton, MA, PSG.

23

Disability, the young and the elderly

Key points

- Disability is anything that impairs normal social, educational or recreational activities.
- Learning disability implies a neurological defect of some kind, often but by no means always brain damage.
- Patients with brain damage often also have physical disabilities such as cerebral palsy, and may be epileptic or have other management problems. Access to care is often their greatest difficulty.
- Down's syndrome, the most common chromosomal anomaly, affects not only learning ability but also stature, craniofacial and dental development, immunity and cardiac development.
- Fragile X syndrome is the next most common chromosomal anomaly; it affects males and manifests mainly by autistic-like behaviour, with learning disability.
- Hydrocephalus is characterized by a very large head. The dilatation of the cerebral ventricles also causes brain damage unless drained with a ventriculo-atrial shunt.
- Cleft lip and palate are common defects, sometimes related to maternal folate deficiency, often seen in isolation but sometimes in syndromes, or with cardiac, renal, skeletal or CNS defects.
- Autism is a failure in interpersonal relationships, development of language and speech in children of normal appearance and sometimes normal intelligence who have ritualistic behaviour.
- Neonates have immature immune defences and craniofacial development is active. Candidosis is easily contracted, and drugs, irradiation and other factors can impair development.
- Hyperkinesia in children may result from psychiatric disorders, foods or additives, or drugs. Poor concentration, restlessness and overactivity are almost uncontrollable.
- Child abuse is any act of omission or commission that endangers or impairs the physical or emotional development of a child. The child must be safeguarded.
- Features suggestive of child abuse include late appearance for medical attention, history inconsistent with injuries, previous trauma, unusual injuries, general neglect and a cowed child.
- Self-inflicted injuries may be seen in psychiatrically ill persons and in some with learning disability, drug abuse or rare pain-insensitivity conditions.
- There is a growing population of elderly persons particularly in the developed world, where the old outnumber the young.
- Mobility and the special senses often become impaired in the elderly, as do immunity and sometimes higher functions.
- Socioeconomic deprivation, loneliness, and medical and physical disorders, are more common in the elderly, and multiple problems are often seen.

DISABILITY

Disability is caused by handicapping conditions that impair normal social, educational or recreational activities. Such patients need dental attention and treatment to at least the same standard as non-handicapped patients and frequently have a greater predisposition to dental disease.

It is important to appreciate, however, that though the treatment of patients with disability is often time-consuming, it is not necessarily more difficult than with normal persons, and can be highly rewarding. Nevertheless, there is evidence of much neglect of such patients by the dental profession. The sad fact is that the institutionalized patient in particular may lead an existence so dreary and emotionally isolated that any sort of friendly personal attention – which must be the essence of dental care – may become a delightful event to be eagerly anticipated and touchingly gratefully received.

Table 23.1   Important handicapping conditions

- Autism
- Cardiac disease
- Cerebral palsy
- Chromosomal anomalies, especially Down's syndrome
- Cleft deformities
- Cystic fibrosis
- Hydrocephalus
- Juvenile arthritis
- Learning disability (mental handicap)
- Muscle diseases
- Spinal cord damage (especially paraplegia) and spina bifida
- Thalidomide deformities
- Visual defects and hearing defects

The main disorders causing disability are shown in *Table 23.1*. Only patients with mental and related handicaps, some specific conditions, children and the elderly will be considered here. Patients with other important specific diseases, such as haemophilia, neurological disorders and muscular dystrophies, are discussed in other chapters.

Table 23.2   Causes of learning disability

Chromosomal anomalies
  Fragile X syndrome

Autosomal trisomies	Edwards' syndrome
	Patau's syndrome
	Down's syndrome
Deletions 5, short arm:	Cri du chat syndrome
Deletions 4, short arm:	Wolf's syndrome
Sex chromosome anomalies	XO Turner's syndrome
	XXX Superfemale
	XXY Klinefelter's syndrome
	XYY XYY syndrome

Inborn errors of metabolism
Protein
  Hypothyroidism (cretinism)
  Phenylketonuria
  Homocystinuria
  Wilson's disease
Carbohydrate
  Galactosaemia
  Mucopolysaccharidosis
Lipids
  Tay–Sachs disease
  Gaucher's disease
Purines
  Lesch–Nyhan syndrome

Phakomatoses
Neurofibromatosis (von Recklinghausen's disease)
Encephalofacial angiomatosis (Sturge–Weber syndrome)
Tuberous sclerosis (epiloia)

Microcephaly
Primary or secondary

Intrauterine damage
Anoxia
Prematurity
Infections
Cytomegalovirus
HIV
Rubella
Syphilis
Toxoplasmosis
Prematurity
Radiation

LEARNING DISABILITY (MENTAL HANDICAP)

Learning disability is usually due to a state of incomplete development of mind, particularly of intelligence, to such a degree that medical treatment or special care or training of the patient is needed. An intelligence

Table 23.3 Acquired causes of learning disability

- Trauma
- Anoxia
- Alzheimer's disease
- Meningitis, encephalitis, HIV
- Metabolic disorders
- Poisons
- Rhesus incompatibility

quotient of less than 70 is the arbitrary dividing line that distinguishes the learning disability from the educationally subnormal. Approximately 3 per cent of the population have learning disability, often with multiple handicaps. *Patients with other neurological defects such as of hearing or speech, may also have learning disability but be of normal intelligence.* Learning disability is frequently the result of brain damage of many types but genetic causes, birth trauma and, later, road traffic accidents are particularly important. The main definable causes of learning disability are outlined in *Tables 23.2* and *23.3* but the cause is usually unknown.

Most patients are 'high grade' (IQ between 50 and 75) and frequently live at home. More severely subnormal patients (IQ below 50), who are totally dependent on others, usually have to be admitted to a long-stay hospital. Brain damage may cause not only mental but also physical handicaps, and epilepsy, visual defects, hearing, speech or behavioural disorders, facial deformities or cardiac defects are also often associated.

Learning disability has three main aspects, namely:

1. Subnormal intelligence.
2. Social incapacities.
3. Abnormal behaviour.

Crime and sexual promiscuity are common, especially in the higher grades. Retribution often follows because, owing to the learning disability, they lack the resources to evade detection and often find themselves pregnant or in court, or both at an early age. Psychiatric disorders are qualitatively little different from those in the non-handicapped, but the symptoms are often modified by poor language development and other defects. However, problems such as hyperkinesis, autism and stereotyped movements are more

frequent. Body-rocking and self-mutilation are common in the severely retarded, especially in the barren environment of an institution. Pica (the ingestion of inedible substances) is also common (*see Fig. 15.2*).

- **General management of those with learning disability**

Learning disability is so varied in severity and character that generalizations cannot be justified. Many patients can be cared for adequately by committed parents or guardians; others are admitted to hostels or institutions at an early age.

Complications may result from over-indulgence by parents, with consequent obesity and its sequelae. Institutionalized patients may develop behavioural disturbances and are prone to infections, particularly viral hepatitis, gastrointestinal infections or infestations, or tuberculosis. Prolonged medication with sedatives, tranquillizers or anticonvulsants often causes adverse effects.

- **Dental aspects of learning disability**

The main questions that must be answered in assessing the possibilities for the dental management of learning disability patients are as follows:

1. Is the patient able to maintain oral hygiene?
2. Is the patient able to give informed consent to treatment?
3. Is the patient able to sit still and cooperate sufficiently to allow conventional dental treatment under local anaesthesia?
4. Is treatment best carried out under general anaesthesia or sedation?
5. Are there any other associated disorders, particularly epilepsy, which need to be anticipated?
6. Can special means be devised to overcome minor physical handicaps to allow maintenance of oral hygiene?
7. Can the patient's interest in maintaining oral hygiene be stimulated in any way such as by simple rewards of various sorts?
8. Has the patient a speech or other communication disorder rather than defective intelligence and is it possible to overcome this communication disorder?

Having solved these problems and decided which patients can be treated by conventional means it is important to appreciate that this is not necessarily more difficult than normal, other than being time-consuming.

Most of those with learning disability, particularly those with Down's syndrome, have low caries activity unless over-indulged with sweets by parents or others. Nevertheless, when caries develops it is frequently untreated or inadequately treated, and the teeth are lost prematurely. Preventive dental care is of paramount importance.

Routine, simple conservative dental treatment should be carried out wherever possible to preserve the teeth. For this purpose, local anaesthesia (if necessary with intravenous or inhalational sedation) is preferable and is usually satisfactory. General anaesthesia certainly makes the work easier for the operator, may permit a higher technical standard of dentistry and, by saving time, may enable more patients to be treated. It is therefore used for most handicapped patients by some operators. However, to do so presupposes the absence of medical contraindications, the assistance of an anaesthetist, as intubation is usually necessary, and other essential facilities.

Poor oral hygiene is the most common problem in handicapped patients and it is frequently impossible for these patients to improve their level of plaque control because of lack of understanding or motivation, associated physical handicaps or other disabilities. In the higher grades of mental defect, electric toothbrushes may be easier to use and effective. Chlorhexidine rinses may also control plaque accumulation to some degree. Regular, routine scaling usually improves the gingival state considerably but there is no indication for sophisticated periodontal surgery. If there are cardiac defects, antibiotic cover may be indicated (Chapter 3).

Other factors contributing to periodontal disease include gingival hyperplasia caused by phenytoin or by one of the genetic syndromes, where gingivectomy may sometimes be justifiable.

Handicapped patients are often made prematurely edentulous. Dentures are often impractical since many patients are incapable of managing them and clinical prosthetic work can be very difficult. Impression-taking is facilitated by using a viscous material (such as composition or a putty-type material) which, if the patient objects violently, can be readily removed without leaving unset material in the oropharynx. If patients will not keep their mouths open, a mouth prop on alternate sides and sectional impressions may overcome the difficulty. Registration of occlusal records can be very trying, but with patience can usually be effected.

Prostheses may also be contraindicated in severe epileptics, who may inhale foreign bodies during a convulsion. Certainly any prosthesis for an epileptic should be constructed of radio-opaque materials. Dentures should be marked with the patient's name typed onto a paper strip. This can be added to the fitting surface at flasking and covered with clear acrylic before processing. Those patients who are incapable of managing full dentures become dental cripples in addition to their other disabilities.

Self-mutilation may involve the oral or orofacial tissues, as in Lesch–Nyhan syndrome (*see* Appendix to Chapter 15) where the lips or tongue may be chewed almost to destruction. Rarely, oral self-mutilation is accidental in patients with congenital indifference to pain, including Riley–Day syndrome (familial dysautonomia) (*see* Appendix to Chapter 15).

CHROMOSOMAL ANOMALIES

Chromosomal anomalies are a common cause of spontaneous abortions and of natal and early neonatal deaths. The sex chromosomes and autosomes are equally frequently affected. Sex chromosome anomalies are usually compatible with life and rarely associated with severe physical disability but autosomal abnormalities are often lethal. Abnormalities of the smaller chromosomes may be compatible with life but can cause multiple handicaps, as in Down's syndrome.

The most common source of major chromosomal anomalies is an error in meiosis (non-disjunction) such that one chromosome too few, or one too many, enters a gamete and subsequently the zygote.

Most of the chromosomal anomalies are rare and many affected individuals survive

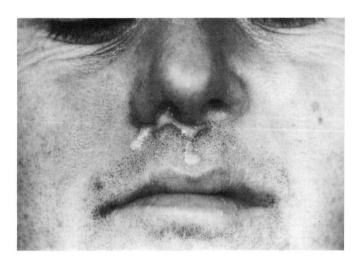

Fig. 23.1 Respiratory infection is one contraindication to general anaesthesia in Down's syndrome. Others include cardiac disease, atlanto-axial instability and anaemia

only for a few years. The most common anomaly of significance in dentistry is Down's syndrome. Medical problems and the main oral manifestations of other chromosomal anomalies are summarized in the Appendix to this chapter.

Down's syndrome (mongolism or trisomy 21)

Down's syndrome is the most common autosomal chromosome abnormality and also the most common of the clinically classifiable categories of learning disability. With an incidence of approximately 1 in 700 live births, Down's syndrome accounts for 5–10 per cent of institutionalized learning disability patients, and about one-third of children with severe learning disability. The trisomic mongol is usually born of an elderly mother: there is a 1 in 2000 chance for a 25-year-old, rising to 1 in 100 at 45 years of age. The other important variant is the translocation type, who is born to a younger mother. In about 50 per cent of the latter patients the condition is inherited from a parent, usually the mother. The risk to these mothers of having a further Down's syndrome baby is 1 in 3 to 1 in 6, so genetic counselling is important.

Congenital cardiac anomalies are found in up to 50 per cent. The main types are atrial septal defect, mitral valve prolapse or, less often, atrioventricular canal and ventricular septal defect. About one-third die in the first few years of life from cardiac disease.

There are typically multiple immunological defects so that infections of the skin, gastrointestinal and respiratory tracts are common, especially in institutionalized patients who are also liable to be hepatitis B carriers.

The risk of acute leukaemia (usually acute lymphoblastic) in Down's syndrome is 20 times greater than in the general population.

• Dental aspects of Down's syndrome

All have learning disability to some degree, but are usually amiable and cooperative most of the time and are generally more easily managed than many other types of patients with learning disability. Epilepsy or cerebral palsy are rare. Most can be treated under local anaesthesia with sedation if necessary. General anaesthesia must be administered by a specialist anaesthetist or is best avoided where possible, in view of other management difficulties which may include:

1. Cardiac defects predisposing to infective endocarditis (rarely).
2. Respiratory disease. There may be difficulty in intubation because of the hypoplastic midface; congenital anomalies of the respiratory tract may be present and there is increased susceptibility to chest infections (*Fig. 23.1*).
3. Anaemia.
4. Possible atlanto-axial subluxation (care when extending neck).
5. Hepatitis B carriage.

There are many oral abnormalities, the most obvious being an open-mouth posture with a protrusive tongue. The tongue may be absolutely or relatively large and is often scrotal, more especially after the age of about 4 years. The circumvallate papillae enlarge but the filiform papillae may be absent. The lips tend to be thick, dry and fissured. There is a poor anterior oral seal and also a strong tongue thrust. Anterior open bite, posterior crossbite and other types of malocclusion are common. The maxillae and malars are small and the mandible is somewhat protrusive. Class III malocclusion is common, but 46 per cent are class I. The orthodontic prognosis is often poor because of learning disability, parafunctional habits and severe periodontal disease. Although the palate often appears to be high, with horizontal palatal shelves (the omega palate), a short palate is more characteristic. There is also an increased incidence of bifid uvula, cleft lip and cleft palate.

As in all other aspects of their development, mongols have retarded tooth formation and eruption. The first dentition may begin to appear only after 9 months and may take 5 years to complete, if ever. The deciduous molars may erupt before the deciduous incisors and deciduous lateral incisors are absent in about 15 per cent. The eruption of the permanent teeth is often also irregular. Missing teeth are common, although, as in the general population, the third molars and lateral incisors are most often absent. Up to 30 per cent have morphological abnormalities in both dentitions, particularly teeth with short, small crowns and roots. The occlusal surfaces of the deciduous molars may be hypoplastic and both dentitions may be hypocalcified.

The most important dental disorder is severe early onset periodontal disease. Lower anterior teeth are usually severely affected and lost early. Acute ulcerative gingivitis is also seen. In contrast, caries incidence is usually low in both dentitions. The cause of the low incidence of caries is unknown but may be related to such factors as the high salivary pH and bicarbonate content.

Fragile X syndrome

Fragile X syndrome is so named because the tip of the X chromosome is susceptible to breakage and appears as a thin thread of chromatin joining two chromosome bands in appropriate preparations of metaphase nuclei. It was earlier thought to be a typical sex-linked recessive disorder but approximately 30 per cent of carrier females have learning disability and there are a few phenotypically normal carrier males. Fragile X syndrome therefore appears to be a sex-linked dominant trait with variable penetrance.

Fragile X syndrome affects 1 in 1000 to 1 in 1500 of the population and is the second most common chromosomal defect associated with learning disability, after Down's syndrome. In addition to learning disability, patients have large testes, a long face and prominent ears.

- ### Dental aspects of fragile X syndrome

Hyperactivity, a short attention span and behavioural disorders similar to those of autism, make dental management difficult.

Earlier descriptions of palatal anomalies in fragile X syndrome have not been confirmed but crossbite and open bite are abnormally frequent. Unlike Down's syndrome, there is no special pattern of frequency of dental caries or periodontal disease.

THALIDOMIDE DEFECT

The teratogenic effects of the hypnotic thalidomide include reduction deformities of the limbs (phocomelia, *Fig. 23.2*) and defects of the eyes, ears, heart, kidneys and gastro-intestinal tract, but normal intelligence. Many affected persons have a globular head with hypertelorism (widely spaced eyes), depressed nasal bridge and a central facial naevus extending from the forehead down to the nose.

Since the withdrawal of thalidomide, those affected are now adults and phocomelia in children is currently a congenital defect of unknown cause.

Oral effects include enamel hypoplasia, cleft palate and abnormalities in tongue morphology.

HYDROCEPHALUS

In the most common type of hydrocephalus, dilatation of the cerebral ventricles is caused

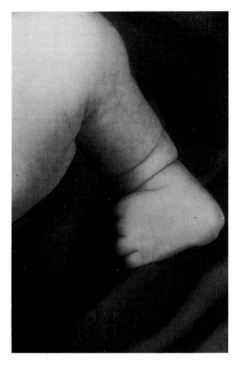

Fig. 23.2 Phocomelia (seal limb) in the thalidomide syndrome

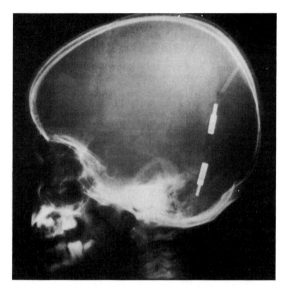

Fig. 23.3 Hydrocephalus: the lateral skull radiograph shows the valve that drains cerebrospinal fluid from the cerebral ventricles to the venous system

by obstruction to the circulation of cerebrospinal fluid and results in compression and atrophy of the brain, and enlargement of the skull. Myelomeningocele may be associated. The main features are outlined in *Table 23.4*. A short-circuit operation with the insertion of a ventriculo-atrial or ventriculo-peritoneal shunt may relieve the intracranial pressure. The cerebrospinal fluid is drained from the cerebral ventricles via a catheter with one-way valves to the right atrium or the peritoneal cavity (*Fig. 23.3*). The valves occasionally can become blocked or detached and are susceptible to infection if there is bacteraemia.

• Dental aspects of hydrocephalus

The weight of the head may be a problem, especially in the anaesthetized patient, and there may be other management difficulties (*Table 23.4*):

1. Infection of ventriculo-atrial shunt. Though infection is rarely from a dental source, antibiotic cover should be given before procedures that might produce bacteraemia.
2. Spina bifida (frequently associated).
3. Epilepsy.
4. Learning disability.
5. Visual impairment.

Table 23.4   Hydrocephalus

- Mechanisms
  Congenital blockage of aqueduct in Arnold–Chiari malformation[a]
  Congenital obstruction of foraminae in Dandy–Walker syndrome[b]
  Acquired blockage of subarachnoid space or cerebral cisterns, e.g. meningitis, haemorrhage, tumour
- Signs
  Large head and bulging fontanelles in children
  Headache, vomiting, mental changes, papilloedema
- Complications
  Epilepsy
  Visual impairment
  Spasticity
  Learning disability or dementia

[a]Downward displacement of medulla and part of cerebellum through the foramen magnum blocks escape of CSF from fourth ventricle.
[a]Congenital obstruction of the foramina of Magendie and Luschka.

CLEFT LIP AND PALATE

The total incidence of cleft deformities is between 2 and 3 per 1000 live births. Cleft lip is more prevalent in males, cleft palate more prevalent in females. There is a family history of clefts in nearly 40 per cent of cases. No teratogens causing clefts have been positively identified in man although thalidomide was, and steroids may be, associated with an increased incidence. In contrast, folic acid given periconceptually may reduce the risk.

Cleft palate may be associated with a wide range of congenital syndromes, especially with chromosome anomalies (Down's syndrome, Edwards' syndrome), and in the Pierre–Robin, Treacher–Collins and Klippel–Feil syndromes (*see* Appendix of Miscellaneous Uncommon or Rare Disorders). There may also be associated congenital defects such as dental, hearing and speech defects.

Systemic complications are more frequent in patients with cleft palate than in those with cleft lip alone. They include especially skeletal, cardiac, renal and central nervous system defects. Up to 20 per cent of patients with clefts have such additional abnormalities which can affect dental management in various ways (Chapters 3, 13 and 17).

One of the first problems for the child is feeding. A Rosti bottle with Gummi teat often helps. Surgical and other technical aspects of management are covered in specialist texts but the usual classification is shown in *Fig. 23.4*. In general, when the lip alone is cleft, initial cosmetic repair is carried out at about 3–6 months of age, though earlier operations are becoming popular. Cleft palate is usually repaired before the child speaks, between 6 and 18 months, typically at about 15 months of age. Surgical revisions of the lip and nose are usually required later.

There can be significant difficulties in management of the airway for anaesthesia in children under the age of 5 years, particularly in young infants and in those with feeding difficulties, bilateral clefts and/or retrognathia. Patients with mandibular dysostoses, or any requiring midface advancement (Le Fort II osteotomy), have the greatest problems. Difficulties are common in Pierre–Robin, Treacher–Collins and Goldenhar's syndromes, and with the cervical spine in Klippel–Feil syndrome. The laryngeal mask

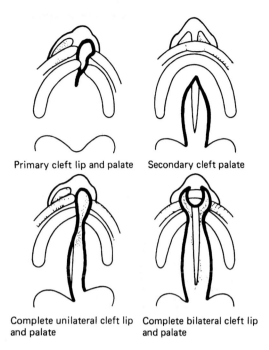

Primary cleft lip and palate   Secondary cleft palate

Complete unilateral cleft lip and palate   Complete bilateral cleft lip and palate

Fig. 23.4 Clefts of the lip and palate. (Adapted from Poswillo, D.E. (1986) in Rowe, A.H.R., Alexander A.G. and Johns R.B. (eds), *Clinical Dentistry*, Oxford, Blackwell Scientific, p. 132)

has been recommended as a guide to fibre-optic endoscopic intubation.

Orthodontic and restorative dental procedures are discussed elsewhere but, as in many other handicapped patients, prevention and continuity of care is of utmost importance and a high rate of success can be achieved. Palatal ulcers seen in neonates with cleft lip and palate appear to result from trauma from the tongue, and resolve if a palatal plate is fitted.

Submucous cleft palate

In this condition, the palatal shelves may fail to join but the overlying mucous membranes are intact and the muscle attachments of the soft palate are abnormal. About 1 in 1200 births are affected and the defect can be recognized by a notched posterior nasal spine, a translucent zone in the midline of the soft palate and a bifid uvula. However, not all these features are necessarily present and a bifid uvula may be seen in isolation.

Feeding difficulties, speech defects and middle ear infections may develop in 90 per cent of affected children. They should, therefore, be referred to a specialist.

AUTISM

Autism is a disorder beginning in the first 30 months of life, in which there is failure to develop interpersonal relationships, delayed development of speech and language, and ritualistic or compulsive behaviour. Autism is seen mainly in first-born males, possibly as a result of some abnormality of pregnancy.

The three main clinical features are:

1. Onset within the first 2–3 years of life.
2. Autism (profound aloneness).
3. Obsessional desire for maintaining an unchanging environment.

These children appear to be isolated from everyone around them and fail to respond to any stimuli, even to being lifted by the parents. They show complete lack of interest in people but are often fascinated with inanimate objects. Some display a combination of lack of response to stimuli, including pain, with abnormal fearlessness. Autistics wander aimlessly about with little creative or imaginative activity. Rages, tantrums and self-directed aggression (which may be reactions to boredom or frustration) are common, or there may be inappropriate giggling.

Most characteristic of the motor abnormalities are finger flicking near the eyes and hand flipping. Facial grimaces, jumping and toe walking are also common and all mannerisms are exaggerated if the autistic is distressed or excited.

Communication disorders such as delayed or immediate echolalia (repetition of words heard) are common. The autistic child rarely uses the pronoun 'I' and frequently uses meaningless words or phrases in a generally immature speech. Some remain mute. Seventy per cent of autistics have an IQ below 70 but some are highly intelligent. Temporal lobe epilepsy develops in about 30 per cent.

• Dental aspects of autism

An essential consideration is to ensure that a routine is developed in which the child is not kept waiting, has a short quiet visit, and always sees the same dental staff. Parental concern is also usually above average. Autistics may be disturbed by noise such as a high-speed aspirator or air rotor and it may be necessary to avoid their use.

Many autistics manage to make dental treatment under local anaesthesia impossible by their lack of response to requests or commands. General anaesthesia or relative analgesia may then be needed, but some may be on medication, such as monoamine oxidase inhibitors or tricyclic antidepressants, which can complicate treatment.

There are no specific dental lesions or medical problems in autism, although there may be trauma from head-banging, and epilepsy.

OTHER HANDICAPPING SYNDROMES

See the Appendix to this chapter and the Appendix to Chapter 15 for inborn errors of metabolism.

Cerebral palsy is discussed in Chapter 17 and rubella syndrome in Chapter 11.

THE YOUNG

There are particular, though uncommon, problems associated with preterm infancy and the neonatal period. There is some evidence that maternal periodontal infection is a risk factor for preterm low birth weight foetuses. Oropharyngeal or orogastric intubation may result in palatal grooving, acquired cleft palate and damage to the deciduous

dentition. Appliances can be constructed to protect the oral tissues from this damage.

The neonate is also in a state of immunological immaturity and may contract candidosis and other infections from other infants, parents or carers, or the environment. Even wooden tongue depressors can be a source of infection. The neonatal period is characterized by rapid development and growth, including the oral tissues which can be damaged by drugs (tetracyclines, immuno-suppressants, cytotoxic agents), and physical agents (irradiation, trauma). Facial, skull, jaw and tooth development can be impaired by radiotherapy, by chemotherapy, and by some immunosuppressants. After the eruption of the teeth, drugs that produce xerostomia, and procedures such as radiotherapy involving the salivary glands predispose to caries, especially in children. Preventive dental care and dietary counselling are of crucial importance.

Informed consent can be difficult to ensure in children too young to understand. All drug doses must be reduced for children and sugar-free preparations should be used. Children may also present behavioural problems in dental treatment, may present some unusual reactions to drugs, and may be the subjects of abuse resulting in orofacial injuries.

Children may react adversely to diazepam and become hyperactive rather than sedated. Similarly, responses to intravenous anaesthetics are unpredictable. Relative analgesia may be difficult or impossible to administer to children with behavioural problems.

THE OVERACTIVE (HYPERKINETIC) CHILD

Although parents not infrequently describe their badly behaved child as 'overactive', the term should be limited to those who demonstrate gross behavioural abnormalities including:

1. Uncontrolled activity.
2. Impulsiveness.
3. Impaired concentration.
4. Motor restlessness and extreme fidgeting.

These activities are seen particularly when orderliness is required, for example in the dental waiting room or surgery. Mischievous children are not, of course, abnormal and overactivity applies to gross misbehaviour such as reckless escapes from parents while on public transport.

Overactivity can be caused by external factors, or factors affecting parents, the child or the child–parent relationship (*Table 23.5*).

Table 23.5 Causes of hyperactivity in a child

- Child
  Hyperkinetic syndrome
  Brain damage
  Low intelligence
  Tartrazine sensitivity
  Anxiety states
  Drug abuse
- Parent
  Child–parent relationship
  Rejection or overprotection
  Inconsistent discipline
  Lack of parental love
- Parental
  Marital disharmony
  Depression
- External
  Institutionalization
  Excessive demands at school

Overactivity is often associated with low intelligence. Extreme overactivity (hyperkinetic syndrome) usually begins in infancy, almost invariably before the age of 5 years.

It is especially common in the mentally handicapped, those with neurological disease, and epileptics (especially in temporal lobe epilepsy). Autism, mania and anxiety states may cause similar abnormal behaviour.

• General management of the overactive child

Psychiatric care, and counselling of the parents are usually necessary. Impaired concentration may respond to stimulants such as amphetamines, pemoline or methylphenidate, but little is known of the adverse effects and dependence is a possibility, although it seems rare.

Sedatives and tranquillizers should be avoided as they may impair learning ability, or cause paradoxical reactions such as aggressive behaviour.

• Dental aspects of the overactive child

Overactive children are often impossible to manage in the dental surgery, and frequently succeed in frustrating all concerned. Any dental treatment is unlikely to be possible unless general anaesthesia is used and such patients are therefore best referred to hospital for dental care. Tranquillizers such as diazepam should be avoided as they usually increase rather than depress overactivity.

CHILD ABUSE (BATTERED CHILD SYNDROME: NON-ACCIDENTAL INJURY)

Child abuse is any act of omission or commission that endangers or impairs the physical or emotional health or development of a child.

Battered children frequently have facial and oral lesions. It is an important condition to be recognized by the dental surgeon, since there is a high risk of further assaults on, or death of, the child and of siblings. Some 35–60 per cent of physically abused children suffer further injury, with a 5–10 per cent mortality. Most affected children are less than 3 years of age and usually less than 1 year of age. Affected families are predominantly of classes IV and V.

The child is often cowed. Most suffer significant neurological, intellectual or emotional damage. The child may also be malnourished and generally neglected, and there may be evidence of previous trauma and delay in seeking care (*Table 23.6*).

The injuries are varied and often multiple. Lacerations, bruising, pinching, bites, abrasions or burns are the main soft-tissue lesions, involve the head and face in over 65 per cent, but can be found in any part of the body. Lacerations of the upper labial mucosa and tearing of the lip from the gingiva are found in about 45 per cent of victims. Other injuries include fractured, missing, displaced or discoloured (dead) teeth, bruising or scars of lips or tongue, binding marks from a gag or lacerations. Fractures of any bone may be seen, but over 33 per cent have fractured ribs or long bones and there may be jaw or head injuries.

Table 23.6   Findings suggestive of child abuse

- Cowed child
- Long interval before attendance for treatment
- Evidence of previous injury (or a previous history of injury)
- Injuries often committed at night
- Multiple injuries incompatible with history at unusual sites

---

Table 23.7   Child abuse: associated factors

- Parental
  Marital disharmony
  Chronic physical illness
  Emotionally deprived, inadequate or impulsive
  Low intelligence
- Child
  Abnormal pregnancy or delivery
  Neonatal separation
  Unwanted
  Hyperactive, ill or aggressive

The injuries are usually inflicted by an adult, often a parent, or by an older sibling. The person responsible may be supported by an inactive partner. Causal factors may be related either to those affecting the parent, or to those affecting the child – often both (*Table 23.7*). It is noteworthy that the person responsible is only rarely psychotic, but the mothers are often emotionally immature or depressed and the fathers often have a psychopathic personality and either or both are frequently of low intelligence.

Child abuse should be suspected if any injuries are incompatible with the history and if any of the features in *Table 23.6* are noted. After genuine accidents, children are usually immediately taken for medical or dental attention; when children are abused, there is often considerable delay.

• Management of child abuse

The child must be fully examined to exclude serious injury, especially subdural haematomas or intraocular bleeding, and must therefore be admitted to hospital. Full records *must* be kept. A skeletal radiographic survey should be undertaken to reveal both new and old injuries and a paediatrician should be consulted. Facial and oral injuries must be carefully recorded, preferably with photographs, and treated appropriately. The differential diagnosis may include osteogenesis imperfecta.

Patients are kept in hospital until the diagnosis is confirmed, since there is a high risk of further injury which may be fatal. If this problem is suspected, the medical practitioner, social services and a child protection society must be involved early on, but strict confidentiality must be observed. Social work departments now keep registers of non-accidental injuries which help identify known offenders.

The dentist should also inform his medical defence society as there may be legal involvement later.

SELF-INFLICTED (FACTITIOUS) ORAL LESIONS

Minor, subconsciously *self-induced* oral lesions are common, the classic examples being bruxism and cheek-biting (morsicatio buccarum). Other lesions may be self-inflicted when the oral mucosa is anaesthetized, such as after a local anaesthetic or surgery to the trigeminal nerve.

Serious deliberate self-inflicted lesions in the mouth are considerably less common than on the skin. This may be due to an underlying need or desire for attention and oral lesions are insufficiently obvious.

Lesions have been classified as follows: (a) injuries superimposed on a pre-existing lesion; (b) injuries secondary to another established habit; and (c) injuries of unknown and/or of complex aetiology.

This last group mainly comprise patients who are emotionally disturbed or with learning disability. Though serious psychiatric disease is less common in children, occasional patients have later committed suicide.

The most common type of self-inflicted oral injuries reported in the past has been so-called self-extraction of teeth. Soft-tissue lesions can be produced, however, typically by picking at the gingivae with the fingernails. In adults injuries may be produced by the use of the pointed end of a nail file, often also at the gingival margins. Other types of injury include the application of caustic substances to the lips or injuries from attempts at suicide.

The diagnosis of self-inflicted injury may be difficult. They should be suspected when the lesions:

1. Do not correspond with those of any recognized disease.
2. Are of bizarre configuration with sharp outlines and in an otherwise healthy mouth.
3. Are in sites accessible to the patient.

In addition, the patient may show signs that suggest emotional disturbance or may be known to be under psychiatric treatment, or may have learning disability.

In spite of such a background, a few patients will admit to injuring themselves. More frequently the diagnosis can be confirmed only by discreet observation after admission of the patient to hospital. However, even when seen to cause the injuries, the patient may still deny having made them.

Once the diagnosis has been made, the patient's family doctor should be told of the necessity for specialist psychiatric assessment.

Rare causes of self-injury include the Lesch–Nyhan syndrome (Chapter 15), and Gilles de la Tourette's syndrome of multiple tics which may affect the face, and coprolalia (involuntary uttering of obscenities) or any cause of sensory loss or pain-insensitivity.

JUVENILE DELINQUENCY

Various orofacial lesions appear to be more common in juvenile delinquents than in the general population: facial and oral tattoos, smoking-related lesions such as keratoses, fellatio lesions on the palate and lip and cheek-chewing and scars are seen more frequently.

THE ELDERLY

A growing proportion of the population is over the age of 65 and the elderly now account for some 15 per cent of the population. The sex differences in life expectancy are resulting in a rise in the proportion of elderly females, many of whom are widows. Some 3 per cent are bedridden, 8 per cent walk with difficulty and 11 per cent are house-bound. Thus many have great difficulty in reaching any facilities for health care.

Very many elderly patients are edentulous and some problems of dental management are thereby greatly reduced. It seems, however, that the proportion of edentulous

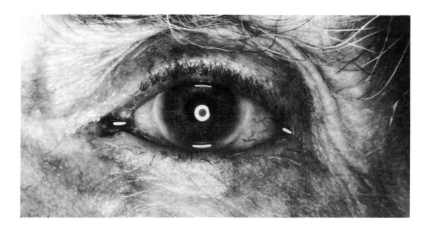

Fig. 23.5 Arcus senilis is a manifestation of old age but may appear prematurely in some hyperlipidaemias

elderly patients is gradually falling and, as a consequence, more of them need restorative dentistry or surgery of various types. Many of the elderly receive no dental attention whatsoever, despite much evidence of their need. It has been found, for example, that 81 per cent of a group of elderly patients had oral lesions and 20 per cent needed further investigation to exclude serious oral disease. Nevertheless, elderly patients are often reluctant to demand attention, especially if they fear consequent hospitalization.

Many physical disorders affect the elderly, particularly a greater incidence and severity of cardiovascular disease, which can affect their dental management. Also important, however, are mental and emotional problems and defects of hearing or sight, as these affect all aspects of treatment, even prosthetic procedures. Dementia from such causes as Alzheimer's disease becomes increasingly common with age. On the other hand, it must not be assumed that an elderly patient is stupid merely because responses are slow.

Multiple disease

There is a rising prevalence with age of many diseases (*Table 23.8*), particularly cardiovascular disease, thromboembolic disease and malignant disease. Up to 75 per cent of those over 65 years of age have one or more chronic diseases. Multiple diseases, atypical symptomatology, polypharmacy and abnormal reactivity towards many drugs further complicate the situation.

Many disorders in the elderly cause non-specific effects such as general malaise, social incompetence, a tendency to fall and mild amnesia. Important causes include Alzheimer's disease, hypothyroidism, anaemia, diabetes, malignant disease and chronic renal failure.

Ataxia, fainting and falls may be due to transient cerebral ischaemic attacks, parkinsonism, postural hypotension, cardiac dysrhythmias or epilepsy.

Intellectual failure

Dementia, particularly as a result of Alzheimer's disease (Chapter 17), is common in the elderly. Mental symptoms in the elderly are often also caused by underlying physical disease, especially if the symptoms are of recent onset. An acute confusional state may result from disorders as widely different as minor cerebrovascular accidents, respiratory or urinary tract infections, or left ventricular failure. A chronic confusional state may result from such conditions as diabetes mellitus, hypothyroidism, carcinomatosis, anaemia, uraemia or drug therapy.

Depression may be an important feature in hypothyroidism or with some drugs. Nutrition may be defective due to poverty, apathy, mental disease or dental defects. Malnutrition may in turn lead to poor tissue healing and predispose to ill health. Ageing is often also associated with declining acuity of many of the senses. Hearing and sight are frequently impaired (*Figs 23.5, 23.6*) as may the sense of smell and taste.

RNID

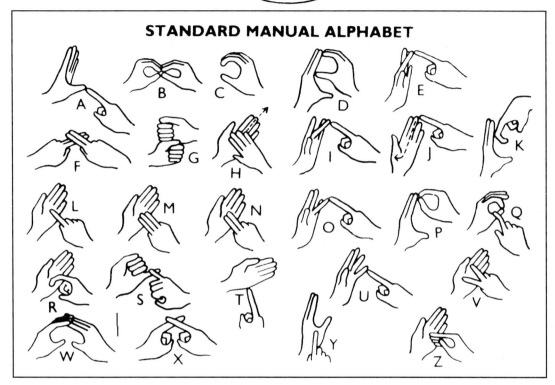

STANDARD MANUAL ALPHABET

Fig. 23.6 Alphabet for the deaf

Social problems

Social disabilities are common as a result of such causes as loss of the spouse, isolation from the family, poverty and lack of mobility. Psychological disorders such as loss of morale are therefore common. Old people tend to be thrifty, careful with food purchasing and heating of accommodation, and often take little exercise.

Temperature regulation may be disturbed so that respiratory, urinary infections or even more serious infections often fail to cause fever. The elderly also readily become hypothermic, especially if thyroid function is poor.

Drug compliance and reactions

About 10 per cent of admissions to geriatric units are caused partly or wholly by drug reactions. Inappropriate treatment, poor supervision, excessive dosage, drug interactions and polypharmacy, or impaired drug metabolism, may all contribute to adverse drug reactions. A further complication is that some drugs may precipitate or aggravate the physical disorders that are more frequent in the elderly. For example, drugs with antimuscarinic activity, such as atropine or antidepressants, may cause urinary retention if there is prostatic enlargement, or may precipitate glaucoma. Phenothiazines may worsen or precipitate parkinsonism, or may cause hypotension, hypothermia, apathy, excessive sedation or confusion.

Drowsiness, excessive sedation or confusional states may also be caused by the benzodiazepines, by barbiturates, or by tricyclic antidepressants, while depression and postural hypotension not uncommonly follow the use of hypotensive agents.

Compliance with drug treatment can be very poor, not least because of forgetfulness.

Altered presentation of disease

Disease may present in a less florid and dramatic way in elderly people. Even severe infections, for example, may cause no fever.

• Dental aspects of care of the elderly

Access to dental care can be a major difficulty for the elderly, who may be frail and have limited mobility. It can take a long time for a patient in a wheelchair, or using a Zimmer frame, to get into the surgery, and onto the dental chair. Domiciliary care may be more appropriate and avoids the physical and psychological problems of a hospital or clinic visit. Handling of elderly patients may demand immense patience. Elderly patients are often extremely anxious about treatment and should therefore be sympathetically reassured and, if necessary, sedated. Remember always to treat the elderly with sympathy and respect and that, while it may be difficult to find the patience to deal with their disabilities, these same ageing processes are operating in us all.

Treatment is often best carried out with the patient sitting upright, as few like reclining for treatment, and some may become breathless and/or panic. It is better to use local anaesthesia where possible, since the risks of general anaesthesia are greater than in the young patient, not least because of associated medical problems.

Benzodiazepines are preferable to opioids for sedation or the induction of general anaesthesia which may be continued with nitrous oxide–oxygen supplemented with halothane or an equivalent. Relative analgesia is preferable. Intravenous sedation in the dental chair is best avoided if there is any evidence of cerebrovascular disease, as a hypotensive episode may cause cerebral ischaemia. After long operations, elderly patients are prone to pulmonary complications, such as atelectasis, and to deep vein thrombosis and pulmonary embolism.

The possibility of physical or mental disorders that may complicate management should always be considered (*see Table 23.8*) and drug treatment should be carefully

Table 23.8 Diseases especially affecting the elderly[a]

* Oral or predominantly oral
  Lichen planus
  Mucous membrane pemphigoid
  Trigeminal herpes zoster and post-herpetic neuralgia
  Carcinoma, premalignant and other white lesions
  Sore tongue
  Sjögren's syndrome
  Candidosis (denture stomatitis and angular stomatitis)
* Cardiovascular disease
  Hypertensive and ischaemic heart disease
  Cardiac failure
  Temporal arteritis
* Neurological or related disease
  Deafness
  Poor vision
  Multi-infarct (cerebrovascular) dementia
  Parkinsonism
  Strokes
  Ataxia
  Trigeminal neuralgia
  Alzheimer's disease
  Respiratory
  Chronic bronchitis and emphysema
  Pneumonia
  Musculoskeletal
  Osteoarthritis
  Osteoporosis
  Paget's disease
  Haematological
  Anaemia (especially pernicious anaemia)
  Chronic leukaemia
  Genitourinary
  Urinary retention or incontinence
  Prostatic hypertrophy
  Renal failure
  Psychiatric
  Insomnia
  Dependence on hypnotics
  Loneliness and depression
  Paranoia
  Dementia
  Acute confusional states
  Atypical facial pain
  Miscellaneous
  Nutritional deficiencies
  Accidents
  Cancer

[a]Multiple conditions are common.

controlled, with the possibility of poor compliance and of adverse reactions always in mind. Polypharmacy must be avoided, not only because of the danger of drug interactions but also because of the practical difficulties that the patient may have in taking the correct doses at the correct times. Elderly patients frequently have difficulties in understanding the medication and in remembering to keep to a regimen. If it appears possible that there is hepatic or renal disease likely to impair drug metabolism or excretion, drug dosage must be reduced appropriately.

Impaired salivation may contribute to a high prevalence of root caries and oral candidosis, which especially affect hospitalized patients. Xerostomia is even more likely if there is medication with neuroleptics or antidepressants.

Some studies have demonstrated mucosal lesions in up to 40 per cent of elderly patients. Most of these are fibrous lumps or ulcers, with a minority of potentially malignant lesions such as keratoses. Oral malignant disease is mainly a problem of the elderly and is a further reason for regular oral examination of these patients. Atypical facial pain (often related to depressive illness), migraine, trigeminal neuralgia, zoster and oral dysaesthesias are more common as age advances.

Many of the elderly are edentulous and of those with remaining teeth, at least 75 per cent have periodontal disease. Dental caries is usually, however, less acute but root caries is more common. Caries may become active if there is xerostomia, especially if there is overindulgence in sweet foods.

By no means all patients complain of oral symptoms or denture-related difficulties but many of the elderly are edentulous with little alveolar bone to support dentures, a dry mouth and a frail, atrophic mucosa. Inability to cope with dentures, or a sore mouth for any reason, readily demoralizes the elderly patient, and may tip the balance between health and disease. The dentist therefore has an important role in supporting morale and contributing to adequate nutrition. Sound teeth should therefore be conserved if they can serve, at least for a few years, as abutments or retainers for prostheses. It may also be unwise to alter radically the shape or occlusion of dentures where they have been worn for years. On the other hand, it is wise to label the dentures with the name of the patient, particularly for those living in sheltered or other residential accommodation, since otherwise dentures can easily be mislaid or mixed up between patients.

Attrition and brittleness of the teeth may complicate treatment, and it may be necessary to provide cuspal coverage in complex or large restorations. Endodontic therapy may be more difficult in view of secondary dentine deposition. Hypercementosis, brittle dentine, low bone elasticity and impaired tissue healing may also complicate surgical procedures.

BIBLIOGRAPHY

Bacher M., Goz G., Pham T., Ney T. and Ehrenfeld M. (1996) Congenital palatal ulcers in newborn infants with cleft lip and palate; diagnosis, frequency and significance. *Cleft Palate J.* **33**, 37–42.

Barnes I. and Walls A. (1994) *Gerodontology.* Oxford, Wright-Butterworth.

Cawson R.A., Spector R.G. and Skelly A.M. (1995) *Basic Pharmacology and Clinical Drug Use in Dentistry*, 6th edn. Edinburgh, Churchill Livingstone.

Cohen B. and Thomson N. (eds) (1986) *Dental Care of the Elderly.* London, Heinemann Medical.

Dick P.T. (1996) Periodic health examination, 1996 update; 1. prenatal screening for and diagnosis of Down's syndrome. *Can. Med. Assoc. J.* **154**, 465–79.

Fleishman R., Peles D.B. and Pisanti S. (1985) Oral mucosal lesions among elderly in Israel. *J. Dent. Res.* **64**, 831–6.

Fontaine A.J. (1985) Managing the cerebral palsy patient. *Dentistry* **85**, 27–8.

Giles D.L. and Murphy W.M. (1980) Dental treatment of the elderly inpatient. *J. Dent.* **8**, 341–8.

Gunawardana R.H. (1996) Difficult laryngoscopy in cleft lip and palate surgery. *Br. J Anaesth.* **76**, 757–9.

Hatch D.J. (1996) Airway management in cleft lip and palate surgery. *Br. J. Anaesth.* **76**, 755–6.

Holt R.D. (1993) Deafness and dentistry. *Br. Dent. J.* **175**, 120–1.

Jorge J.J., Almeida O.P., Bozzo L., Scully C. and Graner E. (1991) Oral mucosal health and disease in institutionalised elderly in Brazil. *Commun. Dent. Oral Epidemiol.* **19**, 173–5.

Kanar H.L (1986) Pharmacologic considerations for patients with disabilities. *Compend. Contin. Educ. Dent.* **7**, 210–21.

MacEntee M.I. and Scully C. (1988) Oral disorders and treatment implications in people over 75 years. *Commun. Dent. Oral Epidemiol.* **16**, 271–3.

MacEntee M.I., Dowell T.B. and Scully C. (1988) Oral health concerns of an elderly population in England. *Commun. Dent. Oral Epidemiol.* **16**, 72–4.

Meechan J.G. and Welbury R.R. (1996) Medical problems affecting the management of children in dentistry. *Dent. Update* **23**, 242–5.

Mitchell S.J., Gray J., Morgan M.E.I., Hocking M.D. and Durbin G.M. (1996) Nosocomial infection with *Rhizopus microsporus* in preterm infants; association with wooden tongue depressors. *Lancet* **348**, 441–3.

Moore R.S. and Hobson P. (1989) A classification of medically handicapping conditions and the health risks they present in the dental care of children. Part I – Cardiovascular, haematological and respiratory disorders. *J. Paediatr. Dent.* **5**, 73–83.

Moore R.S. and Hobson P. (1989) A classification of medically handicapping conditions and the health risks they present in the dental care of children. Part II – Neoplastic, renal, endocrine, metabolic, hepatic, musculoskeletal, neuromuscular, central nervous system and skin disorders. *J. Paediatr. Dent.* **6**, 1–14.

Moss A.L.H., Piggott R.W. and Jones K.J. (1988) Submucous cleft palate. *Br. Med. J.* **297**, 85.

Nunn J.H., Gordon P.H. and Carmichael C.L. (1993) Dental disease and current treatment needs in a group of physically handicapped children. *Commun. Dent. Health.* **10**, 389–96.

Offenbacher S., Katz V., Fertik G., Collins J., Boyd D. *et al.* (1996) Periodontal infection as a possible risk factor for preterm low birth weight. *J. Periodontol.* **67**, 1103–13.

Peak J., Eveson J. and Scully C. (1992) Oral Manifestations of Rett's syndrome. *Br. Dent. J.* **172**, 248–9.

Porter S.R. and Scully C. (1996) *Innovations and Developments in Non-Invasive Oral Health Care.* Northwood, Science Reviews.

Samaranayake L.P., Wilkieson C.A., Lamey P.J. and MacFarlane T.W. (1995) Oral disease in the elderly in long-term hospital care. *Oral Diseases* **1**, 147–51.

Scully C. (1980) The de Lange syndrome. *J. Oral Med.* **35**, 32–4.

Scully C. (1981) Down's syndrome. In Crown S. (ed), *Practical Psychiatry*. London, Northwood Publications, p. 208.

Scully C. (1981) Oral mucosal lesions in association with epilepsy and cutaneous lesions: Pringle–Bourneville syndrome. *Int. J. Oral Surg.* **10**, 68–72.

Scully C. (1981) Special patients. In Manning J. (ed), *General Dental Practice*. London, Kluwer, A.5(9–01)–(9–06).

Scully C. (1988) *The Dental Patient*. Oxford, Heinemann.

Scully C. (1989) *The Mouth and Perioral Tissues*. Oxford, Heinemann.

Scully C. (1989) *Patient Care: a Dental Surgeon's Guide*. London, British Dental Association.

Scully C. (1994) The pathology of orofacial disease. In Barnes I. and Walls A. (eds), *Gerodontology*. Oxford, Wright–Butterworths, pp. 29–41.

Scully C. and Davison M.F. (1980) Orofacial manifestations of the Cri du chat (5p-) syndrome. *J. Dent.* **7**, 313–32.

Scully C. and Welbury R.R. (1994) *Oral Diseases in Children and Adolescents*. London, Wolfe.

Scully C., Cawson R.A. and Griffiths M.J. (1990) *Occupational Hazards to Dental Staff*. London, British Dental Journal.

Shaw G.M., Lammer E.J., Wasserman C.R., O'Malley C.D. and Tolarova M.M. (1995) Risks of orofacial clefts in children born to women using multivitamins containing folic acid periconceptually. *Lancet* **346**, 393–6.

Shellhart W.C., Casamassimo P.S., Hagerman R.J. *et al.* (1986) Oral findings in fragile X syndrome. *Am. J. Med. Genet.* **23**, 179–87.

Steele L. (1982) The delivery of dental care for elderly handicapped patients. *J. Dent.* **10**, 281–8.

Symons A.L., Rowe P.V. and Romanink K. (1987) Dental aspects of child abuse: review and case reports. *Aust. Dent. J.* **32**, 42–7.

Townsend G.C. (1983) Tooth size in children and young adults with trisomy 21 (Down's syndrome). *Arch. Oral Biol.* **28**, 159–66.

Turner G., Daniel A. and Frost M. (1980) X-linked mental retardation, macroorchidism and the (X) (q27) fragile state. *J. Pediatr.* **96**, 836–41.

Van der Bijl P. (1994) Therapeutic considerations in the gerodontic patient. *Compend. Contin. Educ. Dent.* **15**, 478–90.

Van der Waal I. (1983) Disease of the oral mucosa in the aged patient. *Int. Dent. J.* **33**, 319–24.

van Wyck C.W. (1983) An oral pathology profile of a group of juvenile delinquents. *J. Forensic Odonto-Stomatol.* **1**, 3–10.

Von Gonten A.S., Meyer J.B. and Kim A.K. (1995) Dental management of neonates requiring prolonged oral intubation. *J. Prosthodont.* **4**, 222–5.

APPENDIX TO CHAPTER 23

CHROMOSOMAL ANOMALIES

Abnormality	Oral manifestations	Possible management problems
Trisomy 21 (Down's syndrome)	Cranial abnormalities Maxillary hypoplasia Dental abnormalities	Learning disability Cardiac defects in 40% Infections Hepatitis B carriage
Trisomy 13 (Patau's syndrome)	Cranial abnormalities Cleft lip or palate in 75%	Learning disability Cardiac defects in 80% Deafness Epilepsy
Trisomy 18 (Edwards' syndrome)	Cranial abnormalities Microstomia Hypoplastic parotids Gingival cysts	Learning disability Cardiac defects in most Renal disease
Deletion of short arm of chromosome 5 (Cri du chat syndrome)	Cranial abnormalities Malocclusions	Learning disability Cardiac defects Respiratory infections
Deletion of short arm of chromosome 4 (Wolf's syndrome)	Hypodontia	Learning disability
Monosomy X (Turner's syndrome	Small mandible Malocclusions	Cardiac defects Diabetes Keloid formation Renal malformations Learning disability
Trisomy X (Superfemale)	—	Learning disability
Klinefelter's syndrome (XXY)	Taurodontism	Personality defects Diabetes mellitus Asthma

24

Chemical dependence

Key points

- Chemical dependence (substance abuse) is a widespread problem, particularly among teenagers and young adults.
- Crime, violence and medical complications are frequently associated.
- The results of chemical dependence may damage not only the individual but also the family, other members of society and, in the case of the addicted pregnant mother, the fetus.
- Alcohol and solvent abuse and the use of cannabis are the most common habits, followed by abuse of psychedelics (particularly 'Ecstasy'), heroin, methadone and cocaine.
- Injected drug use can be associated with particular problems due to blood-borne infections, notably the hepatitis viruses and HIV, and sometimes infective endocarditis or septicaemia.
- Violent injuries and even death, sexually transmitted diseases and poor compliance with health care are common in the drug-using population.
- Alcohol abuse still causes the most serious drug-related problems for the individual, family and others, particularly because of accidents, trauma, liver disease, cardiomyopathy, infection and CNS damage.
- Alcohol has an additive effect with general anaesthetics, sedatives and other CNS-active drugs, and with metronidazole, when vomiting and headache may result.
- Tobacco use is linked to oral cancer, and cigarette smoking is a major aetiological factor in cancers of the lung, oesophagus and bladder, as well as atherosclerosis and respiratory disease.
- Benzodiazepine abuse is fairly common, the main effect being loss of memory.
- Barbiturates are responsible for many of the deaths of drug abusers since they depress respiration and cause CNS depression, especially if alcohol is also taken.
- Opioids (narcotics) are often used intravenously, with complications that include respiratory depression, malnutrition and depression, sometimes culminating in suicide.
- Amphetamines (including Ecstasy) stimulate, causing excitement, raised pulse rate and blood pressure, anorexia, hallucinations and paranoia, pyrexia and dysrhythmias which may be fatal.
- Cocaine also stimulates and can cause hallucinations, paranoia, dysrhythmias, cerebrovascular accidents, respiratory depression and sometimes death.
- Cannabis may cause tachycardia, and angina in patients with coronary artery disease, and possibly some neurological impairment, bronchitis and impaired fertility.
- Hallucinogens such as LSD and PCP stimulate and have sympathomimetic effects such as raised blood pressure and pulse rate.
- Hallucinogens may cause psychotic reactions leading to accidents, assaults or death.
- Organic solvents such as glue are commonly abused by children and teenagers

and can cause neurological, respiratory and liver damage. Cardiac effects including dysrhythmias may be fatal.
- Anaesthetic abuse has been seen in dental staff who have usually abused nitrous oxide, which can also cause vitamin B_{12} defects leading to neuropathies.

Chemical dependence (substance or drug abuse) is a growing problem worldwide. One recent study from the USA showed that 17 per cent of patients under the age of 60 attending a casualty department with chest pain had used cocaine. Many secondary school children both in the USA and elsewhere have tried drugs of abuse. Drug abuse is particularly troublesome to the community because of drug dependence and the amount of crime committed to obtain money to buy drugs, and the frequency of HIV and hepatitis virus infection in intra-venous abusers.

Abuse of a drug is defined as self-administration in a manner that deviates from the cultural norm and is harmful. The term is therefore not precise and alcohol in particular is often not considered to be a drug of dependence. Addiction is taken to mean the continued use of a specific psychoactive substance despite physical, psychological or social harm. Chemical dependence is a less pejorative term.

In practical terms drug addicts fall into several groups:

Junkies: These are often unemployed, buy illicit heroin (frequently obtaining the money by crime or prostitution) and typically associate with other addicts.

Stables: These addicts are in most ways the opposite of junkies and appear to be respectable members of society. Health care personnel using drugs fall into this category.

Loners: Loners are usually not criminals, do not associate with other addicts but use various non-prescribed drugs.

Two-worlders: These addicts may be in fairly steady employment, like stables, but associate with other addicts, often engage in criminal activities and use both prescribed and illicitly obtained drugs.

Patterns of drug abuse change rapidly, depending on availability, cost, fashion and cultural factors. Currently one of the more common forms of dependence is on caffeine,

---

Table 24.1 Substances abused

- Stimulants (uppers)
  Amphetamine, caffeine, cocaine, dextroamphetamine, diethylpropion, methylphenidate, nicotine, phenmetrazine
- Hypnotic/sedatives (downers)
  Anxiolytics: alprazolam, benzodiazepines (diazepam, flurazepam, temazepam), chlorazepate, chlordiazepoxide, meprobamate
  Barbiturates: amylobarbitone, methohexitone, pentobarbitone, phenobarbitone, secobarbitone, thiopentone
  Ethanol
- Opioids
  Codeine, fentanyl, heroin, hydrocodone, lomotil, meperidine, methyl-phenyl-tetra-hydropyridine (MPTP), morphine, oxycodone, propoxyphene
- Psychedelics (hallucinogens)
  Lysergic acid (LSD), mescaline (peyote), methyl-dimethoxyamphetamine (STP; DOM), methylene dioxyamphetamine (MDA), methylene dimethoxyamphetamine (MDMA; Ecstasy), phencyclidine (PCP), psilocybin
- Cannabinoids
  Marijuana
- Inhalants
  Amyl nitrite, butyl nitrite, enflurane, ether, halothane, isoflurane, nitrous oxide, petrol, solvents (various)

---

in coffee and other beverages, but there is no evidence that there are serious medical or social consequences. In contrast, there can be serious medical, behavioural and social consequences affecting both the user (and any fetus) and others in the community from the use or abuse of other commonly available substances such as alcohol (*Table 24.1*).

Unfortunately, drugs bought on the street are not necessarily pure, and are frequently adulterated, often with unknown ingredients that may be dangerous in their own right, complicating the whole picture of drug abuse. At present, apart from alcohol, solvents, cannabis and Ecstasy, heroin is the main drug of abuse followed closely by methadone and cocaine and these three drugs, together with opioids, barbiturate, psychedelics and some others are restricted by the law in many countries so that possession and trafficking is illegal.

Intravenous injection is frequently used by those who abuse drugs. Frequently, injection technique is filthy, needles or syringes are shared (with the risk of blood-borne infections) and even water from a lavatory pan may be used to dissolve the drug. Assaults, theft and prostitution are often used to fund the drug habit. The life-style of these addicts is thus often such that sexually transmitted disease is common, serious infections are a major complication and there is the frequent risk of maxillofacial and other injuries during assaults or fights. Common complications of intravenous drug abuse therefore include the following:

1. Viral hepatitis (particularly B, C and D) and chronic liver disease.
2. Infective endocarditis and consequent cardiac lesions, usually as a consequence of infected injections – not dental treatment. However, those drug addicts who have had endocarditis as a result of their habits also become susceptible to the disease as a consequence of dental treatment and will need appropriate prophylaxis.
3. Maxillofacial injuries.
4. HIV infection, sexually transmitted and other infectious diseases.
5. Venous thromboses making intravenous injection difficult.

Health care workers are often reluctant to deal with these patients but their numbers are increasing. Many of these drugs alter behaviour or have a potential for or may cause interactions with drugs used for dental purposes (*see* Appendix to Chapter 25) and there may be the possibility of communicable diseases especially in intravenous drug users.

ASPECTS OF CHEMICAL DEPENDENCE

Many drugs and chemicals can cause central nervous system stimulation, depression or hallucinations, or distort perception, thinking or judgement. Abuse of such drugs is increasingly common and presents management difficulties in dentistry, particularly because of behavioural disorders, drug resistance or interactions, hepatitis, HIV infection, other sexually transmitted diseases or social problems. Of extreme concern is the high level of psychoactive drug use in health care workers. One study of medical personnel in the USA in 1986 showed that over half the respondents had used marijuana or cocaine recreationally, or opioids or tranquillizers for self-treatment.

Drugs are abused *experimentally* on only one or two occasions because of curiosity; for *recreation* when they are used in a relatively controlled way; or *in special circumstances*, for example to relieve anxiety or fatigue. *Compulsive drug abuse* is what is generally known as addiction. The drug is taken without any medical indication and despite adverse medical and social consequences. There is intense dependence and there are severe physical or psychological effects if the drug is stopped (withdrawal syndrome).

Identifying the chemically dependent patient can be difficult but certain points in the history and examination may help. Those who abuse drugs not uncommonly abuse several substances, including alcohol and tobacco, and may also neglect their health – general and oral. Alcohol on the breath, nicotine on fingers, the smell of marijuana, tremors, avoidance of eye contact, constricted or dilated pupils, a history of liver disease and irregular attendance for treatment are some possible indicators of dependency.

Common management difficulties are behavioural problems including irregular dental attendance and compliance; anxiety and dental fear and a craving for sweets; and hazards of cross-infection with hepatitis viruses, HIV and increasingly TB. It is important to respect confidentiality. Common oral problems include a high incidence of facial trauma and oral neglect, caries, periodontal disease, smokers' keratoses, gingival and/or buccal ulceration or pigmentation. Some patients may feign oral disease such as pain, or even produce self-inflicted injuries in order to obtain narcotic drugs. Care should thus be taken with any patient who:

1. has subjective symptoms with no objective evidence of the disorder;
2. makes a self-diagnosis and requests a specific drug, especially a psychoactive agent;
3. appears to have a dramatic but unexpected complaint such as trigeminal neuralgia;
4. firmly rejects treatments that exclude psychoactive drugs;
5. has no interest in the diagnosis or investigations or refuses a second opinion.

ALCOHOL

The consumption of alcohol is rising throughout the world and alcohol abuse is still the most common form of drug abuse. As many as 15 per cent of all visits to physicians are alcohol-related, and up to 25 per cent of dental patients may have abused or continue to abuse alcohol.

Alcoholism causes the most serious drug-related effects in many countries, since both affected individuals and others are involved, particularly as a result of road traffic accidents and assaults.

The probability of developing alcoholism is greater in several groups, especially those to whom alcohol is freely available (*Table 24.2*). However, the causes of alcoholism are

Table 24.2 Risk factors for, and findings suggestive of, alcoholism

Occupation	Publicans and other workers in the drinks industry
	Entertainers
	Commercial travellers
	Bored housewives
	Bachelors over 40
	Armed forces
	Doctors
Social problems	Absenteeism
	Frequent job changes
	Marital disharmony
Medical history	Accidents
	Assaults
	Violence
	Cirrhosis
	Macrocytosis
Family history of alcoholism	

obscure and one eminent psychiatrist has stated that nothing useful is known about this aspect of the disease.

Two major difficulties are to define and detect alcoholism. A loose definition is consumption of alcohol to such a degree as to cause deterioration in social behaviour, or physical illness, and the development of dependence, from which withdrawal is difficult or causes adverse effects.

Detection of alcoholism

The effects of alcohol relate to depression of higher centres, initially releasing inhibitions, eventually interfering with the cerebellum and causing ataxia and unconsciousness. After a large alcoholic binge, suppression of protective reflexes such as the cough reflex, can result in inhalation of vomit, and death. The acute effects of alcohol are mainly on judgement, concentration and coordination, and are dose-related as follows:

<100 mg/100 ml	Dry and decent
100–200 mg/100 ml	Delighted and devilish
200–300 mg/100 ml	Delinquent and disgusting
300–400 mg/100 ml	Dizzy and delirious
400–500 mg/100 ml	Dazed and dejected
>500 mg/100 ml	Dead drunk.

A small person, particularly female, is affected at a lower alcohol intake than a larger person or one used to regular alcohol intake.

Signs or symptoms of chronic excessive alcohol drinking include slurred speech, smell of alcohol on the breath, signs of self-neglect whether of the mouth or shabbiness of clothes, an evasive, truculent, over-boisterous or facetious manner, indigestion (particularly heartburn), anxiety (often with insomnia), or tremor of the hands. Later there may be palpitations (and tachycardia) and signs of liver disease, malnutrition, cardiomyopathy, peripheral neuropathy, amnesia and confabulation (in Wernicke's and Korsakoff's CNS syndromes), cerebellar degeneration with ataxia, or dementia.

The difficulties in recognizing whether a patient has been taking alcohol are shown by a survey in a British teaching hospital, where it was found that over 30 per cent of patients attending the casualty department had blood alcohol levels over 80 mg/100 ml. Medical staff, who at the same time were attempting to detect inebriation clinically, underestimated the true extent of the problem by 19 per cent. Recognition of the alcoholic is notoriously difficult and even if the disorder is suspected the history is often a hopelessly unreliable guide to the amount of alcohol consumed. No social class or profession seems to be immune; not only is there a high prevalence of alcoholism amongst vagrants but also among doctors. Women are traditionally even more evasive about their drinking habits, but it is important to bear in mind that women are almost as frequently alcoholic as men.

The CAGE questionnaire may be helpful: a positive response to any of the following questions suggests a diagnosis of alcoholism:

1. Have you ever felt the need to **C**ut down on drink?
2. Have you ever felt **A**nnoyed by criticism of your drinking?
3. Have you ever felt **G**uilty about drinking?
4. Do you drink a morning **E**ye opener?

Laboratory investigations that may be helpful include raised blood levels of alcohol, gamma-glutamyl transpeptidase and other hepatic enzymes. However, raised liver enzyme values can also be found with socially acceptable alcohol consumption. Folate deficiency of no obvious cause is also suspicious. Macrocytosis alone is one of the earliest signs of alcoholism; later there may be macrocytic anaemia.

Laboratory investigations must therefore be interpreted in the light of clinical findings and are of value mainly in the preoperative assessment of patients, or the interpretation of clinical signs.

Many diseases can be caused or aggravated by alcohol. There is a high incidence of alcohol-associated accidents and disease and some 20–30 per cent of those seeking acute medical or surgical attention may be alcoholics.

Complications of alcoholism

1. Injuries, including maxillofacial, from accidents or assaults.
2. Social difficulties.
3. Liver disease.
4. Nutritional defects.
5. Pancreatitis.
6. Alcoholic gastritis and peptic ulcer.
7. Predisposition to infections, especially pneumonia and tuberculosis.
8. Cardiomyopathy.
9. Myopathy.
10. Brain damage and epilepsy.

In one study of alcoholics, the mortality rate over 15 years was about 300 per cent above the norm. Alcohol is an important, if not the main, causal factor in over 25 per cent of road traffic accidents and also in many other accidents or assaults. Many patients presenting with maxillofacial or head injuries have been drinking (*Plate 24*). Alcohol is often a factor in violent or sexual crimes and suicides and also contributes to the spread of sexually transmitted diseases, including HIV. Common social problems include marital difficulties, aggressive behaviour, crime, absenteeism and financial embarrassment.

Acute alcoholic hepatitis may follow binge drinking while cirrhosis commonly results from chronic alcoholism. The inadequate diet of many alcoholics causes nutritional defects which can cause peripheral polyneuropathies (burning hands and feet), pellagra, amblyopia (visual defects) and various organic brain disorders (Wernicke's encephalopathy and Korsakoff's psychosis) or epilepsy. Alcoholism in pregnancy can lead to the fetal alcohol syndrome.

Fetal alcohol syndrome

Alcohol is now the most common teratogen apart from smoking to which the fetus is exposed. Chronic ingestion may cause spontaneous abortion or birth defects (fetal alcohol syndrome, FAS). The prevalence of FAS is similar to that of Down's syndrome.

FAS affects growth, CNS and orofacial features. Most affected children are of short stature. Microcephaly is common and associated with a low IQ, difficulties in eating and speech and muscular incoordination. The FAS patient is irritable as an infant, hyperactive as a child and highly unsociable as an adult.

Facial features include hypoplastic maxillae, low nasal bridge, indistinct philtrum with a hypoplastic upper lip and other features, including small teeth with dysplastic enamel.

Alcohol withdrawal

The features of alcohol withdrawal are similar to, but usually less severe than, the barbiturate withdrawal syndrome. During the first 24 hours there is tremor, anxiety, sweating, weakness, nausea and insomnia. This is followed by vomiting, abdominal cramps and hallucinations and, in severe cases, convulsions (delirium tremens, DTs, rum fits). Hyperthermia is common and there may be exhaustion or cardiovascular collapse. The whole withdrawal syndrome lasts about a week and requires medical supervision and the use of benzodiazepines or chlormethiazole.

The chronic alcoholic needs medical treatment including:

1. Admission to manage rehabilitation and ensure abstinence.
2. Use of drugs to reduce dependence (naltrexone or chlormethiazole) or to cause unpleasant side-effects if alcohol is taken (disulfiram – Antabuse). Reactions can be severe and can be seen when *any* alcohol is used – even the small amounts in medicines or toiletries – for up to one week after disulphiram is taken.

• Dental aspects of alcoholism

Many alcoholics present no dental management problems but complications may include:

1. Erratic attendance for dental treatment.
2. Aggressive behaviour.
3. Liver disease.
4. Cardiomyopathy.
5. Drug interactions (Appendix to Chapter 25).

Alcoholics are best given an early morning appointment, when they are least likely to be under the influence of alcohol. The main relevant medical complications are that liver cirrhosis delays the metabolism of many drugs and there may be a bleeding tendency. Chronic alcoholism may also cause bone marrow depression and possibly anaemia and thrombocytopenia. Care should thus be taken when surgery is contemplated (Chapter 5). General anaesthesia is best avoided, especially if the patient has premedicated himself with alcohol, which increases the risk of vomiting and inhalation of vomit. Alcoholics are especially prone to aspiration lung abscess. Alcoholic heart disease is also a contraindication to general anaesthesia.

Drug interactions with alcohol which may be important in dental management include the following:

Anaesthetics and sedatives: General anaesthetic agents, sedatives or hypnotics generally have an additive effect with alcohol, although these interactions are not entirely predictable. Heavy drinkers, however, become tolerant not only of alcohol but also of other sedatives. Alcoholics are also notoriously resistant to general anaesthesia. Once liver disease develops the position is reversed and drug metabolism is then impaired (Chapter 10) and drugs have a disproportionately greater effect.

Analgesics: Aspirin should be avoided since it is more likely in the alcoholic patient to cause gastric erosions and bleeding, and to precipitate bleeding. The hepatotoxic effects of paracetamol are enhanced, though it is probably the safest analgesic in this group (Chapter 25).

Alcohol: it is important to avoid any alcohol-containing preparations, such as some mouthwashes.

Metronidazole: Metronidazole and alcohol interact to cause widespread vasodilatation, nausea, vomiting, sweating, headache and palpitations similar to the Antabuse reaction. The effects are unpleasant or alarming but rarely dangerous.

One of the most important dental complications of excessive alcohol intake is maxillofacial trauma and head injuries (Chapter 22) and unconsciousness in such patients may be due at least in part to the alcohol itself.

Wound healing may also be impaired in the severe chronic alcoholic and, in a series reported in the USA, alcoholism was found to be a common factor in 22 patients with osteomyelitis following mandibular fractures.

The most common oral effect of alcoholism, however, is neglect leading to advanced caries and periodontal disease, and there is sometimes dental erosion from regurgitation. There may be folate deficiency or other anaemia, with glossitis and sometimes angular stomatitis or recurrent aphthae. Alcoholic cirrhosis may cause a bleeding tendency and a rare manifestation is bilateral painless swelling of the parotids or other major salivary glands (sialosis, Chapter 9). Orofacial features include a smell of alcohol on the breath, telangiectases and possibly rhinophyma ('grog blossom').

Spirit drinking was thought to be a cause of leukoplakia, but this may have applied to the nineteenth century, when alcohol was heavily adulterated, or associated factors operated. The precise relationship of alcohol with oral cancer is contentious.

NICOTINE AND TOBACCO

Cigarette smoking is a major hazard to health and promotes many diseases (*Table 24.3*). Combustion of tobacco gives rise not only to nicotine, tar and carbon monoxide but also about 4000 other compounds, including nitrosamines and aromatic amines, which are known carcinogens. Cigarette smoking is particularly linked to atherosclerotic heart disease, cancers of the lung, oesophagus, mouth and bladder, and chronic obstructive pulmonary disease. Cigarette use also affects the fetus.

There appears to be dependence upon nicotine in chronic smokers. Heavy smokers appear to require a stable blood concentration of nicotine – if they change to a different type of cigarette they also change the pattern of smoking to keep their nicotine levels constant. Smokers metabolize some other drugs more rapidly and require, for example, higher doses of benzodiazepines than non-smokers. Withdrawal leads to nausea, headache, constipation or diarrhoea, irritability, insomnia, poor concentration and increased appetite. The use of nicotine chewing gum or transdermal patches helps reduce the withdrawal symptoms.

- **Dental aspects of smoking and smokeless tobacco**

Difficulties in dental management may include:

1. Chronic obstructive airways disease.
2. Ischaemic heart disease.
3. Resistance to sedation.
4. Associated disorders such as alcoholism or peptic ulcer.

Table 24.3	Diseases associated with cigarette smoking

- Cardiovascular
    Ischaemic heart disease
    Cerebrovascular disease
    Peripheral vascular disease
    Buerger's disease
- Respiratory
    Chronic obstructive airways disease
- Carcinomas
    Oropharyngeal
    Bronchus
    Bladder
    Larynx
    Pancreas
- Fetus
    Increased prevalence of abortion
    Low birthweight
    Increased risk of perinatal and sudden infant deaths
- Gastrointestinal
    Peptic ulcer
- Alcoholism

Smoking may cause mucosal keratinization and pigmentary incompetence and is linked to oral cancer. Smoker's keratosis, in which there is diffuse hyperkeratosis of the palate, is typically caused by pipe smoking. The hyperkeratosis itself is benign and rapidly reversible even after many years of pipe smoking. However, there is some epidemiological evidence of an association between pipe smoking and oral cancer, but when cancer develops in a pipe smoker it is likely to be in the lower retromolar region and not in the area of keratosis.

Oral snuff dipping and chewing tobacco predispose to leukoplakia and oral cancer. Up to 46 per cent of regular users develop leukoplakia. Currently there is particular concern over the mucosal reactions and the carcinogenic potential of the widespread use of smokeless tobacco by children and adolescents, especially in the USA.

Stopping smoking reduces the risk of oral cancer so that by 5 years it is down to that of a non-smoker. However, stopping smoking is not merely difficult but may bring other problems. Aggravation or the onset of recurrent aphthae is noted by some, while others take to eating sweets as a substitute for smoking and may then have increased caries activity, or put on weight.

Smoking also predisposes to periodontal disease, particularly necrotizing gingivitis, to candidosis, and to xerostomia. Cigarette smoking is the most common cause of extrinsic staining of teeth.

Use of nicotine-containing chewing gum may reduce aphthae but may produce hypersalivation.

BENZODIAZEPINES

Dependence on benzodiazepines is becoming common but the effects are considerably less severe than with most other sedatives.

The pattern of dependence on sedatives varies widely. Often neither patient nor doctor realizes that it has developed, since the anxiety, tremor and insomnia that follow the drug's withdrawal are incorrectly attributed to the return of the original anxiety state.

There are two types of medical use for benzodiazepines, as anxiolytics or as hypnotics. The main anxiolytics are diazepam and lorazepam; the main hypnotics are flurazepam, nitrazepam, temazepam and triazolam. Benzodiazepines are very widely prescribed but despite concern, abuse is relatively uncommon. They are widely used, however, by drug-abusers in order to self-medicate opioid withdrawal or to manage adverse effects from cocaine or methamphetamine. They are usually abused orally, or by injecting crushed tablets or the jelly from capsules, sometimes with opioids. Apart from those above, clonazepam, temazepam and bromazepam are sometimes abused. Flunitrazepam, an effective hypnotic, known as roSHAY, roach or roofies, is increasingly abused and has been used to sedate women for sexual assaults.

Fewer than 1 per cent of the population claim to use these sedatives non-medically and then usually infrequently. However, benzodiazepines may be one component of multiple drug abuse. Some patients, mainly housewives, also claim to have become dependent as a result of having been prescribed benzodiazepines for chronic anxiety.

Memory loss is a major feature of benzodiazepine use. Mild physical and psychological dependence on benzodiazepines can develop, and fairly quickly – sometimes within 1 month. Withdrawal symptoms are frequently delayed in onset compared with the barbiturates but may last 8–10 days. Typical effects include insomnia, anxiety, loss of appetite, tremor, perspiration and perceptual disturbances. Sudden withdrawal, particularly of short-acting benzodiazepines, is dangerous since it can cause confusion, fits, toxic psychosis or a condition resembling delirium tremens.

Benzodiazepines should therefore only be prescribed for short periods (not more than 2 weeks). In those that have become dependent, withdrawal should be gradual. The benzodiazepine should be changed to diazepam and this should be reduced by fortnightly decrements of 2.5 mg or less. Complete withdrawal may take several weeks or even months.

Unlike other drugs of abuse at the time of writing only temazepam is a Controlled Drug and benzodiazepines are virtually harmless in overdose.

BARBITURATES

Medically, barbiturates are used for severe insomnia and to control epilepsy. Addiction usually develops in patients who have been prescribed barbiturates for insomnia or anxiety. Two main types of barbiturate addict are recognized and either may also abuse other drugs:

1. Middle-aged women, often living alone, taking large quantities of barbiturates orally and living in a dream world, form the largest group. Chronic toxicity such as rashes and ataxia often develop.
2. Young addicts, who take barbiturates ('sleepers') for immediate effect, by injection, can develop multiple abscesses, gangrene, hepatitis, HIV infection, infective endocarditis or occasionally tetanus. Most of these complications are caused by filthy injection technique.

Barbiturates are also responsible for many of the lethal overdoses taken by addicts to any drugs, since barbiturates are often used to adulterate more expensive drugs such as heroin.

Barbiturates are depressant drugs that produce sedation, and depress respiration and heart rate, as well as impairing thought processes and memory and causing incoordination and ataxia. With chronic use, addicts begin to think slowly, have increasing emotional lability and show signs of self-neglect. Concentration and judgement are increasingly impaired and the barbiturate addict becomes irritable. Although tolerance to barbiturates increases remarkably, the lethal dose remains the same, and with only a small gap between relatively safe and lethal levels, accidental overdose is a relatively common cause of death from respiratory failure and CNS depression, especially if alcohol is also taken. Should barbiturates be withdrawn, the addict initially improves and any ataxia disappears. However, within 12–16 hours a dangerous withdrawal syndrome can develop. Nausea, anxiety, tremor, insomnia, tachycardia, weakness and postural hypotension, are followed by abdominal pain. After 36–48 hours there may, in heavy users, be loss of consciousness and often fits and sometimes death. The syndrome has a slower onset in those who have been using long-acting barbiturates. Barbiturates must only be withdrawn under strict medical supervision. They are Controlled Drugs.

• Dental aspects of barbiturate abuse

Dental management may be complicated by:

1. Altered drug metabolism.
2. Hepatitis B and C.
3. Sexually transmitted disease.
4. Epilepsy.
5. Maxillofacial injuries.
6. Tetanus.
7. HIV infection.

Barbiturates induce liver drug-metabolizing enzymes and cause resistance to anaesthetics, but also enhance the sedative effects of some drugs. Oral complications of barbiturate abuse are rare. A bullous mucosal reaction has been reported but, more common, are manifestations such as atypical facial pain, related to the underlying condition for which the drug was prescribed.

OPIOIDS (NARCOTICS)

Opioids are a group of drugs widely used medically to provide potent analgesia.

Morphine and heroin (diacetyl morphine) are derived from the opium poppy. Others are synthetic such as methadone, dipipanone, dihydrocodeine and pethidine, but many other synthetic analogues or derivatives are also abused. These powerful analgesics appear to act by mimicking the natural brain peptides – enkephalins and endorphins. Opioid abuse develops in three main ways:

1. Use by adolescents in an experimental or recreational way, or as part of a life-style.
2. As a sequel to their medical use for severe pain.
3. Dependence on methadone used for treatment of established drug dependence.

Opioid abuse is widespread in many communities, especially in the USA. Nearly 40 per cent of US army conscripts used narcotics at some time during their year in Vietnam and one-half of them became physically dependent. Abuse of opioids is otherwise mainly in urban areas, particularly the new towns and the major cities.

Opioids can be used orally, sometimes smoked or sniffed, or used intravenously – when maximum effect is obtained. Abuse leads to tolerance at an early stage, and dependence after some months. Withdrawal is then unpleasant though usually not dangerous. Withdrawal of narcotics leads to a withdrawal syndrome within about 8 hours, peaks at about 3–5 days, and fades over 5–14 days. Early features include lacrimation, rhinorrhoea, sweating and persistent yawning. After about 12 hours the addict enters a phase of restless tossing sleep (*yen*) when there is pupil dilatation, tremor, goose-flesh (*cold turkey*), anorexia, nausea, vomiting, muscle spasms, orgasms, diarrhoea and abdominal pains. Pulse rate and blood pressure also rise. Once the main features have subsided, there may be weakness and insomnia for several weeks or months.

Heroin can be sniffed, smoked from a tin-foil (*'chasing the dragon'*) or injected. The use of intravenous heroin is a major drug problem but it is important to note that 'street' heroin contains only about 10 per cent heroin – most is filler such as lactose, fruit sugars, quinine, powdered milk, phenacetin, caffeine, antipyrine, or strychnine. Drugs such as Ecstasy may also have been added.

Methadone is a synthetic agent taken orally as a syrup, usually initially during the treatment of heroin addiction. It is addictive. Use of an illicitly manufactured pethidine – like the drug (MPDP) that caused specific damage to the substantia nigra of the basal ganglia and extreme parkinsonian rigidity – has incidentally led to more detailed understanding of Parkinson's disease and a search for other environmental causes.

Despite widespread belief to the contrary, pentazocine is also used as a drug of dependence, particularly amongst medical and paramedical personnel in the USA. Pentazocine is therefore a Controlled Drug in Great Britain. Pentazocine tablets together with an antihistamine (Ts and Blues, *see* Appendix to this chapter) have been used intravenously as an alternative to the more expensive heroin.

Dipipanone is less sedating than morphine and may therefore be abused, but is available only in tablet form and in combination with an anti-emetic (Diconal). Distalgesic and co-proxamole (because of the dextro-propoxyphene) are also used as drugs of addiction.

Detection of opioid abuse

Early signs of opioid abuse can be difficult or impossible to detect and may remain unsuspected until needle marks are seen, syringes found or medical complications develop. However, lack of concentration, poor performance at work, irritability, desire to be left alone, absences from home or self-neglect are suggestive of abuse. Loss of weight and emaciation, pupil constriction and chronic constipation are more specific signs. Needle marks or thromboses of veins, particularly in the forearms and legs, are common, but addicts are now remarkably adept at finding veins, even lingual or penile veins, that escape casual inspection. Opioids may also be used subcutaneously (skin popping), as snuff or as cigarettes. Many narcotic addicts also abuse alcohol or cocaine or other drugs.

Complications of opioid abuse

Neglect of general health and hygiene is common and the diet is often poor and consists mainly of fast-foods and snacks.

Illegal intravenous drugs are often adulterated with talc, sucrose, baking soda, quinine or starch, and often suspended in dirty water. Syringes and needles are often re-used or shared by several addicts. Infective complications such as septicaemia and pneumonia are therefore common and an acute right-sided endocarditis can be rapidly fatal or may leave substantial cardiac damage. Hepatitis B, C and D are frequently the result of using contaminated injection equipment and indulging in associated activities such as sexual promiscuity or homosexuality (Chapter 10). In some areas addicts are the group at greatest risk from viral hepatitis. Infection with HIV is a growing problem. Sexually transmitted diseases are also prevalent. Constipation, respiratory depression and orthostatic hypotension are common.

The mortality among opioid addicts is 2–6 per cent per annum: deaths are usually from overdose. This is often accidental as a result of impure drugs or the combination with another CNS depressant such as alcohol. Less often, there may be an anaphylactoid reaction to the opioid or impurities in the preparation. Suicide and assaults are other common causes of death, as is AIDS. The morbidity is also high from other infective complications, violence or malnutrition.

Medical supervision and the use of opioid agonists such as oral methadone and levo-alpha-acetylmethadol (LAAM), or antagonists such as naltrexone, or lofexidine are needed in the management of opioid dependence.

• Dental aspects of opioid dependence

The identification of addicts is difficult, especially in view of the different types described earlier. However, abnormal behaviour, persistently constricted pupils or outlining of veins are highly suspicious features. The opioid addict is said to be 'a depressed introvert with constricted pupils'.

Dental treatment can often be given to narcotic addicts without fear of complications, but possible difficulties include:

1. Analgesia (*see below*).
2. Feigning pain or stealing drugs or prescription forms.
3. Behavioural disturbances and withdrawal symptoms.

4. Cardiac lesions
5. Maxillofacial injuries.
6. Hepatitis or chronic liver disease.
7. Infective endocarditis.
8. Sexually transmitted diseases, including HIV infection.
9. Venous thromboses making intravenous injection difficult.
10. Tetanus.
11. Drug interactions.

Simulation of pain is a common manoeuvre to obtain narcotics. Prescription pads may be stolen or drug cabinets raided. Dental drugs that may be attractive to the addict include pethidine, codeine, pentazocine and dextro-propoxyphene (in co-proxamol and distalgesic).

In the established addict, non-narcotic analgesics may be ineffective in controlling dental pain, so that large doses of opioids may have to be given. Needless to say, opioids should not be given or prescribed without first seeking expert advice, and their only indication in dentistry is for severe postoperative pain. Pentazocine, being a narcotic antagonist, should not be used for such patients as it may precipitate a withdrawal syndrome. Perhaps surprisingly, many addicts tolerate pain poorly and complain that local anaesthesia is insufficient for operative procedures. General anaesthesia may therefore be preferred unless there are other medical contraindications. Nausea and vomiting are common if the narcotics are stopped preoperatively.

Furthermore, those under treatment for addiction have a period of several weeks during which they are particularly hypersensitive to pain and stress. If the patient is under treatment for addiction, opioids must be avoided. Local anaesthesia is preferable at this time, since reduced sensitivity to carbon dioxide is a contraindication to general anaesthesia. Although the withdrawal syndrome subsides within about a week, the addict is, for a few weeks thereafter, intolerant of stress and pain. The respiratory response to carbon dioxide is reduced and general anaesthesia may then be hazardous.

There are no specific oral effects of opioid dependence but there is often oral neglect, advanced periodontal disease and caries. Diet and sometimes medications predispose to caries; some agents cause hyposalivation. Caries is often left untreated by the patient who, because of the opioid, may be numbed to the pain. Patients with endocarditis may have oral petechiae. Agents such as lofexidine may produce xerostomia.

AMPHETAMINES

Amphetamines are the main drugs in a group of central stimulants that also include phenmetrazine, methylphenidate and, to a lesser extent, diethylpropion. These drugs, which are eaten, smoked, sniffed or injected, are characterized by their ability to elevate mood. They increase cerebral activity, causing excitement and euphoria, and they dilate the pupils, increase heart rate, blood pressure and sometimes temperature, and cause sleeplessness and anorexia. High doses can cause mood swings, and psychoses – including hallucinations and paranoia. Overdose can cause respiratory failure and death.

Amphetamine addiction may develop in the following ways:

1. Following use for their euphoriant effect.
2. Following their use, for example, by lorry drivers, to stave off fatigue in order to continue their work.
3. As a result of medical use for slimming or for depression.

Amphetamines are taken orally or intravenously (*speed*). They produce a range of effects by stimulating alpha- and beta-adrenergic receptors and thus stimulate the CNS and peripheral nervous system. There is no true withdrawal syndrome and, in this respect, amphetamine addiction is quite different from opioid or barbiturate dependence.

Complications of amphetamine use

Acute toxicity manifests with dry mouth, dilated pupils, tachycardia, aggression, talkativeness, tachypnoea and hallucinations, leading to seizures, hyperpyrexia, dysrhythmias and collapse. Chronic toxicity causes restlessness, hyperactivity, loss of appetite and weight, tremor, repetitive movements and picking at the face and extremities. Eventually with large doses, a paranoid psychosis may develop.

Apart from amphetamine itself, other related drugs include methamphetamine (*ice*), which acts, when inhaled, almost as rapidly as intravenous cocaine but has several hours' duration of action, and *Ecstasy* (methylene–deoxymethamphetamine – MDMA), which has similar properties to the other amphetamines but is more potently hallucinogenic, possibly because of chemical affinities with mescalin and has resulted in a number of deaths. Ecstasy (*E*, *Adam* or *XTC*) is usually taken by mouth, giving effects after 20–60 minutes. Users need to take water or non-alcoholic drinks frequently and in large amounts to avoid hyperthermia ('chill-out'). After long-term use, tolerance develops but there is no physical dependence nor withdrawal symptoms.

- ## Dental aspects of amphetamine dependence

Amphetamine addicts may be remarkably resistant to general anaesthesia and, if using intravenous drugs, may have many of the infective problems of opioid addicts. Monoamine oxidase inhibitors are contraindicated (Appendix to Chapter 25). Bruxism may result from chronic amphetamine use and there can be xerostomia and greater caries incidence.

COCAINE

From being a fashionable drug of abuse for wealthy, apparently respectable members of society in the USA, cocaine has become one of the most widely abused drugs, as a result of smuggling on an enormous scale mainly from South America. A survey in 1991 revealed that almost 1 per cent of the US population over the age of 12 had used cocaine within the previous month.

Cocaine is inhaled (*snorted*), smoked or injected intravenously, intramuscularly or hypodermically. It is also taken orally, sublingually, rectally or vaginally. Free base cocaine (*crack*), obtained by boiling cocaine hydrochloride with sodium bicarbonate, acts so rapidly that, when inhaled or smoked, its effects are similar to intravenous cocaine. Some use cocaine plus heroin intravenously ('*speedballing*'); this is especially dangerous. As a constituent of Brompton cocktail (cocaine, heroin or morphine and alcohol),

cocaine is also sometimes used for the management of patients with terminal disease.

Cocaine has potent effects on dopamine, noradrenaline and 5-hydroxytryptamine neurones in the CNS. Effects start within 5 minutes of intranasal use, and last up to 1 hour. Smoking crack results in effects within 10 seconds. The cocaine addict has aptly been described as a 'sexed-up extrovert with dilated pupils'. Cocaine abuse is characterized by feelings of well-being and heightened mental activity. The cocaine addict is garrulous, witty and the life and soul of the party, but later shows diminished activity.

Long-term inhalation of cocaine can cause, in addition to nasal symptoms similar to those of the common cold, perforation of the nasal septum and ulceration of the palate as a result of ischaemic necrosis. Snorting cocaine predisposes to sphenoidal sinusitis, and occasionally leads to brain abscess. Large doses of cocaine produce paranoia, visual hallucinations (*snowlights*) and tactile hallucinations. The latter are typically of insects crawling over the skin (formication, '*cocaine bugs*'). Toxic reactions to cocaine abuse include angina, coronary spasm, ventricular dysrhythmias, myocardial infarction, cerebrovascular accidents, convulsions, respiratory depression and death. Deaths from cocaine are becoming increasingly common as the drug becomes ever more widely used.

On stopping cocaine, symptoms proceed through a crash phase of depression and craving for sleep, a withdrawal phase of lack of energy and then an extinction phase of recurrence of craving evoked by various external stimuli but of lesser intensity.

- ## Dental aspects of cocaine addiction

Behavioural problems or drug interactions may interfere with dental treatment, and patients who inject cocaine are at risk from the same blood-borne infections as other addicts.

Dental treatment should not be given until 6 hours after the last dose of cocaine has been taken and it may be advisable to avoid adrenaline-containing local anaesthetics because of enhanced sympathomimetic action and subsequent dysrhythmias, acute hypertension or cardiac failure. Where general anaesthesia is needed, isoflurane or sevoflurane are preferred to halothane as this may induce dysrhythmias.

Oral use of cocaine temporarily numbs the lips and tongue and can cause gingival erosions. The main oral effects of cocaine addiction may be a dry mouth and bruxism or dental erosion. Caries and periodontal disease, especially acute necrotizing gingivitis, are increased. Children born to cocaine-using mothers are more prone to have ankyloglossia.

PSYCHEDELIC DRUGS

Psychedelic drugs (hallucinogens, psychotomimetics or psychotogens) induce feelings of enhanced clarity of sensation, higher awareness of sensory input and altered perception, but minimal risk of physical dependence. They include:

1. Cannabis
2. Indolealkylamines such as lysergic acid diethylamide (LSD) and psilocybin.
3. Phenylethylamines such as mescaline.
4. Phenylisopropylamines.
5. Phencyclidine (PCP) and derivatives such as ethyl phenylcyclohexamine (PCE) and thiencylcyclophexyl piperidine (TCP).
6. Ketamine

In addition, as mentioned earlier, the amphetamine Ecstasy (methylene-deoxy-methamphetamine, MDMA) is hallucinogenic as excessive doses of other amphetamines may be.

Cannabis

Cannabis (marijuana) is a widely abused drug; hashish is prepared from cannabis resin. The US 1991 survey suggested 5 per cent of those aged 12 or over had used cannabis in the previous month. It can be taken by many routes but is often smoked as a *reefer*. The effects are prompt, somewhat resemble those of alcohol, but differ with dose and route of administration. Large doses cause dreams, hallucinations, feelings of depersonalization, impaired memory and depressed motor function. Hunger, dry mouth and enhanced sense of taste, smell and

hearing may develop. Conjunctival injection and tachycardia may be seen, and cannabis may induce angina in those with ischaemic heart disease. The only other established health risks are neurological impairment, bronchitis and possibly impaired fertility.

It is controversial whether there are serious medical effects of cannabis abuse, or that the abuse of hard drugs such as narcotics necessarily follows the use of soft drugs such as cannabis. However, the single best predictor of cocaine abuse is frequent use of cannabis during adolescence.

Withdrawal of cannabis can cause tremor, irritability, insomnia, anorexia and fever.

* **Dental aspects of cannabis addiction**

There are no specific aspects of cannabis addiction that influence dental management in most patients, but there is a tendency to a dry mouth, and some concern that cannabis use may predispose to oral cancer.

LSD

Hallucinogens are rarely used over long periods and LSD in particular can cause persistent schizophrenia-like psychosis if it is. Up to 12 per cent of adolescents are estimated to have taken hallucinogenic agents.

These drugs often cause sympathomimetic effects such as pupil dilatation, tremor, nausea and a rise in blood pressure, pulse rate and temperature. *Synaesthesia*, the overflow from one sense to another when, for example, colours are heard, is common. There is often lability of mood, panic ('*bad trip*') and delusions of magical powers, such as being able to fly. Whilst under the influence of these drugs, deaths, accidents and assaults as a result of delusions are therefore common. There is no withdrawal syndrome when psychedelic drugs are stopped, but permanent mental disturbance can follow. Dimethyltryptamine (DMT) has similar actions to LSD.

Phencyclidine (PCP; angel dust)

PCP is a psychedelic frequently abused by smoking, snorting or eating – rarely intravenously. It causes a syndrome closely resembling schizophrenia and manic depressive psychosis, and may produce numbness of the extremities, facial grimacing and flushing, hypersalivation, jaw clenching, expressive dysphasia and memory loss. Nystagmus and hypertension are also prominent features of PCP abuse.

Phencyclidine, which was originally developed as a general anaesthetic, produces a state of dissociative anaesthesia in which the subject becomes detached or dissociated from all bodily sensations and pain. Users may severely injure themselves because of these dissociative effects and the psychotic reactions cause violently aggressive behaviour towards others. PCP in overdose may cause hyperthermia, respiratory depression, seizures, and intracerebral haemorrhage and death. Phencyclidine is therefore now regarded as one of the most dangerous drugs of addiction. Because of its low price and availability, it is often sold with, or as a misrepresentation of, other drugs of abuse. Addicts to the latter may therefore be unknowingly exposed to phencyclidine. The closely related anti-parkinsonian drug procyclidine may sometimes also be abused.

Ketamine (special K)

Ketamine is an anaesthetic agent related to PCP and causing similar reactions. It is taken orally as a tablet, snorted or smoked, or by injection as a liquid. Effects come on and recede faster than those of LSD but include aggression, as with PCP.

• Dental aspects of psychedelic drug abuse

Grossly abnormal behaviour can develop from abuse of any of the psychedelic drugs and a psychiatric opinion should be obtained. Hallucinogen-induced crises often respond to diazepam 10–20 mg orally, but intravenous diazepam or intramuscular chlorpromazine may be needed.

If general anaesthesia is required, intravenous barbiturates should be avoided because they may induce convulsions, respiratory distress or coma. Opioids are also contraindicated.

ORGANIC SOLVENT ABUSE

A range of volatile substances is available over the counter. Adhesives, aerosols, cleaning and degreasing agents and solvents such as petrol, gas lighter fuels and fire extinguishers are abused. Drugs such as amyl and butyl nitrite may also be similarly abused. Solvent sniffing is increasingly common and has led to many deaths of children and young adults. The sniffers are usually male teenagers who are predominantly glue-sniffers. Glue is squeezed into a paper or plastic bag, placed around the mouth and inhaled. Those who sniff petrol or other organic liquids inhale them from a cloth soaked in the liquid or directly from the container. Abusers of aerosol sprays often inhale through a cloth which traps the particulate matter but permits the propellant to pass, but some spray the aerosol directly into the mouth. Used in the latter way these aerosols are highly dangerous and can cause severe respiratory damage or death.

Sniffing solvents produces an effect somewhat between that of alcohol and a psychotomimetic. Toxic effects include hypoxia, cardiac dysrhythmias and sometimes sudden death, liver damage and neurological damage and delusions. Chronic abuse can impair memory and concentration and a small number of cases of permanent damage to brain, liver or kidneys have been reported. If liver function is impaired, it can interfere with drug metabolism. Signs of solvent abuse include slurred speech, euphoria, anorexia and a circumoral (glue sniffers') rash. Jaundice may be seen and the pulse may be irregular.

Specific chemicals may also have additional side-effects. Chronic abuse of petrol, for example, can cause respiratory damage, anaemia, lead poisoning and cranial nerve palsies. A syndrome of mental handicap, hypotonia, scaphocephaly and high malar bones has also been reported in children of mothers who inhaled petrol during pregnancy (fetal gasoline syndrome).

ANAESTHETIC ABUSE

Nitrous oxide has all the properties of a drug of dependence, in that it induces impaired consciousness with a sense of dissociation and often of exhilaration (laughing gas). The reason that it has not become a widely abused drug is simply the practical problem of carrying the heavy cylinders around. However, addiction to nitrous oxide is an occupational hazard of anaesthetists and dental surgeons. Chronic abuse of nitrous oxide can lead to interference with vitamin B_{12} metabolism and neuropathy. Sixteen of a series of 18 patients with this type of polyneuropathy were dentists, most of whom had abused nitrous oxide for periods exceeding 3 months. Vague neurological symptoms have also been reported by dentists and dental staff working in environments contaminated by nitrous oxide. Occasionally patients have died as a result of drowsiness of an anaesthetist abusing nitrous oxide.

Cases of nitrous oxide abuse have been reported in the USA among dental and medical students who obtained supplies by stealing large hospital cylinders.

Abuse of halothane is a hazard, particularly in the USA. A particularly remarkable case is that of a nurse who developed skeletal fluorosis, hypertension and renal damage as a consequence of secretly sniffing another fluorinated hydrocarbon anaesthetic, methoxyflurane.

Ether and chloroform are rarely abused, as they were in the past, as other agents are more readily available. Ketamine abuse is discussed above.

ANABOLIC STEROIDS

Anabolic steroids are synthetic derivatives of testosterone (*Table 24.4*) used to promote tissue repair and growth and are used or abused by some athletes to increase muscle mass and performance. About 10 per cent of secondary school children in USA use anabolic steroids.

Adverse effects may be seen on the liver, gonads, cardiovascular system, blood coagulation, skeleton and behaviour. Those relevant to dentistry include impaired ability to metabolize drugs, hypertension, dysrhythmias, hypercoagulability and disturbed behaviour with aggression, irritability, paranoia, headache and psychoses. In relation to the use of general anaesthesia, gastrointestinal inflammation may predispose to

Table 24.4 Some anabolic steroids

- Ethylestronol
- Fluoxymesthone
- Methyltestosterone
- Nandrolone
- Oxandrolone
- Oxymetholone
- Stanozolol
- Testosterone

vomiting, and there may be scoline sensitivity. Low plasma cortisol levels might be an indication for a corticosteroid cover before operation.

Gamma hydroxybutyrate is used by some body-builders.

The International Olympic Committee (IOC) prohibits the use of various drugs by athletes. Antimicrobials are allowed, and analgesics such as aspirin and paracetamol are permitted alone, but codeine and dextropropoxyphene are banned. Anxiolytics may sometimes be banned, and ephedrine and systemic corticosteroids are best avoided. Topical corticosteroids are permitted.

BIBLIOGRAPHY

Anderson H.R., MacNair R.S. and Ramsey J.D. (1985) Deaths from abuse of volatile substances; a national epidemiological survey. *Br. Med. J.* **290**, 304–7.

Barnett R. and Shusterman S. (1985) Fetal alcohol syndrome. *J. Am. Dent. Assoc.* **111**, 591–3.

Barrett G. (1989) *Treating Drug Abusers.* London, Routledge.

Caracci G. and Miller N.S. (1991) Epidemiology and diagnosis of alcoholism in the elderly. *Int. J. Geriat. Psychiatry* **6**, 511–15.

Cawson R.A., Spector R.G. and Skelly A.M. (1995) *Basic Pharmacology and Clinical Drug Use in Dentistry*, 6th edn. Edinburgh, Churchill Livingstone.

Clarren S.K. (1981) Recognition of fetal alcohol syndrome. *J. Am. Med. Assoc.* **245**, 2436–9.

Committee on the Review of Medicines (1980) Systematic review of the benzodiazepines. *Br. Med. J.* **1**, 910–2.

Ernsert V.L., Grady D.G., Green J.C. *et al.* (1990) Smokeless tobacco use and health effects among baseball players. *J. Am. Med. Assoc.* **264**, 218–24.

Fortenberry I. D. (1985) Gasoline sniffing. *Am. J. Med.* **79**, 740–2.

Friedlander A.H. and Gorelick D.A. (1988) Dental management of the cocaine addict. *Oral Surg. Oral Med. Oral Pathol.* **65**, 45–8.

Friedlander A.H., Mills M.J. and Gorelick D.A. (1987) Alcoholism and dental management. *Oral Surg. Oral Med. Oral Pathol.* **63**, 42–6.

Gawin F.H. and Ellinwood E.H. (1988) Cocaine and other stimulants. *N. Engl. J. Med.* **318**, 1173–82.

Harris E.F., Friend G.W. and Tolley E.A. (1992) Enhanced prevalence of ankyloglossia with maternal cocaine use. *Cleft Palate Craniofac. J.* **29**, 72–6.

Haverkos H.W. and Lange W.R. (1990) Serious infections other than human immunodeficiency virus among intravenous drug abusers. *J. Infect. Dis.* **161**, 894–902.

Hollander J., Todd K., Green G. *et al.* (1995) Chest pain associated with cocaine: an assessment of prevalence in suburban and urban emergency departments. *Ann. Emerg. Med.* **26**, 671–6.

Holt S., Stewart I.C., Dixon I.M.I. *et al.* (1980) Alcohol and the emergency service patient. *Br. Med. J.* **281**, 638–9.

Iosub S., Fuchs M., Bingo N. *et al.* (1981) Fetal alcohol syndrome revisited. *Pediatrics* **68**, 475–9.

Isaacs S.O., Martin P. and Washington I.A. (1986) Phencyclidine (PCP) abuse; a close-up look at a growing problem. *Oral Surg. Oral Med. Oral Pathol.* **61**, 126–9.

Krutchkoff D.J., Eisenberg E., O'Brient J.E. *et al.* (1990) Cocaine-induced dental erosions. *N. Engl. J. Med.* **320**, 408.

Leonard R.H. (1991) Alcohol, alcoholism and dental treatment. *Compend. Contin. Educ. Dent.* **12**, 274–83.

Medical Research Council (1994) *The Basis of Drug Dependence.* London, Medical Research Council.

Ong T.K., Rustage K.J., Harrison K.M. *et al.* (1988) Solvent abuse: an anaesthetic management problem. *Br. Dent. J.* **164**, 150–1.

Parry J., Porter S.R., Scully C., Flint S.F. and Parry M.G. (1996) Mucosal lesions due to oral cocaine use. *Br. Dent. J.* **180**, 462–4.

Pickworth W.B. (1995) Caffeine dependence. *Lancet* **345**, 1066.

Porter S.R. and Scully C. (1996) *Innovations and Developments in Non-Invasive Oral Health Care.* Northwood, Science Reviews.

Quartey J.B. (1992) Dentistry and the chemically dependent patient. *Dentistry* **92**, 14–16

Ratcliff J.S. and Collins G.B. (1987) Dental management of the recovered chronically dependent patient. *J. Am. Dent. Assoc.* **114**, 601–3.

Rosenbaum C.E. (1980) Dental precautions in treating drug addicts: a hidden problem among teens and preteens. *Pediatr. Dent.* **2**, 94–6.

Schukit M.A. (1989) *Drug and Alcohol Abuse: A Clinical Guide to Diagnosis and Treatment.* New York, Plenum Press.

Scully C. (1988) *The Dental Patient.* Oxford, Heinemann.

Scully C. (1989) *The Mouth and Perioral Tissues.* Oxford, Heinemann.

Scully C. (1989) *Patient Care: a Dental Surgeon's Guide.* London, British Dental Association.

Scully C., Cawson R.A. and Griffiths M.J. (1990) *Occupational Hazards to Dental Staff.* British Dental Journal, London.

Smith B.K., Haug R.H., Shepard L. and Indresano A.T. (1991) Management of the oral and maxillofacial surgery patient on anabolic steroids. *J. Oral Maxillofac. Surg.* **49**, 627–32.

Committee to the Surgeon General (1986) *The Health Consequences of Using Smokeless Tobacco.* Bethesda, Md, NIH, N086-2874.

Waldman H.B. (1989) Fetal alcohol syndrome and the realities of our time. *J. Dent. Child.* Nov., pp. 435–7.

Wesson D.R. and Ling W. (1996) Addiction medicine. *J. Am. Med. Assoc.* **275**, 1792–3.

Woods J.H., Katz J.L. and Winger G. (1988) Use and abuse of benzodiazepines. *J. Am. Med. Assoc.* **260**, 3476–80.

APPENDIX TO CHAPTER 24

SOME STREET NAMES AND OTHER TERMS FOR DRUGS OF ABUSE

Street names	*Drug*
Acapulco gold	Cannabis
Acid	LSD
Angel dust/mist	Phencyclidine
Animal tranquillizer	Phencyclidine
Base	Cocaine
Beans	Amphetamine
Bennies	Amphetamine
Bhang*	Cannabis
Billy	Amphetamine
Biscuits	Ecstasy
Black tar	Heroin
Blanco	Heroin
Blow	Cannabis

continued

Blue angel/devil/heaven	Amylobarbitone
Bolivian	Cocaine
Booze	Alcohol
C	Cocaine
Cadillac	Cocaine
Candy	Barbiturates
Charas	Cannabis
Charlies	Cocaine
Chip	Heroin
Christmas trees	Barbiturates
Coke	Cocaine
Co-pilot	Methamphetamine
Crack	Cocaine free base
Crystal	Methamphetamine
Crystal joints	Phencyclidine
Cubes	LSD
Dagga*	Cannabis
Dennis the Menace	Ecstasy
Dexies	Dexamphetamine
Disco (disco biscuit)	Ecstasy
Doe	Methamphetamine
Dope	Heroin
Dot	LSD
Downers	Barbiturates
Drinamyl	Amphetamines
E	Ecstasy
Ecstasy	Methylene deoxymethamphetamine
Edwards	Ecstasy
Elephant	Phencyclidine
Freebase	Cocaine
Ganga*	Cannabis
GHB	Gamma hydroxy butyrate
Girl	Cocaine
Gold dust	Cocaine
Goofballs	Barbiturates
Goon	Phencyclidine
Grass	Cannabis
Gunk	Morphine
H	Heroin
Hash (hashish*)	Cannabis
Hocus	Morphine
Hog	Phencyclidine
Horse	Heroin
Horse tranquillizer	Phencyclidine
Ice	Methamphetamine
Jack up	Amylobarbitone
Jellies	Tranquilizers
Junk	Cocaine
K (Special K)	Ketamine
KJ	Phencyclidine
Lady	Cocaine
Lilly	Secobarbitone
Love drug/dove	Methamphetamine or Ecstasy
Ludes	Methaqualone
(Marihuana)* marijuana	Cannabis
Mesc	Mescaline
Microdot	LSD

continued

Mist	Phencyclidine
Monkey	Morphine
Mushroom	Psilocybin
Nebbies	Pentobarbitone
Panama gold	Cannabis
Paris	Methaqualone
PCP	Phencyclidine
Peace pills	Phencyclidine
Peaches	Amphetamine
Pink	Morphine
Poppers	Amylnitrite
Pot	Cannabis
Purple haze	LSD
Purple hearts	Dexamphetamine and amylobarbitone
Quads	Methaqualone
Red devils	Secobarbital
Reefer	Cannabis
Rhubarb and custard	Ecstasy
Rock	Cocaine
Rocket fuel	Phencyclidine
Scuffle	Phencyclidine
Sensi	Cannabis
Shit	Heroin
Silly putty	Psilocybin
Skunk	Cannabis
Smack	Heroin
Snow	Cocaine
Soapers	Methaqualone
Soma	Phencyclidine
Speed	Amphetamine (intravenously)
Speedball	Opioids and amphetamine (or cocaine and heroin)
Spliff	Cannabis
Strawberry	LSD
Sulphate	Amphetamine
T	Phencyclidine
TCP	Thiencylcyclohexyl piperidine
Tea	Cannabis
Tic tac	Phencyclidine
Ts and Blues	Pentazocine and tripelannamine
Vitamins	Ecstasy
Wash	Cocaine
Weed	Cannabis
White lightning	LSD
Yellow jackets	Pentobarbitone

*Correct name in country of origin

25

Reactions to drugs and materials, and drug interactions

Key points

- Drugs may influence dental treatment or cause oral adverse reactions.
- The use of drugs may be the only indication to dental staff of underlying systemic disease in the patient.
- All drugs taken should be checked against a formulary for the type, action, contraindications, potential drug interactions and adverse effects.
- The most serious drug interactions in dentistry are with general anaesthetic agents, drugs with activity on the CNS, and antihypertensive agents.
- There are virtually no serious drug interactions with local anaesthetics used in normal doses.
- Allergic reactions are possible with any drug but are most common with antibiotics (especially penicillin), anaesthetics, analgesics and antiseptics.
- All allergens should be avoided if possible, and an alternative drug used.
- Penicillin allergy is a real problem though many 'allergies' to it are not true allergic responses. A minority of patients may also cross-react with cephalosporins.
- Halothane should not be used repeatedly on any patient.
- Aspirin may be a hazard in children, persons with a bleeding tendency, peptic ulceration, and diabetes, and those with aspirin allergy.
- Iodine sensitivity is a contraindication to the use of iodine-containing preparations such as some radiological contrast media, and povidone-iodine.
- Patients and staff may react to dental materials such as resins, latex and many other materials, including restorative metals and resins.
- Provided local anaesthesia is used, there are few significant contraindications to, or adverse reactions or interactions from, drugs used in routine dentistry.
- Drugs may adversely affect oral health. Common effects are of xerostomia and gingival hyperplasia, but lichenoid reactions, ulcers and other lesions may result.

Drugs used routinely in dentistry rarely cause significant adverse effects unless used recklessly. The chief dangers are those of general anaesthesia, particularly with intravenous agents, and occasionally of allergic reactions, particularly to penicillin (Chapters 1, 16 and 18). Drug use in the medically compromised patient, however, may carry risks, such as the epileptogenic effects of some agents.

Local anaesthetic agents, such as lignocaine (lidocaine) with adrenaline, the most widely used drugs in dentistry, have proved in practice to be remarkably safe. However, *noradrenaline* is dangerous and able to cause potentially lethal hypertension. Furthermore, gross overdose of local anaesthetics can be dangerous. One dentist has been found guilty of manslaughter, having given 16 cartridges of lignocaine with adrenaline local anaesthetic solution to an elderly patient who subsequently died.

Many drugs can cause oral side-effects or can affect salivary gland function. Dental amalgams and other dental materials have few proven toxic effects if used appropriately. Possible toxic effects of mercury on the nervous system have been discussed in Chapter 12 and possible local effects of dental materials have been discussed in Chapter 17.

The main problems caused by drugs in dentistry may therefore be summarized as follows:

1. Substance (chemical) dependence and abuse.
2. Drug reactions and interactions.
3. Adverse effects of drugs used in dentistry.
4. Oral side-effects of drugs.

Few of the drugs commonly used in general dental practice cause significant adverse reactions. Even in patients with cardiac disease, the lack of evidence of inter-actions of local anaesthetics with tricyclic or other antidepressants, and the rarity of hyper-sensitivity reactions, must be stressed. Furthermore, the introduction of parabens-free local anaesthetics has further reduced side-effects. The use of general anaesthetic or sedative techniques, however, is more likely to produce adverse reactions.

The excessive use of *any* drug, however, can cause harm. Aspirin readily causes platelet dysfunction, and excessive doses have led to post-extraction bleeding. Paracetamol (acetoaminophen) is also a safe analgesic but, given in repeated doses for dental pain, it has produced severe liver damage. The use of excessive amounts of local anaesthetic agents can be dangerous (Chapter 2).

Drug interactions are also more common in the elderly or in medically handicapped patients (Appendix to this chapter).

Drug absorption and metabolism can be affected by food and some drugs: grapefruit juice for example can produce toxicity from cyclosporin and terfenadine.

HYPERSENSITIVITY TO DRUGS USED IN DENTISTRY

Those with atopic disease or from an affected family, or those with HIV disease or Sjögren's syndrome may be more likely to develop hypersensitivity to drugs. The drugs causing the most severe and potentially lethal reactions are the penicillins and intravenous anaesthetic agents, but frequently patients without any atopic tendency are affected.

Hypersensitivity to penicillins

Hypersensitivity reactions to beta-lactams (penicillins and cephalosporins) are the most frequent type of immunological reactions to drugs. Allergic reactions are more likely to follow parenteral rather than oral penicillin. The common reactions are urticarial and irritating rashes (*Plate 25*), but sometimes a serum sickness type of reaction with joint pains and fever can follow some days or weeks after administration.

The most dangerous type of reaction is acute anaphylaxis, which has been estimated to have caused approximately 300 deaths a year in the USA.

Mechanism of penicillin allergy: The major antigenic determinant appears to be the penicilloyl group which forms as a result of metabolic cleavage of the beta-lactam ring. This product acts as a hapten and binds to body proteins to become antigenic.

Most persons receiving penicillin develop IgG or IgM antibodies but these only occasionally cause reactions. Specific IgE antibodies to penicillin form rarely, but are the cause of anaphylactic reactions by binding to mast cells and triggering release of media-tors. Contrary to traditional belief and surprisingly, there appears to be no associa-tion between penicillin anaphylaxis and atopic disease even though the latter is mediated by the same mechanisms.

On the very rare occasions when no other antibiotic than a penicillin is indicated for a life-threatening infection, it may be possible to predict the possibility of an IgE mediated response and an anaphylactic reaction, by skin testing with benzylpenicilloyl polylysine, which gives a wheal and flare reaction within 10 minutes. Fewer than 10 per cent of those who claim to be allergic to penicillin react positively in this way. Anaphylaxis is virtually unknown in those who give negative reactions to this test.

A history of previous reactions to penicillin suggests a greater risk of acute anaphylaxis but there is no completely reliable method of prediction. Patients allergic to penicillin can usually react to any other penicillin except aztreonam, and sometimes also react to cephalosporins. However, some allergic reactions can be selective for certain semi-synthetic penicillins, and some patients tolerant of benzylpenicillin can show delayed reactions to aminopenicillins.

Unfortunately anaphylaxis can occasionally also be the first manifestation of sensitivity to penicillins and, rarely, a patient who has had penicillins on several occasions without ill-effect can suddenly develop acute anaphylaxis. A negative history therefore reduces the chances but does not totally exclude the possibility of anaphylaxis. From the practical and medicolegal viewpoints therefore, reliance has to be placed on the history and an alternative antimicrobial – but *not* one of the many penicillin derivatives except aztreonam – given, when the patient claims to be allergic to penicillin. A patient should of course be lying down when injections are given as fainting after injections is common and may be confused with anaphylaxis.

• Management of anaphylaxis

An anaphylactic reaction can be recognized by the onset of symptoms within a few minutes of injection. Reactions after oral administration are delayed by the time taken for the drug to be absorbed.

The first symptoms are likely to be anxiety, usually followed by such changes as paraesthesiae around the mouth or of the extremities, and wheezing. Loss of consciousness and pallor caused by a precipitous and dangerous fall in blood pressure follow almost immediately. The blood pressure may fall so low as to be difficult to measure and the pulse may be impalpable. Ashen cyanosis quickly follows in severe cases. Oedema of the face or larynx may be associated. Death can follow within 5 minutes, and immediate treatment is essential.

The patient should be laid flat with legs raised, and given oxygen. Adrenaline 1 mg (10 ml of 1:10 000 or 1 ml of 1:1000), is given intramuscularly and the plunger of the syringe withdrawn before injection to make sure that the needle is not in a vein. Although there is a risk of inducing dysrhythmias, the hazards from adrenaline are less than that of the acute hypotension which can precipitate cardiac arrest.

Intramuscular adrenaline should be followed by an antihistamine such as diphenhydramine or hydroxyzine and at least 200 mg intravenous hydrocortisone succinate.

Cardiopulmonary resuscitation should be started if the heart stops. There is no evidence that antihistamines alone (by any route) are effective (*see* Chapter 26).

Medical assistance should be obtained and the patient should be removed to hospital as soon as possible for observation or further treatment if necessary since relapses may follow over up to 24 hours.

Since a negative history of reactions to penicillin does not exclude the possibility of anaphylaxis it is arguable that penicillin should not be given immediately before a general anaesthetic. Admittedly the chances are small but acute anaphylactic reactions during anaesthesia have been reported and, clearly, their recognition under such circumstances could be difficult. If penicillin has to be given, half an hour should be allowed to elapse before induction of anaesthesia. After such a period a severe reaction is unlikely.

Sensitivity to any of the penicillins confers sensitivity to all members of this group of antibiotics. Depot penicillins, which are slowly excreted, can maintain the antigenic challenge so that treatment of a reaction may have to be continued until all the antigen is used up. Procaine penicillin can occasionally cause vertigo, hallucinations and acute anxiety reactions if given intravenously or if it accidentally enters a vein. Such reactions, though rare, may be mistaken for anaphylaxis.

Cephalosporins

Cephalosporins have a somewhat similar chemical structure to penicillins and about 10 per cent of those sensitized to penicillin are also sensitive to the cephalosporins. Equally, a patient sensitive to penicillin is more likely to become sensitized to the cephalosporins than an unsensitized person. Cefaclor may produce a serum sickness-like reaction. A cephalosporin should preferably not be given to a patient allergic to penicillin unless there is a specific bacteriological indication. However, this is rarely a consideration in dentistry.

Reactions to intravenous anaesthetic agents

Intravenous anaesthetic agents can cause anaphylactic-type reactions, either as a result of hypersensitivity and/or by inducing histamine release. These agents are, in order of risk, propanidid, Althesin, methohexitone and thiopentone. These reactions have sometimes been fatal, probably because of failure to recognize their nature, and both propanidid and Althesin have now been withdrawn in the UK as a result.

The level of risk is unclear, but it has been estimated that reactions complicated more than 1 per 1000 administrations of propanidid and its fatalities have put this drug out of use. Althesin may have caused reactions in 1 in 10 000–20 000 administrations. In one report it was estimated that allergic reactions to methohexitone developed in 1 per 7000 administrations but this is probably an overestimate. Similarly, in a survey of 100 anaphylactic reactions to anaesthetic agents the only fatal cases (four in number) were apparently caused by thiopentone. This, however, is probably more likely to be a reflection of the enormous scale of use of thiopentone than an indication of the true prevalence of allergy to this drug.

Allergic reactions to intravenous anaesthetic agents can take several forms. In the most severe type there is bronchospasm, flushing of the skin and a sharp fall in blood pressure. The loss of consciousness that results must be distinguished from the onset of anaesthesia.

Fatal reactions of this type have now been reported for virtually all the intravenous agents in current use (Propofol is the exception) and one of the most important aspects of management is their recognition.

Treatment is then by the same means as for penicillin anaphylaxis.

Halothane hepatitis

This reaction appears to be mediated at least in part by some form of hypersensitivity, as discussed in Chapters 2 and 10.

Allergic reactions to muscle relaxants and related compounds

Certain muscle relaxants appear responsible for about 50 per cent of adverse reactions during general anaesthesia. Suxamethonium is the agent most commonly responsible, but alcuronium, tubocurarine and other relaxants are sometimes implicated. Although some are allergic reactions with serum IgE antibodies detectable, there is also direct release of mediators such as histamine from mast cells, so that some use the term 'anaphylactoid' rather than anaphylaxis. There does not need to be previous exposure to the agent; presumably cross-reacting antigens are implicated. Tachycardia, vascular collapse and skin reactions (flushing, oedema or urticaria) are the most frequent signs.

Allergic reactions to other drugs

Adverse reactions to the administration of local anaesthetic agents are rare (Chapter 2).

Aspirin can rarely also provoke allergic reactions. Aspirin-induced asthma is a recognized but rare side-effect, mainly in patients with nasal polyps ('triad asthma' – asthma, nasal polyps and aspirin sensitivity). Again, in relation to the scale of use of aspirin (an estimated 6 000 000 000 tablets annually), the incidence of such complications is almost negligible. If, however, there is a history of allergy to aspirin, it should not be given.

Other non-steroidal anti-inflammatory analgesics may, even more rarely, induce allergic reactions. Morphine by contrast, directly triggers histamine release from mast cells and very occasionally causes anaphylactoid reactions.

Antiseptics such as iodine may elicit allergic responses. Iodine-containing preparations can be found in some radiological contrast media and antiseptics such as povidone-iodine.

Table 25.1	Dental materials that may cause contact reactions

- Mercury amalgams
- Gold alloys
- Methylmethacrylate monomer
- Epoxy resins
- Composite resins
- Rubber base materials
- Latex
- Periodontal dressings
- Denture fixatives
- Essential oils
- Toothpastes
- Mouthwashes

Table 25.2 Typical components of dental methyl methacrylate

Liquid	Powder
Methyl methacrylate	Polymethyl methacrylate
Organic amines (accelerator)	Pigments
Hydroquinone (inhibitor)	Organic peroxides
Dimethacrylate (cross-linker)	(initiators)
Ultraviolet absorber	Titanium dioxide

REACTIONS TO MATERIALS USED IN DENTISTRY (*Table 25.1*)

Resins

Though it is virtually impossible to prove that any material is totally non-antigenic, there is little evidence that polymethyl methacrylate (PMMA) denture base causes contact sensitization. Occasionally there are isolated reports of persons who appear to have had allergic reactions to polymethyl methacrylate. However it is difficult to assess the significance of such cases in view of the widespread use of PMMA as a wool substitute (Acrylic) for clothing and as a denture base without trouble. Nevertheless, these materials contain a wide range of components which are potentially sensitizing (*Table 25.2*) and there are undoubted cases, particularly in dental staff, of allergic contact reactions to methyl methacrylate, dimethacrylates such as butanediol- or ethylene glycol-dimethacrylates (used in cross-linked resins), accelerators such as dimethyl-toluidine or tolydiethanolamine, inhibitors such as hydroquinone, and epoxy resins.

Affected persons should avoid exposure to these materials. Surgical rubber or vinyl gloves offer little if any protection as they are quickly penetrated by the chemicals. Commercial laminated disposable protective gloves are available (4H glove; Safety 4 A/S Denmark).

Latex

Allergic reactions to latex and rubber products have become increasingly common since the widespread use of protective medical gloves following the advent of AIDS. The most common products containing latex include medical gloves (now increasingly worn), balloons, condoms, carpets, textiles and foam rubber. Latex itself is the fluid obtained from the rubber tree; processing involves the use of several chemicals including thiurams, carbamates and mercaptobenzothiazoles – which may be the main allergens for contact dermatitis to latex. Rubber elongation factors such as prenyltransferase and hevein may be important allergens. Some of the latex proteins may also be associated with the glove lubricating powder, and may become aerosolized, causing respiratory, ocular or nasal symptoms. The sensitizer to latex allergy is often rubber in the soles of shoes. Features of a type 1 or immediate allergic reaction range from pruritus to urticaria and, rarely, anaphylaxis.

Repeated exposure to latex products predisposes to allergies which are commonly seen in patients frequently exposed to medical gloves during care, or chronically exposed because of urethral catheterization. Medical conditions associated with latex allergy include persons with spina bifida, those with urogenital anomalies, imperforate anus, tracheo-oesophageal fistula, VATER association (vertebral defects, imperforate anus, tracheo-oesophageal fistula, radial and renal dysplasia), pre-term infants, ventriculoperitoneal shunts, paraplegia, mental handicap, cerebral palsy, multiple surgery and atopy. Up to 60 per cent of patients with spina bifida may be allergic. Latex allergy is also more common in atopic individuals.

Latex allergy is a growing problem for health care workers. The allergen is often also present in the glove powder, and can thus be discharged into the air. Starch glove powder can also cause direct skin irritation, can interfere with wound healing and impair implant osseo-integration and composite bonding.

Contact dermatitis to latex is a type IV delayed response, appearing after 24–48 hours from exposure, and can be revealed by patch-testing, skin prick tests or RAST assays.

Items used in dentistry that may contain latex include:

- Rubber gloves
- Rubber dam
- Rubber sleeves on props, and bite blocks
- Prophylaxis cups and polishing wheels and points
- Induction masks
- Tourniquets and blood pressure cuffs
- Orthodontic elastics
- Some bandages and tapes
- Headgear and head positioners

Avoidance of exposure is the best course and affected persons should only contact latex-free vinyl, neoprene, tactylon or styrene butadiene medical or dental products.

Other materials

Contact dermatitis, an eczema-like, cell-mediated reaction that differs from atopic eczema in being caused by some readily identifiable substance with which the susceptible individual comes into repeated contact and which produces a reaction restricted to the site of contact, is fairly common in dentistry and elsewhere. A typical example is dermatitis of the hands of housewives using detergents, particularly those containing enzymes. A variety of dental materials, particularly mercury, are also potential causes (*Table 25.1*).

Nevertheless, contact dermatitis affecting either dentist or patient was surprisingly uncommon before the increase in latex reactions. Like eczema, there is little convincing evidence for the existence of an oral equivalent of contact dermatitis. In those sensitized to mercury, amalgam restorations can safely be inserted, provided that no stray amalgam is allowed to reach the patient's skin.

Dental amalgam has been reported to cause mucosal reactions, such as lichenoid lesions.

However, the evidence is conflicting and mercury can be absorbed from amalgams into the mucosa without causing any reaction.

Illustrative of the difference in response between skin and mucosa to sensitizing agents is that occasionally a substance to which the patient is sensitized, when put in the mouth, can induce the typical rash on the skin. This has been reported in the case of nickel sensitivity when a nickel-containing denture caused a rash but not an oral reaction.

As mentioned earlier, methylmethacrylate monomer is sensitizing and irritant, but its low antigenicity is shown by the fact that even those who are habitually handling undiluted monomer rarely develop allergy to it. There is also little evidence that monomer leaks out of dentures but, if it does, it rarely causes local irritation or allergy.

Contact dermatitis can occasionally affect the vermilion border of the lips or, more frequently, the perioral skin. Causes include components of lipsticks (such as fluorescein, oleyl alcohols and cinnamon or other essential oils), toothpastes and some foods, notably mangoes and oranges. Some food additives are thought occasionally to cause granulomatous oral reactions. Components of toothpastes can also cause inflammation of the gingivae or other parts of the oral mucosa but there is no convincing evidence that most such reactions are caused by hypersensitivity rather than chemical irritation.

Perioral dermatitis, cheilitis, gingivitis and other lesions have been described in patients using tartar control toothpastes which contain pyrophosphates or cinnamonaldehyde.

The main consideration in the management of contact dermatitis is strict avoidance of the sensitizing agent or, if it must be handled, gloves should be used.

ADVERSE EFFECTS OF DRUGS USED IN DENTISTRY IN THE MEDICALLY COMPROMISED PATIENT

Possible contraindications to the main drugs prescribable by the dental surgeon are tabulated in Appendix 2 to this chapter. Dental surgeons will encounter some of the conditions rarely, if at all, in general practice but the danger is much increased where general anaesthesia is used or where medically compromised patients are seen. Any suggestion of previous drug reaction or allergy, and particularly any adverse reaction during anaesthesia, should be taken seriously. Patients with allergy to one drug, and probably those patients with Sjögren's syndrome or HIV disease, may be particularly liable to drug allergies (Chapters 9 and 20). Other patients who are at particular risk from drug reactions are those with cardiovascular, hepatic or renal disease and the elderly. Drug doses should be reduced in the elderly, and those with liver or kidney dysfunction. Possible drug interactions are uncommon in general dental practice but are more likely when general anaesthesia is used (Appendix 3 to this chapter).

The pharmacology, advantages and disadvantages of anaesthetic agents and other drugs used in dentistry and the legal aspects of prescribing are discussed more fully in texts of dental pharmacology (*see* Bibliography).

ORAL SIDE-EFFECTS OF DRUGS

Oral side-effects caused by drugs are relatively uncommon but may be important. The most common drug-induced oral disorders are candidosis (usually caused by tetracyclines, ampicillin or corticosteroids), gingival hyperplasia (caused by phenytoin, cyclosporin and calcium-channel blockers), lichenoid reactions (from NSAIDs and many others) and dry mouth caused by many drugs with an atropinic action. Some drugs almost invariably cause oral side-effects, for example oral ulcers with some of the cytotoxic agents, while other drugs have few reported oral complications. Some newer habits, such as the use of oral snuff (smokeless tobacco), can cause gingival recession and leukoplakia and possibly predispose to oral cancer. Oral use of cocaine can cause gingival ulceration or desquamation. Some drugs that may occasionally cause oral complications are tabulated in Appendix 4 to this chapter.

BIBLIOGRAPHY

Anneroth G., Ericson T., Johansson I. *et al.* (1992) Comprehensive medical examination of a group of

patients with alleged adverse effects from dental amalgams. *Acta Odont. Scand.* **50**, 101–11.

Assem E.S.K. and Punnia-Moorty A. (1988) Allergy to local anaesthetics: an approach to a definitive diagnosis. *Br. Dent. J.* **164**, 44–7.

Basker R.M., Hunter A.M. and Highe A.S. (1990) A severe asthmatic reaction to polymethylmethacrylate denture base resin. *Br. Dent. J.* **169**, 250–1.

Beacham B.E., Kurgansky D. and Gould W.M. (1990) Circumoral dermatitis and cheilitis caused by tartar control dentifrices. *J. Acad. Dermatol.* **22**, 1029–32.

Blanca M. (1995) Allergic reactions to penicillins; a changing world? *Allergy* **50**, 777–82.

Bochner B.S. and Lichtenstein L.M. (1991) Anaphylaxis. *N. Engl. J. Med.* **324**, 1785–90.

Cawson R.A., Spector R.G. and Skelly A.M. (1995) *Basic Pharmacology and Clinical Drug Use in Dentistry*. Edinburgh, Churchill-Livingstone.

Curley R.K., Macfarlane A.W. and King C.M. (1986) Contact sensitivity to the amide anesthetics lidocaine, prilocaine and mepivicaine. *Arch. Dermatol.* **122**, 924–6.

Dodson M.E. (1982) Adverse reactions and anaesthesia. *Adverse Drug Reaction Bull.* No. 96.

Donaldson D. and Gibson G. (1980) Systemic complications with intravenous diazepam. *Oral Surg. Oral Med. Oral Pathol.* **49**, 126–30.

Douidar S.M., Al-Khalil I. and Habersang R.W. (1994) Severe hepatotoxicity, acute renal failure, and pancytopenia in a young child after repeated acetoaminophen overdosing. *Clin. Pediatr.* **33**, 42–5.

Engibous P.J., Kittle P.E., Jones H.L. and Vance B.J. (1993) Latex allergy in patients with spina bifida. *Pediatr. Dent.* **15**, 364–6.

Fisher M. (1995) Treatment of acute anaphylaxis. *Br. Med. J.* **311**, 731–3.

Grogono A.W. and Seltzer I.L. (1980) A guide to drug interactions in anaesthetic practice. *Drugs* **19**, 271–9.

Holgate S.T. (1988) Penicillin allergy; how to diagnose and when to treat. *Br. Med. J.* **296**, 1213–14.

Kanerva L., Estlander T., Jolanki R. and Tarvainen K. (1993) Occupational allergic contact dermatitis caused by exposure to acrylates during work with dental prostheses. *Contact Derm.* **28**, 268–75.

Lamey P-J. and Lamb A.B. (1988) Prospective study of aetiological factors in burning mouth syndrome. *Br. Med. J.* **296**, 1243–6.

Lamey P-J., Lewis M.A.O., Rees T.D. *et al.* (1990) Sensitivity reaction to the cinnamonaldehyde component of toothpaste. *Br. Dent. J.* **168**, 115–18.

Leading Article (1985) Drug reactions during anaesthesia. *Lancet* **i**, 1222–3.

Lin R.Y. (1992) A perspective on penicillin allergy. *Arch. Intern. Med.* **152**, 930–7.

Mitchell J.R. (1988) Acetominophen toxicity. *N. Engl. J. Med.* **319**, 1601.

Nelson L.P., Sporowski N.J. and Shusterman S. (1994) Latex allergies in children with spina bifida: relevance for the pediatric dentist. *Pediatr. Dent.* **16**, 18–22.

Porter S.R. and Scully C. (1996) *Innovations and Developments in Non-Invasive Oral Health Care.* Northwood, Science Reviews.

Schatz M. (1992) Adverse reactions to local anesthetics. *Immunol. Allerg. Clin. North Am.* **12**, 585–609.

Scully C. (1988) *The Dental Patient.* Oxford, Heinemann.

Scully C. (1989) *The Mouth and Perioral Tissues.* Oxford, Heinemann.

Scully C. (1989) *Patient Care: a Dental Surgeon's Guide.* London, British Dental Association.

Scully C., Cawson R.A. and Griffiths M.J. (1990) *Occupational Hazards to Dental Staff.* London, British Dental Journal.

Task Force on Allergic Reactions to Latex. (1993) Committee report. *J. Allerg. Clin. Immunol.* **92**, 16–18.

Vale J.A. and Proudfoot A.T. (1995) Paracetamol (acetoaminophen) poisoning. *Lancet* **346**, 547–52.

Vervloet D. (1985) Allergy to muscle relaxants and related compounds. *Clin. Allerg.* **15**, 501–8.

Walker D.M. (1982) Adverse reactions to drugs and materials in dentistry. *Dent. Update* **20**, 537–45.

Walls R.S. (1996) Latex allergy; a real problem. *Med. J. Aust.* **164**, 707–8.

APPENDIX 1 TO CHAPTER 25

ADVERSE REACTIONS: ADVICE TO DENTAL PRACTITIONERS

- Almost any drug may produce unwanted or unexpected adverse reactions; never use any drug unless there are good indications.
- The true incidence of adverse drug reactions is often not known, and many adverse reactions are probably not, at present, recognized as drug-related.
- Always take a full medical history and ask specifically about adverse drug reactions, since the medical status may influence the choice of drugs used.
- Avoid polypharmacy, and use only drugs with which you are familiar.
- Drugs can cause a wide range of adverse reactions affecting the mouth. Patients should be warned if serious adverse reactions are liable to occur (e.g. systemic corticosteroids), and provided with the appropriate warning card to carry.

APPENDIX 2 TO CHAPTER 25

DRUGS TO BE AVOIDED OR USED ONLY IN REDUCED DOSES FOR SPECIFIC CONDITIONS

Condition	Drug that may be contraindicated[a]	Condition	Drug that may be contraindicated[a]
Addison's disease (hypoadrenocorticism)	Any general anaesthetic Methohexitone Thiopentone	Allergies	Aspirin Methohexitone Penicillin
		Anorexia	Paracetamol
Alcoholism	Antidepressants Any general anaesthetic Aspirin Baclofen Carbamazepine Cephamandole Chlorpropamide Metronidazole Paracetamol Salicylate Tinidazole	Asthma	Aspirin NSAIDs Opiates
		Bleeding disorders	Aspirin Corticosteroids
		Burns	Suxamethonium
		Carcinoid syndrome	Opiates
		Cardiovascular diseases	Adrenaline Chloral hydrate Halothane Methohexitone Pentazocine

continued

Condition	Drug that may be contraindicated[a]	Condition	Drug that may be contraindicated[a]
Cardiovascular diseases *continued*	Propanidid Thiopentone Tricyclics	Hypertension *continued*	Adrenaline Corticosteroids Ketamine Pentazocine
Cerebrovascular disease	Diazepam[b]	Hyperthyroidism	Adrenaline Atropinics
Children under 12 years	Aspirin Tetracyclines	Hypothyroidism	Any general anaesthetic Codeine Diazepam Dihydrocodeine Methohexitone Opiates Pethidine Thiopentone
Chronic lymphocytic leukaemia	Amoxycillin Ampicillin		
Constipation	Codeine		
Diabetes mellitus	Aspirin Corticosteroids		
Diarrhoea	Clindamycin Mefenamic acid	Infectious mononucleosis	Amoxycillin Ampicillin
Drug addiction	Pentazocine	Liver disease	Any general anaesthetic Antidepressants Aspirin Carbamazepine Carbenoxolone Chloral hydrate Clindamycin Corticosteroids Co-trimoxazole Dextropropoxyphene Diazepam Erythromycin estolate Etretinate Flumazenil Halothane Ketoconazole Methohexitone Opiates or codeine Paracetamol/ acetoaminophen Pentazocine Phenothiazines Rifampicin Suxamethonium Thiopentone Tricyclics
Dystrophia myotonica (myotonic dystrophy)	Methohexitone Suxamethonium Thiopentone		
Elderly	Atropinics Diazepam Dihydrocodeine Ketamine NSAIDs Tricyclics		
Epilepsy	Enflurane Flumazenil Fluoxetine Ketamine Methohexitone Phenothiazines 4-quinolones Tricyclics		
Glaucoma	Atropinics Carbamazepine Diazepam[b] Steroids Tricyclics		
Glucose-6-phosphate dehydrogenase deficiency	Aspirin Co-trimoxazole Sulphonamides	Malignant hyperpyrexia	Halothane Ketamine Suxamethonium
Gout	Amoxycillin Ampicillin Aspirin	Neuromuscular diseases	Diazepam Methohexitone Suxamethonium Tetracyclines Thiopentone
Head injury	Ketamine Opiates		

continued

Condition	Drug that may be contraindicated[a]	Condition	Drug that may be contraindicated[a]
Parkinsonism	Benzodiazepines	Renal disease *continued*	Aspirin Carbamazepine Cephaloridine Cephalothin Chloral hydrate Clindamycin Co-trimoxazole Diazepam Dihydrocodeine Mefenamic acid Metronidazole Opiates Paracetamol/ acetoaminophen Sulphonamides Suxamethonium Tetracyclines
Peptic ulcer	Aspirin Chloral hydrate Corticosteroids Mefenamic acid		
Phaeochromocytoma	Adrenaline Barbiturates Enflurane		
Porphyria	Carbamazepine Co-trimoxazole Dextropropoxythene Diazepam Erythromycin MAOI Metronidazole Sulphonamides Thiopentone		
		Respiratory disease	Any general anaesthetic Dextropropoxyphene Diazepam Dihydrocodeine Methohexitone Opiates Thiopentone
Pregnancy	Care with all drugs Aspirin Co-trimoxazole Diazepam Epsilon amino caproic acid Etretinate Flumazenil Mefenamic acid[c] Opiates Sulphonamides Tetracyclines		
		Suxamethonium sensitivity	Suxamethonium Local anaesthetics
		Systemic lupus erythematosus	Tetracyclines
		Teenagers	Metoclopramide
Psychiatric disease	Ketamine	Thrombotic disease	Epsilon amino caproic acid Tranexamic acid
Raised intracranial pressure	Ketamine Opiates		
Renal disease	Any general anaesthetic or CNS depressant or NSAID Aciclovir (systemic)	Thyroid disease	Povidone-iodine
		Tuberculosis	Corticosteroids
		Urinary retention (prostatic disease)	Atropinics Opiates

[a]Contraindications are often relative, or of theoretical interest only; other drugs may also be contraindicated.
[b]Midazolam may be safer but should still be used with caution.
[c]And breast feeding.

POSSIBLE CONTRAINDICATIONS TO DRUGS USED IN DENTISTRY

Drug	Possible contraindications	Possible reaction
Aciclovir (systemic)	Renal disease	Urea rises
Adrenaline	Hypertension Hyperthyroidism	Hypertension Dysrhythmias

continued

Drug	Possible contraindications	Possible reaction
Adrenaline *continued*	Ischaemic heart disease Phaeochromocytoma	Dysrhythmias Hypertension
Ampicillin (or amoxycillin)	Allergy to penicillin Chronic lymphocytic leukaemia Gout Infectious mononucleosis	Anaphylaxis Rash Rash Rash
Antidepressants	Alcoholism	Potentiated
Aspirin	Allergy to aspirin including aspirin-induced asthma Alcoholism Bleeding disorders Breast feeding Children under 12 years Diabetes mellitus Glucose-6-phosphate dehydrogenase deficiency Gout Liver disease Peptic ulcer Pregnancy Renal disease	Anaphylaxis Gastric bleeding Gastric bleeding Reye's syndrome Reye's syndrome Interferes with control Haemolysis Gout worse Bleeding tendency Gastric bleeding Haemorrhage Fluid retention and gastric bleeding
Atropinics	Elderly Glaucoma Hyperthyroidism Urinary retention or prostatic hypertrophy	Confusion Glaucoma exacerbated Tachycardias Urine retention
Carbamazepine	Alcoholism Elderly Glaucoma Liver disease Porphyria	Sedation Agitation or confusion Raised intraocular pressure Hepatotoxic Acute porphyria
Carbenoxolone	Liver disease	Toxicity
Cephalosporins	Allergy to cephalosporins Allergy to penicillins Renal disease	Anaphylaxis Allergy Nephrotoxic
Chloral hydrate	Cardiovascular disease Gastritis Liver disease Renal disease	Fluid retention Gastric irritation Coma CNS depression
Clindamycin	Diarrhoea Liver disease Renal disease	Aggravated Increased toxicity Increased toxicity
Codeine	Colonic disease Hypothyroidism Liver disease	Constipation Coma Respiratory depression
Corticosteroids	Diabetes mellitus Glaucoma Hypertension	Diabetes worsened Glaucoma exacerbated Increased hypertension

continued

Drug	Possible contraindications	Possible reaction
Corticosteroids *continued*	Liver disease	Increased side effects
	Peptic ulcer	Perforation
	Tuberculosis	Possible dissemination
Co-trimoxazole	Elderly	Agranulocytosis
	Glucose-6-phosphate-dehydrogenase deficiency	Haemolysis
	Liver disease	Enhanced toxicity
	Porphyria	Acute porphyria
	Pregnancy	Folate deficiency
	Renal disease	Increased toxicity
Dextropropoxyphene	Liver disease	Potentiated paralysis
	Porphyria	
	Pregnancy	Fetal depression
	Respiratory disease	Respiratory depression
Diazepam	Cerebrovascular disease	Cerebral ischaemia
	Chronic obstructive airways disease	Respiratory depression
	Elderly	Cerebral ischaemia
	Glaucoma	Increased intraocular pressure
	Hypothyroidism	Coma
	Neuromuscular disorders	Condition deteriorates
	Porphyria	Acute porphyria
	Pregnancy	Fetal hypoxia/dependence
	Severe kidney disease	Increased diazepam effect
	Severe liver disease	Increased diazepam effect
Dihydrocodeine	Elderly	Increased toxicity
	Hypothyroidism	Coma
	Renal disease	Increased toxicity
	Respiratory disease	Respiratory depression
Enflurane	Epilepsy	Epileptogenic
	Phaeochromocytoma	Hypertension
Epsilon amino caproic acid	Haematuria	Renal tract obstruction
	Pregnancy	Thrombosis
	Thrombotic disease	Thrombosis
Erythromycin estolate	Liver disease	Hepatotoxic
	Porphyria	Paralysis
Etretinate	Liver disease	Hepatotoxic
	Pregnancy	Teratogenic
Flucomazole	Pregnancy	Teratogenic
Flumazenil	Allergy	Allergy
	Epilepsy	Epileptogenic
	Liver disease	Delayed excretion
	Pregnancy	Teratogenic
Fluoxetine	Epilepsy	Epileptogenic
Halothane	Cardiac dysrhythmias	Increased dysrhythmias
	Halothane hepatitis	Hepatitis
	Malignant hyperpyrexia	Pyrexia

continued

Drug	Possible contraindications	Possible reaction
Halothane *continued*	Recent anaesthesia with halothane	Hepatitis
Ketamine	Elderly	Hallucinations
	Epilepsy	Fits
	Hypertension	Hypertension
	Malignant hyperpyrexia	Pyrexia
	Psychiatric disease	Psychotic reactions
	Raised intracranial pressure	Increased intracranial pressure
Ketoconazole	Liver disease	Hepatotoxic
Lincomycin	(as for Clindamycin)	
Local anaesthetics	Suxamethonium sensitivity	Respiratory depression
Mefenamic acid	Asthma	Bronchospasm
	Diarrhoea	Diarrhoea worse
	Peptic ulcer	Bleeding
	Pregnancy and lactation	?Teratogenic
	Renal disease	Renal damage
Methohexitone	Addison's disease	Coma
	Allergies	Anaphylaxis
	Barbiturate sensitivity	Anaphylaxis
	Cardiovascular disease	Cardiovascular depression
	Dystrophia myotonica	Increased weakness
	Epilepsy	Epileptogenic
	Hypothyroidism	Coma
	Liver disease	Increased anaesthesia
	Myasthenia gravis	Increased weakness
	Porphyria	Acute porphyria
	Post-natal drip	Laryngeal spasm
	Respiratory disease	Respiratory depression
Metoclopramide	Teenagers	Dystonic reactions
Metronidazole	Blood dyscrasias	Leucopenia
	CNS disease	Neuropathy
	Liver disease	Toxicity
	Porphyria	Acute porphyria
	Pregnancy	?Teratogenic
	Renal disease	Increased drug effect
Midazolam	(as for Diazepam)	
NSAIDs	Asthma	Bronchospasm
	Elderly	Toxicity
	Peptic ulcer	Gastric bleeding
	Pregnancy	Patent ductus arteriosus
	Renal disease	Nephrotoxic
Opiates	Asthma	Bronchospasm
	Carcinoid tumour	Increased toxicity
	Chronic obstructive airways disease	Respiratory depression
	Head injury	Confuse 'eye signs'
	Hypothyroidism	Coma
	Liver disease	Increased respiratory depression

continued

Drug	Possible contraindications	Possible reaction
Opiates *continued*	Pregnancy	Fetal depression
	Renal disease	Increased respiratory depression
	Urinary retention or prostatic enlargement	Urinary retention
Paracetamol/ acetoaminophen	Alcoholism	Hepatotoxicity
	Anorexia	Hepatotoxicity
	Liver disease	Hepatotoxicity
	Renal disease	Nephrotoxicity
Penicillins	Allergy to penicillin	Anaphylaxis
	Renal disease	Hyperkalaemia with i.m. benzyl penicillin
Pentazocine	Hypertension	Hypertension
	Liver disease	Enhanced activity
	Myocardial infarct (recent)	Cardiac arrest
	Narcotic addict	Withdrawal syndrome
	Pregnancy	Fetal depression
Pethidine	Hypothyroidism	Coma
Povidone-iodine	Lactation	Toxicity
	Pregnancy	Toxicity
	Thyroid disease	Toxicity
Promethazine	Liver disease	Coma
4-quinolones	Epilepsy	Epileptogenic
Rifampicin	Liver disease	Hepatotoxic
Sulphonamides	Glucose-6-phosphate dehydrogenase deficiency	Haemolysis
	Liver disease	Toxicity
	Porphyria	Acute porphyria
	Pregnancy	Fetal haemolysis
	Renal disease	Crystalluria
Suxamethonium	Burns	Dysrhythmias
	Dystrophia myotonica	Increased muscle weakness
	Liver disease	Apnoea
	Malignant hyperpyrexia	Pyrexia
	Myasthenia gravis	Increased muscle weakness
	Renal disease	Apnoea
	Suxamethonium sensitivity	Apnoea
Tetracyclines	After gastrointestinal surgery	Enterocolitis
	Children under 7	Tooth staining
	Myasthenia gravis	Increased muscle weakness
	Pregnancy	Tooth staining (fetus)
	Renal disease	Nephrotoxicity
	Systemic lupus erythematosus	Photosensitivity
Thiopentone	Addison's disease	Coma
	Barbiturate sensitivity	Anaphylaxis
	Cardiovascular disease	Cardiovascular depression

continued

Drug	Possible contraindications	Possible reaction
Thiopentane continued	Dystrophia myotonica	Increased weakness
	Hypothyroidism	Coma
	Liver disease	Increased anaesthesia
	Myasthenia gravis	Increased weakness
	Porphyria	**Acute porphyria**
	Post-natal drip	**Laryngeal spasm**
	Respiratory disease	**Respiratory depression**
Tranexamic acid	Haematuria	Renal tract obstruction
	Pregnancy	Thromboses
Triclofos	Thromboembolic disease	Thromboses
Tricyclics	(*see* Chloral hydrate)	Postural hypertension
	Cardiovascular disease	Dysrhythmias
	Elderly	Hypotension
	Epilepsy	Increased fits
	Glaucoma	Glaucoma exacerbated
	Liver disease	Increased drug effect

Note: Many of these reactions are likely to be of more theoretical interest than clinical significance, so that reference should also be made to the appropriate chapters for particular diseases.

APPENDIX 3 TO CHAPTER 25

POSSIBLE DRUG INTERACTIONS IN DENTISTRY

Drug used in dentistry	Interaction with	Possible effects
Aciclovir	Zidovudine	Lethargy
Adrenaline	Halothane	Dysrhythmias
	Tricyclics	Pressor response in overdose
Amphotericin	Aminoglycosides	Enhanced nephrotoxicity
	Cyclosporin	Enhanced nephrotoxicity
Anaesthetics (general)	Antihypertensives	Hypotension
	MAOI	Enhanced hypotension; anaesthetics potentiated
Antibiotics	Oral anticoagulants	Enhanced anticoagulant effect
	Oral contraceptive	Reduced contraceptive effect
Aspirin	Alcohol	Increased risk of gastric bleeding
	Corticosteroids	Peptic ulceration
	Lithium	Lithium toxicity
	Methotrexate	Enhanced methotrexate activity
	Metoclopramide	Potentiation
	Oral anticoagulants	Enhanced anticoagulant effect

continued

Drug used in dentistry	Interaction with	Possible effects
Aspirin continued	Oral hypoglycaemics	Enhanced hypoglycaemic effect
	Phenylbutazone	Increased liability of peptic ulceration
	Probenecid	Uricosuric action reduced
	Sodium valproate	Bleeding tendency
	Sulphinpyrazone	Uricosuric action reduced
Atropine	Metoclopramide	Antagonism
Azathioprine	Allopurinol	Toxicity
	Rifampicin	?Transplant rejection
Baclofen	ACE inhibitors	Enhanced hypotension
	Alcohol	Sedation
Barbiturates	Alcohol	May be increased sedation or resistance
	Antihistamines	Enhanced sedation
	Antihypertensives	Hypotension
	Corticosteroids	May precipitate hypotensive crises
	Cyclosporin	Reduced effect of cyclosporin
	MAOI	Enhanced sedation
	Oral anticoagulants	Reduced anticoagulant activity
	Phenothiazines	Tremor
	Phenytoin	Reduced phenytoin effect
	Tricyclics	Cardiac arrest
Carbamazepine	Cyclosporin	Reduced effect of cyclosporin
	Dextropropoxyphene	Carbamazepine enhanced
	Doxycycline	Reduced doxycycline effect
	Erythromycin	Carbamazepine toxicity
	Fluoxetine	Confusion
	Lithium	Lithium toxicity
	MAOI	Possible hypertension
	Oral anticoagulants	Reduced anticoagulant effect
	Oral contraceptive	Reduced contraceptive effect
	Paracetamol	Liver damage
	Phenytoin	Reduced phenytoin effect
	Sodium valproate	Reduced effect of valproate
Cephalosporins	Diuretics	Increased nephrotoxicity
	Oral anticoagulants	Increased bleeding tendency
Codeine	MAOI	Coma
Colchicine	Cyclosporin	Nephrotoxicity and myotoxicity
Corticosteroids	ACE inhibitors	Reduced hypotensive effect
	Aminoglycosides	Reduced steroid effects
	Aspirin or other analgesics	Increased liability of peptic ulceration
	Cyclosporin or other immunosuppressives	Increased immuno-suppression
	Oral anticoagulants	Gastric bleeding
	Oral antidiabetics	Reduced effect
Co-trimoxazole	Methotrexate	Possible fetal deficiency
	Oral anticoagulants	Increased bleeding

continued

Drug used in dentistry	Interaction with	Possible effects
Co-trimoxazole continued	Oral contraceptive	Reduced contraceptive effect
	Oral hypoglycaemic	Enhanced hypoglycaemia
	Phenytoin	Phenytoin toxicity
Cyclosporin	ACE inhibitors	Hyperkalaemia
	Allopurinol	Nephrotoxicity
	Colchicine	Nephrotoxicity and myotoxicity
	Erythromycin	Cyclosporin toxicity
Danazol	Oral anticoagulants	Potentiated anticoagulation
Dextropropoxyphene	Alcohol	Central nervous system depression
	Carbamazepine	Carbamazepine enhanced
	Oral anticoagulants	Enhanced anticoagulant effect
	Orphenadrine	Tremor, anxiety and confusion
Diazepam and other sedatives	Antihistamines	Enhanced sedation
	Cimetidine	Enhanced sedation
	Halothane	Halothane enhanced
	L-dopa	Antagonism
	Lithium	Hypothermia
	Pentazocine and opiates	Respiratory depression
	Phenytoin	Phenytoin toxicity
	Suxamethonium	Activity of suxamethonium reduced
	Tricyclics	Enhanced sedation
Ephedrine	MAOI	Hypertension
	Tricyclics	Hypertension
Erythromycin	Carbamazepine	Carbamazepine toxicity
	Cyclosporin	Increased cyclosporin absorption
	Oral anticoagulants	Increased bleeding
	Terfenadine	Dysrhythmias
	Theophyllines	Toxicity
Fluconazole	Astemizole	Dysrhythmias
	Cisapride	Dysrhythmias
	Terfenadine	Dysrhythmias
	Oral anticoagulants	Enhanced anticoagulant effect
	Oral antidiabetics	Enhanced antidiabetic effect
	Oral contraceptive	May impair contraception
	Rifampicin	Fluconazole effect reduced
	Zidovudine	Myelotoxicity
Flumazenil	Tricyclics	Sedation
Fluoxetine	Alcohol	Enhanced alcohol effect
	Antiepileptics	Antagonized
	Carbamazepine	Confusion
	MAOI	CNS effects
	Warfarin	Enhanced anticoagulant effect
Gentamicin	Frusemide	Toxicity and nephrotoxicity
Halothane	Aminophylline	Dysrhythmias
	Anticonvulsants	Phenytoin toxicity

continued

Drug used in dentistry	Interaction with	Possible effects
Halothane *continued*	Antihypertensives	Hypotension
	Diazepam	Enhanced activity of halothane
	Fenfluramine	Dysrhythmias
	Isoprenaline	Dysrhythmias
	L-dopa	Dysrhythmias
	Lithium	Dysrhythmias
	Opiates	Respiratory depression
	Phenothiazines	Respiratory depression; hypotension
Itraconazole	(as for Fluconazole)	
Ketamine	CNS depressants	Increased sedation
Ketoconazole (*see also* Fluconazole)	Cyclosporin	Nephrotoxicity
	Simvastatin	Risk of myopathy
Monoamine oxidase inhibitors (MAOI)	Antihypertensives	Reduced or increased hypotensive effect
	Codeine	Hypertension
	General anaesthesia	Hypertension
	L-dopa	Hypertensive crisis
	Methohexitone	Hypotension
	Opiates	Respiratory depression
	Oral anticoagulants	Enhanced anticoagulant effect
	Oral hypoglycaemics	Enhanced hypoglycaemia
	Pethidine	Hypertensive crisis
	Propranolol	Hypertensive crisis
	Tricyclics	Excitation and other interactions
	Tyramine-containing foods	Hypertensive crisis
Mefenamic acid	Oral anticoagulants	Enhanced anticoagulant effect
	Oral hypoglycaemics	Enhanced hypoglycaemia
Methohexitone	Alcohol	Increased sedation
	Antihypertensives	Hypotension
	MAOI	Coma
	Opiates including pentazocine	Respiratory depression
	Phenothiazines	Respiratory depression or hypotension; tremor
Metronidazole	Alcohol	Headache and hypotension
	Oral anticoagulants	Increased bleeding tendency
Miconazole	(as for Fluconazole)	
Midazolam	(Erythromycin and as for Diazepam)	
Noradrenaline	Tricyclics	Hypertension
NSAIDs	Antihypertensives	Hypotension, hyperkalaemia

continued

Drug used in dentistry	Interaction with	Possible effects
NSAIDs continued	Cyclosporin	Nephrotoxicity
	Lithium	Lithium toxicity
	Oral anticoagulants	Increased bleeding tendency
	Oral antidiabetics	Enhanced antidiabetic activity
Opiates	Halothane	Respiratory depression
	MAOI	Respiratory depression or coma
	Methohexitone	Respiratory depression
Paracetamol/ acetoaminophen	Alcohol	Hepatotoxicity
	Anticonvulsants	Hepatotoxicity
	Carbamazepine	Hepatotoxicity
	Cholestyramine	Reduced absorption of paracetamol
	Isonicotinic acid hydrazide (INAH)	Enhanced hepatotoxicity
	Metoclopramide	Potentiation
	Oral anticoagulants	Increased bleeding tendency
	Zidovudine	Increased myelosuppression
Pentazocine	Diazepam	Respiratory depression
Pethidine	MAOI	Hypertensive crisis
	Phenothiazines	Respiratory depression
Phenothiazines	Alcohol	May be increased sedation
	Antihistamines	Enhanced sedation
	Antihypertensives	Hypotension
	Barbiturates	Tremor
	Oral anticoagulants	Enhanced anticoagulant effect
	Pethidine	Respiratory depression
	Tricyclics	Convulsions
Phenylbutazone	Aspirin	Increased liability of peptic ulceration
Phenytoin	Carbamazepine	Reduced carbamazepine effect
	Disulphiram	Disulphiram potentiated
	INAH	INAH potentiated
	Phenylbutazone	Phenylbutazone potentiated
Promethazine	Methohexitone	Increased side-effects of methohexitone
Rifampicin	Antacids	Reduced rifampicin absorption
	Antifungals	Increased metabolism of antifungals
	Cyclosporin	Reduced effect of cyclosporin

continued

Drug used in dentistry	Interaction with	Possible effects
Rifampicin *continued*	Oral anticoagulant	Reduced bleeding tendency
	Oral contraceptive	Reduced contraceptive effect
Sulphonamides	Methotrexate	Increased methotrexate toxicity
	Oral anticoagulants	Enhanced anticoagulant effect
	Oral hypoglycaemics	Enhanced hypoglycaemia
	Phenytoin	Phenytoin toxicity
Suxamethonium	Cytotoxic drugs	Prolonged muscle paralysis
	Diazepam	Activity of suxamethonium reduced
	Diethylstilboestrol	Prolonged muscle paralysis
	Digitalis	Digitalis toxicity enhanced
	Ecothiopate	Prolonged muscle paralysis
	Lithium	Onset of suxamethonium delayed; action prolonged
	Propanidid	Enhanced muscle paralysis
	Spironolactone	Plasma potassium rises; potential dysrhythmias
Tetracyclines	ACE inhibitors	Reduced absorption of tetracyclines
	Antacids	Lower serum levels of tetracyclines
	Barbiturates	Reduced doxycycline blood levels
	Cimetidine	Reduced serum tetracycline levels
	Iron	Reduced serum tetracycline levels
	Methoxyflurane	Renal damage
	Milk	Reduced tetracycline absorption
	Oral anticoagulants	Bleeding tendency
	Oral contraceptive	Reduced contraceptive effect
Thiopentone	Alcohol	Increased sedation
	Antihypertensives	Hypotension
	MAOI	Coma
	Opiates	Respiratory depression
	Phenothiazines	Respiratory depression
	Sulphonamides	Barbiturate potentiated
Tricyclics	Adrenaline	Hypertensive response in overdose

continued

Drug used in dentistry	Interaction with	Possible effects
Tricyclics continued	Alcohol	Enhanced central nervous system
	Anaesthetics	Cardiac arrest
	Antihypertensives	Impaired blood pressure control
	Atropinics	Enhanced atropinic effect
	Carbamazepine	Confusion
	Cimetidine	Tricyclic enhanced
	Contraceptive pill	Tricyclic effect reduced
	Diazepam	Enhanced sedation
	MAOI	Excitation and other interactions
	Oral anticoagulants	Enhanced anticoagulant effect
	Phenothiazines	Convulsions

Note: Many of these drug interactions are of little more than theoretical importance in dentistry, or are the result of overdose of one or both agents. However, there can be a wide range of individual variations in response to drugs, especially sedating agents.

APPENDIX 4 TO CHAPTER 25

ORAL SIDE-EFFECTS OF DRUG TREATMENT (MOST ARE RARE, BUT MORE COMMON CAUSES ARE PRINTED IN ITALIC)

Angio-oedema
ACE inhibitors
Aspirin
Cervical lymph node enlargement
Phenytoin
Phenylbutazone
Primidone
Disturbed taste
Anti-thyroids
Aurothiomalate
Aztreonam
Baclofen
Biguanides
Calcitonin
Captopril
Cilazapril
Erythema multiforme
(and Stevens–Johnson syndrome)
Barbiturates
Busulphan
Carbamazepine
Clindamycin
Codeine
Frusemide
Penicillin
Phenylbutazone

Phenytoin
Sulphonamides
Tetracyclines
Facial pain
Phenothiazines
Stilbamidine
Vinca alkaloids
Gingival hyperplasia
Cyclosporin
Diltiazem
Felodipine
Lacidipine
Nifedipine
Oral contraceptive
Phenytoin
Amlodipine
Verapamil
Halitosis
Dimethyl sulphoxide (DMSO)
Disulfiram
Isorbide dinitrate
Hypersalivation
Anticholinesterases
Buprenorphine
Clonazepam
Clozapine
Ethionamide

continued

Haloperidol
Iodides
Ketamine
Mercurials
Nicardipine
Niridazole
Remoxipride
Triptorelin
Involuntary facial movements
Butyrophenones
Carbamazepine
L-dopa
Lithium
Methyldopa
Metirosine
Metoclopramide
Phenothiazines
Phenytoin
Trifluoroperazine
Labial crusting
Etretinate
Lichenoid reactions
Amiphenazole
Captopril
Carbimazole
Chloroquine
Chlorpropamide
Clofibrate
Dapsone
Dipyridamole
Ethionamide
Gaunoclor
Gold
Griseofulvin
Labetalol
Lincomycin
Lithium
Mepacrine
Metformin
Methyldopa
Metronidazole
Niridazole
Non-steroidal anti-
inflammatory drugs
(NSAIDs)
Oxprenolol
Para-aminosalicylate
Penicillamine
Phenindione
Phenothiazines
Practolol
Propranolol
Prothionamide
Quinidine
Quinine
Streptomycin
Tetracycline

Thiazides
Tolbutamide
Triprolidine
Lupoid reactions
Ethosuximide
Gold
Griseofulvin
Hydralazine
Isoniazid
Methyldopa
Para-aminosalicylate
Penicillin
Phenytoin
Procainamide
Streptomycin
Sulphonamides
Tetracyclines
Oral candidosis
Broad spectrum
antimicrobials
Corticosteroids
Drugs causing xerostomia
Immunosuppressives
Oral mucosal pigmentation
ACTH
Amodiaquine
Anticonvulsants
Busulphan
Chlorhexidine
Chloroquine
Heavy metals
Mepacrine
Minocycline
Oral contraceptive
Phenothiazines
Smoking
Oral ulceration
Aztreonam
Aurothiomalate
Clarithromycin
Cocaine
Cytotoxics
DDc
Emepromium
Gold
Indomethacin
Isoprenaline
Naproxen
Nicorandil
Pancreatin
Penicillamine
Phenindione
Phenylbutazone
Phenytoin
Potassium chloride
Proguanil
Pemphigoid-like reactions

continued

Clonidine
Frusemide
Penicillamine
Psoralens
Pemphigus-like reactions
Captopril
Penicillamine
Rifampicin
Red saliva
L-dopa
Rifabutin
Rifampin
Salivary gland pain
Bethanidine
Clonidine
Cytotoxics
Guanethidine
Methyldopa
Tetrabenazine
Tricyclics
Salivary gland swelling
Anti-thyroid agents
Chlorhexidine
Cimetidine
Clonidine
Clozapine
Ganglion-blocking agents
Insulin
Interferon
Iodides
Isoprenaline
Methyldopa
Nitrofurantoin
Oxyphenbutazone
Phenothiazines
Phenylbutazone
Ritodrine
Sulphonamides
Scalded mouth sensation
Captopril
Sinusitis
Quinapril
Tooth discoloration
Chlorhexidine
Clarithromycin
Enalapril
Essential oil
Etidronate
Fluorides
Fosinopril
Imipenem
Iron
Lisinopril

Metronidazole
Penicillin
Pentamidine
Perindopril
Propafenone
Quinapril
Ramipril
Terbinafine
Tetracyclines[a]
Trandolopril
Zopiclone
Trigeminal paraesthesia
Acetazolamide
Colistin
Ergotamine
Hydralazine
Isoniazid
Labetalol
Methysergide
Monoamine oxidase inhibitors
Nalidixic acid
Nitrofurantoin
Phenytoin
Propofol
Propranolol
Stilbamidine
Streptomycin
Sulphonylureas
Sulthiame
Tricyclics
Trilostane
Xerostomia
Amphetamines
Antihistamines
Atropinics
Benzhexol
Benztropine
Biperiden
Clonidine
Cyclobenzaprine
DDI
L-dopa
Fenfluramine
Fluoxetine
Ganglion-blocking agents
Ipratropium
Isotretinoin
Lithium
Monoamine oxidase inhibitors
Opiates
Orphenadrine
Phenothiazines
Propantheline
Selegiline

[a]Minocycline can cause tooth staining in adults; any tetracycline can discolour developing teeth.

26

Socioeconomic, ethnic and geographical health issues

Key points

- Poverty, malnutrition, and poor water, food and personal hygiene underlie many diseases.
- Infections and infestations are prevalent in areas of poverty.
- Many infections and infestations are found predominantly in the developing world, especially in the tropics.
- Some infections are transmitted from animals, their excreta, or parasites.
- Exotic diseases are now being seen in the developing world in those who have travelled to, or lived in, the developing world, and in immunocompromised persons.
- Some diseases, such as haemoglobinopathies, are seen mainly in specific ethnic groups.
- Some diseases are common, others rare in certain groups because of lifestyle.

Many diseases and other problems such as malnutrition are more prevalent in poverty stricken areas, particularly in the developing world, in war zones and in some tropical regions. Prevalent amongst these problems are accidents and violence, and many caused by micro-organisms and parasites. Several of these problems have been discussed elsewhere in this text. Hepatitis viruses (Chapter 10), HIV (Chapter 20) and tuberculosis (Chapter 8) are examples of major infections worldwide, especially in the developing world. These and other infections and infestations are increasingly being encountered in the developed world, or during work or travel in the developing world. The infections and infestations are too many to mention.

A number of diseases can also be contracted from animals. Wild animals can, for example, cause Lyme disease, an infection with *Borrelia burgdorferi*, transmitted via ticks

from deer. Pet animals may bite or scratch, and cause infections such as cat scratch disease p. 218, toxoplasmosis p. 539 and many others.

Though imported diseases are still rare in the developed world, it must be appreciated that millions of people are now travelling by air and many travel in areas hitherto largely regarded as remote. Many others emigrate to other countries, either legally or otherwise. As a consequence, these exotic diseases, problems related to cultural habits (such as betel nut or paan use) and problems related to weather (such as actinic cheilitis) are appearing increasingly in the developed world.

This chapter discusses mainly the relevant imported diseases, problems related to social deprivation and those which religious or ethnic groups may present during oral health care. There are many others which space precludes.

INFECTIONS

This section highlights infections that are especially prevalent in the developing world. They are prevalent mainly in the tropics, but appear elsewhere, particularly in war zones or where there are other disasters that lead to falling water and food hygiene, and the proliferation of rodents and other pests. Protection is mainly by improved food, water and personal hygiene and nutrition, and often immunization, as well as avoidance of contact with the organism, such as by the use of barrier precautions (Chapter 11) where possible.

BACTERIAL INFECTIONS

Diphtheria (Chapter 11)

Tetanus (Chapter 11)

Tuberculosis (Chapter 11)

Meningitis (Chapter 11)

Typhoid

Typhoid fever is caused by *Salmonella typhi*, caught from contaminated water or food. Fever, rash, splenomegaly and leukopenia result, and it may lead to intestinal bleeding or perforation.

S. typhi may survive freezing and may thus persist in frozen but contaminated food. *S. typhi* is excreted in the faeces of convalescent persons and carriers.

Vaccination against typhoid is indicated when travelling to the developing world, especially where sanitation is poor. Chloramphenicol is the usual treatment but *S. typhi* may be resistant in India, the Middle East and South East Asia, when ciprofloxacin is indicated.

Paratyphoid

Paratyphoid is a disease similar to typhoid, but usually less severe. It is caused by *Salmonella cholerae-suis* or *enteritidis*.

Cholera

Cholera is caused by *Vibrio cholerae*, caught mainly from contaminated water, occasionally from food. Cholera is endemic in Bangladesh and may occur in epidemics throughout the tropics, currently in South America, the Middle East, Africa and Asia. Cholera causes massive diarrhoea with depletion of water and electrolytes, and can be fatal. Some persons are chronic carriers of the bacterium.

Cholera is uncommon in travellers to areas of risk, provided clean water only is ingested. The vaccine gives little protection; water, food and personal hygiene are crucial.

Non-venereal treponematoses (endemic treponematoses)

Bejel (endemic syphilis)
Bejel, a non-venereally acquired chronic childhood infection caused by *T. pallidum*, is prevalent among nomads in the Arabian peninsula and sub-Saharan Africa.

Poverty, overcrowding and unhygienic practices facilitate the transmission of infection. Unlike syphilis, bejel does not usually have an obvious primary stage. Secondary and tertiary stages are encountered, mainly manifesting on skin and mucosa. Mucous patches, angular stomatitis, rashes, pigmentary changes and tenderness of long bones may be seen.

About one-third of patients develop lesions of the late or tertiary stage of the disease which are mainly gummatous. Skin lesions are usually extensive, chronic, destructive, healing with scarring and depigmentation. Gummatous destruction of the nasal septum, lips, soft palate and nasopharynx may lead to facial deformity (rhinopharyngitis mutilans).

Diagnosis and management: Dark ground microscopy and serology are needed to confirm the diagnosis. Penicillin is the drug of choice; tetracycline and erythromycin are alternatives.

Pinta
Pinta, caused by *T. carateum*, is almost exclusively confined to Central and South America. The mode of transmission is either by direct or indirect contact.

The incubation period is usually 2–3 weeks. The primary lesion is a slowly developing subcutaneous granulomatous lesion on the trunk, leg or face usually in young adults of 15–30 years of age.

Secondary lesions (pintides) are papules which develop into plaques with scaly and centrally pigmented areas tending eventually to become depigmented and atrophic. Hyperkeratosis of the palms and soles may be seen and facial skin is extensively affected but there are no oral lesions.

Diagnosis and management: Clinical examination together with dark ground microscopy and serology are needed for the diagnosis. Penicillin is the drug of choice.

Yaws (framboesia; pian; bouba)

Yaws is a contagious disease caused by *T. pertenue*, seen throughout Equatorial Africa, Asia, Central and South America, the South Pacific Islands and Australia.

Yaws is transmitted either by contact with the early infectious lesions or via contaminated utensils or possibly insects. The incubation period is between 9 and 90 days. The primary stage may be of very short duration. A papule appears and may ulcerate. One to three months later painless papillomas or framboesial granulomas appear in the axilla, groin or around the body orifices. Skin lesions may spontaneously heal in about 3–6 months. Bone and cartilage lesions are frequently found, including osteitis, periostitis and dactylitis. In infected growing children 'sabre tibia' may develop.

Most patients then have a stage of latency which may last a lifetime, but in some, about 5 years after the primary infection, gummatous nodular ulcerative lesions may develop.

During the secondary and tertiary stages of yaws, bone involvement may result in thickening of the face on either side of the nose giving rise to a characteristic facial appearance called 'goundou'. The other type of lesion is a destructive lesion of the palate, eventually destroying parts of the nose (Gangosa) and causing a 'saddle-nose' defect.

Diagnosis and management: Dark field microscopy, biopsy and serology are useful. Treatment is with penicillin, erythromycin or tetracycline.

Granuloma inguinale (donovanosis)

Granuloma inguinale is a chronic, ulcerative granulomatous disease caused by *Calymmatobacterium granulomatis*, a Gram-negative bacillus probably transmitted by sexual intercourse. Granuloma inguinale has been reported in the Americas, the Far East and Africa.

After an incubation period of 1–4 weeks, a papule or nodule appears usually in the inguinal or anogenital region. This progresses to a locally destructive granulomatous ulcer.

Three main types of donovanosis have been described, ulcerative, exuberant and cicatricial. Almost any oral site may be involved and the clinical appearance of the lesions is variable. Oral lesions are often misdiagnosed as actinomycosis.

Diagnosis and management: Direct examination of a piece of granulation tissue compressed between two slides and stained by Giemsa for the presence of Donovan bodies (clusters of bacilli lying within leucocytes) is the best method. Tetracycline, ampicillin or trimethoprim-sulphamethoxazole are first line therapy.

Lymphogranuloma venereum

Lymphogranuloma venereum (LGV) or lymphogranuloma inguinale is a sexually transmitted disease caused by *Chlamydia trachomatis*, seen worldwide but particularly common in Central and South America, India, Indonesia and Africa.

LGV primarily affects the external genitalia, the inguinal lymph nodes and lymphatics. About 10 days after exposure a small vesicle appears and then ruptures and heals without scarring. About one week to two months later there may be swelling and tenderness of the regional lymph nodes and suppuration. Healing involves scarring which blocks lymphatic channels causing oedema (elephantiasis).

Cervical lymphadenopathy is common. The tongue is the oral site most frequently affected in primary LGV infections, usually with a painless vesicle. As the disease progresses, the tongue enlarges with areas of scarring and deep groves on the dorsum which are intensely red with loss of superficial epithelium.

Diagnosis and management: Laboratory confirmation of diagnosis includes isolation of *C. trachomatis* and serological tests. A skin test (Frei test) is available but not specific. LGV is treated by sulphonamides, tetracycline, erythromycin or rifampicin.

Other bacterial infections (*Table 26.1*)

VIRAL INFECTIONS

Poliomyelitis (Chapter 11)

Blood-borne viruses

HIV and hepatitis viruses are especially prevalent in the developing world (Chapters 10 and 20).

Arboviruses

Arboviruses are viruses transmitted to man by arthropods, mostly mosquitoes, sandflies, or ticks. These viral infections are thus seen principally in the tropics and wooded areas. Latin America, the southern USA, South East Asia and Africa are the areas of greatest prevalence but arboviruses have been reported worldwide. Protection is best achieved by avoiding insect bites (wearing protective clothing and using insect repellants), and using prophylactic measures such as vaccination where available.

There are many arboviruses described, most infections resulting in fever, some with rashes and arthralgias, others also with lymphadenopathy, and some with CNS involvement or haemorrhagic features. Tick-borne encephalitis is seen in forested areas of Austria, Northern Europe and Scandinavia, but yellow fever, Japanese encephalitis and dengue fever are probably the best known arbovirus infections. A vaccine against tick-borne encephalitis is available for those walking or camping in forests in areas at risk. Travellers to the tropical areas of Africa and South America require immunization against yellow fever. Travellers to monsoon areas of South East Asia may require immunization against Japanese encephalitis. There is no vaccine against dengue.

Arenaviruses

Various haemorrhagic fevers are caused by arenaviruses. *Lassa fever*, the most infamous, is called after the Nigerian town where this infection was first recorded in 1969. Cases have since been reported from Liberia, Sierra Leone and adjacent countries. The virus spreads via rats and possibly close contact, and produces fever, oral ulceration, shock, vomiting and facial and neck oedema. The infection is self-limiting but the mortality rate is high. Other arenavirus infections include Korean, Argentinian and Bolivian fevers.

Rhabdoviruses

There has also been increasing concern about more serious viral pathogens also causing haemorrhagic fevers. One group, the filoviruses, have caused considerable concern as they have high transmissibility, morbidity and mortality.

Ebola virus is the best known of these, first reported in Zaire and Sudan in 1976 but causing several outbreaks in Africa since. Ebola fever has now been reported from Zaire, Sudan, Gabon and Nigeria. The virus spreads mainly in blood or by the sexual route; airborne transmission appears unlikely. There is no specific treatment and no vaccine, and there is a very high mortality rate.

Others such as Marburg virus have also been of concern since the first reports in 1967 in persons working with monkeys in Germany and Yugoslavia.

Rabies is an acute viral infection of the CNS, transmissible in saliva mainly by bites, and is widespread among dogs, cats, foxes, racoons, wolves and similar animals. Rabies is endemic in Europe and North America, as well as in less developed countries. A few days after the bite of a rabid animal there are paraesthesiae and fasciculations around the area of the bite, followed by an encephalitic phase, followed by brain stem dysfunction with dysphagia and hypersalivation. The disease is usually fatal.

Prophylaxis is vital. Vaccine before travel is only indicated for those at high risk, such as on long journeys in remote areas. Avoid contact with animals, whether wild or apparently tame. Any bite should be cleansed, and rabies vaccine given immediately, with rabies immune globulin.

Table 26.1 Bacterial infections which occasionally have implications in dentistry

Infecting organism	Main features	Orofacial lesions	Treatment
Neisseria meningitidis	Meningitis	Petechiae Occasionally: herpes labialis Facial palsy	Penicillin
Haemophilus influenzae	Cellulitis Pneumonia Meningitis	Buccal cellulitis	Penicillin
Streptococcus pyogenes	Acute pharyngitis Cellulitis Scarlet fever Erysipelas	Peritonsillar abscess Cellulitis Palatal punctiform erythema or petechiae Raspberry tongue	Penicillin
Clostridium perfringens (Cl. welchii), Cl. sporogenes, Cl. oedematiens, Cl. septicum	Gas gangrene	Gas gangrene	Antitoxin Penicillin
Clostridium botulinum	Botulism	Xerostomia Parotitis Muscle weakness	Antitoxin
Pseudomonas aeruginosa	Skin and lungs		Sulphadiazine Aminoglycosides
Pseudomonas mallei	Glanders (acute pneumonia)	Ulceration from nasal glanders Ulcers	Penicillin Cephalosporins
Pseudomonas pseudomallei	Melioidosis (lung or other or other localized infections or septicaemia)	Oral abscesses, or other infections Parotitis	Tetracycline
Escherichia coli	Enteric infections mainly Also urinary tract wound and other infection	Found in some oral infections, especially in denture-wearers and immunocompromised	Ampicillin Cephalothin Cefalexin Co-trimoxazole
Proteus vulgaris		Occasional infections	
Salmonellae typhi, paratyphi, choleraesuis and enteritidis	Typhoid and paratyphoid fever	Occasional infections	Co-trimoxazole Ampicillin
Francisella tularensis	Tularaemia	Pharyngitis Stomatitis (often ulcerative) Faucial membrane Cervical lymphadenopathy	Streptomycin
Brucella, melitensis, suis and abortus	Brucellosis	Rare infections Cervical lymphadenopathy	Tetracycline with streptomycin
Mycoplasma hominis and pneumoniae	Pneumonia	Rare infections or cranial nerve palsies ? Reiter's syndrome	Tetracyclines
Rickettsia rickettsiae	Rocky mountain spotted fever	Petechiae Faucial gangrene	Tetracycline
Rickettsia akari	Rickettsialpox	Vesicles	Tetracycline
Bacillus anthracis	Anthrax	Painful or ulcerated swellings mainly on palate	Penicillin
Nocardia asteroides, brasiliensis and caviae	Nocardiosis	Ulceration Cheek or gingiva	Co-trimoxazole

SYSTEMIC MYCOSES

Systemic infection of healthy individuals with fungi is common in endemic areas, but is often asymptomatic, and may resolve spontaneously. Even acute pulmonary and primary mucocutaneous symptomatic lesions, in otherwise healthy persons, may resolve without treatment. However, chronic pulmonary infection tends to progress and disseminated infections can be fatal. Immunocompromised persons, however, are at particular risk from these mycoses (*Tables 20.3* and *26.2*); conversely, clinical infection

Table 26.2 Factors predisposing to mycoses

Predisposing factor	Aetiologic agent(s)
Impaired cell-mediated immunity	Candida spp.[a]
	Cryptococcus neoformans
	Histoplasma capsulatum
	Coccidioides immitis
	Paracoccidioides brasiliensis
	Blastomyces dermatitidis
Traumatized skin	Candida spp.
	Torulopsis glabrata
	Malassezia furfur[b]
Ketoacidosis	Agents of zygomycosis
Therapy with desferoxamine	Agents of zygomycosis
Intravenous drug abuse	Candida spp.
	Agents of zygomycosis
Malnutrition	Candida spp.
	Agents of zygomycosis
Neutropenia	Candida spp.
	Aspergillus spp.
	Agents of zygomycosis
	Pseudallescheria boydii
	Trichosporon spp.
	Fusarium spp.
Chronic granulomatous disease	Aspergillus spp.
	Candida albicans
	Torulopsis glabrata

[a]Infections tend to be limited to mucocutaneous involvement without dissemination.
[b]In patients who are receiving lipid emulsions intravenously.

with these mycoses may be an indication of an underlying immune defect. The increase in mycoses in immunocompromised persons is accompanied by significant morbidity and mortality and 'new' opportunists are appearing – including new Candida species *Candida krusei, Torulopsis glabrata, Fusarum* and *Trichosporon beigelii*. Patients at greatest risk from these mycoses include those with leukaemia, leukopenia, solid tumours, transplant patients, burns patients, premature infants and those with HIV disease.

Orofacial lesions caused by the main systemic mycoses may occasionally be seen in isolation but they are typically associated with lesions elsewhere, often in the respiratory tract. A tumour-like nodule or mass, chronic oral ulceration, chronic maxillary sinus infection, or bizarre mouth lesions, especially in immunocompromised patients, or in those who have been in endemic areas, or where there is granuloma formation on biopsy, may suggest the diagnosis. Tissue forms of the fungus may be visible but special stains are often required. Patients should be

managed in consultation with a physician with appropriate expertise.

Most of these mycoses are diagnosed on the basis of a history of foreign travel or an immunocompromising state, and investigations including smear, biopsy, culture, sometimes serodiagnosis, physical examination and chest radiograph.

Most systemic mycoses can be treated with systemic amphotericin given orally, liposomally, or slowly intravenously. Adverse effects to intravenous amphotericin include thrombophlebitis, nephrotoxicity, chills, nausea, anaemia and hypokalaemia. The azoles are often considered better but the cost is prohibitive where they are most needed – in the developing world.

Given orally, the adverse effects of ketoconazole include nausea, gynaecomastia and liver damage. The main adverse effects of miconazole include thrombophlebitis and ventricular tachycardia. Fluconazole and itraconazole are now being used but fluconazole resistance can be a significant problem.

Though the above generalizations hold true for most mycoses, each has individual characteristics.

Aspergillosis

Aspergillus species are the most common environmental fungi, being prolific saprophytes in soil and decaying vegetation. Inhalation of the spores must be common but disease is rare. Nevertheless, aspergillosis is found worldwide, is increasing and is the most prevalent mycosis, second only to candidosis.

Aspergillus spores colonize the respiratory tract. *Aspergillus fumigatus* is the most common pathogen but *A. flavus* and others are encountered. The most common disease is allergic bronchopulmonary aspergillosis. Invasive aspergillosis is less common: it affects the lungs mainly but may spread to brain, bone or endocardium. Aspergillomas are fungus balls that grow in pre-existing cavities such as tuberculous lung cavities.

Invasive sinus aspergillosis is rare and affects mainly immunocompromised hosts, though it is also seen in some apparently healthy individuals in subtropical countries, such as Sudan, Saudi Arabia or India. Though *A. fumigatus* is the usual cause of invasive sinus aspergillosis, *A. flavus* appears to predominate in immunocompromised individuals. There is destruction of the antral wall which may be characterized by antral pain, swelling or sequelae from orbital invasion (impaired ocular motility, exophthalmos, or impaired vision) or intracranial extension (headaches, meningism).

Chronic sinus aspergillosis is uncommon and presents as a diffusely opaque antrum on radiography, sometimes with dense punctate radio-opacities, and is unresponsive to treatment used for bacterial sinusitis.

Allergic fungal sinusitis is also uncommon, and is usually due to fungi other than aspergillus.

Aspergilloma of the maxillary antrum is uncommon, presenting typically in a healthy host as a hyphal ball in a chronically obstructed sinus.

Occasional cases of sinus aspergillosis arise as a result of metastasis from pulmonary aspergillosis or iatrogenically following dental procedures such as extractions, endodontics or implants in the maxilla.

Oral lesions of aspergillosis are seen predominantly in some immunocompromised patients with invasive aspergillosis. Yellow or black necrotic ulcers appear typically in the palate or occasionally the tongue.

The main differential diagnoses are from mucor and from pseudomonas infections. MR and CT imaging are more sensitive than conventional radiography in detecting bone erosion. Diagnosis is confirmed by smear and lesional microscopy, staining with periodic acid Schiff (PAS) or Gomori methenamine silver. Immunostains may help definitive diagnosis.

Topical ketoconazole or clotrimazole may clear superficial infections but if there is no resolution in 72 hours, a course of systemic amphotericin should be tried. Antifungals alone are not of proven efficacy and prolonged conservative therapy may worsen the prognosis.

Non-invasive antral forms are treated by antral debridement and drainage, though corticosteroids may also be indicated in allergic sinusitis. Invasive aspergillosis should be treated by surgical debridement supplemented with amphotericin and, some suggest, hyperbaric oxygen. Oral lesions of aspergillosis are treated with amphotericin. Miconazole is not active, and ketoconazole not particularly active against Aspergillus, but itraconazole may have a place in treatment. Fluconazole is under trial.

Blastomycosis

Blastomyces dermatitidis causes North American blastomycosis, seen predominantly in North America. *Paracoccidioides brasiliensis* causes the South American form. Spores may be inhaled to produce respiratory and sometimes disseminated disease. Outdoor workers are particularly affected, but it is increasingly recognized in HIV disease.

Ulcer may affect the oral mucosa. Definitive diagnosis is based on biopsy, smear or culture. Ketoconazole is highly effective treatment as are amphotericin, miconazole and itraconazole.

Coccidioidomycosis

Coccidioidomycosis is seen mainly in South West USA, Mexico, Central America and parts of South America. Inhalation of spores of *Coccidioides immitis*, found in soil, produces subclinical infection in up to 90 per cent of the population. Clinical illness presents typically as acute pulmonary disease and fever (San Joaquin valley fever), sometimes with erythema nodosum or erythema multiforme. Chronic pulmonary disease is less common. Pregnant women, blacks, Filipinos and Mexicans and immunocompromised persons are prone to disseminated coccidioidomycosis. Oral lesions of coccidioidomycosis are rare and typically secondary to lung involvement.

Diagnosis is mainly by history and examination supported by histology and the spherulin or coccidioidin skin tests. Management is with systemic amphotericin, sometimes supplemented with ketoconazole, itraconazole or fluconazole.

Cryptococcosis

Cryptococcosis is seen worldwide. Aspiration of spores of *Cryptococcus neoformans*, a yeast found especially in pigeon faeces and soil, may lead to infection.

In healthy persons, infection with cryptococcus is typically subclinical. Dissemination to the meninges, heart, spleen, pancreas, adrenals, ovaries, muscles, bones, liver and gastrointestinal tract is especially liable in immunocompromised persons. Most patients with disseminated cryptococcosis have meningoencephalitis at the time of diagnosis and, untreated, this is fatal in over 70 per cent.

Oral cryptococcus infection has presented mainly with non-healing extraction wounds, or chronic ulcers in AIDS. Diagnosis is confirmed by microscopy. Culture and assay of serum or CSF for capsular antigen and antibody may help.

Systemic amphotericin is effective, best supplemented with flucytosine. Ketoconazole and itraconazole may be effective.

Histoplasmosis

Histoplasmosis is the most frequent systemic mycosis in the USA and has now been recorded in many countries worldwide. *Histoplasma capsulatum*, the causal organism, is a soil saprophyte found particularly in the Ohio and Mississippi valleys, in Latin America, India, the Far East and in Australia.

Histoplasma is found especially in bird and bat faeces. In endemic areas, over 70 per cent of adults are infected, typically subclinically, by inhaling spores. Clinical presentations include acute and chronic pulmonary and cutaneous histoplasmosis. Disseminated and potentially lethal histoplasmosis which can affect the reticuloendothelial system, lungs, kidneys and gastrointestinal tract is rare and seen typically in immunocompromised persons.

Oral lesions have been mostly chronic ulcers recorded mainly in persons with HIV infection. Diagnosis is confirmed by microscopy, culture and serotests.

Amphotericin is given first for treatment, followed by ketoconazole. Fluconazole and itraconazole are under trial.

Mucormycosis (zygomycosis; phycomycosis)

Fungi of the order Mucorales (of the class Zygomycetes) are responsible for most mucormycosis. However, not only *Mucor* and *Rhizopus* mainly, but also *Absidia*, *Apophysomyces*, *Mortierella*, *Saksenaea*, *Rhizomucor* and *Cunninghamella* (Table 26.3)

Table 26.3 The more common pathogenic members of the Mucorales

Family	Species	Synonyms
Cunninghamellaceae	*Cunninghamella elegans*	—
	C. bertholletiae	
Mortierellaceae	*Mortierella wolfii*	—
Mucoraceae	*Absidia corymbifera*	*A. ramosa*
	Mucor circinelloides	—
	M. miehei	*Rhizomucor miehei*
	M. pusillus	*Rm. pusillus*
	Rhizopus microsporus	—
	R. oryzae	*R. arrhizus*
	R. rhizopodiformis	*R. cohnii,* *R. equinus*
Saksenaeaceae	*Saksenaea vasiformis*	—
Syncephalastraceae	*Syncephalastrum* spp.	—

may be involved and the condition is probably, therefore, better termed zygomycosis.

These fungi are ubiquitous worldwide in soil, manure and decaying organic matter and can commonly be cultured from the nose, throat, mouth and faeces of healthy individuals. Infection is rare in otherwise healthy individuals. Immunocompromising conditions underlie most zygomycosis. Rhinocerebral zygomycosis is especially predisposed to by diabetes mellitus but cases are now appearing in HIV disease and malnutrition. Leukaemia predisposes to rhinocerebral, pulmonary and disseminated zygomycosis. Desferoxamine therapy predisposes to disseminated zygomycosis.

Rhinocerebral and pulmonary zygomycosis are the most common forms. Rhinocerebral zygomycosis is usually caused by *Rhizopus oryzae*, typically commences in the nasal cavity or paranasal sinuses with pain and nasal discharge, and fever, and may then invade the palate. Orbital invasion may produce orbital cellulitis, impaired ocular movements, proptosis and ptosis. Intracranial invasion follows penetration of ophthalmic vessels or the cribriform plate.

Diagnosis is confirmed by smear, and histologic demonstration of tissue invasion by hyphae. Radiography or MRI typically show thickening of the antral mucosa with patchy destruction of the walls. MRI or computerized axial tomography may demonstrate the extent of the lesion.

Zygomycosis used to be almost uniformly fatal and still has a mortality approaching 20 per cent. Control of underlying disease is essential if possible, together with systemic amphotericin and surgical debridement.

Rhinosporidiosis

Rhinosporidiosis, caused by *Rhinosporidium seeberi*, affects the nasal and other mucosae. Particularly common in India and Sri Lanka, it is also found in Latin America, Africa and South East Asia. Oral lesions are usually proliferative lumps on the palate. Diagnosis is by biopsy; surgery is required for treatment.

Sporotrichosis

Sporothrix schenckii is found throughout the world mainly as a saprophyte on various plants and shrubs. Disease is seen almost exclusively in visitors to tropical and subtropical countries. Infection follows an injury to the epithelium, and progresses in some to the lymphatic form. The primary lesion is a sporotrichotic chancre which may ulcerate if in the mouth. Lesions may also then arise in lymphatics. Pulmonary and disseminated sporotrichosis are rare and of uncertain origin: antral and oral involvement has been described.

Diagnosis is confirmed by histology and culture. Potassium iodide is effective treatment for superficial sporotrichosis, itraconazole or amphotericin for other forms.

Systemic candidosis

Candidosis is typically a superficial mycosis. Nevertheless, Candida increasingly frequently causes invasion of deep organs. Candida species implicated now include *C. albicans*, *C. tropicalis*, *C. parapsilosis*, *C. guilliermondii*, *C. krusei* and *C. lusitania*. Some are resistant to fluconazole.

Other less common mycoses (Table 26.4)

Antral infections with various unusual fungi are increasingly reported in immunocompromised persons.

Table 26.4 Cutaneous and other less common mycoses: increasingly reported – mainly in immunocompromised patients

- Predominantly cutaneous mycoses
  Dermatophytes
    Epidermophyton
    Microsporum
    Trichophyton
  Others
    Malassezia (pityrosporum or pityrosporan)
    Trichosporon
- Hyalohyphomycoses
  Fusarium spp.
  Penicillium spp.
  Paecilomyces spp.
  Other species
- Phaeohyphomycoses
  Alternaria spp.
  Exophiala jeanselmei (Phialophora gougerotii)
  Wangiella dermatitidis
  Bipolaris (Drechsclera) spicifera
  Other species

PARASITIC INFESTATIONS

Parasitic infestations are endemic in the developing world and are now being seen increasingly in the developed world, in travellers or immigrants, individuals having usually acquired infections from zoonotic parasites, water, or improperly prepared food. There are many other parasitic infestations, the most common being scabies, fleas and lice, which are increasing even in developed countries. Many can be avoided by good hygiene, avoidance of insect bites (using protective clothing and insect repellants), and avoiding high-risk areas.

Malaria is one of the more serious parasitic infections worldwide, and is seen in the many parts of the tropics where the Anopheline mosquito survives. Many hundreds of cases are imported into the West in travellers; not all survive. Toxoplasmosis is not uncommon in the developed world, and is endemic in the developing world.

Many exotic parasitic infestations are known but few are relevant to oral health care (*Tables 26.5* and *26.6*). However, oral lesions have been described in ancylostomiasis, ascariasis, cysticercosis, echinococcosis, filariasis, gnathostomiasis, gongylonematosis,

Table 26.5   Worms (helminths) that may affect the oral tissues

Usual helminth	Geographical distribution	Oral lesions
Cestodes		
Cysticercus cellulosae (Taenia solium larvae)	Worldwide	Painless swellings
Echinococcus granulosus	Middle East North and East Africa Asia Latin America Australasia	Cystic lesions
Nematodes		
Ancylostoma duodenale	Mediterranean littoral Middle East China India South America	Creeping lesions
Filariae	South East Asia India East Africa South America	?
Gnathostoma spinigerum	South East Asia	Transient swelling
Gongylonema pulchrum	Former USSR China Sri Lanka	Creeping lesions
Onchocerca volvulus	Africa Central America	Nodules
Trichinella spiralis	Worldwide	Painful swellings
Ascaris lumbricoides	Worldwide	Submandibular swelling
Trichuris trichiuria	South East Asia	? Ulcerative stomatitis

Table 26.6   Abbreviated taxonomy and classification of main tropical parasitic organisms and related oral diseases

I **PROTOZOA** (unicellular)
Flagellates (class)
Sarcomastigophora (genus)
   Leishmania spp.　　　　　Leishmaniasis
　　　　　　　　　　　　　　(*Table 26.7*)

II **Metazoa** (multicellular with differentiated tissues)
HELMINTHS (worms)
Nematodes/round worms (class)
   Trichinella spiralis　　　Trichinosis
   Gnathostoma spinigerum　Gnathostomiasis
   Ancylostoma spp.　　　　Larva migrans
   Onchocerca spp.　　　　　Onchocerciasis
Platyhelminths/flat worms (class)
Cestodes/tapeworms
   Echinococcus　　　　　　Hydatid disease/
　　　　　　　　　　　　　　Echinococcosis
   Taenia solium　　　　　　Cysticercosis

INSECTS
Diptera (order)
   Calliphoridae　　　　　　Myiasis
   Oestridae　　　　　　　　Myiasis
   Sarcophagidae　　　　　　Myiasis

mucocutaneous leishmaniasis, myiasis, onchocerciasis, trichinosis and trichuriasis and, though uncommonly reported, these may be under-diagnosed. Furthermore, since the appearance of the HIV pandemic, cases of HIV-related parasitic infestations are now being reported.

Many of these exotic parasitic infestations are difficult to diagnose unless there is a high index of suspicion. Clinicians and pathologists should be vigilant therefore, especially when examining lesions in travellers or immigrants. Patients should be managed in consultation with a specialist physician.

Scabies

Scabies is a common infestation with the mite *Sarcoptes scabiei*, which is transmitted by close contact, particularly in bed. The mite burrows into the superficial skin and lays eggs which excite an inflammatory response. An itchy rash develops at the sites, typically interdigitally and on the wrists. Scabies is treated in the patient and family/partners with malathion or permethrin, and improved hygiene.

Lice

There are three main types of lice. Head lice (*Pediculosis humanis* var. *capitis*) infest hair; *P. corporis* infests the body and clothes; *Phthirius pubis* (crab lice) infest the pubic hair area. Lice are transmitted by close contact or via discarded clothing. They feed off the host's blood and the puncture wounds can become itchy and bleed. Lice infestations are increasing in many areas, especially in vagrants, and head lice are particularly common in school children.

Lice can, under appropriate circumstances, also transmit disease such as typhus (*Rickettsia prowazeki*), relapsing fever (*Borrelia recurrentis*) and trench fever (*R. quintana*). Treatment is with improved hygiene and the use of malathion and carbaryl.

Fleas

Fleas are parasites of man and other animals, living mainly on the hairy parts of the body, depositing eggs that can cause an itchy rash. They are transmitted to those in close proximity. Rodent fleas in particular can act as vectors of plague (*Pasteurella pestis*) and typhus, and have been responsible for recent outbreaks of disease in India and other areas. Improved hygiene and malathion are indicated.

Malaria

Malaria is the main parasitic infection; it still infects over 100 million persons in the world, mainly in tropical areas of Africa, Latin America and Asia, and in some cases can be fatal. Transmitted by the bite of an infected mosquito, there are four main species of the protozoon, namely *Plasmodium vivax*, *P. ovale*, *P. malariae* and *P. falciparum*. These infect erythrocytes and damage them, causing haemolysis, as well as fever, myalgia, headaches and in some cases cerebral involvement. Infection with *P. falciparum* is usually the most dangerous, while *P. vivax* is usually benign.

Diagnosis is made from the history of travel to a malarial area and confirmed by demonstrating the parasite in a blood smear. Repeated smears may be required.

Prophylactic chemotherapy significantly reduces the risk of contracting malaria, and this should be continued for 6 weeks after leaving the malarial area. The usual drugs used are chloroquine and/or proguanil, but mefloquine is recommended where the malaria risk is high and chloroquine resistance likely. Specialist advice should always be sought before travel to the tropics. Insect repellants and nets reduce the risk of mosquito bites.

Treatment of malaria is usually with chloroquine though there is now often drug resistance, particularly in Asia and Latin America. Quinine, mefloquine or halofantrine are used for *P. falciparum* infections

Toxoplasmosis (*see* p. 231)

Toxoplasma gondii is a common intestinal parasite of many animals, particularly cats. Infection is contracted mainly from the ingestion of the organism, either from the animal faeces or in inadequately cooked food. For example, up to 10 per cent of lamb and pork can contain cysts. Toxoplasma may also occasionally be transmitted in infected blood or blood products.

T. gondii may cause a glandular fever type of illness with fever, and lymphadenopathy. This often causes cervical lymphadenopathy, sometimes with fever, rash, hepatosplenomegaly, myalgia and other minor features. There are usually no other untoward sequelae, unless the patient is immunocompromised or pregnant, though some patients may develop chorioretinitis, which threatens sight.

Toxoplasmosis in immunocompromised patients may cause severe pneumonia or necrotizing encephalitis, or myocarditis. CNS involvement is common, and can cause changes in mental status, headache, neurological defects and epilepsy. CT scans may demonstrate the lesions.

Transplacental spread in pregnancy may lead to fetal toxoplasmosis, with resultant congenital defects and blindness TORCH syndrome.

Diagnosis is confirmed serologically by the Sabin–Feldman dye test, ELISA, indirect fluorescent antibody test or indirect haemagglutination test. The organism may be

Table 26.7 Types of leishmaniasis

Form of leishmaniasis	Main leishmania spp.	Main endemic geographic distribution
Visceral	L. donovani–L. infantum	Mediterranean littoral, south-west Asia, China, Latin America, India, East Africa
Cutaneous		
Old World cutaneous (Oriental sore)	L. tropica	Central Asia and Afghanistan
	L. tropica and L. major	Middle East, India, Afghanistan, sub-Saharan Africa
	L. aethiopica	East Africa
New World cutaneous		
Pian bois (bush yaws)	L. brasiliensis guyanensis	Guyana, Surinam, French Guyana, Brazil (Amazon)
Panamanian	L. brasiliensis panamensis	Panama, Costa Rica
('Chiclero ulcer' or 'Bay sore')	L. mexicana mexicana	Mexico, Guatemala, Belize
Venezuelan montane ('Uta')	L. mexicana venezuelensis	Venezuela
	L. peruviana	Peru
Enzootic rodent	L. mexicana amazonensis	Panama, Brazil (Amazon)
Diffuse cutaneous	L. mexicana amazonensis	Latin America
	L. mexicana pifanoi	Venezuela
	L. aethiopica	Ethiopia and Kenya
Mucocutaneous		
South American (Espundia)	L. brasiliensis brasiliensis Possibly L.b. panamensis and L.b. guyanensis	Latin America
Sudanese	L. donovani	Sudan

demonstrable in tissue sections or smears. Treatment is not required for asymptomatic healthy persons who are not pregnant. For immunocompromised patients, treatment is a combination of pyrimethamine and sulphadiazine, together with folic acid, since pyrimethamine is a folate antagonist. Treatment may need to be carried on for at least one month after clinical resolution. Weekly full blood counts are essential.

Sulphadiazine alone is used for pregnant patients with toxoplasmosis, since pyrimethamine may be teratogenic. Clindamycin, clarithromycin and azithromycin are alternatives.

Leishmaniasis

Leishmaniasis is the main tropical parasitic disease in which oral lesions may be found, typically in mucocutaneous leishmaniasis, and in Latin America.

Life cycle
The life cycle of leishmania comprises a bloodsucking sandfly as intermediate host and humans or other vertebrates, including dogs and cats, as the definitive hosts. The developmental stage of leishmania is the amastigote in the vertebrate host and promastigote in the arthropod host. After inoculation into the skin, leishmanias multiply within histiocytes.

Leishmania species
Human *Leishmania* species, although similar in morphology and life cycle to each other, produce different types of infections (*Table 26.7*). **Visceral** leishmaniasis or kala-azar is caused by three species belonging to the *L. donovani.–L. infantum* complex in Latin America, Africa, Asia, southern Russia and the Mediterranean basin. **Mucocutaneous** leishmaniasis is seen in Latin America and caused by *L. brasiliensis* complex. **Cutaneous** (and mucocutaneous) forms of Leishmaniasis are caused by *L. tropica, L. major, L. aethiopica, L. mexicana* complex and *L. brasiliensis* complex (*L.b. brasiliensis, L.b. panamensis* and *L.b. guyanensis*) present in tropical Africa, the Mediterranean area including Italy, Spain, Southern France, the Middle East and North Africa, and Central and South America.

• Clinical features and diagnosis

The incubation of mucocutaneous leishmaniasis is usually 2–8 weeks but can be as long as 3 years. The lesion begins at the site of the sandfly bite, usually on the face. An itching papule develops and becomes surrounded by gradually spreading erythema and induration. In a few days, the surface crusts and then breaks down to a slowly extending ulcer which discharges fluid. Healing usually begins in 3–12 months, leaving a scar.

Secondary lesions develop at the mucocutaneous junctions many years after the primary infection, and are destructive. The nose is the site of predilection.

Oral lesions are most frequent in mucocutaneous leishmaniasis, when the hard palate is typically involved (espundia). A mid-facial granulomatous destructive lesion may result. It has been suggested that loosening and spontaneous shedding of teeth may represent the initial symptoms of oral disease and that fungating lesions are rather frequent in the oral mucosa.

Investigations: Clinical and serologic tests are useful but the demonstration of the parasite in biopsies or smears is the most definitive. A leishmanin skin test is also available.

• Management

Mucocutaneous leishmaniasis may heal spontaneously but, since there can be extensive destruction of tissue, chemotherapy is indicated, using pentavalent antimony as sodium stibogluconate (Pentostam) or meglumine antimonate. If the patient fails to respond, amphotericin is usually effective. Pentamidine isethionate by deep intramuscular injection is an alternative.

Trichinosis

Trichinosis is the most frequent roundworm infestation to affect the oral tissues, mainly muscles.

Life cycle
Trichinella spiralis is a helminth, a nematode. Infestation is acquired through the ingestion of contaminated meat. Pigs and rats are the most important reservoir and most infections are related to eating pork products. Trichinosis is more prevalent in Central Europe and North America, where pork is widely consumed, than it is in Islamic or Jewish cultures or tropical countries. Many infestations are subclinical.

Both larval and adult forms of *T. spiralis* may parasitize humans, which are then the definitive host and later become the intermediate host when the larvae are established in the muscles. Therefore the same host sustains the adult worm temporarily and the larvae for a long period of time. After ingestion of the infective larvae in infected meat, they mature to adult forms in the intestine in approximately one week. Adult female nematodes then deposit larvae in the mucosal epithelium. The larvae penetrate the mucosa and subsequently enter the bloodstream and pass to the muscles such as the tongue, masseter, gastrocnemius, deltoid and diaphragm where they grow and develop, and become encapsulated. The capsules can calcify and appear as radio-opaque nodules.

• Clinical features and diagnosis

In mild infections, symptoms are often vague and transient. Acute trichinosis is characterized by a triad known as Beeson's signs of myalgia, facial and palpebral oedema and fever with eosinophilia. Myocarditis is present in up to 20 per cent of patients and there may be involvement of lungs, kidneys, pancreas and central nervous system. Rare cases have involved the tongue and masseter as painful chronic swellings.

The diagnosis is clinical, supported by a history of ingestion of poorly cooked meat, and by investigations. There is eosinophilic leucocytosis and serodiagnosis is feasible after the third week. There are also increased serum levels of muscle enzymes (such as creatine phosphokinase). However, the definitive diagnosis relies on biopsies from affected muscle or blind biopsies from the deltoid or gastrocnemius.

• Prevention and management

Prevention requires meat to be cooked throughout at a temperature above 65 °C. The treatment is mebendazole or thiabendazole.

Echinococcosis (echinococciasis)

Echinococcosis is the presence of hydatid cysts from tapeworms of the genus *Echinococcus* in human tissues. It is typically contracted by the ingestion of ova excreted in dog faeces. Echinococcosis has been a serious problem in many sheep-raising regions.

Life cycle
Echinococcosis (hydatid disease or hydatidosis) is caused most often by larvae (Cestodes) of *E. granulosus*. It remains most prevalent in Australia, New Zealand, South, East and North Africa, Mediterranean countries and in some parts of the former USSR, Middle East and the Americas.

The adult tapeworm lives in the small intestine. Many mammals can serve as intermediate hosts, but sheep are the most common. The eggs hatch in the sheep's intestine, releasing oncospheres that penetrate the intestinal mucosa, enter the blood stream and develop into hydatid cysts in various organs, particularly the liver and the lungs. Daughter cysts pass in the faeces and are swallowed by the intermediate host, other sheep. Dogs and wolves are infected by eating the discarded offal of sheep. Man is an accidental intermediate host, infected by ingestion of eggs in the faeces of dogs. Most of the time, contamination is related to improper hand-washing and less often by ingestion of contaminated water or food. Only the larval stage, the hydatid cyst, develops in humans.

• Clinical features and diagnosis

The incubation is very long, from 10 to 30 years, and there are no specific clinical signs. However, when a hydatid cyst reaches a large volume it can act as a space-occupying lesion causing compression of adjacent structures. Typically the liver and sometimes the lungs, bone or brain are affected and the lesions can sometimes be demonstrated radiographically or by ultrasound. A skin test (Casoni test) is available but not specific. Serology may be helpful.

Oral lesions: Hydatid cysts in the oral tissues are usually firm, round swellings of several months' duration, mainly in the tongue. A history of possible exposure to infection may be elicited. A hydatid cyst may show a smooth, round outline on radiography. Eosinophilia is merely suggestive of a parasitic disease and not specific. However, a definitive diagnosis is often made only by identifying the hydatid cyst at operation.

• Prevention and management

Prevention relies on the protection of definitive hosts (dogs) as well as intermediate hosts (sheep) from becoming contaminated. The elimination of contact with potentially contaminated dogs, thorough hand-washing and washing of vegetables and wild berries located close to the ground are the best protection for man.

High doses of mebendazole, albendazole or flubendazole interfere with growth of larvae but are *not curative* in humans. The only curative treatment is surgery.

Cysticercosis

Taeniasis is the condition caused by adult tapeworms in the small intestine of humans. Cysticercosis, the presence of larvae of the pork tapeworm *Taenia solium* in human tissues, is seen worldwide.

Life cycle
The encysted larva of *Taenia solium*, called *Cysticercus cellulosae*, may cause cysticercosis. Pork is the usual intermediate host and thus cysticercosis prevails in regions of poverty and where hygiene is insufficient, particularly in Africa, the Far East, India, Latin America, Eastern Europe and in the Iberian peninsula. It is rare in peoples such as Jews and Muslims who avoid pork.

The adult *Taenia solium* lives in the intestine of man, the only definitive host, and the stools release eggs which, if they contaminate the ground, can be swallowed by pigs. The eggs hatch in the pig's intestine releasing oncospheres that enter the bloodstream, and become encysted as cysticerci in muscle. The life cycle is completed when man ingests inadequately cooked pork containing cysticerci (measly pork). Upon reaching man's intestine, the oncospheres are released, penetrate the mucosa and are distributed to various tissues and organs where they develop into cysticerci, mainly in muscles.

• Clinical features and diagnosis

Cysticerci are most common in the brain and eye, striated muscles in the tongue, neck and trunk, and skin and subcutaneous tissues.

Oral lesions of cysticercosis are rare, typically well-circumscribed, soft, elastic and fluctuant submucosal swellings present for many years.

Diagnosis usually relies upon surgical removal of the parasite, the appearance of the translucent membrane, with its central milky spot, being characteristic.

• Prevention and management

Prevention relies on thorough cooking of pork meat and good hygiene procedures. There is no reliable medical treatment but albendazole or, better, praziquantel (plus prednisolone) can be curative. Single or even multiple parasites may be excised from the various tissues and organs.

Myiasis

Myiasis is the condition when fly maggots invade living tissue, or when they are harboured in the intestine or any part of the body and feed on the host's organs. Human myiasis is most common in the tropics.

Life cycle
Three main families of flies – Calliphoridae, Oestridae and Sarcophagidae – have been reported to cause human myiasis. The ova are most commonly deposited in the nose. Most troublesome to man in the New World is *Cochliomyia hominovorax* (screwworm, Calliphoridae). The related *Chrysomyia bezziana* (Calliphoridae) is seen in Africa, Asia, the Pacific Islands and the Old World.

• Clinical features and diagnosis

Larvae are able to burrow through either necrotic or healthy tissue. Some produce a type of larva migrans creeping eruption (*see below*). When the larvae mature, they migrate out of the host in an effort to reach soil to pupate and may then be visible.

Oral lesions: Oral myiasis is a rare entity, seen mainly in people who are in the habit of sleeping with their mouth open, have incompetent lips or are mouth-breathers. Lesions are thus mainly in the anterior maxilla or mandible.

• Prevention and management

A few drops of turpentine oil or 15 per cent chloroform in light vegetable oil should be instilled in the lesion and larvae should be removed with blunt tweezers.

Larva migrans

Nematodes that are not normally parasitic to man can, if they infect humans, often fail to develop fully and may wander in the tissues, causing one of several forms of 'larva migrans' before they die. Oral lesions have been recorded in relation to various worms, including *Ancylostoma* and *Gongylonema* species.

Life cycle
The syndrome of *visceral* larva migrans is synonymous with toxocariasis – infection by larvae from roundworms of dogs, cats or wild carnivores.

The syndrome of *cutaneous* larva migrans (creeping eruption) is caused by larvae from hookworms mainly of dogs, cats and other mammals; it is this type that may affect the mouth.

Adult hookworms live mainly in the intestines of animals and they release ova into the faeces. The ova are thus found in sand or soil contaminated by animals and, under favourable conditions of temperature and humidity, hatch into infective larvae. Larva migrans is thus common in tropical climates, in the US along the coast from Southern New Jersey to Florida, around the Caribbean and around the Mediterranean, but may also occur elsewhere during warm weather. It is seen especially in those working or playing in warm, moist, shaded sandy places.

• Clinical features and diagnosis

Cutaneous larva migrans is characterized by itching serpiginous tracks, mainly on the feet, hands or buttocks. The disease is self-limiting but nearly 50 per cent of patients can develop transient migratory pulmonary infiltrates with eosinophilia (Loeffler's syndrome).

Table 26.8   Main religions and their relevance (*see also Table 26.9*)

Religion	Main festival or religious occasion(s)	Dietary points	Medical problems	Other comments
Buddhism	Wesak	Often vegetarian		
Christianity	Christmas, Easter	–	Jehovah's Witnesses refuse blood transfusions	–
Hinduism	Mahashivaratri, Ram Navami, Janmastami	Often eat no meat or meat products, eggs or fish. Some drink no tea, coffee or alcohol, and eat no garlic or onions	–	–
Islam (Muslim)	Ramadan, Mawlid, al-Nabi	Eat no pork, drink no alcohol. Eat halal meat. During Ramadan, between sunrise and sunset eat and drink nothing, and smoke nothing, unless ill, young, old or pregnant	–	Often cover much of the body and head/face
Judaism	Rosh Hashanah, Yom Kippur, Pesach	Eat no pork or shellfish, and only kosher meat. Fast for 25 hr from eve of Yom Kippur	Orthodox Jews may refuse organ transplants	No work on Sabbath (Saturday)
Sikhism	Vaisakhi, Diwali, Hola	Eat no fish or eggs, usually no beef or pork. Often vegetarian	–	Invariably cover head

• Prevention and management

Larva migrans can at least partly be prevented by stopping dogs, cats and other animals contaminating play areas. Local application of 10 per cent thiabendazole, ethyl chloride, chloroform, electrocoagulation and cryotherapy have been tried. If the lesions are multiple, particularly in the mouth, thiabendazole is indicated but can produce adverse effects such as anorexia, nausea and rashes. Albendazole or mebendazole are alternatives.

Filariasis

Filariae are a group of helminthic parasites whose adult and larval forms are found in man and are transmitted by the bite of blood-sucking insects – usually mosquitoes or black flies.

Onchocerciasis is seen mainly in tropical Africa, but also in Saudi Arabia, the Yemen and Latin America. Onchocerciasis is caused by the filariae *Onchocerca volvulus* (in Africa) and *O. caeutiens* (in Latin America). Oncocerciasis may involve the face or, rarely, the mouth as a rubbery nodule, but eye lesions remain a major problem in Africa (river blindness). The diagnosis is made by identifying the worm in biopsies. Treatment is with Ivermectin.

Lymphatic filariasis is infestation by Filarioidea nematodes (*Wuchereria bancrofti*, *Brugia malayi* or *B. timori*) transmitted by blood-sucking mosquitoes and particularly seen in India, South East Asia and the South Pacific, and also Latin America, East Africa and Egypt. The lymphatics are affected with various obstructive sequelae usually presenting as oedema or elephantiasis. Brugia species tend to affect only the lower limbs. *W. bancrofti* have rarely been found in the mouth. Diagnosis is from blood examination for filariae. Diethylcarbamazine is the treatment of choice but requires close medical supervision.

Trichuriasis

Trichuriasis, infestation of the large intestine by the whipworm *Trichuris trichiura*, is common in the Caribbean islands and South East Asia, especially in children, who contract the condition by ingesting eggs from contaminated soil. No specific oral lesions have been recorded but anaemia is common. Trichuriasis is diagnosed by faecal examination for the worms and is treated with mebendazole, albendazole or exantel.

Table 26.9 Ethnic groups: their main language, religion, habits and medical problems

Ethnic group	Main language(s)	Main religion(s)	Diet and habits[a]	Medical problems[b]
Afro-Caribbean	English	Christian	Seventh Day Adventists consume no pork, tea or coffee. Rastafarians often use marijuana, but may be vegan or eat no pork	Sickle cell disease, hypertension, cerebro-vascular accidents, rheumatic carditis, diabetes, G6PD deficiency, schizophrenia. Carcinomas of cervix, liver and prostate. Jehovah's Witnesses refuse blood transfusions
Arabs	Arabic	Muslim		Diabetes, thalassaemia, haemophilia, pemphigus Behçet's syndrome
Armenians	Armenian	Christian	–	Thalassaemia
Bangladeshi	Bengali, Urdu	Muslim	Healthy diet, dislike oral medication, and females prefer female health care workers. Often smoke or use pan	Tuberculosis, ischaemic heart disease, diabetes, peptic ulcer, hypertension, submucous fibrosis, carcinomas of cervix, breast and mouth
Chinese	Cantonese	Taoism, Confucianism, Buddhism	Often eat rice diet, and smoke. May not like venepuncture	Hepatitis B, G6PD deficiency, thalassaemia, carcinoma of nasopharynx, oesophagus, stomach. Kimura's disease
Cypriots (*see* Greeks, Turks)				
Eritreans	Tigrinya, Arabic	Muslim, Christian		
Ethiopians	Amharic	Muslim, Christian		
Ghanaian	Twi	Muslim, Christian		Sickle cell disease
Greeks	Greek	Christian	Healthy diet	Thalassaemia, pemphigus, Behçet's syndrome
Gujaratis	Gujarati	Hindu	Often eat no meat, eggs or fish	Ischaemic heart disease, lactose intolerance hypertension, submucous fibrosis, carcinomas of cervix, breast and mouth
Iranian	Farsi	Muslim		Coeliac disease
Irish	English	Christian	May be high alcohol intake	Gastric ulcer, stomach
Japanese	Japanese	Buddhism, Shintoism	Diet often of rice, raw fish and eggs.	cancer, Behçet's syndrome, Kawasaki disease, Kikuchi–Fujimoto disease
Kurds	Kurdish	Muslim		
Nigerians	Yoruba, Ibo, Hausa	Muslim, Christian		Sickle cell disease
Pakistanis	Punjabi	Muslim		Ischaemic heart disease, diabetes, thalassaemia, lactose intolerance, hypertension, submucous fibrosis, carcinomas of cervix, breast and mouth
Somalis	Somali	Muslim	May use qat	
South Africans (whites)	English, Dutch	Christian		Ischaemic heart disease, porphyria
Sudanese	Arabic	Muslim, Christian		
Tamil	Tamil	Hindu	Vegetarian	Ischaemic heart disease, lactose intolerance
Turks	Turkish	Muslim		Thalassaemia, pemphigus, Behçet's syndrome
Vietnamese	Vietnamese, Cantonese	Buddhism	Vegetarian	Hepatitis B

[a]*See* Table 26.8 for religious points.
[b]The problems may depend on the generation, and degree of integration with the indigenous community. Many immigrant groups suffer social deprivations and have related medical problems such as accidents and high perinatal mortality rates. Some also suffer from psychiatric disorders consequent on persecution or racism. Some have imported infectious diseases prevalent in their home countries, such as viral hepatitis, HIV or exotic diseases.

Gnathostomiasis

Gnathostomiasis is a rare benign infestation, seen mainly in Southern and South East Asia, caused by larvae of the nematode *Gnathostoma spinigerum*, harboured in chicken, snails or fish. The worm may produce swellings in the skin or mouth, or occasionally bleeding. Skin tests and sero-diagnosis help the diagnosis. Metronidazole may be of some benefit, or the worm can be excised.

ETHNIC AND CULTURAL FACTORS

Hereditary and lifestyle factors are important in the predisposition to some disorders and to the lack of others. Hereditary factors clearly result in significant disease such as sickle cell disease, thalassaemia, glucose-6-phosphate dehydrogenase deficiency and other haemo-globinopathies (Chapter 5), and porphyria and some types of amyloidosis (Chapter 15). Genetic factors are also at play in pemphigus (Chapter 12), Behçet's syndrome (Chapter 21) and many other relevant disorders. Some cultural and lifestyle factors are also important in health and disease, and in the management of patients. These points are summarized in *Tables 26. 8* and *26.9*, but one of the most relevant disorders seen virtually exclusively in a particular ethnic group is submucous fibrosis.

Oral submucous fibrosis

Oral submucous fibrosis (OSMF), though not regarded as a connective tissue disease, has pathological changes closely similar to those of scleroderma (Chapter 21). Unlike the latter, which has severe effects on the skin but minimal effects on the oral mucosa, OSMF causes severe and often disabling fibrosis of the oral tissues alone.

Oral submucous fibrosis affects virtually only those from the Indian Subcontinent. Serum immunoglobulin IgG, IgA and IgM levels are raised. No consistent specific immunological abnormalities appear to be associated, although there is a greater prevalence of connective tissue diseases. The condition appears to be related to the chewing of areca nut.

There is some evidence that it is premalignant. Iron deficiency anaemia may be present but this is not uncommon in Asians in the absence of submucous fibrosis.

Clinically, OSMF causes symmetrical fibrosis of such sites as the cheeks, soft palate or inner aspects of the lips. The fibrosis is often so severe that the affected area is almost white and so hard that it literally cannot be indented with the finger. Frequently the buccal fibrosis causes such severe restriction of opening that dental treatment becomes increasingly difficult and finally impossible. Ultimately tube feeding may become necessary.

Intra-lesional corticosteroids and regular stretching of the oral soft tissues with an interdental screw may delay fixation in the closed position. Failing this, operative treatment may become necessary.

BIBLIOGRAPHY

Abbas K., El Toum I.A. and El Hassan A.M. (1992) Oral leishmaniasis associated with kala-azar. A case report. *Oral Surg. Oral Med. Oral Pathol.* **73**, 583–4.

Al-Ismaily M.I. and Scully C. (1995) Oral myiasis: report of two cases. *Int. J. Paediatr. Dent.* **5**, 177–9.

Almeida O.P.D. and Scully C. (1991) Oral lesions in the systemic mycoses. *Curr. Opin. Dent.* **1**, 423–8.

Andrew J., Bernard M., Ledaux M. and Achten G. (1988) Larva migrans of the oral mucosa. *Dermatologica* **176**, 296–8.

Assal A.M. and Arafat M.S. (1984) Hydatid disease of the maxilla. *J. Laryngol. Otol.* **98**, 1027–9.

Bakilana P.B. (1985) Microfilaria in oral cytological smears – report of 2 cases. *Odontostomatologie Tropicale* **VIII**, 133–4.

Balarajan P.R. and Raleigh V.S. (1995) *Ethnicity and Health in England*. London, HMSO.

Bedi R., Bahl V. and Rayan R.R. (1996) *Dentists, Patients and Ethnic Minorities*. London, Faculty of General Dental Practitioners.

Borzoni F., Gradoni L., Gramicia M., Maccioni A., Valdes E. and Loddo S. (1991) A case of lingual and palatine localization of viscerotropic Leishmania infantum zymodene in Sardinia, Italy. *Trop. Med. Parasitol.* **42**, 193–4.

Bozzo L., Lima I.A., Almeida O.P.D. and Scully C. (1992) Oral myiasis caused by sarcophagidae in an extraction wound. *Oral Surg. Oral Med. Oral Pathol.* **74**, 733–5.

Curphey J.E. (1971) Trichiniasis of the mandible. *Oral Surg. Oral Med. Oral Pathol.* **31**, 19–24.

El-Safi S.H., Peters W. and Evans D.A. (1991) Studies on the leishmaniases in the Sudan. 3. Clinical and parasitological studies on visceral and mucosal leishmaniasis. *Trans. R. Soc. Trop. Med. Hyg.* **85**, 465–70.

Ettinger R.L. (1993) Demography and dental needs in international perspective. *Gerodontology* **10**, 3–9.

Fazakerley M.W. and Woolgar J.A. (1991) Cysticercosis cellulosae. An unusual cause of labial swelling. *Br. Dent. J.* **170**, 105–6.

Goto H., Sotto M.N., Corbett C.E.P. *et al.* (1990) A case of multiple lesion mucocutaneous leishmaniasis caused by Leishmania (Viannia braziliensis) infection. *J. Am. Dent. Assoc.* **93**, 48–51.

Hansen L.S. and Allard R.H.B. (1984) Encysted parasitic larvae in the mouth. *J. Am. Dent. Assoc.* **108**, 632–6.

Health Education Authority (1994) *Health and Lifestyles; Black and Minority Ethnic Groups in England.* London, HEA.

Indira C., Ramesh V. and Misra R.S. (1990) Association of oral cysticercosis and post kala-azar dermal leishmaniasis. *Int. J. Oral Maxillofac. Surg.* **9**, 266–7.

Jain R.K., Gupta O.P. and Aryya N.C. (1989) Cysticercosis of the tongue. *J. Laryngol. Otol.* **103**, 1227–8.

Kalovidouris A., Gouliamos A., Andreou I. *et al.* (1985) Primary hydatid disease of the infra-temporal fossa and the parotid gland. *Radiology* **25**, 235–6.

Karmi G. (1996) *The Ethnic Health Handbook.* Oxford, Blackwell.

Lopes M.A., Zaia A.A., Almeida O.P.D. and Scully C. (1994) Larva migrans affecting the mouth. *Oral Surg. Oral Med. Oral Pathol.* **77**, 362–7.

Marsden P.D. (1986) Mucosal leishmaniasis ('espundia' Escomel, 1911) (1986) *Trans. R. Soc. Trop. Med. Hyg.* **80**, 859–76.

Mattin D. and Smith J.M. (1991) The oral health status, dental needs and factors affecting utilisation of dental services in Asians aged 55 years and over, resident in Southampton. *Br. Dent. J.* **170**, 369–72.

Nandakumar H. and Shankaramba K.B. (1989) Hydatid cyst of the mandible: a case report. *J. Oral Maxillofac. Surg.* **47**, 759–61.

Onerci M., Turan E. and Ruacan S. (1991) Submandibular hydatid cyst. A case report. *J. Craniomaxillofac. Surg.* **19**, 359–61.

Ostrofsky M.K. and Baker M.A. (1975) Oral cysticercosis: three case reports. *Tydskrif Van Die Tandheelkrundige Vereniging Sui-Afrika* **30**, 535–7.

Patel S.K. and Gelbier S. (1991) The UK Panch Gam Patidar community and dentistry. *Comm. Dent. Hlth* **8**, 25–30.

Piette E.M.G. (1989) Revue generale des mycoses d'interet maxillofacial. *Acta Stomatol. Belg.* **86**, 87–140.

Prabhu S.R., Wilson D.F., Daftary D.K. and Johnson N.W. (eds) (1992) *Oral Diseases in the Tropics.* Oxford, Oxford University Press.

Rakprasitkul S. and Tongnoi D. (1982) Cysticercosis of the lower lip (a case report). *J. Dent. Assoc. Thailand* **32**, 223–36.

Rao P.L., Radhakrishna K. and Kapadia R.D. (1990) Cysticercosis of the tongue. *Int. J. Paediatr. Otorhinolaryngol* **20**, 159–61.

Rivera F., Maximo Castillo I.R., Chavez M. *et al.* (1986) Pathogenic and free-living protozoa cultured from the nasopharyngeal and oral regions of dental patients. *Env. Res.* **39**, 364–71.

Sampaio R.N.R., Sampaio R.H.B. and Marsden P.D. (1985) Pentavalent antimonial treatment in mucosal leishmaniasis. *Lancet* **i**, 1097.

Scully C. (1988) *The Dental Patient.* Oxford, Heinemann.

Scully C. (1989) *Patient Care: a Dental Surgeon's Guide.* London, British Dental Association.

Scully C. (1989) *The Mouth and Perioral Tissues.* Oxford, Heinemann.

Scully C. and Almeida O. (1992) Orofacial manifestations of the systemic mycoses. *J. Oral Pathol. Med.* **21**, 289–94.

Sookasam M. and Reichart P.A. (1992) Migratory facial swelling due to gnathostomiasis. *Int. J. Oral Maxillofac. Surg.* **21**: 176–7.

Sposto M.R., Mendes-Gianini M.J., Moraes R.A., Branco F.C. and Scully C. (1994) Paracoccidioidomycosis manifesting as oral lesions: a clinical, cytological and serological investigation. *J. Oral Pathol. Med.* **23**, 85–7.

Spostos R., Scully C., Almeida O.P.D., Jorge J., Graner E. and Bozzo L. (1993) Oral paracoccidioidomycosis: a study of 36 South American patients. *Oral Surg. Oral Med. Oral Pathol.* **75**, 461–5.

Webb D.J., Seidel J. and Correll R.W. (1986) Multiple nodules on the tongue of a patient with seizures. *J. Am. Dent. Assoc.* **112**, 701–2.

Williams H.K., Edwards M.B. and Adekeye E.O. (1986) Onchocerciasis of the face and mouth. *Oral Surg. Oral Med. Oral Pathol.* **62**, 560–3.

Zegarelli E.V., Kutscher A.H. and Osipow J. (1965) Trichinosis found during examination of oral inflammatory tumor: report of case. *J. Oral Surg.* **23**, 655–6.

Zeltser R. and Lustmann J. (1988) Oral myiasis. *Int. J. Oral Maxillofac. Surg.* **17**, 288–9.

27

Emergencies

This chapter summarizes the emergencies that may arise in dentistry; greater detail can be found in the relevant preceding chapters.

The collapse of a patient in the dental surgery is a disturbing experience for all concerned – even if the outcome is complete recovery. Life-threatening emergencies in the dental surgery are fortunately rare but their very rarity makes it likely that unwise dental staff may be caught by surprise. Reducing the element of surprise and training all staff in preparation for such unwanted events are the best means of preventing and managing emergencies.

Emergencies should be prevented wherever possible by careful assessment of the patient and care in treatment, particularly when general anaesthesia is used, when there are invasive or painful procedures, or when medically compromised patients are being treated. Pulse oximetry to detect hypoxia in the early stages can be particularly valuable to prevent complications, especially when sedation or general anaesthesia are used.

PREVENTION

Forewarned is forearmed applies especially to emergencies. Confidence and satisfactory management of emergencies can be increased by the following precautions.

1. *Always have readily available* a telephone and the number of the local hospital and patient's general medical practitioner (or another helpful local practitioner) written by the phone. Train staff how to call for assistance.
2. *Train ancillary staff in emergency procedures.* All dental staff should know how to clear and maintain the airway, and how to

Table 27.1   Suggested emergency kit

- **Portable apparatus for administering oxygen**
  British Oxygen Company or Medical and Industrial Equipment Ltd
  or for administering air
  Air-viva resuscitator (B.O.C.)
- **Oral airway**
  Portex disposable Guedel airways sizes 1–4
- **Aspirator**
  Any high vacuum aspirator
- **Tourniquet**
  Any
- **Disposable syringes**
  2 ml and 10 ml sizes
- **Disposable needles**
  Sizes 19 and 21
- **Drugs**
  Adrenaline
  Adrenaline injection (0.5 ml ampoules of 1 in 1000 solution)
  Corticosteroid
  Hydrocortisone sodium succinate injection BP or hydrocortisone sodium phosphate (100 mg vials)
  Diazepam
  Diazepam for injection (10 mg vials)
  Glucose
  Dextrose injection (20% or 50% solution)
  Nitrous oxide/oxygen
  Anaesthetic machine, relative analgesia machine or Entonox
  Flumazenil
  Flumazenil for injection (500 μg vials)

carry out cardiopulmonary resuscitation. All dentists should also be able to perform venepuncture. Training should be repeated at least annually.
3. *Have a readily available emergency kit* that is frequently checked and working, as suggested in *Table 27.1*. Only a few emergencies can be treated definitively in the dental surgery.

Suggestions in some texts that 20 or more drugs should be kept for the management of emergencies are not practicable; so large a number of drugs could be a source of confusion and, if incorrectly used, dangerous.

4. *Never work alone.*
5. *Keep abreast of changes in practice,* by continuing education.

Unfortunately, recent surveys have shown that many practices have woefully inadequate facilities, and many staff are ill-equipped to deal with emergencies.

The chief emergencies are as follows.

1. Fainting and other causes of sudden loss of consciousness.
2. Anaesthetic emergencies (particularly respiratory obstruction or arrest).
3. Acute chest pain, particularly myocardial infarction.
4. Cardiac arrest.
5. Anaphylactic shock.
6. Collapse in a patient with a history of corticosteroid therapy.
7. Strokes.
8. Fits.
9. Asthmatic attacks.
10. Drug reactions and interactions.
11. Maxillofacial injuries.
12. Psychiatric emergencies.
13. Haemorrhage.
14. Inhaled foreign bodies.

Fuller discussion of these conditions can be found in the relevant chapters; this section is limited to the tabulation of the main diagnostic and management points in these emergencies for easy reference. For all, however, the basic principles are **ABC**:

Airway
Breathing
Circulation

SUDDEN LOSS OF CONSCIOUSNESS

Fainting

Fainting is the most common cause of sudden loss of consciousness. Up to 2 per cent of patients faint before or during dental treatment. Predisposing factors include:

1. Anxiety.
2. Pain.
3. Fatigue.

4. Fasting (possibly).
5. High temperature and relative humidity.

Young fit adult males in particular are prone to faint in the dental surgery, especially after injections.

- **Signs and symptoms**

1. Premonitory dizziness, weakness or nausea.
2. Pallor.
3. Cold moist skin.
4. Pulse initially slow and weak, then rapid and full.
5. Loss of consciousness; limp patient.

- **Management of a faint**

1. Lower the head (preferably by laying patient flat or putting head between knees).
2. Tight clothing should be loosened at the neck but smelling salts are of no value unless the patient is already recovering.
3. Recovery is usually rapid and the patient should be reassured. If there is no recovery, consider other causes of collapse – especially anaphylaxis, bradycardia, myocardial infarction or hypoglycaemia (diabetic). Monitor the pulse.
4. Defer further treatment where possible.

- **Differential diagnosis**

Fainting often simulates the early stages of more serious emergencies such as:

1. Myocardial infarction.
2. Stroke.
3. Corticosteroid insufficiency.
4. Epilepsy.
5. Drug reactions.
6. Hypoglycaemia.
7. Bradycardia or heart block.

The cause of sudden loss of consciousness may be suggested by the patient's history. Collapse of a diabetic at lunchtime, for example, is likely to be caused by hypoglycaemia. Collapse of a patient with angina or previous myocardial infarction may be caused by a myocardial infarct. Collapse at the sight of a needle or during an injection is likely to be a simple faint, but if it follows some minutes after an injection of penicillin, is likely to be anaphylaxis. The simple precaution of laying patients flat before giving injections will prevent fainting. The clinical features of the episode, for example severe chest pain, may also aid the diagnosis.

Collapse of uncertain cause

In the absence of an obvious diagnosis of the cause of sudden loss of consciousness:

1. The patient should be laid flat. Recovery is almost instantaneous if the patient has simply fainted. If there is not immediate recovery, then take the pulse. An absent pulse means cardiac arrest – in which case cardiopulmonary resuscitation is immediately indicated.
2. If the pulse is palpable, give glucose – orally (4 sugar lumps) if the patient has not completely lost consciousness, or 20 ml of 20–50 per cent sterile glucose intravenously if unconscious. A hypoglycaemic patient will rapidly improve with this regimen. If there is still no improvement, medical assistance should be summoned.
3. In the meantime, maintain the airway and give oxygen.
4. Give hydrocortisone sodium succinate 200 mg intravenously.

Collapse of a diabetic patient

Hypoglycaemia is the most dangerous complication of diabetes since the brain is starved of glucose. Glucose but *not insulin* should be given to the diabetic who collapses, unless it is certain that the cause is hyperglycaemia. Remember also that collapse may be caused by other disease, for example myocardial infarction, since ischaemic heart disease is a common complication of long-standing diabetes.

• Diagnosis of hypoglycaemia

Increasing drowsiness, disorientation, excitability or aggressiveness in a diabetic, especially if it is known that a meal has been missed, suggests hypoglycaemia.

• Management of hypoglycaemia

1. Lay the patient flat.

2. If conscious, give glucose orally (at least 4 sugar lumps). If unconscious, give sterile glucose intravenously (20 ml of 20–50 per cent solution) or intramuscular glucagon 1 mg.
3. Call an ambulance.

The differences between hypo- and hyperglycaemic coma, discussed in Chapter 14, are summarized again here:

Hypoglycaemia	*Hyperglycaemia*
Rapid onset	Slow onset
Irritability or aggressiveness	Drowsiness or disorientation
Moist skin	Dry skin, dry mouth, deep breathing, Hypotension Pulse weak
Pulse full and rapid	Blood sugar raised
Blood sugar low	Urine sugar usually
Urine sugar absent	present

ANAESTHETIC EMERGENCIES

Anaesthetic emergencies include:

1. Respiratory failure.
2. Respiratory obstruction.
3. Anaesthetic overdose, or drug interactions.
4. Cardiac arrest.
5. Anaphylaxis (intravenous agents).
6. Circulatory failure in corticosteroid-treated patient.

Respiratory failure

• Causes

Anaesthetic overdose or hypoxia.

• Diagnosis

1. Breathing stops.
2. Ashen cyanosis.
3. Pulse initially rapid and weak; later irregular or impalpable.
4. Cardiac arrest follows.

• Management

1. Stop anaesthetic.

2. Inspect and clear airway and give oxygen.
3. Lay patient flat.
4. Inflate chest rhythmically with oxygen or by mouth-to-mouth resuscitation (1 inflation about every 5 seconds).
5. Call an ambulance.

Respiratory obstruction

- **Causes**

Causes of respiratory obstruction are laryngeal spasm or foreign material in the airway. Prevention of inhalation of a foreign body such as a tooth or endodontic instrument is far better than cure. At the least such an occurrence causes great embarrassment, at worst respiratory obstruction, lung abscess or death.

- **Diagnosis**

1. Breathing stops or is irregular with crowing or croaking on inspiration.
2. Violent respiratory efforts.
3. Deepening cyanosis.

- **Management**

1. If patients cannot cough the object out, do not slap them on the back, rather use the Heimlich manoeuvre to clear the airway. Give oxygen.
2. Inspect and clear airway by suction. If obstruction is not in the pharynx but lower in respiratory tract, endoscopy, laryngotomy or tracheostomy may be needed.
3. After recovery, if a foreign body is lost, refer for plain radiographs – two views at right-angles – of abdomen and of chest. If the foreign body is in the chest, refer the patient immediately to a casualty unit and then a chest surgeon. Bronchoscopy may be required as the object may not be visible on radiography.

If a foreign body is lost and its location unknown and there is no respiratory obstruction, check the area around the patient first, but then act as in (3) above.

Anaesthetic overdose or drug interaction

- **Diagnosis**

1. Pallor.
2. Bradycardia (halothane) or tachycardia (other anaesthetic agents).
3. Hypotension.
4. Respiratory depression (barbiturates especially).

- **Management**

1. Stop anaesthetic; give oxygen and ventilate artificially if necessary.
2. Give cardiopulmonary resuscitation if necessary.
3. Call an ambulance.

ACUTE CHEST PAIN

Acute severe chest pain is usually caused by angina or myocardial infarction.

- **Diagnosis**

1. Severe crushing retrosternal pain.
2. Breathlessness, vomiting and loss of consciousness if there is an infarct.
3. Pulse may be weak or irregular if there is an infarct.

- **Management**

1. If the patient has a history of angina give anti-anginal drugs if the patient has them (glyceryl trinitrate 0.5 mg sublingually). If there is no relief of pain in 3 minutes – it is probably an infarct.
2. Summon assistance.
3. Do not lay the patient flat if this increases breathlessness.
4. Give nitrous oxide and oxygen (50/50) to relieve pain and anxiety.
5. Reassure the patient.
6. Call an ambulance.

CARDIAC ARREST

Recognition is difficult in the anaesthetized patient unless the pulse is continuously monitored. Suggestive features are sudden pallor and respiratory arrest: only later do the pupils dilate. Asystole and ventricular fibrillation account for most cardiac arrests.

- **Causes**

Causes are myocardial infarction, hypoxia, anaesthetic overdose, anaphylaxis or severe hypotension.

- **Diagnosis**

1. Loss of consciousness.
2. Absence of arterial pulses (feel carotid artery, anterior to sternomastoid).

After about 15 seconds of complete cerebral anoxia, the patient may start to convulse. Other signs too late to be of use include:

1. Respiratory arrest and eventual cyanosis.
2. Pupil dilatation and absence of light reaction.
3. No measurable blood pressure.

- **Management**

Cardiopulmonary resuscitation (CPR): the initial management depends on the availability or otherwise of a cardiac monitor and defibrillator. In their absence:

1. Summon assistance and note the time.
2. Lay the patient on the floor.
3. Clear the airway.
4. Give external cardiac compression at 60/minute. Depress sternum 2 inches at each compression.
5. Artificially ventilate once every five chest compressions, if two operators are present. Use an airway with face mask and oxygen, or mouth-to-mouth. The risk of transmission of infection is very small. Two main types of device are available to give external air resuscitation (EAR); the anaesthetic face-mask type, and the oropharyngeal airway, but if use of these is unsuccessful, intubation will be required. Face-mask types of airway are easy to use (Laerdal pocket mask; MTM resuscitator; Seal-Vent Easy). The oropharyngeal airway type can achieve better airway patency (Brook airway; Dual Aid; Hi-Tilt airway; Sussex Valve airway; Safar S airway). Airway maintenance

may require the use of an oral airway (Guedel), a nasopharyngeal airway, laryngeal mask, or oesophageal obturator.
6. If a competent person is present, instruct them to set up an intravenous infusion and infuse 100 ml of 8.4 per cent sodium bicarbonate, continued at 10 ml/min. Defibrillation may also be indicated if there is ventricular fibrillation or asystole. Drugs may help. Intravenous adrenaline 0.01 mg/kg or another alpha-adrenergic agent are of value.
7. Persist until there is restoration of good spontaneous pulse, of blood pressure, purposive movements (not twitches), reflex activity or of consciousness. The patient should be admitted to hospital.

If the patient is not resuscitated after 15 minutes, recovery is unlikely. The duration of resuscitation should not be assessed subjectively as, in these alarming circumstances, a few seconds may seem like minutes or hours.

ANAPHYLACTIC SHOCK

- **Causes**

Penicillin is most often the cause, but also muscle relaxants and (rarely) methohexitone, cephalosporins, sulphonamides, vancomycin, NSAIDs, radiographic contrast media, vaccines, immunoglobulins, various foods and insect stings.

- **Prevention**

Strict avoidance of the cause; slow administration of suspected agents and avoidance of the intravenous route. Where there is a previous history, the patient should carry an adrenaline aerosol such as Medihaler-epi, for use in an emergency.

- **Diagnosis**

1. The patient may complain of facial flushing, itching, paraesthesiae or peripheral coldness.
2. Wheezing, abdominal pain, nausea.
3. Loss of consciousness.
4. Pallor going on to cyanosis.

5. Cold clammy skin.
6. Rapid, weak or impalpable pulse.
7. Facial oedema or sometimes urticaria.

- **Management**

1. Lay the patient flat with the legs raised.
2. Give 0.5 ml of 1 in 1000 adrenaline intramuscularly (adult). Repeat every 10 minutes until recovery starts.
3. Give oxygen.
4. Give 10–20 mg chlorpheniramine slowly intravenously.
5. Give 200 mg of hydrocortisone sodium succinate or 50 mg methylprednisolone intravenously every 6 hours up to four times.
6. Call an ambulance.
7. Hospitalize the patient, as anaphylaxis may recur within the next 24 hours.

COLLAPSE OF A PATIENT WITH A HISTORY OF CORTICOSTEROID THERAPY

- **Causes**

Collapse is caused by adrenal insufficiency in general anaesthesia, trauma, infections or other stress.

- **Diagnosis**

1. Pallor.
2. Pulse: rapid, weak or impalpable.
3. Loss of consciousness.
4. Rapidly falling blood pressure.

- **Management**

1. Lay patient flat and raise legs.
2. Give at least 200 mg hydrocortisone sodium succinate intravenously.
3. Call ambulance.
4. Give oxygen.
5. Consider other possible reasons for collapse.

STROKE

The patient is usually hypertensive.

- **Diagnosis**

Varies with size and site of brain damage.

1. Loss of consciousness.
2. Weakness of arm and leg on one side.
3. Side of face may droop.

- **Management**

1. Maintain clear airway.
2. Call ambulance.

FITS

- **Causes**

1. In a known epileptic, starvation, menstruation and some drugs such as methohexitone, tricyclics or alcohol may precipitate a fit.
2. Fits may also follow loss of consciousness for other reasons – especially a deep faint.

- **Diagnosis of grand mal attack**

1. Loss of consciousness with rigid, extended body. Sometimes preceded by brief cry.
2. Widespread jerking movements.
3. Incontinence sometimes.
4. Slow recovery with the patient sometimes remaining dazed.

- **Management**

1. Put patient prone in head-injury ('recovery') position. Most fits terminate spontaneously. All that can be done is to stop patients damaging themselves.
2. If the convulsions do not stop within 5 minutes, or if another attack starts, give an adult 10–20 mg diazepam intravenously (or intramuscularly, but absorption is slow and unpredictable).
3. Maintain the airway and give oxygen.
4. Call an ambulance.
5. Repeat diazepam if no recovery within 5 minutes.

ASTHMATIC ATTACKS

• Causes

Anxiety, infection or exposure to an allergen can precipitate asthma attacks.

• Diagnosis

1. Breathlessness.
2. Expiratory wheezing, but may not be apparent because of shallow breathing.
3. Accessory muscles of respiration in action.
4. Rapid pulse (usually over 110 per minute).

• Management

1. Reassure the patient.
2. Do not lay the patient flat.
3. Give the anti-asthmatic drugs normally used (such as salbutamol nebulizer), and then immediately –
4. Give hydrocortisone sodium succinate 200 mg intravenously.
5. Give oxygen.
6. If there is no response within 2–3 minutes, give salbutamol or terbutaline rather than aminophylline, by slow i.v. injection. If these drugs are unavailable, give 1 ml 1 in 1000 adrenaline, intramuscularly.
7. Call an ambulance.

DRUG REACTIONS AND INTERACTIONS

These include particularly:

1. Anaphylaxis (*see above*).
2. Reactions to local anaesthetics (rarely).
3. Overdose of intravenous barbiturates.
4. Hypotension resulting from interaction of intravenous barbiturates with antihypertensive drugs.
5. Hypertension from interaction of pethidine with monoamine oxidase inhibitors.

Local anaesthetic reactions

These include:

1. Fainting (unrelated to the anaesthetic agent).
2. Intravascular injection of local anaesthetic.
3. Temporary facial palsy or diplopia.
4. Local anaesthetic allergy.
5. Cardiovascular reactions.

All, except minor reactions such as fainting, are exceedingly rare.

Intravascular injection of local anaesthetic

• Cause

1. Failure to use aspirating syringe.
2. Rapid injection.

• Diagnosis

Possible effects may include agitation, confusion, drowsiness, fits or loss of consciousness.

• Management

1. Lay the patient flat.
2. Reassure the patient.
3. Maintain the airway.

Most patients recover spontaneously within half an hour.

Temporary facial palsy, diplopia or localized facial pallor

These can occasionally result when the anaesthetic tracks towards the facial nerve or orbital contents but effects will wear off with the anaesthetic. The eyelids should be closed and a protective dressing worn until the anaesthetic abates.

Local anaesthetic allergy

Allergy to local anaesthetics is managed as for anaphylaxis.

Cardiovascular reactions

Usually only palpitations are experienced. Reassure the patient and await natural subsidence of symptoms. If reaction is severe, such as myocardial infarction (probably coincidental), treat as above.

Overdose of intravenous barbiturates

1. Clear the airway, lay the patient flat and artificially ventilate.
2. Summon assistance.

Hypotension resulting from interaction of intravenous barbiturates with antihypertensive drug

1. Clear the airway, lay the patient flat and artificially ventilate if necessary.
2. Summon assistance.

Hypertension resulting from interaction of pethidine with monoamine oxidase inhibitors

This reaction is difficult to manage, but an alpha-blocker such as phentolamine should be given if there is severe hypertension. Medical help is needed.

PSYCHIATRIC EMERGENCIES

Such emergencies may be occasioned by an underlying psychiatric disorder or:

1. Drugs: especially barbiturates, alcohol, or other drugs of addiction, or drug withdrawal, or corticosteroids.
2. Pain or discomfort.
3. Infections, particularly in the elderly.
4. Hypoglycaemia or endocrine disorders.
5. Temporal lobe epilepsy.
6. Cerebral tumours.

- **Management**

1. Summon psychiatric assistance or call an ambulance.
2. Do not sedate the patient; this may confuse the diagnosis and may occasionally be fatal. Diazepam is likely also to worsen the excitement of a psychotic patient.
3. If the patient is violent and uncontrollable, call the police.

HYPERVENTILATION SYNDROME

The textbook picture of hyperventilation syndrome is that of an anxious or hysterical

Table 27.2	Hyperventilation syndrome: symptoms

- **Neurological and psychological**
  Anxiety
  Weakness
  Lightheadedness
  Dizziness
  Disturbed consciousness
  Paraesthesia
  Tetany
  Muscle pain or stiffness
- **Cardiovascular and respiratory**
  Palpitations
  Chest pain
  Breathlessness
- **Other**
  Dry mouth

young woman overbreathing until carbon dioxide washout results in tetany and paraesthesia. However, the clinical features vary widely (*Table 27.2*) and males are often affected. Organic causes include pain and cardiovascular or nervous system disease. Hyperventilation is also a response to acidosis (either metabolic or drug-associated) and to poor respiratory exchange, but in this case hyperventilation is a compensatory physiological response.

The common denominator underlying hyperventilation syndrome is usually anxiety, but this in turn can either cause or result from cardiovascular symptoms such as extrasystoles or tachycardia.

- **Management**

The diagnosis is obvious in typical cases as described above, but in less well-defined cases patients should be reassured and then encouraged to rebreathe into a paper bag to overcome the alkalosis. Patients should later, between attacks, be encouraged to overbreathe to show them how the symptoms develop. Any underlying cause should be investigated and if necessary treated. Otherwise the most important aspect of treatment, if reassurance is ineffective, is sedation, usually with diazepam. If, however, there is obvious sympathetic overactivity as shown particularly by tachycardia or dysrhythmias, a cardiologist's opinion should be obtained as treatment with a beta-blocker may be necessary. In patients with hysterical personalities, however, the response to treatment may be poor.

HAEMORRHAGE

• Causes

Usually local, particularly traumatic extractions. Uncommonly caused by haemorrhagic disease, but this must always be considered (Chapter 4). Post-extraction bleeding often worries the patient excessively because a little blood makes a lot of mess.

• Management

1. Reassure the patient.
2. Get fussing relatives out of the way.
3. Gently clean the mouth and locate the source of bleeding.
4. Suture the socket under local anaesthesia.
5. Enquire into the patient's history, especially family history.
6. If bleeding is persistent or severe and there has been loss of more than about 500 ml, or if the patient is severely anaemic or debilitated, then the patient should be admitted to hospital. Tranexamic acid (500 mg in 5 ml, by slow intravenous injection) may be effective in the interim.
7. Call an ambulance if the bleeding is uncontrollable.

BIBLIOGRAPHY

Anon (1989) Drugs for the doctor's bag. *Drug and Therapeutics Bulletin* **29**, 17–19.

Association of Anaesthetists of Great Britain and Ireland (1990) *Anaphylactic Reactions Associated with Anaesthesia.* London, AAGB.

Baskett P.J.F. (1989) *Resuscitation Handbook.* Philadelphia, Lippincott.

Bochner B.S. and Lichtenstein L.M. (1991) Anaphylaxis. *N. Engl. J. Med.* **324**, 1785–90.

Cawson R.A. Spector R.G. and Skelly A.M. (1995) *Basic Pharmacology and Clinical Drug Use in Dentistry,* 6th edn. Edinburgh, Churchill Livingstone.

Douglas D.M., Sukenick E., Andrade W.P. and Brown J.S. (1994) Biphasic systemic anaphylaxis; an inpatient and outpatient study. *J. Allerg. Clin. Immunol.* **93**, 977–85.

Editorial (1981) Inhaled foreign bodies. *Br. Med. J.* **282**, 1649–51.

Edmondson H.D. and Frame J.W. (1986) Medical emergencies in general practice. *Dent. Update* **11**, 263–73.

Ewan P.W. (1997) Treatment of anaphylactic reactions. *Prescriber's J.* **37**, 125–32.

Fisher M. (1995) Treatment of acute anaphylaxis. *Br. Med. J.* **311**, 731–3.

Hussain I., Matthews R.W. and Scully C. (1992) Cardiopulmonary resuscitation skills of dental personnel. *Br. Dent. J.* **173**, 173–4.

Leading Article (1988) Intratracheal drugs. *Lancet* **i**, 743–4.

Malamed S.F. (1993) Managing medical emergencies. *J. Am. Dent. Assoc.* **124**, 40–51.

Niemann J.T. (1992) Cardiopulmonary resuscitation. *N. Engl. J. Med.* **327**, 1075–80.

Roberts J.R. (1998) *Emergency Medicine and Surgery.* Philadelphia, W.B. Saunders.

Scully C. (1988) *The Dental Patient.* Oxford, Heinemann.

Scully C. (1989) *The Mouth and Perioral Tissues.* Oxford, Heinemann.

Scully C. (1989) *Patient Care: a Dental Surgeon's Guide.* London, British Dental Association.

Scully C. (1997) The prevention and management of emergencies. *Br. Dent. J. Launchpad* **4**, 18–22.

Scully C., Epstein J. and Wiesenfeld D. (1998) *Oxford Handbook of Postgraduate Dentistry.* Oxford, Oxford University Press (in press).

Shirlaw P.J., Scully C., Griffiths M.J. *et al.* (1986) General anaesthesia, parenteral sedation and emergency drugs and equipment in general dental practice. *J. Dent.* **14**, 247–50.

Wakeen L.M. (1993) Dental office emergencies; do you know your legal obligations? *J. Am. Dent. Assoc.* **124**, 54–7.

Further reading

Cawson R.A., Binnie W. and Eveson J.W. (1995) *Colour Atlas of Oral Disease*. London, Mosby–Wolfe.

Eveson J.W. and Scully C. (1995) *Colour Atlas of Oral Pathology*. London, Mosby–Wolfe.

Porter S.R. and Scully C. (1991) *Radiograph Interpretation in Dentistry*. Oxford, Oxford University Press.

Porter S.R. and Scully C. (1995) *Oral Health Care for Those with HIV and Other Special Needs*. Northwood, Science Reviews.

Porter S.R. and Scully C. (1996) *Innovations and Developments in Non-Invasive Orofacial Health Care*. Northwood, Science Reviews.

Porter S.R., Scully C., Welsby P. and Gleeson M. (1993) *Colour Guide of Medicine and Surgery for Dentistry*. London, Churchill Livingstone.

Scully C. (1989) *Patient Care: a Dental Surgeon's Guide*. London, British Dental Journal.

Scully C. and Cawson R.A. (1992) *Colour Guide to Oral Medicine*. London, Churchill Livingstone.

Scully C. and Samaranayake L.P. (1992) *Clinical Virology in Oral Medicine and Dentistry*. Cambridge, Cambridge University Press.

Scully C. and Shepherd J.P. (1986) *Slide Interpretation in Oral Diseases and the Oral Manifestations of Systemic Diseases*. Oxford, Oxford University Press.

Scully C. and Welbury R. (1994) *A Colour Atlas of Oral Diseases in Children and Adolescents*. London, Mosby–Wolfe.

Scully C., Almeida O.P., Bozzo L., Vizioli M.R. and Jorges J. (1992) *An Atlas of Oral Diagnosis (Atlas de diagnostico bucal)*. Sao Paulo, Livraria Santos editora.

Scully C., Cawson R.A. and Griffiths M.J. (1990) *Occupational Hazards to Dental Staff*. London, British Dental Journal.

Scully C., Epstein J. and Wiesenfeld D. (1988) *Oxford Handbook of Postgraduate Dentistry*. Oxford, Oxford University Press (in press).

Scully C., Flint S. and Porter S.R. (1996) *Oral Diseases*. London, Dunitz.

Appendix

Miscellaneous uncommon or rare disorders of possible relevance to dentistry not included elsewhere

Disorder	Manifestations	Oral features	Management problems
Acanthosis nigricans	Pigmented papillomatous skin lesions	Papillomatous lesions	Adenocarcinoma (usually gastrointestinal)
Acrodermatitis enteropathica (zinc deficiency)	Skin vesicles Hair loss Diarrhoea	Perioral or oral erosions	Malabsorption syndrome
Alstrom's syndrome	Nerve deafness Retinitis pigmentosa	—	Diabetes mellitus
Ataxia telangiectasia	Mental handicap Ataxia Immunodeficiency	Occasional telangiectasia	Learning disability Diabetes mellitus Hypoadrenocorticism
Beckwith's syndrome	Gigantism Omphalocele or umbilical hernia	Macroglossia Hypoplastic middle third of face	Hypoglycaemia Hyperlipidaemia
Biemond's syndrome	Obesity Hypogonadism	—	Diabetes mellitus Obesity
Blackfan–Diamond syndrome	Red cell aplasia	—	Anaemia
Bloom's syndrome	Telangiectasia Depigmentation Short stature	Chronic cheilitis Carcinoma	50% develop neoplasia, particularly lymphoreticular
Cerebrohepatorenal syndrome (Lowe)	Hypotonia Flexion contractures	Micrognathia	Bleeding tendency Epilepsy
Chondroectodermal dysplasia (Ellis–van Creveld syndrome)	Polydactyly Dwarfism Ectodermal dysplasia	Midline defect in upper lip Natal teeth Conical or bicuspid teeth	Cardiac defects Learning disability
Cockayne's syndrome	Neuropathy Premature ageing Dwarfism Deafness	Prognathism	Deafness Learning disability blindness
Coffin–Lawry syndrome	Mental handicap Osteocartilaginous anomalies	Hypoplastic zygoma and maxilla	Learning disability
Congenital indifference to pain	Self-mutilation Bone fractures and infections	Self-mutilation	Patient incapable of perceiving pain

Disorder	Manifestations	Oral features	Management problems
Cowden's syndrome	Multiple hamartomas	Papillomatosis	Breast or thyroid carcinoma
Darier's disease	Papular skin lesions	Papules	—
Dyskeratosis congenita	Skin pigmentation Alopecia Nail defects Aplastic anaemia	Leukoplakia Carcinoma	Pancytopenia Multiple oral carcinomas
Fabry's disease (Angiokeratoma corporis diffusum)	Angiokeratomas Extremity pain Hypertension Fever	Angiokeratomas	Hypertension Renal disease Myocardial infarction
Fanconi's anaemia	Abnormalities of radius	Rarely squamous carcinoma Dental defects	Anaemia, leukaemia Renal defects Diabetes mellitus Hypoadrenocorticism
Focal dermal hypoplasia (Goltz syndrome)	Fatty deposits in skin Anomalies of extremities Skin atrophy	Labial papillomas ± cleft lip–palate Enamel hypoplasia Large pulp horns	—
Fragile X syndrome	Long face Large ears	High arched palate Cross bite	Learning disability
Froehlich's syndrome	Obesity Hypogonadism	Open bite	± Learning disability Obesity
Hallermann–Streiff syndrome	Hypotrichosis Cranial anomalies Micro-ophthalmia Cataracts	Mandibular hypoplasia TMJ abnormal position Dental anomalies	Visual defects
Hermansky–Pudlak syndrome	Albinism Bleeding tendency	Gingival haemorrhage	Bleeding tendency
Hyalinosis cutis et mucosae	Waxy skin nodules Hoarseness	Oral plaques and infiltration Dental hypoplasia	Laryngeal involvement Epilepsy
Incontinentia pigmenti (Bloch–Sulzberger syndrome)	Pigmented skin lesions Skeletal defects Neurological defects	Hypodontia Conical teeth	Learning disability Epilepsy Visual defects
Kartagener's syndrome	Sinusitis Dextrocardia	—	Immunodeficiency
Klippel–Feil deformity	Abnormalities of cervical vertebrae	—	Syringomyelia Fainting attacks
Laurence–Moon–Biedl syndrome	Retinitis pigmentosa Polydactyly Obesity	—	Learning disability Blindness Obesity
Maffuci syndrome	Haemangiomas Enchondromas 20% develop chondro sarcomas	Haemangiomas	Anaemia
Marcus–Gunn syndrome	Ptosis Lid winking in conjunction with jaw movement	—	—
Moebius syndrome	Congenital facial palsy Skeletal and muscular anomalies	Facial palsy May be hypoglossal palsy	Facial palsy
Noonan's syndrome	Webbed neck Short stature	Micrognathia Dental defects	Cardiac defects Pulmonary stenosis Thyroid disease
Papillon–Lefevre syndrome	Palmar and plantar hyperkeratosis	Periodontosis	—

Disorder	Manifestations	Oral features	Management problems
Pierre Robin syndrome	—	Micrognathia Cleft palate Glossoptosis	Cardiac defects Airways obstruction
Prader–Willi syndrome	Mental handicap Obesity Hypogonadism	Dental defects	Diabetes mellitus
Progeria (Werner or Hutchinson–Gilford syndrome)	Alopecia, dwarfism, senile appearance, hydro-cephalic appearance	Mandibular hypoplasia, Delayed eruption Crowding	Early atheroma with coronary and cerebro-vascular insufficiency
Rieger's syndrome	Hypodontia Ocular anomalies	Hypodontia Maxillary hypoplasia	Blindness
Rothmund–Thomson syndrome	Poikiloderma, cataracts, hypogonadism, dwarfism	Microdontia, dental hypoplasia	Visual defect
Ruvalcaba–Myrhe–Smith syndrome	Macrocephaly Intestinal polyps Penile pigmented macules	Tongue polyps	Learning disability
Schmidt's syndrome	Hypoadrenocorticism Hypoparathyroidism	Candidosis	Diabetes mellitus Autoimmune diseases Malabsorption syndrome
Scurvy	Purpura	Gingival swelling and haemorrhage	Bleeding tendency
Seckel's syndrome	Microcephaly Mental handicap	Zygomatic hypoplasia Mandibular hypoplasia	Learning disability
Sjögren–Larsson syndrome	Ichthyosis Mental handicap Cerebral palsy	Dental hypoplasia, Indifference to pain	Learning disability Cerebral palsy
Smith–Lemli–Opitz syndrome	Short stature Mental handicap Urogenital anomalies Syndactyly	Maxillary abnormalities	Learning disability Cerebral palsy
Takayasu's disease	Pulseless large arteries from aortic arch	Pain in muscles of mastication, ulcers	Syncope Steroid therapy
Treacher–Collins syndrome	Downward sloped palpebral fissures	Mandibulofacial dysostosis	Deafness Airways obstruction Cardiac defects
Tylosis	Palmar and plantar hyperkeratosis	—	Oesophageal carcinoma
Vitiligo	Depigmented area of skin	Rarely depigmentation	Thyrotoxicosis Hypoadrenocorticism
Waardenburg's syndrome	Deafness Heterochromia iridis White forelock	Prognathism	Deafness (20%)
Werner's syndrome	Cataracts Osteoporosis Thyroid cancer	–	Diabetes mellitus
Xeroderma pigmentosum	Hyperpigmentation Mental handicap	Squamous cancer of lip at early age	Tendency to skin malignancy

Index